Acquired Aphasia

Acquired Aphasia

Edited by

MARTHA TAYLOR SARNO

Department of Rehabilitation Medicine
New York University School of Medicine
New York, New York

ACADEMIC PRESS

A Subsidiary of Harcourt Brace Jovanovich, Publishers

New York   London   Toronto   Sydney   San Francisco

ACADEMIC PRESS, INC.
111 Fifth Avenue, New York, New York 10003

United Kingdom Edition published by
ACADEMIC PRESS, INC. (LONDON) LTD.
24/28 Oval Road, London NW1 7DX

Library of Congress Cataloging in Publication Data
Main entry under title:

Acquired aphasia.

    Bibliography: p.
    Includes index.
    1. Aphasia.   I. Sarno, Martha Taylor.   [DNLM:
1. Aphasia.   WL 340.5 A186]
RC425.A26   616.85'52   81-12890
ISBN 0-12-619320-7   AACR2

PRINTED IN THE UNITED STATES OF AMERICA

    83 84   9 8 7 6 5 4 3 2

Contents

4

Assessment of Aphasia   67
OTFRIED SPREEN and ANTHONY RISSER

5

Phonological Aspects of Aphasia   129
SHEILA BLUMSTEIN

6

Syntactic Aspects of Aphasia   157
RITA SLOAN BERNDT and ALFONSO CARAMAZZA

7

Lexical and Semantic Aspects of Aphasia   183
HUGH W. BUCKINGHAM, JR.

8

Auditory Comprehension in Aphasia 215
KAREN RIEDEL

9

Explanations for the Concept of Apraxia of Speech 271
HUGH W. BUCKINGHAM, JR.

10

Aphasia-Related Disorders 303
EDITH KAPLAN and HAROLD GOODGLASS

11

Intelligence and Aphasia 327
KERRY HAMSHER

Contributors

Numbers in parentheses indicate the pages on which the authors' contributions begin.

MARTIN L. ALBERT (385), Department of Neurology, Boston University School of Medicine, and Aphasia Research Center, Veterans Administration Medical Center, Boston, Massachusetts 02130

ARTHUR BENTON (1), Departments of Neurology and Psychology, University of Iowa, Iowa City, Iowa 52242

RITA SLOAN BERNDT (157), Department of Psychology, The Johns Hopkins University, Baltimore, Maryland 21218

SHEILA BLUMSTEIN (129), Department of Linguistics, Brown University, Providence, Rhode Island 02912, and Aphasia Research Center, Veterans Administration Medical Center, Boston, Massachusetts 02130

HUGH W. BUCKINGHAM, JR. (183, 271), Interdepartmental Program in Linguistics and Department of Speech, Louisiana State University, Baton Rouge, Louisiana 70803

CAROL BULLARD-BATES (399), Department of Psychology, Royal Ottawa Rehabilitation Centre, Ottawa, Ontario, Canada K1H 8M2

ALFONSO CARAMAZZA (157), Department of Psychology, The Johns Hopkins University, Baltimore, Maryland 21218

HANNA DAMASIO (27), Division of Behavioral Neurology, University of Iowa College of Medicine, Iowa City, Iowa 52242

ANTONIO DAMASIO (51), Division of Behavioral Neurology, University of Iowa College of Medicine, Iowa City, Iowa 52242

HOWARD GARDNER (361), Psychology Department, Boston University Medical School, and Aphasia Research Center, Veterans Administration Medical Center, Boston, Massachusetts 02130, and Harvard Project Zero, Harvard University, Cambridge, Massachusetts 02138

HAROLD GOODGLASS (303), Psychology Service, Boston Veterans Administration Medical Center and Department of Neurology, Boston University School of Medicine, Boston, Massachusetts 02130

KERRY HAMSHER (327), Section of Neurology, University of Wisconsin Medical School, Mount Sinai Medical Center, Milwaukee, Wisconsin 53201

EDITH KAPLAN (303), Department of Neurology, Boston University School of Medicine, and Aphasia Research Center, Veterans Administration Medical Center, Boston, Massachusetts 02130

HARVEY S. LEVIN (427), Division of Neurosurgery, University of Texas Medical Branch, Galveston, Texas 77550

LORAINE K. OBLER (385), Department of Neurology, Boston University School of Medicine, and Aphasia Research Center, Veterans Administration Medical Center, Boston, Massachusetts 02130

KAREN RIEDEL (215), Institute of Rehabilitation Medicine, Speech Pathology Services, New York University Medical Center, New York, New York 10016

ANTHONY RISSER (67), Department of Psychology, University of Victoria, Victoria, British Columbia, V8W 2Y2 Canada

JOHN SARNO (465), Department of Rehabilitation Medicine, New York University School of Medicine, and Institute of Rehabilitation Medicine, New York, New York 10016

MARTHA TAYLOR SARNO (485), Department of Rehabilitation Medicine, New York University School of Medicine, and Institute of Rehabilitation Medicine, New York, New York 10016

PAUL SATZ (399), Department of Psychology, University of California, Los Angeles, Los Angeles, California 90024, and Neuropsychiatric Institute, Camarillo State Hospital, Camarillo, California 93010

OTFRIED SPREEN (67), Department of Psychology, University of Victoria, Victoria, British Columbia, V8W 2Y2 Canada

ELLEN WINNER (361), Department of Psychology, Boston College, Boston, Massachusetts 02167, and Project Zero, Harvard Graduate School of Education, Harvard University, Cambridge, Massachusetts 02138

Preface

During the past two decades, aphasia has been a subject of increasing interest to a variety of disciplines beyond those of speech pathology, medicine, and psychology. Once the exclusive province of the neurologist, to whom we owe a great debt for pioneer work, aphasia is now studied as well by speech and language pathologists, linguists, cognitive psychologists, neuropsychologists, and others. The burgeoning of clinical and academic activity is the primary impetus for this volume, whose purpose it is to provide an authoritative text and reference book for graduate students, clinicians, and research workers in the many fields now concerned with aphasia.

The contents and roster of contributors reflect the view that no single discipline or author can be expert in all of the areas that contribute to our knowledge of aphasia. It is the editor's intent, therefore, to provide to the student of aphasia a comprehensive, almost exhaustive text by bringing together the writing of some of the most prolific and knowledgeable workers in the field of aphasia. Many of the contributors are pioneers in the areas of their special interest. The result is that all aspects of aphasia are treated in depth; indeed, each chapter is a review of the subject under discussion. The fact that the authors come from a diversity of disciplines adds to the richness and authority of the text.

The breadth of the book may also be judged by the fact that there are chapters on artistry and aphasia, aphasia in children, in closed-head injury, and in the elderly, as well as the emotional aspects of aphasia. Topics relevant to a comprehensive understanding of the disorder are included. "Trendy" subjects have been avoided. A textbook cannot be all things to all people, but the experience and sophistication of the authors of this volume have resulted in a work of broad applicability. Issues and problems, diversity and controversy are liberally represented.

Though the physiology of communication in health and disease remains an enigma at the most basic level, there is a large body of information on the subject reflecting a century of hard work and creative energy. It is another purpose of this volume to provide the student a distillation of that great effort and a thorough review of our knowledge to date.

The volume is logically organized for courses in aphasia. Chapters on the history, anatomy, and nature of aphasia set the stage for reviews of other dimensions of the disorder (e.g., phonology, auditory comprehension, etc.). The "special" chapters alluded to above add to the completeness and uniqueness of the work and reflect the fact that certain populations require different insights and management.

It should be noted that the scope of this volume does not permit a review of the techniques and practice of aphasia therapy. Broad principles have been outlined but to cover that subject in detail would require another textbook equal to this in length. Aphasia therapy cannot be conducted by formula; it is a process that grows out of the specific needs of the patient and the knowledge and imagination of the therapist.

The text makes no assumptions about previous knowledge of aphasia, linguistics, or neuroanatomy, and it includes a glossary of those terms not normally found in medical dictionaries.

I am deeply grateful to the authors whose chapters comprise this book. My special thanks to Hanna Damasio for the anatomical illustrations which she created for her chapter, to the patients and staff of the Speech Pathology Service of the Institute of Rehabilitation Medicine, to Karen Riedel, Eric Levita, and Margaret Naeser for their invaluable help, and to Rae Dorin and Esther Toledo for typing assistance. I am indebted to my father, Abril Lamarque, for his guidance in the overall graphic design, and to Antonia Buonaguro for her dedicated help with all stages of the project. I am especially grateful to my husband, John, for pointing up the need for such a text and for his support, encouragement, and incisive criticism.

Glossary

AGRAMMATISM: Speech characterized by generally preserved use of nouns and verbs or substantive words and a relative reduction in low information parts of speech.

ANOSOGNOSIA: Impaired recognition of one's own disease processes.

ANTEROGRADE AMNESIA: Inability to learn and retain new information reflected by impaired recall of events subsequent to the onset of the deficit.

COMPUTERIZED TOMOGRAPHY: Computer generated reconstruction of slices of brain and skull, made up of a series of points, each representing the absorption value of brain tissue, bone, and cerebrospinal fluid to an x-ray beam.

CONTIGUITY DISORDER: Contiguity refers to the inability to combine units making up language. Broca's aphasics are said to manifest primarily a contiguity disorder that affects their ability to construct phonological and grammatical contexts (e.g., at the phonological level, it refers to the chaining of sounds making up a word. The Broca's aphasic does not select any phoneme at random, but unifies the chain by omitting more phonological contrasts than he can cope with).

CROSSED APHASIA: Aphasia secondary to a lesion in the hemisphere ipsilateral to the preferred hand.

DISCONNECTION SYNDROME: Language behavior that is similar to aphasia resulting from the partial isolation of the two hemispheres through injury or sectioning of the corpus callosum.

EQUIPOTENTIALITY: When used with reference to brain function, this word refers to the theoretical concept that all cerebral cortical tissue has an equal capacity for differentiation based upon developmental imperatives.

FUNCTIONAL COMMUNICATION: Communication that is useful in the everyday activities of life, appropriate to the needs of the individual user, but not representative of the full range of communication of which the individual may be capable.

GRAMMATICAL MORPHEMES: The class of bound and free morphemes that provide structural information about sentence organization. These include the function words (e.g., articles, conjunctions, pronouns, auxiliary verbs and prepositions) and inflectional suffixes (e.g., tense and number markers).

IDEOMOTOR APRAXIA: Impaired execution of symbolic gestures (e.g., military salute) and/or gestures descriptive of object use (e.g., hammering) not attributable to motor weakness, incoordination, akinesia, abnormal movement, or incomprehension.

PARAPHASIA (LITERAL; PHONEMIC): The substitution or rearrangement of sounds or syllables in otherwise correct words (e.g., tevelision for television), which is often one of the symptoms of fluent aphasia.

PARAPHASIA (VERBAL): The substitution of one correct English word or phrase for another usually unrelated in meaning (e.g., girl for boy). When the substituted word is in the same meaning category as the intended word, it is referred to as a semantic aphasia.

RADIONUCLIDE BRAIN SCAN: Imaging of the brain obtained through detection of photon emission from radioactive Technetium previously injected intravenously.

SEGMENTAL FEATURES: The individual components of the speech stream (e.g., the sound of speech).

SUBSTANTIVE WORDS: Those words which carry the meaning: nouns, verbs, adjectives, and adverbs. Sometimes referred to as high information or content words.

SUPRASEGMENTAL COMPONENT: That component of the sound stream which spans individual segments (e.g., melody).

SURFACE STRUCTURE: The syntactic organization of a sentence that is closest to its actual spoken or written form.

VISUAL FIELDS: Refers to those parts of the field of vision which are indirect, therefore imprecise, as opposed to the limited area that is direct and precise; located in a large area peripheral to the central, direct field of vision.

Acquired Aphasia

1

Aphasia: Historical Perspectives

ARTHUR BENTON

The origins of aphasic disorder no doubt go back to the distant past. The association between disturbed speech and traumatic head injury must have been quite familiar to all primitive people who enjoyed the gift of speech. In any case, references to speechlessness as a sign or form of disease can be found in the earliest medical writings, for example, the Edwin Smith Surgical Papyrus, an Egyptian manuscript that dates back to 1700 B.C. and that is believed to be a copy of a still older manuscript (Breasted, 1930).

Early Contributions

Aphasia in Greek Medicine

The Hippocratic writings (ca. 400 B.C.) include many descriptions of speech disturbances, usually within the setting of protracted and often fatal illness. However, it is not clear exactly what was meant by such terms as *aphōnos* and *anaudos*; translators have given them various meanings depending upon their context. Thus, whether distinctions were made between aphasia, dysarthria, muteness, and aphonia is not known. A passage in the Coan Prognosis (No. 353 in the translation of Chadwick & Mann, 1950) associates speechlessness following convulsions "with paralysis of the tongue, or of the arm and right side of the body [p. 248]." Another passage in the Coan Prognosis (No. 488 in the Chadwick–Mann translation) states that "an incised wound in one tem-

1

ple produces a spasm in the opposite side of the body [p. 263]." Taken in combination, the two observations provide a basis for relating speech disorder to injury of the left hemisphere. There is no evidence that the correlation was made.

Aphasia in Roman Medicine

Some developments during the Roman period deserve mention. The Latin author and commentator, Valerius Maximus (ca. A.D. 30), described the first case of traumatic alexia (Benton & Joynt, 1960). Soranus of Ephesus and other medical writers of the period differentiated loss of speech due to paralysis of the tongue from that resulting from other causes (Creutz, 1934). However, the other causes were not specified, and whether these physicians had in mind a distinction between an articulatory and an amnesic type of aphasia is uncertain. It was also in this period that physicians and philosophers localized specific cognitive functions in different regions of the brain, more often in the cerebral ventricles than in the substance of the brain itself (Benton, 1976; Pagel, 1958). Perception was assigned to the lateral ventricles, reasoning to the third ventricle, and memory to the fourth ventricle. The ventricles and their connections were conceived as forming the structural basis for a dynamic process in which sensory information is received and integrated in the lateral ventricles, reflected upon in the third ventricle, and placed into a memory store in the fourth ventricle.

Aphasia in the Renaissance

One development during the Renaissance consisted in the application of this schema of ventricular localization to specific problems of diagnosis and treatment. Antonio Guainerio, a fifteenth-century physician, mentioned two aphasic patients; one could say only a few words and the other showed paraphasic misnaming. Reasoning deductively, he ascribed their condition to an excessive accumulation of phlegm in the fourth ventricle with consequent impairment of "the organ of memory" (Benton & Joynt, 1960). Direct surgical intervention to alleviate traumatic aphasia was another feature of Renaissance medicine. Reports describing cases of depressed skull fracture in which removal of bone fragments in the brain led to restoration of speech in the patient were published by Nicolò Massa and Francisco Arceo (Benton & Joynt, 1960; Soury, 1899).

The following statement by Johann Schenck von Grafenberg (1530–1598) indicates that at least some physicians of the time understood that brain disease could cause a nonparalytic type of speech disorder.

I have observed in many cases of apoplexy, lethargy and similar major diseases of the brain that, although the tongue was not paralyzed, the patient could not speak because, the faculty of memory being abolished, the words were not produced [Benton & Joynt, 1960, p. 209].

Later writers made the same point. For example, in 1742 Gerard Van Swieten wrote that he had seen "many patients whose cerebral functions were quite sound after recovery from apoplexy, except for this one deficit—in designating objects, they could not find the correct names for them [Benton & Joynt, 1960, p. 211]." These observations formed the basis for the classification of motoric and amnesic types of aphasic disorder that was made in the early nineteenth century.

Credit for the first explicit, albeit very brief, description of the syndrome of alexia without agraphia goes to Gerolamo Mercuriale (1530–1606). In the course of discussing cerebral localization of function, he cited the case of a printer who had lost the ability to read after sustaining an epileptic seizure. He could still write but could not read what he had written. Mercuriale regarded the deficit as symptomatic of a partial loss of memory (Meunier, 1924).

Seventeenth-Century Contributions

Relatively detailed descriptions of cases that leave no doubt that the patient was truly aphasic are first encountered in the seventeenth century. Two of these case reports are of particular interest. One, published in 1676 by Johann Schmidt, is entitled "Loss of Reading Ability following Apoplexy with Preservation of Writing." In it Schmidt describes a patient who suffered from a paraphasic expressive speech disorder after a stroke. Eventually he recovered oral speech but was still completely alexic. He could write to dictation but "could not read what he had written even though it was in his own hand.... No teaching or guidance was successful in inculcating recognition of letters in him [cited in Benton & Joynt, 1960, p. 209]."

The second case report, entitled "On a Rare Aphonia," described a patient with a nonfluent expressive speech disorder and an equally severe incapacity for repetition. She was unable to repeat even short phrases, such as "God will help." However, within this context of grossly defective conversational and repetitive speech, she showed remarkably preserved capacity for serial speech. Once she was started off, she could recite the Lord's Prayer, Biblical verses, and the like. It was this dissociation that led Peter Rommel, the author of the paper published in 1683, to designate his case as an instance of a "rare aphonia" (see Benton & Joynt, 1960, for translations of the Latin texts of Schmidt and Rommel).

Eighteenth-Century Descriptions

Many allusions to different forms of aphasic disorder appeared during the eighteenth century. Among them was the first description, in 1745 by Olaf Dalin, of preservation of the capacity to sing in a patient with a severe expressive speech disorder (see Benton & Joynt, 1960, for a translation of the Swedish text).

The 1770 monograph of Johann Gesner entitled "Speech Amnesia" was the first major study of the disorder (see Benton, 1965). It was a landmark contribution on a number of counts. From a clinical standpoint, the six case reports in it provided a wealth of information about such diverse features of aphasia as jargonaphasia and jargonagraphia, inability to read aloud with preserved ability to read silently for understanding, differential impairment in reading one language as compared to another, and preservation of the ability to recite familiar prayers within the setting of defective conversational speech. Moreover, in contrast to most earlier authors, Gesner emphasized that word-finding difficulties and paraphasic speech reflect not a loss of memory in general but a specific type of memory loss, namely, speech amnesia. Finally, and perhaps most importantly, Gesner was the first to advance a theory of the nature of aphasic disorders in terms of "speech amnesia." In discussing jargonaphasia, he insisted that it did not signify a dementia but only a specific type of forgetting. He pointed out that ideation and the memory for words must be distinguished from each other. Ideation is evoked by the perception of physical objects and the action of the sensory nerves. The evocation of words follows ideation, and hence additional neural energy or action is required for it to take place. Therefore, it is understandable that brain disease could impair the memory for words but leave ideation intact so that a patient might be able to recognize an object and know its significance, yet misname it or not be able to name it at all. The physical basis for such a disturbance in verbal memory was a sluggishness (Trägheit) in the relationships among the different parts of the brain.

Thus, in a rather vague way, Gesner advanced an associationist theory of aphasia, which stated that the disorder consisted of a failure to connect a perception or idea with its appropriate linguistic sign. He called the disorder SPEECH AMNESIA, as had his predecessors, but he went a step further by ascribing to what today we would call ASSOCIATIVE PROCESSES. Some 25 years later, Alexander Crichton (1798) ex-

TABLE 1.1
Knowledge of Aphasia in 1800

Clinical Descriptions
    Nonfluent aphasia: Speechlessness
    Fluent aphasia: Anomia, paraphasia, jargonaphasia (Van Swieten, 1742; Gesner, 1770)
    Agraphia (Gesner, 1770; Linné, 1745)
    Alexia without agraphia (Mercuriale, ca. 1580; Schmidt, 1676)
    Preserved capacity for serial speech (Rommel, 1683)
    Preserved capacity for singing (Dalin, 1745)
    Dissociation in reading different languages (Gesner, 1770)
    Unawareness of defect (Van Goens, 1789; Crichton, 1798)
    Lack of emphasis on comprehension defects (Morgagni, 1762)

Theory
    Defective "organ of memory" (Guiainerio, 1481; Schenck von Grafenberg, 1583)
    Defective associational processes (Gesner, 1770; Crichton, 1798)

Neuropathologic Concepts
    Ventricular localization: Fourth ventricle (Guainerio, 1481)
    Disease of the brain

---

pressed the idea with greater clarity. Writing about paraphasic speech, he suggested that this "very singular defect of memory . . . ought rather to be considered a defect of that principle, by which ideas, and their expressions, are associated, than of memory; for it consists in this, that the person, although he has a distinct notion of what he means to say, cannot pronounce the words which ought to characterize his thoughts [Crichton, 1798, p. 371]."

    Table 1.1 presents a summary of the knowledge of aphasia that had been gained by 1800. It is evident that a substantial amount of information about the disorder was available to the well-informed physician or layman. For the most part, this knowledge was of a clinical nature. However, little had been written about the basic nature of the aphasic disorders although brief statements of an associationist theory had been made by Gesner and Crichton. The neurological bases of aphasia remained quite obscure.

Aphasia: 1800–1860

    During the first decades of the nineteenth century, further advances were made along all lines: clinical knowledge, theoretical formulation, and neuropathology. With regard to clinical study, there were a number of contributions to knowledge of the phenomenology of aphasia. Osborne (1833) described a highly educated patient with severe jargonaphasia who nevertheless was able to understand oral speech and to read. He could even read foreign languages, and, in contrast to his grossly defective speech, his writing was only mildly affected. Lordat (1843) reported what appears to be the first case of dissociation of language loss in a polyglot. The patient could hardly say a word in French but could speak fluently in his native Languedoc. Bouillaud (1825) described involuntary echolalia in aphasic patients and called attention to the extreme verbosity of some patients. Marcé (1856) wrote a paper on agraphia in which he showed that the severity of the impairment in writing could vary independently of that in oral speech. He therefore postulated the existence of a cerebral center for writing that was distinct from the center for oral speech. A decade later, Ogle (1867) confirmed the independence of the two forms of expressive language disability and employed the term AGRAPHIA to designate impairment in writing.

More sophisticated theoretical formulations of the nature of aphasia were also advanced. The most important was that made by Jean-Baptiste Bouillaud (1796–1881), who classified aphasic disorders into two basic types, one being articulatory and the other amnesic in nature. Bouillaud (1825a) insisted that it was necessary "to distinguish two different phenomena in the act of speech, namely the power of creating words as signs of our ideas and that of articulating these same words. There is, so to speak, an internal speech and an external speech [p. 43, translation by author]." He then pointed out that "it is not uncommon to observe suspension of speech sometimes solely because the tongue and its congenerous organs refuse the pronunciation of words and sometimes because the memory of these words escapes us [p. 43]." Thus, one must distinguish between "two causes which can lead to loss of speech, each in its own way; one by destroying the organ of memory of words, the other by an impairment in the nervous principle which directs the movements of speech [Bouillaud, 1825b, pp. 285–286]."

The validity of Bouillaud's division of aphasic disorders into an articulatory, apraxic, aphemic category and an amnesic category is still generally accepted under the rubric of "nonfluent" and "fluent" types of aphasia. Lordat (1843) proposed essentially the same classification when he distinguished between "verbal asynergy," or loss of the ability to pronounce words, and "verbal amnesia," or loss of memory for words. His concept of verbal asynergy was based on his observation of cases of aphasia "in which the patient has a clear idea of the words he should utter and in which the muscles of speech are completely free from paralysis [cited in Benton, 1964, p. 323]." Lordat also discussed the relationship between intelligence and language and concluded that they were essentially independent; aphasia was neither a sign nor a cause of dementia.

The problem of the neuropathological basis of the aphasic disorders was first brought into prominence by the anatomist and phrenologist Franz Joseph Gall (1758–1828). His theory held that the human brain was an assemblage of organs, each of which formed the material substrate of a specific cognitive ability or character trait. Among the approximately 30 traits localized in his system were two cerebral "organs" of language, one for speech articulation and the other for word memory, which he placed in the orbital region of the frontal lobes.

Gall's hypothesis that the brain is not a unitary equipotential organ, but instead consists of an aggregate of functionally specialized areas, attracted both loyal supporters and vigorous opponents. No issue was more hotly debated than his localization of speech and language in the frontal lobes, and there was no more ardent champion of the concept than Jean-Baptiste Bouillaud, who marshaled clinical as well as pathological evidence to support the contention. However, Bouillaud's evidence was not altogether convincing, and, in any case, empirical testing of the hypothesis by others did not support it. For example, the clinical pathologist Gabriel Andral (1797–1876) reported on the clinical status during life of 37 patients in whom he had found lesions of the frontal lobes on autopsy. Speech disturbances had been present in 21 patients, while 16 had shown no sign of speech disorder. Moreover, Andral had seen 14 cases of aphasia with lesions confined to postrolandic areas and not involving the frontal lobes. He therefore concluded that "loss of speech is not a necessary result of lesions in the anterior lobes and furthermore it can occur in cases in which anatomical investigation shows no changes in these lobes [Andral, 1840, T.5 p. 368; translation by author]."

Aphasia: 1861–1900

Paul Broca

The protracted controversy over the validity of Gall's placement of language centers in the frontal lobes was no nearer resolution in 1860 than in 1830, but it did serve a most important function. It provided the impetus for the surgeon and the physical anthropologist Paul Broca (1824–1880) to examine the brains of two aphasic patients who had been under his care during the last months of their lives. The autopsy findings showed that the lesion that was ostensibly responsible for the nonfluent aphasic disorder shown by these patients during life was situated in both cases in the posterior part of the left frontal lobe. At the time, Broca interpreted his findings as supporting the Gall–Bouillaud thesis that the seat of language was in the frontal lobes, and he made no particular reference to the fact that the lesions were left sided. However, as he collected additional cases, his attention was drawn to the unilateral nature of the lesion causing the nonfluent impairment of speech to which he gave the name APHEMIA. Reporting in 1863 on the autopsy findings in eight aphasic patients, he noted that all had lesions on the left frontal lobe. He rather cautiously added, "I do not dare to draw a conclusion and I await new findings." The "new findings" were soon forthcoming, and in 1865 Broca enunciated his famous dictum, "We speak with the left hemisphere."

The validity of Broca's generalization was readily confirmed, and the doctrine of hemispheric cerebral dominance for language was born. At practically the same time, a number of clinicians added the qualification that left hemisphere dominance for speech held only for right-handed persons; in left handers the right hemisphere appeared to be dominant for language function.

Broca's discovery led to a major revolution in medical and physiological thinking. From a medical standpoint, aphasia was tranformed from a minor curiosity to an important symptom of focal brain disease. From a physiological standpoint, the reality of cerebral localization was established, and this led to a period of intense investigation of functional localization in both animals and human subjects (Benton, 1977; Young, 1970).

The place of Marc Dax (1771–1837) in this history deserves mention. In the 1860s his son, Gustav Dax (1815–1893), asserted that in 1836 Marc Dax had written a paper in which he assembled a mass of evidence to show that aphasia was related to disease of the left hemisphere. This unpublished paper, entitled "Lesions of the Left Hemisphere Coinciding with Forgetfulness of the Signs of Thought," was then published by Gustav Dax in 1865. There followed a minor controversy over whether Dax or Broca should be accorded priority for the discovery of left hemisphere dominance for speech (see Critchley, 1964). Analysis of the question indicates that, although Marc Dax did write the remarkable paper that his son published three decades later, there is no evidence that he presented it at a regional medical meeting in Montpellier, as was claimed (Joynt & Benton, 1964). Apparently the paper remained a private document. Thus, it seems that Dax did discover the special relationship between left hemisphere disease and aphasia about 25 years before Broca's first observation. However, he did not make his discovery known to the medical world other than through the distribution of copies of his paper to two or three friends.

The Contribution of Carl Wernicke

When Broca made his localization, he emphasized that he did not mean to imply that all forms of aphasia were related to left frontal lobe disease but only the motoric type, which he called aphemia and which was essentially the same as the articulatory and asynergic types of the disorder described by Bouillaud and Lordat. It remained for a German neuropsychiatrist, Carl Wernicke (1848–1905), to demonstrate that the occurrence of the other major type of aphasic disorder, that is, the amnesic type, was related to disease of the left temporal lobe. In a monograph published in 1874 (when he was 26 years old), Wernicke described the major features of what he called SENSORY APHASIA, now called WERNICKE'S APHASIA. These features were fluent but disordered speech, analogous disturbances in writing, impaired understanding of oral speech, and impairment in both oral and silent reading. The crucial, or at least most frequently occurring, lesion associated with this aphasic syndrome was situated in the hinder part of the first temporal gyrus of the left hemisphere, the region now known as WERNICKE'S AREA.

Wernicke's contribution was by no means limited to this discovery, important as that was (Geschwind, 1967). He pointed out the danger of mistaking sensory aphasia, characterized as it is by disordered speech and impaired understanding, with a confusional or even a psychotic state. He also emphasized the necessity for distinguishing between an aphasic impairment in naming objects from an agnosic (or asymbolic) failure to recognize objects, a point made by Freud (1891) some 15 years later. Moreover, as will be seen, he not only accounted for known aphasic syndromes from the rather simple neural model that he developed but also correctly predicted the existence of syndromes that had not been described at the time.

The Associationist School

Broca and Wernicke were not only localizationists but also "associationists." That is to say, like Gesner and Crichton, they thought of aphasic disorders as disturbances in attaching appropriate verbal labels to ideas, objects, or events, with basic intellectual capacity remaining essentially intact. In addition, their discoveries provided a basis for classifications of aphasic disorders as well as schematic models to explain their nature. For the most part, these models depicted the anatomic structures and neural mechanisms that were presumed to underlie language performances. The typical formulation was in terms of interconnected cortical centers that served as depositories for the auditory and visual memories of words and of the movement patterns of speech and writing. Models of this type were proposed by most of the leading aphasiologists of the late nineteenth century, such as Wernicke, Lichtheim, Charcot, and Bastian.

The schema of Lichtheim (1885), an elaboration of a simpler model proposed by Wernicke, postulated the existence of five interconnected cortical centers, four of which serve different aspects of language: a center of the memory-images of the movement patterns of oral speech (M); a center of the memory-images of word sounds (A); a center of the memory-images of the movement patterns of writing (W); and a center of the memory-images of written words (V). A fifth cortical area (C) was designated as a center in which concepts or ideas to be expressed were formulated. Lichtheim was not alone in postulating such a center, but most of the "diagram makers," to use Head's (1926) derisive term, regarded intellectual activity as a function of large areas of the cerebral cortex outside the region bounded by the language centers. The five centers were connected not only with each other but with other cortical and subcortical areas. For example, the auditoverbal and visuoverbal centers were intimately associated with the corresponding cortical receiving areas for audition and vision. Arrows in his diagram indicated the direction of flow of information from one center to another.

Reasoning deductively from his models, Lichtheim predicted the existence of seven major aphasic syndromes. Some of them were familiar to clinicians; others were still of a hypothetical nature. He reasoned that a lesion of Center M would produce the clinical picture of Broca's aphasia as then conceived: pervasive impairment in oral speech expression with preservation of the ability to understand oral speech and to read silently. Writing to dictation and spontaneous writing would be impaired because, as the diagram indicates, the underlying neural mechanisms involve Center M, these performances being typically mediated by "speaking to onself." On the other hand, writing from copy, a purely visuographic performance not involving "speaking to oneself," would be preserved.

The already familiar syndrome of Wernicke's sensory aphasia was, of course, produced by a lesion in Center A. In addition to defective understanding of oral speech and defective silent reading, the patient would also show inability to repeat and to read aloud, since the neural mechanisms underlying these performances involve transmission of information from the primary auditory and visual cortical receiving centers to Wernicke's area, in which Center A is located. Oral speech expression would be paraphasic, because the lesion of Center A prevented appropriate transmission of sound-images to the center for speech utterance.

Both Broca's aphasia and Wernicke's aphasia could be classified as "central" aphasic disorders in the sense that they were produced by lesions in the cortical centers in which memory-images or representations were stored. In his original formulation, Wernicke (1874) considered what the outcome of a lesion interrupting the connection between Centers A and M (i.e., impairing the conduction of information from Wernicke's area to Broca's area) would be. Since Center A was intact, the patient's understanding of oral speech as well as his silent reading would be preserved. Moreover, his oral speech expression would be fluent, since Center M was also intact. Nevertheless, his oral speech expression would be disordered, that is, paraphasic, because the break in the connection between Centers A and M prevented effective translation of sound-images into spoken sounds. Wernicke called this aphasic syndrome, which had not been described clinically up to that time and was therefore of a hypothetical character, CONDUCTION APHASIA to distinguish it from syndromes due to lesions in the cortical centers. Lichtheim agreed with this formulation and added an important defining feature to the syndrome, namely, the inability to repeat spoken utterances. Subsequent clinical observation has confirmed the existence of the syndrome of conduction aphasia that Wernicke had deduced from his model (Benson, 1979; Benson & Geschwind, 1971; Benson, Sheremata, Buchard, Segarra, Price, & Geschwind, 1973; Damasio & Damasio, 1980).

Another syndrome postulated by Lichtheim concerned the consequences of a break in the connection between the concept center (C) and the expressive speech center (M). He predicted that spontaneous speech would be impoverished since ideas could not reach verbal expression. On the other hand, since the basic mechanisms of speech are intact, strictly linguistic performance such as repetitive speech and reading aloud would be preserved. The understanding of speech would also be spared, since both Center A and its connection with Center C remain intact. The real existence of this syndrome, designated by Wernicke (1886) as TRANSCORTICAL MOTOR APHASIA, has also been confirmed by subsequent clinical observation (Benson, 1979; Benson & Geschwind, 1971).

These were (in rather oversimplified terms) some of the aphasic syndromes deduced by Wernicke, Lichtheim, and other "diagram makers" from their models of the neural mechanisms underlying normal and pathological language performances. Their approach was notably successful in some respects, and it possessed the merit of linking aphasic disorders with brain function. However, there was general agreement that it was only partially successful in accounting for the diverse phenomena of aphasia and the curious combinations of symptoms often encountered in aphasic patients. Moreover, serious objections to this associationist–anatomical approach were advanced by clinicians who viewed aphasia as being more than a linguistic disorder in the narrow sense and considered that it was as much a defect in thinking as in speech.

The Cognitive School

The influential French clinician Armand Trousseau (1801–1867) was the first major figure to challenge the assumption that thinking per se is not impaired in uncomplicated aphasic disorder. Attacking Broca's concept of aphemia, he cited cases from the literature and his own practice to show that aphasic patients, whose disability appeared on superficial examination to be of a purely linguistic nature, in fact showed numerous intellectual defects. He concluded categorically that "intelligence is always lamed" in aphasia (Trousseau, 1865).

This theme was then developed in greater depth by the English neurologist John Hughlings Jackson (1835–1911), who may be considered to be the founder of the "cognitive school" in the field of aphasia. Following an earlier brief formulation by the French physician Jules Baillarger (1809–1890), he distinguished between two levels of speech: emotional (or automatic) and intellectual. It is the intellectual level of utterance, involving the statement of "propositions," that is impaired in the aphasic patient, who may show considerable preservation of automatic language in the form of interjections, oaths, clichés, and recurring utterances. Jackson (1878) then pointed out that the basic unit of language is not the word but the meaningful proposition.

> To speak is not simply to utter words, it is to propositionise. A proposition is such a relation of words that it makes one new meaning; not by a mere addition of what we call the separate meanings of the several words; the terms of the proposition are modified by each other. Single words are meaningless, and so is any unrelated succession of words. The unit of speech is the proposition. A single word is, or is in effect, a proposition, if other words in relation are implied [p. 311].

Thus, the essential defect in aphasia, according to Jackson, consisted of a loss of this ability to "propositionise," that is, to use words in the service of thought. At the same time, the capacity to use words as a form of emotional expression might well be retained. The capacity for propositional speech is an intellectual, not a narrowly linguistic, ability, and consequently the aphasic patient of necessity "will be lame in his thinking" since "speech is a PART of thought" (Jackson, 1874).

A somewhat different formulation of aphasia as a cognitive disorder was reflected in the concept of "asymbolia," introduced by Finkelnburg (1870) to denote a general impairment of symbolic thinking. Such a defect might be manifested in dealing with nonverbal, as well as verbal, types of information, for example, failing to recognize the symbolic import of pantomimed actions, the value of coins, or the meaning of environmental sounds, such as the ring of a doorbell or the bark of a dog. Aphasia could then be regarded as a particular manifestation of asymbolia rather than as simply an instrumental disorder of language.

There was also resistance to accepting a basic assumption associated with the localizational models of the "diagram makers," namely, that a limited cortical region, such as Broca's area or Wernicke's area, was the repository of memory-images of speech movements or word sounds. It seemed incomprehensible to some students of brain function that the nervous elements comprising these cortical centers could be endowed with such extraordinary functional properties (Benton, 1976). It was not that these critics believed in the functional equipotentiality of all regions of the hemisphere or denied the facts of clinical localization of lesions, but they were convinced that the "diagram makers" had fallen into the error of confusing symptom with function. Jackson (1874) made this point succinctly when he warned that "to locate the lesion which destroys speech and to locate speech are two different things."

Finally, the creation by Pitres (1898) of the category of AMNESIC APHASIA, a syndrome characterized by difficulty in naming and in retrieving words in conversation, with essential preservation of the basic expressive and receptive language capacities, posed difficulties for the proposed models. Some neurologists (e.g., Mills, 1899) tried to meet the problem by postulating the existence of a "naming" center in the temporal lobe, but this simplistic solution was not taken seriously.

Nevertheless, despite the attacks on it, the concept that aphasia was a group of disorders produced by breaks in the connection of objects, events, and ideas with their appropriate verbal signs was the one held by most neurologists as of 1900. However, as will be seen, there was a significant change in thinking over the following 25 years in France and Britain as a result of the influential contributions of Pierre Marie and Henry Head, both of whom were vigorous proponents of the cognitive position and of a unitary theory of the nature of aphasia.

Early Twentieth-Century Developments

Associationist Models

During the early twentieth century, there were further elaborations of the concept that discrete cortical and subcortical centers and their interconnections provided the neurological basis of language functions. Joseph-Jules Dejerine (1849–1917) was a major figure in this development. Among his notable achievements was his demonstration of the anatomical substrate of the syndrome of pure alexia without agraphia and his interpretation of it as a "disconnection syndrome" (see Geschwind, 1965; Lecours & Lhermitte, 1979). S. E. Henschen (1847–1930) undertook a monumental analysis of all the clinicopathological reports in the literature on aphasia and formulated a detailed model that postulated the existence of numerous separate cortical centers for almost every aspect of language function as well as for such allied activities as calculation and musical appreciation and expression (Henschen, 1919–1922). Still another important figure was Karl Kleist (1870–1962), who, on the basis of detailed examination of soldiers with penetrating brain wounds, believed that it was possible to make a precise localization of the cortical regions underlying diverse language performances (Kleist, 1934).

Cognitive Models

The development of explicit cognitive theories of the nature of aphasia was an important feature in the development of thought about the disorder during the first quarter of the twentieth century. In large part this development was due to the contributions of Pierre Marie (1853–1940) and Henry Head (1861–1940). Both of these neurologists viewed aphasia as a single disorder that necessarily incorporated the component of intellectual defect.

The first of Marie's papers on the subject bore the provocative title "The Left Frontal Convolution Plays No Special Role in Language Function" (Cole & Cole, 1971; Marie, 1906). In it he flatly denied that Broca's area was a center of expressive speech and cited clinical evidence to support this negative conclusion. Specifically, he pointed to cases in which a lesion in Broca's area had caused no speech disturbance and, conversely, cases of Broca's aphasia in which no lesion in Broca's area was found. Subsequent papers in the series vigorously attacked the pluralistic concept of discrete types of aphasic disorder and proposed that there was in fact one basic disorder, the syndrome of disturbed fluent speech expression and impaired understanding of speech known as Wernicke's aphasia. This disorder ALWAYS involved impairment in general intelligence. Marie did not offer an explicit definition of the nature of this impairment. Apparently what he had in mind was the aphasic patient's intellectual passivity and his frequent inability to cope with practical tasks that made no obvious demands on the understanding or expression of speech. In consonance with his unitary conception of the nature of aphasia, Marie proposed a single broad localization of the lesion causing the disorder. Later he modified his opinion to some degree, but at the time when he advanced his famous "Revision of the Question of Aphasia," he implicated a single extensive territory that included the posterior parts of the first and second temporal gyri, the supramarginal gyrus, and the angular gyrus.

The work of Henry Head (1926) in England was equally influential in fostering a significant change in attitude about the role of cognitive factors in aphasia. Defining the disorder as a loss of capacity for symbolic formulation and expression, he insisted that it involved an impairment in thinking that was reflected in the patient's nonverbal performances as well as in his verbal behavior. Consequently, the extensive test battery that he developed for the assessment of aphasic disorder included nonverbal tasks that are not ordinarily considered to be measures of language functions. But Head maintained that performance on such tasks as imitating the posture of the confronting examiner, drawing pictures, or setting the hands of a clock involved the manipulation of symbols and concepts and that, therefore, they were valid measures of the fundamental cognitive capacity that was impaired in aphasia.

Another figure deserving mention in this context is Kurt Goldstein (1878–1965), who applied cognitive theory with particular force to the category of amnesic aphasia, with its defining features of impairment in object naming and difficulty in finding words in conversation. Goldstein insisted that these linguistic defects were a direct expression of a loss of the abstract attitude that was also reflected in defective performance on such nonverbal tasks as the sorting of colors and the classification of objects, which also made demands on the capacity for abstract reasoning (Goldstein, 1924).

The Modern Period

To divide the history of a topic into periods or stages is necessarily a somewhat arbitrary procedure. I have designated 1935 as the beginning of the "modern period" because this was the year of publication of the comprehensive study by Weisenburg and McBride that generated a substantial amount of new information about aphasia and at the same time provided a methodological model for subsequent investigations.

Cognitive Factors in Aphasia

Weisenburg and McBride (1935) gave an extensive battery of verbal and nonverbal tests to 60 aphasic patients and compared their performances with those of 38 nonaphasic patients with unilateral brain disease and 85 control patients (i.e., without evidence of brain disease). The nonverbal component of their test battery included drawing, visuoperceptual, and block-assembling tasks. They found that, although inferior performance on varying numbers of the nonverbal tasks was shown by a majority of the aphasic patients, there was considerable interindividual variability, some patients performing on a defective level on many tests and others performing adequately on all tests. They also found that there was a positive relationship of moderate degree between the extent of the observed cognitive impairment on the nonverbal tests and the estimated severity of the patient's aphasic disability.

Despite their finding that cognitive defects were extraordinarily frequent in aphasic patients, Weisenburg and McBride concluded that aphasia did not necessarily involve impairment in intellectual function since even some severely aphasic patients performed adequately on nonverbal tests. Nor could they support Head's contention that the essential cognitive defect in aphasia was a disturbance of symbolic thinking, since in many instances defective performance did not seem to be related to faulty symbolic understanding or formulation. On the other hand, they emphasized the considerable variation in performance from case to case and ascribed at least a part of this variability to differences in the role of language in the thinking of different individuals. As they phrased it:

> It cannot be doubted that verbal symbols and language formulations have permeated mental functioning to a far greater extent in some persons than in others, and that the more firmly established they are as types of reactions and means of attacking problems the greater will be the consequences of the language disorder [Weisenburg & McBride, 1935, p. 461].

Thus, the premorbid intellectual makeup of an aphasic patient was invoked as a possible determinant of the cognitive changes observed in association with his linguistic disability. Weisenburg and McBride also insisted that the "definition of the changes in intelligence in aphasia must be determined in the individual case, with due regard not only for the decreased efficiency but for the qualitative characteristics of the changes [p. 462]."

Subsequent studies of cognitive function in asphasia generally followed the pattern established by Weisenburg and McBride of comparing the performances of aphasics with those of nonaphasic patients with unilateral brain disease and control patients or normal subjects. These studies produced a broad spectrum of results that did not permit a simple interpretation and that confirmed the position of Weisenburg and McBride that interindividual variability is an overriding feature of the performances of aphasic patients.

A number of studies have utilized the Wechsler–Bellevue Scales (Wechsler, 1944) and the Wechsler Adult Intelligence Scale (Wechsler, 1958) to assess the intelligence of aphasic patients. In line with expectations, the patient's Verbal Scale IQs were generally lower than their Performance Scale IQs. The majority of patients had subnormal Performance Scale IQs as well, testifying to a decline in intellectual function that extended beyond strictly linguistic performances. Alajouanine and Lhermitte (1964) reported that 25% of a group of unselected aphasic patients had a Performance Scale IQ of 79 or lower. Orgass, Hartje, Kerchensteiner, and Poeck (1972) found the mean Wechsler Performance Scale IQ of a group of 30 aphasic patients to be 79, which is far below normal standards. However, interindividual variation was wide, the scores ranging from an IQ of 50, indicative of frank dementia, to an IQ of 113, reflecting intactness of the cognitive skills measured by the performance scale.

Symbolic thinking and abstract reasoning have been studied on the assumption that these capacities are particularly likely to be impaired in patients with aphasic disorder (Bay, 1962, 1964; Goldstein, 1948). Classification tests, such as color and object sorting (Goldstein & Scheerer, 1941), and the Progressive Matrices of Raven (1938, 1963) have been among the tasks utilized to investigate the question. The results have been much the same as those found in studies of nonverbal "intelligence" with the Wechsler scales. Defective performance was shown by many aphasic patients, whereas most nonaphasic patients with left hemisphere disease performed normally (Basso, De Renzi, Faglioni, Scotti, & Spinnler, 1973; Colonna & Faglioni, 1966; De Renzi, Faglioni, Savoiardo, & Vignolo, 1966; De Renzi, Faglioni, Scotti, & Spinnler, 1972). However, interindividual variability was high, and the correlation between performance level and the severity of the aphasic disorder, as measured by naming ability and level of oral language comprehension, was never high and indeed sometimes absent (Basso et al., 1973). Thus, the general conclusion has been that the inferior performances of some aphasic patients could not be ascribed to their language impairment.

Other types of cognitive deficit have been found to occur with notable frequency in aphasic patients, particularly those with defects in oral and written language comprehension. Among these are impairment in facial discrimination (Benton, 1980; Hamsher, Levin, & Benton, 1979), constructional apraxia (Benton, 1973), and defective grasp of the meaning of pantomimed actions (Duffy, Duffy, & Pearson, 1975; Varney, 1978).

Neurolinguistics

An important development in recent decades has been a concerted effort to describe in precise terms the alterations of speech shown by aphasic patients and to relate these changes to the anatomic substrate of the disorder as well as to the cognitive status of aphasic patients. Dealing with such questions as the nature of AGRAMMATISM, PARAGRAMMATISM, "word-finding disturbance," SYNTACTIC APHASIA, and other disturbances, this effort obviously required expertise in the field of linguistics. As a consequence, a number of linguists became actively engaged in the undertaking, which has come to be known as NEUROLINGUISTICS.

Although some neurologists and psychologists (e.g., Alajouanine, Ombredane, & Durand, 1939; Kleist, 1934; Ombredane, 1926, 1933; Pick, 1913) had dealt with neurolinguistic problems in earlier years, the seminal figure in the field was Roman Jakobson. His monograph (Jakobson, 1941) comparing the phonemic disturbances in the utterances of aphasic patients to the speech of children and relating both to more general aspects of phonology had a profoundly stimulating effect on subsequent investigative work. Even more important was the fundamental distinction that he made between disorders of "similarity" or selection and disorders of "contiguity" or combination in aphasic speech (Jakobson, 1956). Word-finding difficulties, anomia, and paraphasic utterances reflect impairment of the similarity component in normal speech, that is, application of the appropriate verbal symbol to an idea or intention. Telegraphic speech and defective syntactic utterances reflect impairment of the contiguity component of normal speech, that is, the temporal organization of words into meaningful, syntactically correct propositions. Jakobson maintained that these two distinctive processes constituted fundamental dimensions along which the speech of aphasics could be classified.

More recent research in neurolinguistics has followed the lines of Jakobson's thinking and expanded beyond it to address other problems. One important advance has been the demonstration of the nature and significance of the fluency–nonfluency dimension in aphasic speech

(Benson, 1967; Goodglass, Quadfasel, & Timberlake, 1964; Kerchensteiner, Poeck, & Brunner, 1972). This dimension, which had been described by Bouillaud, Jackson, and Wernicke and which is related in some respects to Jakobson's dichotomy, has been shown to have a bimodal distribution so that a majority of aphasic patients can be validly classified as "fluent" or "nonfluent." Among other linguistic topics that have been the subject of study are agrammatism and paragrammatism (Cohen & Hécaen, 1965; Goodglass & Mayer, 1958), the analysis and measurement of disorders of auditory comprehension (Boller & Dennis, 1979; De Renzi & Vignolo, 1962; Goodglass, Gleason, & Hyde, 1970; Orgass & Poeck, 1966), the stylistic analysis of aphasic speech (Spreen & Wachal, 1973; Wachal & Spreen, 1973), and disturbances in reading (Lesser, 1978; Marshall & Newcombe, 1966).

Anatomical Basis of Aphasia

The extreme localizationist approach to the "anatomy" of the aphasic disorders was carried forth by the California neurologist Joannes Nielsen (1890–1969), whose thinking followed the lines laid down by Henschen (1919–1922) and Poetzl (1928). His monograph (Nielsen, 1936) appeared at a time when concern with identifying the neural mechanisms underlying language function and language disorder had diminished somewhat as compared to earlier decades. Interest in the area revived after World War II, however, with the expanded opportunities for study afforded by the large number of casualties produced by that conflict and by advances in the development of neuroradiologic diagnostic procedures.

One topic that engaged the attention of researchers was the question of the relationship between hand preference and hemispheric cerebral "dominance" for language. The rule that the relationship between handedness and the cerebral hemisphere controlling language function was symmetric in nature (i.e., that the "language" hemisphere was opposite in side to the preferred hand) was accepted for many decades after its original formulation in the 1860s. The generalization was first questioned by Chesher (1936), who pointed out that "crossed" aphasia (i.e., following a lesion in the hemisphere IPSILATERAL to the preferred hand) occurred with too high a frequency in left-handed patients to be considered exceptional. Chesher concluded that hemispheric specialization for language in these patients must be different in nature from that in right-handed patients. Subsequent studies by Conrad (1949), Goodglass and Quadfasel (1954), Humphrey and Zangwill (1952), and Russell and Espir (1961) of aphasic and nonaphasic patients with unilateral brain lesions demonstrated conclusively that hemispheric specialization differed markedly in right handers and left handers. For example, Russell and Espir recorded the side of lesion in 189 right-handed and 13 left-handed patients who presented an aphasic disorder after having sustained a unilateral penetrating brain wound. Of the 189 right handers, 186 proved to have a left hemisphere lesion and only 3 (1.6%) had a right hemisphere wound, indicating the rarity of "crossed" aphasia in right-handed persons. But of the 13 left handers, 9 (69%) had left hemisphere wounds and 4 (31%) had right hemisphere wounds. Thus, they confirmed the earlier findings of Conrad and others that the traditional rule linking the language hemisphere with hand preference held for right handers but not for left handers, who were at least as likely to be left hemisphere dominant as right hemisphere dominant for speech. Further, a number of observers recorded their impression that aphasic disorders tended to be milder and more transient in left handers and inferred from this that some left handers have bilateral representation of language functions (Hécaen & Ajuriaguerra, 1963; Subirana, 1969), a conclusion that was supported by Milner, Branch, and Rasmussen (1966), who showed that a small proportion of left handers were rendered aphasic after pharmacologic inactivation of EITHER hemisphere by the Wada test (Wada & Rasmussen, 1960).

At the same time, it became clear the mediation of language function in right-handed persons is not an exclusive property of the left hemisphere and that the right hemisphere also possesses some linguistic capabilities, however limited they may be. Gazzaniga and Sperry (1967; Gazzaniga, 1970) were able to show that some patients who had undergone section of the corpus callosum for relief of intractable epilepsy could understand the meaning of simple words presented in the left visual field although they were unable to read the words aloud. Since the visuoverbal information was processed by the disconnected right hemisphere, it was reasonable to infer that the successful recognition of the meaning of the words was mediated by neural mechanisms in that hemisphere. Even more convincing evidence that the right hemisphere does possess some capacity to mediate language was furnished by Smith (1966; Burkland & Smith, 1977) in studies of right-handed patients who had undergone complete left hemispherectomy in an effort to arrest the growth of malignant cerebral neoplasm. Although both of the patients studied were severely aphasic postoperatively, they nevertheless showed some ability to respond appropriately to oral and written verbal commands and some expressive speech. Similar findings were reported by Gott (1973) in her study of a 12-year-old girl who had undergone complete left hemispherectomy at the age of 10 years.

A first step toward achieving some degree of understanding of the anatomical basis of hemispheric cerebral dominance for language was made by Geschwind and Levitsky (1970), who demonstrated that the planum temporale, that is, the superior surface of the posterior temporal lobe, is larger on the left side than on the right in a majority of human brains. This morphological asymmetry of an area involved in the mediation of language function was, of course, consistent with the rule of left hemisphere dominance. Wada (1969; Wada, Clarke and Hamm 1975; Witelson & Pallie, 1973) found that this hemispheric difference is already evident in infant brains, and subsequent studies showed that there are interhemispheric architectonic differences as well (Galaburda, Sanides, & Geschwind, 1978).

A path-breaking and influential paper by Geschwind (1965), in which agnosic, apraxic, and aphasic disorders were interpreted as products of neural disconnection, provided the impetus for a fresh approach to the anatomical study of aphasic syndromes. Investigative work exemplifying the approach includes studies of conduction aphasia (Benson *et al.*, 1973; Damasio & Damasio, 1980), mixed transcortical aphasia (Geschwind, Quadfasel, & Segarra, 1968), and transcortical motor aphasia (Rubens, 1976). Analyses of the current state of anatomical knowledge with respect to some aspects of aphasia will be found in the chapters by A. Damasio, H., Damasio, and Levin in this volume.

References

Alajouanine, T., & Lhermitte, F. 1964. Non-verbal communication in aphasia. In A. V. S. de Reuck & M. O'Connor (Eds.), *Disorders of language*. Boston: Little, Brown.

Alajouanine, T., Ombredane, A., & Durand, M. 1939. *Le syndrome de désintégration phonétique dans l'aphasie*. Paris: Masson.

Andral, G. 1840. *Clinique médicale* (4th ed.). Paris: Fortin, Massonet Cie.

Basso, A., De Renzi, E., Faglioni, P., Scotti, G., & Spinnler, H. 1973. Neuropsychological evidence for the existence of cerebral areas critical to the performance of intelligence tests. *Brain, 96*, 715–728.

Bay, E. 1962. Aphasia and non-verbal disorders of language. *Brain, 85*, 411–426.

Bay, E. 1964. Classifications and concepts of aphasia. In A. V. S. de Reuck & M. O'Connor (Eds.), *Disorders of language*. Boston: Little, Brown.

Benson, D. F. 1967. Fluency in aphasia: Correlation with radioactive scan localization. *Cortex, 3*, 258–271.

Benson, D. F. 1979. *Aphasia, alexia and agraphia*. New York: Churchill Livingstone.

Benson, D. F., & Geschwind, N. 1971. Aphasia and related cortical disturbances. In A. B. Baker & L. H. Baker (Eds.), *Clinical neurology*. New York: Harper.

Benson, D. F., Sheremata, W. A., Buchard, R., Segarra, J., Price, D., & Geschwind, N. 1973. Conduction aphasia. *Archives of Neurology, 28*, 339–346.

Benton, A. L. 1964 Contributions to aphasia before Broca. *Cortex, 1*, 314–327.

Benton, A. L. 1965. J. A. P. Gesner on aphasia. *Medical History, 9*, 54–60.

Benton, A. L. 1973. Visuoconstructive disability in patients with cerebral disease: Its relationship to side of lesion and aphasic disorder. *Documenta Ophthalmologica, 34,* 67–76.

Benton, A. L. 1976. Historical development of the concept of hemispheric cerebral dominance. In S. F. Spicker & H. T. Engelhardt, Jr. (Eds.), *Philosophical dimensions of the neuromedical sciences.* Dordrecht, Holland: Reidel.

Benton, A. L. 1977. The interplay of experimental and clinical approaches in brain lesion research. In S. Finger (Ed.), *Recovery from brain damage: Research and theory.* New York: Plenum.

Benton, A. L. 1980. The neuropsychology of facial recognition. *American Psychologist, 35,* 176–186.

Benton, A. L., & Joynt, R. J. 1960. Early descriptions of aphasia. *Archives of Neurology, 3,* 205–221.

Boller, F. & Dennis, M. 1979. *Auditory comprehension: Clinical and experimental studies with the Token Test.* New York: Academic Press.

Bouillaud, J. B. 1825a. Recherches cliniques propres à démontrer que la perte de la parole correspond à la lésion des lobules antérieurs du cerveau. *Archives générales de Médecine, 8,* 25–45.

Bouillaud, J. B. 1825b. *Traité clinique et physiologique de l'encéphalite.* Paris: J. B. Baillière.

Breasted, J. H. 1930. *The Edwin Smith Surgical Papyrus.* Chicago: Univ. of Chicago Press.

Broca, P. 1863. Localisation des fonctions cérébrales: Siège du langage articulé. *Bulletin de la Société d'Anthropologie, 4,* 200–203.

Broca, P. 1865. Du siège de la faculté du langage articulé. *Bulletin de la Société d'Anthropologie, 6,* 337–393.

Burkland, C. W., & Smith, A. 1977. Language and the cerebral hemispheres. *Neurology, 27,* 627–633.

Chadwick, J., & Mann, W. N. 1950. *The medical works of Hippocrates.* Oxford: Blackwell.

Chesher, E. C. 1936. Some observations concerning the relationship of handedness to the language mechanism. *Bulletin of the Neurological Institute of New York, 4,* 556–562.

Cohen, D., & Hécaen, H. 1965. Remarques neurolinguistiques sur un cas d'agrammatisme. *Journal de Psychologie Normale et Pathologique, 62,* 273–296.

Cole, M. F., & M. Cole, 1971. *Pierre Marie's papers on speech disorders.* New York: Hafner.

Colonna, A., & Faglioni, P. 1966. The performance of hemisphere damaged patients on spatial intelligence tests. *Cortex, 2,* 293–307.

Conrad, K. 1949. Ueber aphasische Sprachstoerungen bei hirnverletzten Linkshaendern. *Nervenarzt, 20,* 148–154.

Creutz, W. 1934. *Die Neurologie des 1.-7. Jahrhunderts n. Chr.: Eine historisch-neurologische Studie.* Leipzig: Thieme.

Crichton, A. 1798. *An inquiry into the nature and origin of mental derangement.* London: T. Cadell, Jr. & W. Davies.

Critchley, M. 1964. Dax's law. *International Journal of Neurology, 4,* 199–206.

Damasio, H., & Damasio, A. R. 1980. The anatomical basis of conduction aphasia. *Brain, 103,* 337–350.

De Renzi, E., Faglioni, P., Savoiardo, M., & Vignolo, L. A. 1966. The influence of aphasia and of the hemispheric side of lesion on abstract thinking. *Cortex, 2,* 399–420.

De Renzi, E., Faglioni, P, Scotti, G., & Spinnler, H. 1972. Impairment of color sorting behavior after hemispheric damage: An experimental study with the Holmgren skein test. *Cortex, 8,* 147–163.

De Renzi, E., & Vignolo, L. A. 1962. The Token Test: A sensitive test to detect receptive disturbances in aphasics. *Brain, 85,* 665–678.

Duffy, R., Duffy, J., & Pearson, K. 1975. Pantomime recognition in aphasic patients. *Journal of Speech and Hearing Research, 18,* 115–132.

Finkelnburg, F. C. 1870. Niederrheinische Gesellschaft: Sitzung von 21 März 1870 in Bonn. *Berliner Klinischer Wochenschrift, 7,* 449–450; 460–462. (Also published as Finkelnburg's 1870 lecture on aphasia with commentary, R. J. Duffy & B. Z. Liles [trans.]. 1979. *Journal of Speech and Hearing Disorders, 44,* 156–168.)

Freud, S. 1891. *Zur Auffassung der Aphasien.* Leipzig & Vienna: Deuticke. (Also published as *On aphasia,* E. Stengel [Trans.]. 1953. New York: International Universities Press.)

Galaburda, A. M., Sanides, F., & Geschwind, N. 1978. Human brain: Cytoarchitectonic right–left asymmetries in the temporal speech region. *Archives of Neurology, 35,* 812–817.

Gazzaniga, M. S. 1970. *The bisected brain.* New York: Appleton.

Gazzaniga, M. S., & Sperry, R. W. 1967. Language after section of the cerebral commissures. *Brain, 90,* 131–148.

Geschwind, N. 1965. Disconnexion syndromes in animals and man. *Brain, 88,* 237–294; 585–644.

Geschwind, N. 1967. Wernicke's contribution to the study of aphasia. *Cortex, 3,* 449–463.

Geschwind, N., & Levitsky, W. 1970. Human brain: Left–right asymmetries in temporal speech region. *Science, 161,* 186–187.

Geschwind, N., Quadfasel, F. A., & Segarra, J. M. 1968. Isolation of the speech area. *Neuropsychologia, 6,* 327–340.

Goldstein, K. 1924. Das Wesen der amnestischen Aphasie. *Schweizer Archiv fuer Neurologie und Psychiatrie, 15,* 163–175.

Goldstein, K. 1948. *Language and language disturbances.* New York: Grune & Stratton.

Goldstein, K., & Scheerer, M. 1941. Abstract and concrete behavior: An experimental study with special tests. *Psychological Monographs, 43,* 1–151.

Goodglass, H., Gleason, J. B., & Hyde, M. 1970. Some dimensions of auditory language comprehension in aphasics. *Journal of Speech and Hearing Research, 13,* 595–606.

Goodglass, H., & Mayer, J. 1958. Agrammatism in aphasia. *Journal of Speech and Hearing Disorders, 23,* 99–111.

Goodglass, H., & Quadfasel, F. A. 1954. Language laterality in left-handed aphasics. *Brain, 77,* 521–548.

Goodglass, H., Quadfasel, F. A., & Timberlake, W. H. 1964. Phrase length and type and severity of aphasia. *Cortex, 1,* 133–153.

Gott, P. S. 1973. Language after dominant hemispherectomy. *Journal of Neurology, Neurosurgery and Psychiatry, 36,* 1082–1088.

Hamsher, K., Levin, H. S., & Benton, A. L. 1979. Facial recognition in patients with focal brain lesions. *Archives of Neurology, 36,* 837–839.

Head, H. 1926. *Aphasia and kindred disorders of speech.* London: Cambridge Univ. Press.

Hécaen, H., & Ajuriaguerra, J. de. 1963. *Les gauchers: Prévalence manuelle et dominance cérébrale.* Paris: Presses Universitaires de France.

Henschen, S. E. 1919–1922. *Klinische und anatomische Beiträge zur Pathologie des Gehirnes,* 7 vols. Stockholm: Nordiska Bokhandlen.

Humphrey, M. E., & Zangwill, O. L. 1952. Dysphasia in left-handed patients with unilateral brain lesions. *Journal of Neurology, Neurosurgery and Psychiatry, 15,* 184–193.

Jackson, J. H. 1874. On the nature of the duality of the brain. *Medical Press and Circular.* 1, 19, 41, 63. (Reprinted in *Brain,* 1915, *38,* 80–103.)

Jackson, J. H. 1878. On affections of speech from disease of the brain. *Brain, 1,* 304–330.

Jakobson, R. 1941. *Aphasie, Kindersprache und allgemeine Lautgesetze.* Uppsala: Almquist & Wiksell. (Also published as: *Child language, aphasia and language universals,* A. R. Keiler [Trans.]. 1968. The Hague: Mouton.)

Jakobson, R. 1956. Two aspects of language and two types of aphasic disturbances. In R. Jakobsen & M. Halle (Eds.), *Fundamentals of language.* The Hague: Mouton.

Joynt, R. J., & Benton, A. L. 1964. The memoir of Marc Dax on aphasia. *Neurology, 14,* 851-854.

Kerchensteiner, M., Poeck, K., & Brunner, E. 1972. The fluency-nonfluency dimension in the classification of aphasic speech. *Cortex, 8,* 233-247.

Kleist, K. 1934. *Gehirnpathologie.* Leipzig: Barth.

Lecours, A. R., & Lhermitte, F. 1979. *L'aphasie.* Paris: Flammarion.

Lesser, R. 1978. *Linguistic investigations of aphasia.* London: Arnold.

Lichtheim, L. 1885. [On aphasia.] *Brain, 7,* 433-485. (Originally published in *Deutsches Archiv fuer Klinische Medizin,* 1885, *36,* 204-268.)

Lordat, J. 1843. Analyse de la parole pour servir à la theorie de divers cas d'alalie et de paralalie. *Journal de la Société de Médecine Pratique de Montpellier, 7,* 333-353, 417-433; *8,* 1-17.

Marcé, L. V. 1856. Sur quelques observations de physiologie pathologique tendant à démontrer l'existence d'un principe coordinateur de l'écriture. *Mémoires de la Société de Biologie, 3,* 93-115.

Marie, P. 1906. La troisième circonvolution frontale gauche ne joue aucun rôle spécial dans la fonction du langage. *Semaine Médicale, 26,* 241-247.

Marshall, J. C., & Newcombe, F. 1966. Syntactic and semantic errors in paralexia. *Neuropsychologia, 4,* 169-176.

Meunier, M. 1924. *Histoire de la médecine.* Paris: Le François.

Mills, C. K. 1899. Anomia and paranomia with some considerations regarding a naming center in the temporal lobe. *Journal of Nervous and Mental Disease, 26,* 757-758.

Milner, B., Branch, C., & Rasmussen, T. 1966. Evidence for bilateral speech representation in some non-right handers. *Transactions of the American Neurological Association, 91,* 306-308.

Nielsen, J. M. 1936. *Agnosia, apraxia, aphasia: Their value in cerebral localization.* New York: Hoeber.

Ogle, W. 1867. Aphasia and agraphia. *St. George's Hospital Reports, 2,* 83-122.

Ombredane, A. 1926. Sur le méchanisme de l'anarthrie et sur les troubles associés due langage intérieur. *Journal de Psychologie Normale et Pathologique, 23,* 940-955.

Ombredane, A. 1933. Le langage. In G. Dumas (Ed.), *Nouveau traité de psychologie* (Vol. 3). Paris: Alcan.

Orgass, B., Hartje, W., Kerchensteiner, M., & Poeck, K. 1972. Aphasie und nichtsprachliche intelligenz. *Nervenarzt, 43,* 623-627.

Orgass, B., & Poeck, K. 1966. Clinical evaluation of a new test for aphasia: An experimental study of the Token Test. *Cortex, 2,* 222-243.

Osborne, J. 1833. On the loss of faculty of speech depending on forgetfulness of the art of using the vocal organs. *Dublin Journal of Medical and Chemical Science, 4,* 157-170.

Pagel, W. 1958. Medieval and Renaissance contributions to knowledge of the brain and its functions. In F. N. L. Poynter (Ed.), *The history and philosophy of knowledge of the brain and its functions.* Oxford: Blackwell.

Pick, A. 1913. *Die agrammatischen sprachstörungen.* Berlin: Springer-Verlag.

Pitres, A. L. 1898. *L'aphasie amnésique et ses variétés cliniques.* Paris: Alcan.

Poetzl, O. 1928. Die optisch-agnostischen Stoerungen. Leipzig: Deuticke.

Raven, J. C. 1938. *Progressive matrices.* London: H. K. Lewis.

Raven, J. C. 1963. *Guide to using the Coloured Progressive Matrices.* London: H. K. Lewis.

Rubens, A. 1976. Transcortical motor aphasia. In H. Whitaker & H. A. Whitaker (Eds.), *Studies in neurolinguistics* (Vol. 1). New York: Academic Press.

Russell, W. R., & Espir, M. L. E. 1961. *Traumatic aphasia*. Oxford: Oxford Univ. Press.
Smith, A. 1966. Speech and other functions after left (dominant) hemispherectomy. *Journal of Neurology, Neurosurgery and Psychiatry, 29,* 467–471.
Soury, J. 1899. *Le système nerveux central*. Paris: Carré & Naud.
Spreen, O., & Wachal, R. S. 1973. Psycholinguistic analysis of aphasic language. *Language and Speech, 16,* 130–146.
Subirana, A. 1969. Handedness and cerebral dominance. In P. J. Vinken & G. W. Bruyn (Eds.), *Handbook of clinical neurology* (Vol. 4). Amsterdam: North Holland.
Trousseau, A. 1865. *Clinique medicale de l'Hôtel-Dieu de Paris* (2nd ed.). Paris: J. B. Baillière.
Varney, N. R. 1978. Linguistic correlates of pantomime recognition in aphasic patients. *Journal of Neurology, Neurosurgery and Psychiatry, 41,* 564–568.
Wachal, R. S., & Spreen, O. 1973. Some measures of lexical diversity in aphasic and normal language performance. *Language and Speech, 16,* 169–181.
Wada, J. A. 1969. Interhemispheric sharing and shift of cerebral speech function. *Excerpta Medica International Congress Series, 193,* 296–297.
Wada, J. A., Clarke R., & Hamm, A. 1975. Cerebral hemispheric asymmetry in humans. *Archives of Neurology, 32,* 239–246.
Wada, J., & Rasmussen, T. 1960. Intra-carotid injection of sodium amytal for the lateralization of cerebral speech dominance. *Journal of Neurosurgery, 17,* 262–282.
Wechsler, D. 1944. *The measurement of adult intelligence* (3rd ed.). Baltimore: Williams & Wilkins.
Wechsler, D. 1958. *The measurement and appraisal of adult intelligence* (4th ed.). Baltimore: Williams & Wilkins.
Weisenburg, T., & McBride, K. E. 1935. *Aphasia*. New York: Commonwealth Fund. (Reprinted in 1964, New York: Hafner.)
Wernicke, C. 1874. *Der aphasische Symptomenkomplex*. Breslau: Cohn and Weigert.
Wernicke, C. 1886. Einige neuere Arbeiten über Aphasie. *Fortschritte der Medizin, 4,* 371–377.
Witelson, S. F., & Pallie, W. 1973. Left hemisphere specialization for language in the newborn: Neuroanatomical evidence of asymmetry. *Brain, 96,* 641–646.
Young, R. M. 1970. *Mind, brain, and adaptation in the nineteenth century*. Oxford: Oxford Univ. Press (Clarendon).

2

Cerebral Localization of the Aphasias[1]

HANNA DAMASIO

The history of cerebral localization of the aphasias begins with Broca's discovery of a relation between a disturbance of language and damage to the lower posterolateral aspect of the left frontal lobe (Broca, 1861a, 1861b). Broca was not only calling attention to the asymmetry of the brain in relation to language, in what became the first modern study in cerebral dominance, but preparing the ground for further correlations between acquired aphasia and cerebral lesions. The next historical step came with Wernicke's report of the association between the symptom complex of Wernicke's aphasia and damage to the posterior aspect of the first left temporal gyrus (Wernicke, 1874). The notion of left cerebral dominance acquired strength, and the concept that different pathological behaviors could be related to different brain lesions established itself. Wernicke proceeded to predict the anatomical lesion responsible for a third aphasia type, conduction aphasia. The lesion, he thought, would fall between those found in Wernicke's aphasia and in Broca's aphasia, most probably in the insular region. It is currently apparent that, in essence, the prediction was correct.

The next major step came with Déjerine's description of the syndromes of alexia with agraphia (1891) and alexia without agraphia (1892). His reports established a connection between written language and the brain, just as Broca's and Wernicke's had established a link between the brain and aural language. Alexia with agraphia was associated with damage to the parietal lobe, in structures interposed be-

---

1. See Figures 2.14–2.19 at the end of this chapter for diagrams of left hemisphere, basal ganglia, ventricular system, and normal CT scan.

ACQUIRED APHASIA

tween Wernicke's area and the visual association cortex. On the other hand, alexia without agraphia was found to be the result of a lesion exclusively located in the left occipital lobe. The location of the lesion was such that it would prevent access of visual information to those structures of the parietal and temporal lobe with which impairments of reading, writing, and aural comprehension had previously been associated. The lesion had to be strategically located at a crossroads of visual information traffic. It interrupted the flow of information from the right to the left visual cortices, by means of damaging either the corpus callosum proper or its outflow (the *forceps major*). It also severed crucial connections between the left visual cortex itself and left parietal and temporal language cortex.

A further step in the anatomical mapping of the aphasias should be noted. Wernicke, and later on Goldstein (cf. Goldstein, 1948), reported on the appearance of peculiar forms of aphasia, different from the ones described until then and also associated with different lesions. Two major varieties of aphasia, designated transcortical motor and transcortical sensory, were thus added, both hallmarked by a lack of impediment in verbal repetition. Significantly, the anatomical correlates of those aphasias were located both anteriorly and posteriorly to the ones associated with the other varieties. For transcortical motor aphasia, the lesion was in frontal lobe structures rostral to Broca's area. For transcortical sensory aphasia, damage was found in parietal and occipitotemporal structures posterior to Wernicke's area. (Figure 2.1 illustrates the gross localization of these fundamental syndromes of aphasia.)

The decades that followed consolidated knowledge of aphasia localization. Numerous case reports of all the principal types of aphasia, accompanied by more or less expert description of clinical symptomatology, confirmed the essential correctness of the discoveries of the founders of aphasiology. Occasionally such case reports gave rise to conflicting evidence but rarely if ever shattered the foundations provided by the work of Broca, Wernicke, Dejerine, and Goldstein. More often than not, they refined the gross mapping of the earlier days, rendering knowledge of the anatomical localization of the aphasias more complex.

In 1965 Geschwind drew on this remarkable body of morphological evidence to interpret the aphasias and associated disorders in modern anatomical and physiological terms. In the years that followed, stimulated by Geschwind's seminal monograph, the anatomical correlation of the various aphasic syndromes was reassessed. New tools were added, too: the radionuclide brain scan made its appearance permitting new anatomical insights, and the Boston Aphasia Research Center's classi-

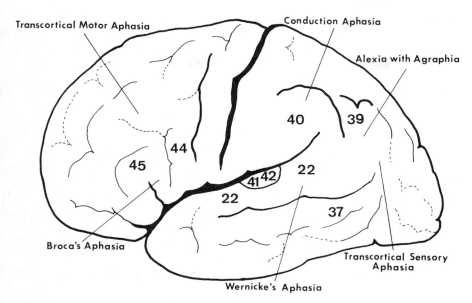

FIGURE 2.1. *Diagrammatic representation of the major loci of lesions in the principal types of aphasia. Brodmann's areas 44 and 45 correspond to the classic Broca's area, area 22 to Wernicke's area. Areas 41 and 42 correspond to the primary auditory cortex; these extend into the depth of the sylvian fissure. Area 40 = supramarginal gyrus. Area 39 = angular gyrus. Area 37, principally located in the posterior sector of the second temporal gyrus, does not have correspondence in gyral nomenclature.*

fication key became widely known, permitting a better comparison of cases originating in different centers. The notion of fluency as a useful variable for correlation was also introduced. Using radionuclide brain scans, Benson demonstrated a consistent association between nonfluent speech and prerolandic lesions, and between fluent speech and post-rolandic lesions (Benson *et al.*, 1968). The nonfluent aphasias were those of the Broca and transcortical motor types. Within the limits of brain scan resolution, they correlated as expected with left frontal lobe lesions. The fluent aphasias included Wernicke's, conduction, and transcortical sensory, which tended to cluster in the posterior left quadrant as expected. For a variety of reasons, some exceptions to this pattern were found. But the adherence to this rule was more impressive than the departure from it. Only a partially conflicting study came to light (Karis & Horenstein, 1976), whereas a more extensive study corroborated the results of Benson (Kertesz, Lesk, & McCabe, 1977).

The advent of computerized tomography (CT) in 1973 changed the panorama of the anatomical study of higher behavior in the human. For the aphasia field, CT was particularly beneficial. Unlike radionuclide brain scan, CT provided the possibility of studying with considerable anatomical detail not only a large variety of cerebral lesions but also the surrounding intact cerebral tissue. After the first few years of technological upgrading and methodological pathfinding, CT studies have now reached a stage that permits the *in vivo* description of cerebral changes necessary both for comprehensive clinical evaluation and for research.

The first study of CT correlations with aphasia came from Naeser and Hayward (1978). Their localization of Broca's, Wernicke's, conduction, and global aphasias conformed to classical anatomical localizations. Kertesz and his co-workers (Kertesz, Harlock, & Coates, 1979) replicated Naeser and Hayward's findings, adding data on the differences produced by acute and chronic stages of aphasia. Later, by establishing a correspondence between gross brain anatomy and Brodmann's cytoarchitectonic map, other authors attempted to further the localizational information of CT scan studies (H. Damasio & A. Damasio, 1979a; Gado, Hanaway, & Frank, 1979) by developing templates of the CT cuts. Using bony structures and the ventricular system as landmarks, the lesions seen in the CT scan were plotted into the best-fitting templates and then read as a three-dimensional reconstruction. Using this method we have studied the CT scan correlates of the major types of aphasia (A. Damasio & H. Damasio, 1980, 1981; A. Damasio, H. Damasio, & Chui, 1980; A. Damasio, Yamada, H. Damasio, & McKee, 1980; H. Damasio & A. Damasio, 1979b, 1980).

Fluent Aphasias

Conduction Aphasia

The anatomical correlates of conduction aphasia have been well documented with postmortem studies (Benson, Sheremata, Buchard, Segarra, Price, & Geschwind, 1973) and CT scan (H. Damasio & A. Damasio, 1980) studies.

Conduction aphasia is associated with left perisylvian lesions involving the primary auditory cortex (areas 41 and 42), a portion of the surrounding association cortex (area 22), and to a variable degree the insula and its subcortical white matter as well as the supramarginal gyrus (area 40). In some cases with lesser or no involvement of auditory and insular regions, the compromise of area 40 is extensive. In Figure 2.2 the pathological changes in six cases of conduction aphasia are superimposed in a composite diagram. The lesions appear at template levels 4–10, but they cluster preponderantly in levels 4–7. Each level represents a CT scan cut and is separated from the next by approximately 1 cm. The extent to which such lesions project to the left lateral surface of the brain is variable. Some are so well contained within the sylvian fissure (where areas 41, 42, and a good portion of 22 are located) that they would not be visible

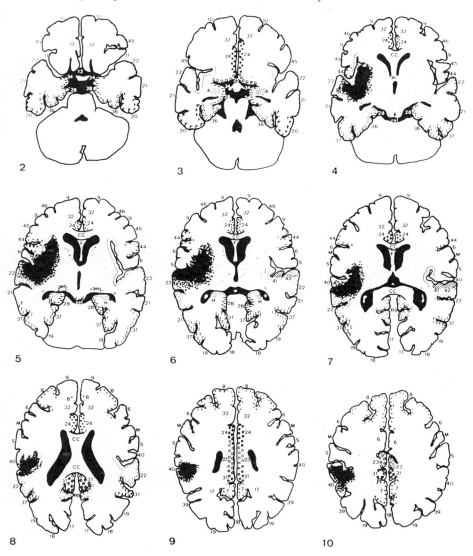

FIGURE 2.2. *Composite diagram of the lesions in six cases of conduction aphasia.*

on the surface. However, the ones involving supramarginal gyrus would be seen in the suprasylvian region.

Wernicke's Aphasia

Wernicke's aphasia is generally associated with lesions of the posterior region of the left superior temporal gyrus. But the lesions often extend into the second temporal gyrus and into the nearby parietal region, particularly the angular gyrus. A typical example is shown in Figure 2.3. We have studied the CT scan correlates of patients with Wernicke's aphasia. All our patients had fluent paraphasic speech, with semantic and phonemic paraphasias, and severe impairment in aural comprehension, visual naming, and sentence repetition. A composite diagram of the lesions found in those cases can be seen in Figure 2.4. It indicates some involvement of the primary auditory cortex (areas 41 and 42) and a particularly extensive compromise of the surrounding area 22 (Wernicke's area). The latter corresponds both to the lateral aspect of 22 as well as to its reflection in the planum temporale. In addition there is

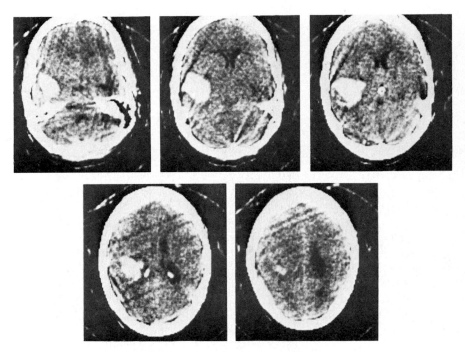

FIGURE 2.3. *CT scan of a patient with Wernicke's aphasia.*

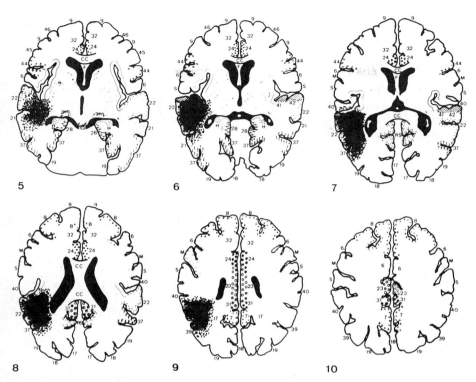

FIGURE 2.4. *Composite diagram of lesions found in cases of Wernicke's aphasia.*

extension into the second temporal gyrus (in which part of area 37 and area 21 are located), and some involvement of the angular gyrus (area 39). Most lesions extend into the cerebral depth compromising cortical and subcortical white matter. Some reach the left lateral ventricle at the level of the trigone. Rarely the lesion may be exclusively in the white matter and spare the cortex. No lesion extends into the insula. Although a lateral surface view of the brain would fail to indicate the real extent of some of these lesions, it would provide a more comprehensive view than with conduction aphasia.

Transcortical Sensory Aphasia

We have analyzed the CT scan correlates of six patients with transcortical sensory aphasia. Two were women and four were men, with ages ranging from 46 to 71 years (mean of 61 years). All these patients had fluent paraphasic speech and defective aural comprehension, but sentence repetition was either normal or minimally impaired.

The plotting of the lesions on the corresponding templates can be seen in Figure 2.5. Damage involves area 37 but extends into portions of area 22. The lesions also reach into area 39 (angular gyrus) and occasionally into the visual association cortex (area 19). Areas spared in these cases include the primary auditory cortex (areas 41 and 42) and most of area 22, both in its anterior sector as well as in the planum temporale.

In summary, transcortical sensory aphasia is associated with left hemisphere lesions involving the posterior portion or the middle temporal gyrus (area 37) and extending into both visual and auditory association cortices as well as occasionally into the angular gyrus.

Comparing these three types of aphasia, it is evident that there are some areas of anatomical overlap. Nevertheless, the core of each anatomical pattern is quite distinctive. Along a rostro-caudal axis, the anatomical core of Wernicke's aphasia seems to occupy the midsector, with involvement of the planum temporale (the posterior portion of area 22, contained in the sylvian fissure) plus some anterior and posterior

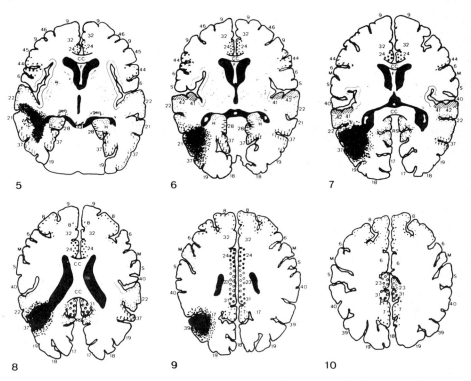

FIGURE 2.5. *Composite diagram of lesions found in six cases of transcortical sensory aphasia.*

extension. The core of conduction aphasia is more anterior, often extending into the insula. Overlap with Wernicke's takes place in the anterior portions of area 22. Transcortical sensory aphasia occupies the more posterior sector, clearly encompassing area 37, and extending into visual association cortex and angular gyrus. Overlap takes place in the more posterior portion of area 22. But none of these three syndromes overlaps anatomically with the nonfluent aphasias discussed in the next section.

If the clinical picture of these three types of aphasia are considered, a similar situation is found. There is some clinical overlap, and yet the core of each syndrome is remarkably distinctive.

Nonfluent Aphasias

Broca's Aphasia

Broca's aphasia is associated with lesions of the left frontal lobe, which generally involve Broca's area (field 44 of Brodmann, located in the third frontal gyrus) and to a variable degree can also involve the nearby lower portion of the motor strip, or other cortical fields anterior or superior to area 44. Variable extension into the underlying white matter is seen in many cases. Mohr (Mohr, Pessin, Finkelstein, Funkenstein, Duncan, & Davis, 1978) has pointed up the wide ranging anatomical correlates of this syndrome and noted that severity of the syndrome with respect not only to the speech defect itself but also to the accompanying neurological and behavioral signs can be related to the location and extent of the lesion. We will illustrate this point with two examples.

Case 1 is that of a 40-year-old, right-handed woman, with a thrombotic infarction. Initially she had a complete inability to utter single words or sentences but had remarkably intact aural comprehension and gestural communication. A right central facial paresis completed the neurological picture. Speech improved rapidly to a nonfluent halting discourse in which connectives were missing. Repetition of sentences was impaired and so was writing. The CT scan showed a small area of gray matter enhancement, suggestive of a lesion in the left frontal lobe, that would involve (*a*) area 45 and 44 (Broca's area); (*b*) the portion of area 6 immediately above (the so-called Exner's area); and (*c*) the nearby facial motor region. Subcortical extension was minimal (see Figure 2.6). This patient continued to recover so well that one year later she had only minimal signs of impairment. Her speech is now slow but grammatically correct.

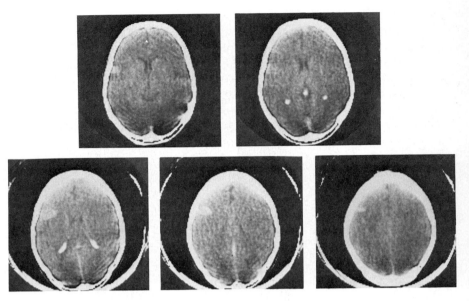

FIGURE 2.6. *CT scan of a patient with Broca's aphasia.*

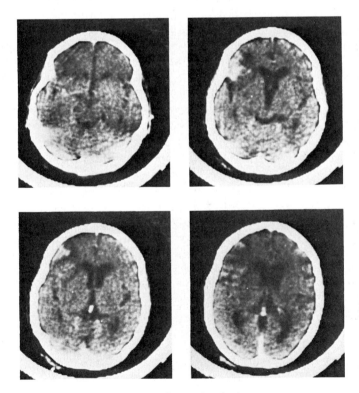

FIGURE 2.7. *CT scan of another patient with Broca's aphasia.*

Case 2 represents the other extreme of Broca's aphasia. A 74-year-old right-handed woman suffered a thrombotic infarction. In the acute phase, she had minimal speech output, inability to repeat words or sentences, a defect in aural comprehension, impaired reading and writing, and right-sided neglect. The CT scan of this woman also showed a lesion in the left frontal lobe, but it included far more than Broca's area. Areas 45 and 44 were involved, but the lesion extended into areas 6 and 9 as well as into the motor cortex. Furthermore, it extended deep into the white matter reaching close to the anterior horn of the left lateral ventricle, damaging part of the head of the caudate nucleus as well as part of the lenticular nucleus (see Figure 2.7). It should be noted, however, that regardless of being an extensive lesion, it does not reach posteriorly into the insula or temporal lobe region; that is, it never overlaps areas related to the fluent aphasias. The evolution of this case was quite different from the previous one. Speech, as it emerged, was nonfluent, with the usual characteristics of Broca's aphasia. But recovery was modest in comparison to the first case.

Transcortical Motor Aphasia

The principal difference between transcortical motor aphasia and Broca's aphasia is in verbal repetition, which is possible in the former and impaired in the latter. Patients with transcortical motor aphasia often have echolalia in the setting of an otherwise nonfluent speech. Lesions are invariably located outside Broca's area, either deep in the left frontal substance or else in the cortex but anteriorly or superiorly to Broca's area. Figure 2.8 shows the CT scan template of a case of transcortical motor aphasia. The lesion is small, located deep in the white matter of the left frontal lobe. It lies anteriorly but close to the anterior horn of the left lateral ventricle. It does not involve cortical areas. It most certainly disrupts connections between mesial structures of the frontal lobe, namely the supplementary motor area, and structures of Broca's area and the motor area.

Mutism

The syndromes of mutism are not, in the strict sense, part of the aphasias. In mutism, speech output is minimal or absent at all times, unlike the aphasias, in which it is only absent during the acute phase. However, the place of mutism in a discussion of localization of the aphasias is justified and necessary, since it is often mistaken for transcortical motor aphasia and even for Broca's aphasia. The clinical dif-

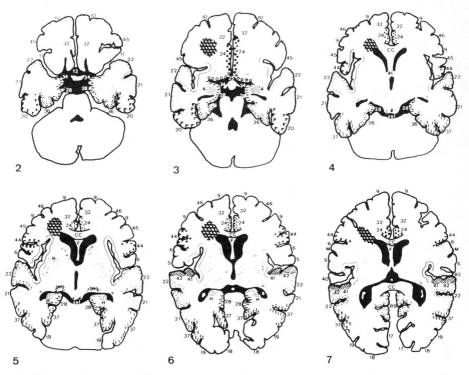

FIGURE 2.8. *Template of CT scan of a patient with transcortical motor aphasia.*

ferences, however, are clear, and the anatomical localization distinct for both. Patients with mutism are aspontaneous both in relation to their nonexistent speech as well as in relation to other motor behaviors, for example, gestural communication and motor drive toward new stimuli. However, if stimulated enough, they can repeat words and sentences normally, and their comprehension of aural and written language is intact. The recovery of these patients is also different from that of patients with Broca's aphasia or transcortical motor aphasias, since the improvement is usually speedier (in fact it can be sudden) and proceeds into grammatically correct speech with normal fluency without an intervening agrammatical stage. True mutism is associated with lesions in the mesial aspect of the frontal lobe, which involves the supplementary motor area (the mesial portion of area 6), its connections, and the nearby anterior cingulate (area 24).

Figure 2.9 is a composite diagram of lesions in three cases of mutism. The lesions appear in the very high portion of the left frontal lobe, above

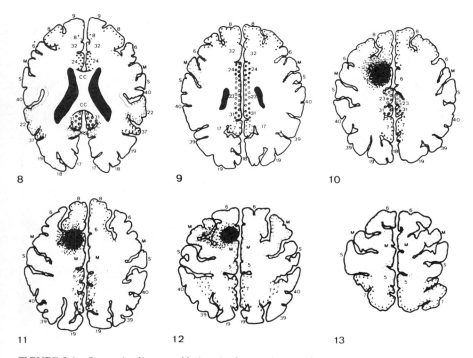

FIGURE 2.9. *Composite diagram of lesions in three patients with mutism.*

the level of the lateral ventricles. The core of damage involves the white matter immediately underneath the mesial portion of area 6. The nearby anterior cingulate cortex and its connections are involved to a variable extent. The damage can extend to involve motor areas mainly in their mesial aspect (corresponding to the cerebral representation of the lower limb) but also in their lateral portion (related to upper limb representation). This generally correlates with the presence or absence of paralysis of the foot and leg or of the arm. The lesion does not extend into the frontal regions, which we have previously seen affected in the aphasias.

Global Aphasia

Patients with global aphasia, like those with Broca's aphasia, may have variable lesions, both in extent and in location. The expected lesion in a patient with the typical clinical picture will involve the whole left perisylvian region, affecting all areas correlated to the different types of

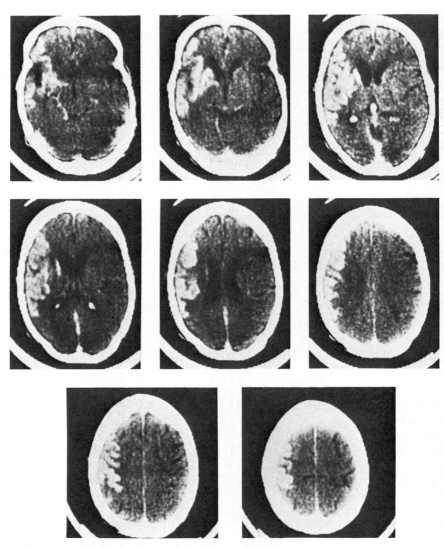

FIGURE 2.10. *CT scan of a patient with global aphasia.*

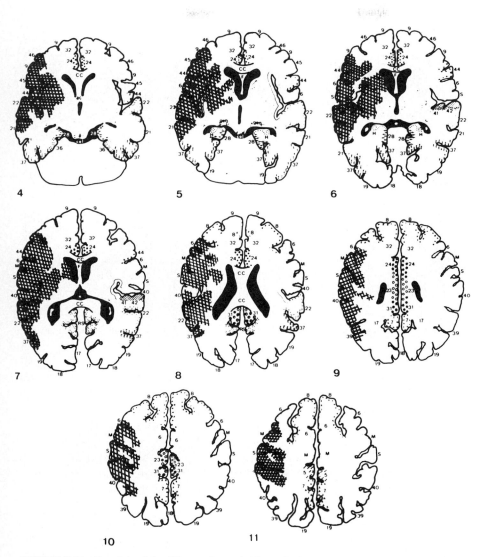

FIGURE 2.11. *Template of the CT scan shown in Figure 2.10.*

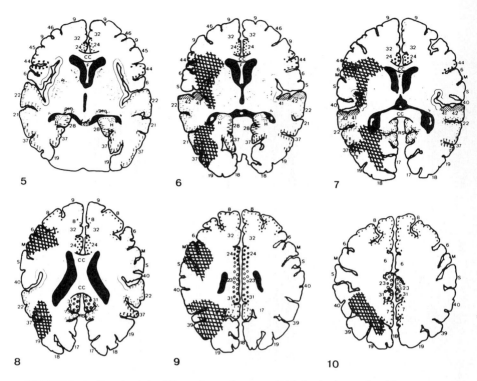

FIGURE 2.12. *Template of a CT scan in another case of global aphasia, produced by two separate lesions.*

aphasia. Figure 2.10 shows the lesions of such a case. The lesion is the result of an infarction in the territory of the middle cerebral artery. All the perisylvian language areas are involved. As can be seen in Figure 2.11, the damage extends from areas 45 and 44 anteriorly, to the insula, to the auditory areas 41, 42, and 22, to area 40, and in part to areas 39 and 37. The motor and somatosensory areas 4,3,1, and 2 are also involved. But the damage is not limited to the cortex: There is involvement of the underlying white matter as well as of the lenticular and the caudate nuclei.

A similar clinical picture can be seen with the combination of two lesions in the left hemisphere, one anterior and one posterior. This possibility is illustrated in Figure 2.12. In this case the anterior lesion involves area 44 as well as the underlying white matter and extends into the insula. The posterior lesion involves white matter close to the wall of the left lateral ventricle at the level of the trigone, extending into areas

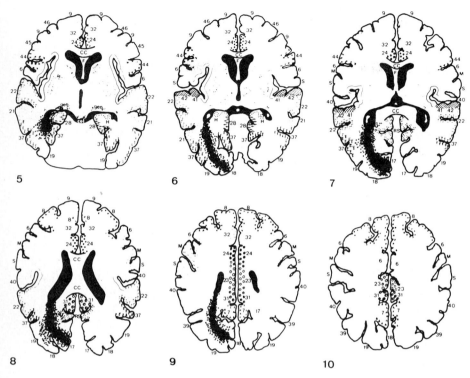

FIGURE 2.13. *Composite diagram of CT scans obtained in patients presenting with alexia without agraphia.*

37, 19, 39, and 40. The patient had a global aphasia with severe impairment in all linguistic abilities.

It is hoped that in the future these different anatomical localizations will be correlated either with subtle differences in the clinical features of global aphasia or with different patterns of recovery from this type of aphasia. So far not enough data are available to permit a prediction of the different localizations on the basis of clinical evaluation.

Alexia without Agraphia (Pure Alexia)

Alexia without agraphia is not an aphasic disorder as such, since speech output and aural comprehension are intact. However, these patients are unable to comprehend written language and are, in that sense, aphasic. The syndrome is associated with a remarkably consistent anatomical localization. Figure 2.13 gives the composite of nine cases of alexia without agraphia. In general the lesion extends from the occipital cortex deep into the white matter, reaching the left lateral ventricle at the level of the trigone and occipital horn. It involves both the primary visual cortex (area 17) and the visual association cortices (areas 18 and 19). In a few cases it can extend into the white matter underlying areas 37 and 21. The optic radiations are compromised in some way in all cases. Only in one of these cases does the lesion involve the corpus callosum proper at the level of the splenium. In all cases, however, the lesions disrupt the fibers coming from the splenium of the corpus callosum, in the forceps major. Hence, callosal output is interrupted before it can reach multimodal association areas (e.g., 39 and 37) of the left hemisphere.

Atypical Aphasias

We have had the opportunity to identify some cases of atypical aphasia syndromes and to discover their anatomical locus. These aphasias are generally of the fluent type, resembling Wernicke's aphasia, but unlike what is seen in typical fluent aphasias, there are disturbances of articulation and often right hemiparesis.

The lesions are located deep in the left hemisphere and invariably include the anterior limb of the internal capsule. In addition, portions of the putamen and caudate can be variably compromised. Such cases present no evidence of cortical damage and represent an entirely new variety of aphasia (A. Damasio & H. Damasio, 1981).

In conclusion, a large variety of acquired aphasic syndromes and of closely associated disturbances (mutism, pure alexia) can be related to relatively specific brain lesions, located throughout the left cerebral hemisphere. More than 100 years of study of anatomoclinical correlations, using autopsy material as well as radionuclide brain scans and CT scans, have proven that, in spite of the inevitable variability from patient to patient, the correlation between aphasic syndromes and cerebral localization is extremely consistent. But numerous exceptions exist, which can be found, in particular, in left-handed subjects, whose cerebral dominance for language is variable and even in a minority of right-handed subjects who have right cerebral dominance for language and therefore give rise to "crossed" aphasia syndromes when their right hemispheres are injured.

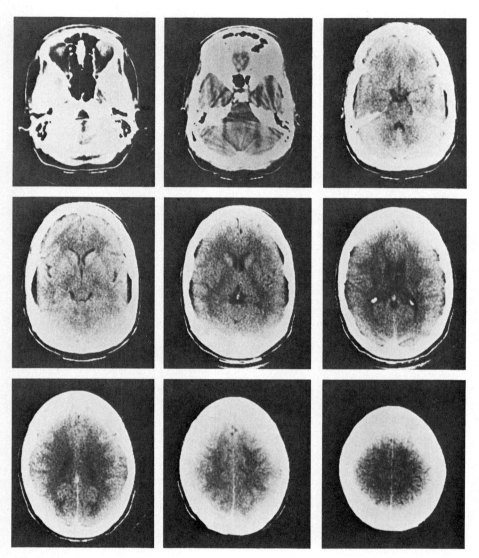

FIGURE 2.14. *Normal CT scan image. The white shading corresponds to maximum absorption of X rays (e.g., calcium in bone); the black shading to minimal absorption (OH$_2$ in cerebrospinal fluid). The white matter has a lower degree of absorption than the gray matter and is therefore darker. CT scan cuts are usually made at an angle of 15–25° to the inferior cantomeatal line. Cuts should be read from left to right and from top to bottom, the first one representing the lowest brain cut, the last one, the highest cut. Unless otherwise marked, the brain is observed from the top; therefore the left hemisphere is on the left.*

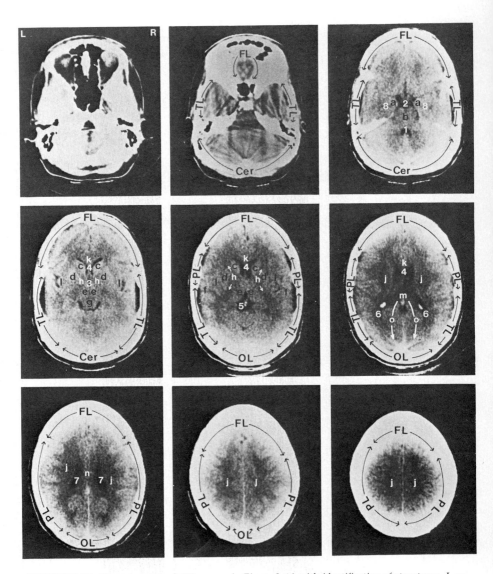

FIGURE 2.15. *The same normal CT scan as in Figure 2.14 with identification of structures. L =* *left; R = right; FL = frontal lobe; TL = temporal lobe; PL = parietal lobe; OL = occipital lobe;* *Cer = cerebellum; l = insula limited laterally by the sylvian fissure; a = amygdala; b = brain* *stem; c = head of the caudate nucleus; d = lenticular nucleus; e = thalamus; f = primary* *auditory area; g = colliculi; h = internal capsule at the genu (the arrows are placed in the anterior* *and posterior limb of the internal capsule); j = centrum semi ovale (the bulk of the white matter in* *each hemisphere); l = genu of corpus callosum; m = splenium of corpus callosum; n = body of corpus* *callosum; o = the arrows indicate the outflow of the splenium of the corpus callosum toward visual* *cortex—the forceps major; 1 = fourth ventricle; 2 = suprasellar cistern; 3 = third ventricle; 4 =* *anterior horns of the lateral ventricles; 5 = superior cerebellar cistern; 6 = occipital horn of lateral* *ventricles; 7 = body of lateral ventricles; 8 = temporal horn of lateral ventricle seen only as a slit.*

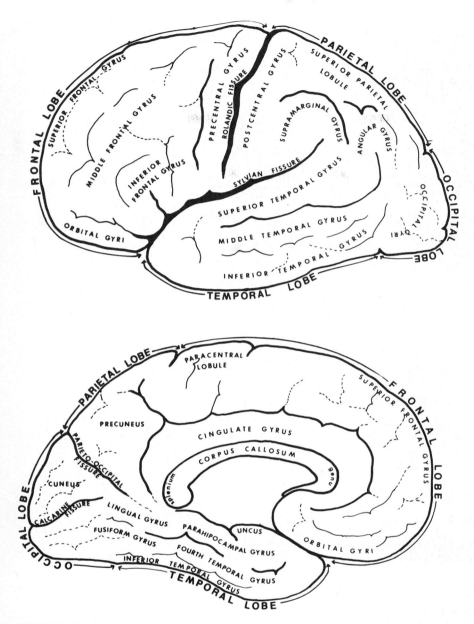

FIGURE 2.16. *Left hemisphere, lateral and mesial aspects, with identification of the four lobes, major fissures, and gyri. Note that the insula cannot be seen on a lateral view since it is buried in the depth of the sylvian fissure, in its anterior portion, and is covered by the frontal operculum (the more posterior and inferior portion of the inferior frontal gyrus and the inferior portion of the precentral gyrus).*

47

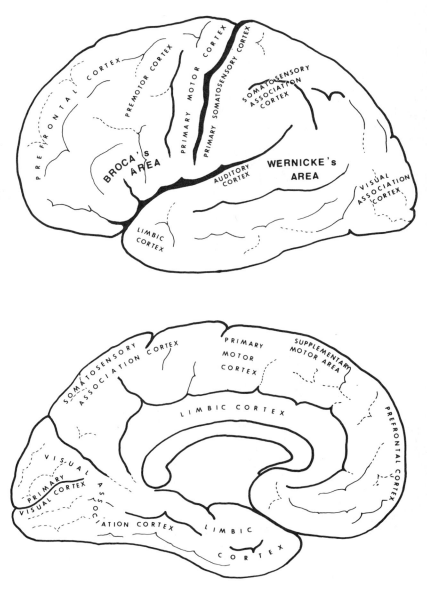

FIGURE 2.17. *Left hemisphere, lateral and mesial aspects, with identification of the major functional areas. Note that the auditory cortex occupies both the lateral aspect of the superior temporal gyrus and the superior aspect, inside the sylvian fissure (not seen in this lateral view) where the transverse temporal gyri (the primary auditory areas) and the planum temporale are located.*

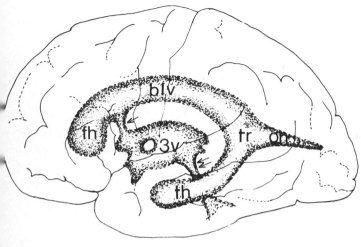

fh + blv + tr + oh + th = left lateral ventricle; fh = frontal horn; blv = body; tr = trigone; oh = occipital horn; th = temporal horn; 3v = third ventricle which connects with both lateral ventricles through the foramina of Monro (the left one is marked with an arrow) and continues caudally into the aqueduct (double arrow).

FIGURE 2.18. *Left hemisphere with the ventricular system.*

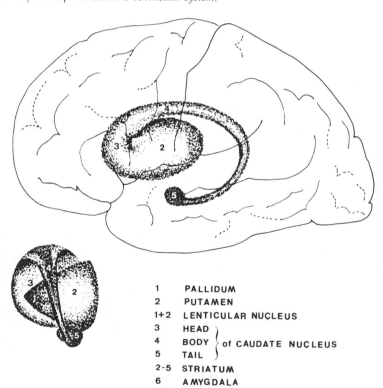

1	PALLIDUM
2	PUTAMEN
1+2	LENTICULAR NUCLEUS
3	HEAD ⎫
4	BODY ⎬ of CAUDATE NUCLEUS
5	TAIL ⎭
2-5	STRIATUM
6	AMYGDALA

FIGURE 2.19. *Left hemisphere with the basal ganglia seen in lateral view. The insert shows the basal ganglia seen from the occipital pole.*

49

References

Benson, D. F. 1967. Fluency in aphasia: Correlation with radioactive scan localization. *Cortex, 3,* 373–394.

Benson, D. F., Sheremata, W. A., Buchard, R., Segarra, J., Price, D., & Geschwind, N. 1973. Conduction aphasia. *Archives of Neurology, 28,* 339–346.

Broca, P. 1861. Portée de la parole. Ramollisement chronique et destruction partielle du lobe antérieur gauche du cerveau. *Paris Bulletin de la Société d'Anthropologie, 2,* 219. (a)

Broca, P. 1861. Remarques sur le siège de la faculté du langage articulé, suivies d'une observation d'aphémie. *Paris Bulletin de la Société d'Anatomie, 2,* 330–357. (b)

Damasio, A., & Damasio, H. 1981. Aphasia with nonhemorrhagic lesions in the basal ganglia and internal capsule. *Archives of Neurology* (in press).

Damasio, A., & Damasio, H. 1980. Prosopagnosia: Anatomical basis and neurobehavioral mechanism. *Neurology, 30,* 390.

Damasio, A., Damasio, H., & Chui, H. 1980. Neglect following damage to frontal lobe or basal ganglia. *Neuropsychologia, 18,* 123–132.

Damasio, A., Yamada, T., Damasio, H., & McKee, J. 1980. Central achromatopsia: Behavioral, anatomical, and physiologic aspects. *Neurology, 30,* 1064–1071.

Damasio, H., & Damasio, A. 1979. *A computerized tomography guide to the identification of cerebral structures.* Department of Neurology, University of Iowa College of Medicine. (a)

Damasio, H., & Damasio, A. 1979. "Paradoxic" extinction in dichotic listening: Possible anatomic significance. *Neurology, 29,* 644–653. (b)

Damasio, H., & Damasio, A. 1980. The anatomical basis of conduction aphasia. *Brain, 103,* 337–350.

Déjerine, J. 1891. Sur un cas de cécité verbale avec agraphie, suivi d'autopsie. *Memoires Société Biologique, 3,* 197–201.

Déjerine, J. 1892. Contribution à l'étude anatomo-pathologique et clinique des différentes variétés de cécité verbale. *Memoires Société Biologique, 4,* 61–90.

Gado, M., Hanaway, J., & Frank, R. 1979. Functional anatomy of the cerebral cortex by computed tomography. *Journal of Computer Assisted Tomography, 3,* 1–19.

Geschwind, N. 1965. Disconnexion syndromes in animals and man. *Brain, 88,* 237–294, 585–644.

Goldstein, K. 1948. *Language and language disturbances.* New York: Grune & Stratton.

Karis, R., & Horenstein, S. 1976. Localization of speech parameters by brain scan. *Neurology, 26,* 226–230.

Kertesz, A., Harlock, W., & Coates, R. 1979. Computer tomographic localization, lesion size, and prognosis in aphasia and nonverbal impairment. *Brain and Language, 8,* 34–50.

Kertesz, A., Lesk, D., & McCabe, P. 1977. Isotope location of infarcts in aphasia. *Archives of Neurology, 34,* 590–601.

Mohr, J. P., Pessin, M. S., Finkelstein, S., Funkenstein, H. H., Duncan, G. W., & Davis, K. R. 1978. Broca aphasia: Pathologic and clinical aspects. *Neurology, 28,* 311–324.

Naeser, M. A., & Hayward, R. W. 1978. Lesion localization in aphasia with cranial computed tomography and the Boston Diagnostic Aphasia Exam. *Neurology, 28,* 545–551.

Wernicke, K. 1874. *Der aphasische symptomkomplex.* Breslau: Cohn and Weigert.

3

The Nature of Aphasia: Signs and Syndromes

ANTONIO DAMASIO

Aphasia is a disturbance of one or more aspects of the complex process of comprehending and formulating verbal messages that results from newly acquired disease of the central nervous system (CNS). We shall begin by considering this operational definition of aphasia, analyzing each of its components.

Newly Acquired Disease. It is important to note that the disease that produces aphasia is both acquired and recent (e.g., cerebral infarction, tumor, or contusion) rather than congenital and long standing (e.g., genetic or environment induced prenatal cerebral defect). The former (acquired disease) befalls individuals previously capable of using language appropriately. The latter may produce developmental language defects in young individuals whose ability to use language will never attain a normal level.

Of the Central Nervous System. The reference to the central nervous system is also important (although it is quite clear that all mental activity and communication stems from the activity of the central nervous system) because aphasia is not the result of a peculiar utilization of language related to psychogenic or social deviations. Furthermore, in true aphasia, the CNS disease compromises certain structures in a focal rather than in a generalized fashion; for example, aphasia is not the result of widespread cerebral disease but rather the consequence of a concentrated, well-targeted insult to the brain.

51

Verbal Messages. Throughout this chapter we will refer to VERBAL COMMUNICATION and to LANGUAGE almost interchangeably. On the other hand, LANGUAGE and SPEECH are not interchangeable terms. The latter should be reserved for the act of "speaking a verbal message" independently of the process of formulating the message itself. In the above definition, we used VERBAL MESSAGES to call attention to the fact that aphasia relates exclusively to a disturbance in verbal language as opposed to other forms of language, for example, the language of gestures or of facial expression.

Disturbance of One or More Aspects of the Complex Process of Comprehending and Formulating Verbal Messages. Aphasia can affect the comprehension of the language the patient either hears spoken or sees written, or both. It can also affect the formulation of his oral language production, his writing, or both. Often, aphasia disturbs both reception and expression of language, in both visual (written) and auditory (spoken) modes. Yet, each of the several fundamental types of aphasia (syndromes) compromises one or two of these modes preponderantly. It is a grave mistake to ignore the marked differences in each syndrome between the verbal communicative abilities that remain intact and those that become either moderately or severely impaired. Indeed, in some instances, (e.g., in PURE ALEXIA or in PURE WORD DEAFNESS), only one of those several abilities will suffer while all others remain unaffected. More about this particular question later.

The emphasis on the terms COMPREHENDING and FORMULATING verbal messages is particularly pertinent. Aphasics have trouble comprehending verbal messages, that is, deciphering their meaning, as opposed to hearing or seeing those messages. Neither deafness (peripheral or central) nor blindness is the problem. Although a deaf or blind person cannot be expected to comprehend within the particular mode of his perceptual impairment, he will comprehend the same verbal message normally if processed by an intact sensory channel, for example, Braille (tactile) reading in the blind. Aphasics have trouble formulating verbal messages for example, choosing the lexical and syntactical items necessary to convey meaning and ordering them in such a way that meaning is indeed imparted on the person who receives the message. But an impediment of phonation that will prevent the production of speech has nothing to do with formulation of verbal messages (people can still write what they cannot say), nor does the loss of the two hands interfere with language formulation (people can still say it if they have formulated it, and they can certainly write with a pen held between the teeth or the toes).

In order to characterize the nature of the disturbance, stating what aphasia is not becomes just as important as stating what it is. For instance, aphasia is not a disturbance of articulation. Many patients suffer from speech disturbances, also acquired and due to novel disease of the central nervous system affecting the cerebral cortex or the basal ganglia, the brain stem or the cerebellum, and, in any case, the left or the right sides of the CNS. Yet few of those patients will have an aphasia also, and it is possible to prove that, although the speech sounds are poorly formed in themselves or are inappropriately repeated in time, the choice of words and the structure of sentences are grammatically correct, appropriate to the intentions of their author, and understandable to the attentive listener or reader. That is to say, such patients have a motor disturbance affecting speech. Stating that they have a speech disturbance is quite acceptable, but it does not follow that they have a verbal language disturbance: Their language formulation is normal, their communication is linguistically correct, and hence, they do not have an aphasia.

Patients with mutism, who can be entirely silent, are not aphasic either, although occasionally their absence of speech does conceal an aphasia. Often these patients fail to indicate any desire to communicate by gesture, mimicry, or writing. Consequently, little is known about what they do or do not comprehend of the environment and what they may or may not want to say (or think, for that matter) about it. However, as most of them awake from these peculiar states of apparent indifference, they resume language communication using proper grammar and showing no evidence of aphasia. When probed about their abnormal behavior, they clearly give testimony to a strange experience of avolition but not to any problem with the actual composition of contents for verbal communication. Most such patients have CNS disease in areas of the brain quite different from those that produce aphasias, for example, in the supplementary motor area or cingulate gyrus, as opposed to the region around the sylvian fissure. A few have acute psychotic states and no gross brain disease, although they suffer from profound changes in neurochemical mediators in certain regions of the brain.

Also not aphasic are patients with aphonia. They are mute, in the narrow sense of the word, but in reality are suffering from an impediment in their phonatory apparatus that prevents them from speaking. (Many acute diseases of the larynx and pharynx can produce aphonia.) They should be able to comprehend language (and indicate so by nodding or pointing responses), and they should be able to turn their thoughts into language by writing, in addition to being able to mouth words. The exception (other than malingering, of course) is a conversion reaction, the currently uncommon psychiatric diagnosis of HYSTERICAL APHONIA.

Finally, it should be clear that the language disorder noted in altered states of consciousness is not an aphasia either. Any patient with a confusional state, that is to say, with a profound disorder of attentional mechanisms, will produce disturbed language and fail to comprehend verbal communication. But such patients have a concomitant disorder of their thought processes that parallels their language disturbance. Unlike the patient with aphasia, who struggles to turn properly organized meanings into language and fails to do so (or tries, without success, to turn the message he heard into internal meaning), patients with confusional states communicate their disorder thought processes verbally, with remarkable success. Confusional states are most commonly produced by metabolic disturbances and intoxications but can be the result of cerebral tumors (either directly affecting the CNS structures that sustain vigilance and the process of attention, or acting by remote mechanisms).

The picture of a patient with aphasia should begin to emerge now.

1. An aphasic produces some speech, or even abundant speech, which is grammatically incorrect. The errors include omission of crucial words (such as connective words and other functors of speech), erroneous choice of words (substitution of the intended word for another that may or may not be related in sound or meaning), or disturbance of word order. The rule that aphasic patients always produce some speech can be violated during the first few hours postonset of disease (or, more rarely, during the first couple of days) in some acute cerebrovascular accidents. But even during that speechless phase, most aphasic patients will attempt to communicate by gesture or facial expression.

2. An aphasic often has difficulty in comprehending a purely verbal command (that is, a verbal message given through auditory or visual means, without accompanying gestures, facial expressions, or meaningful emotional intonation). The errors of comprehension may range from an almost complete inability to comprehend any but the most elementary questions, to mild defects of comprehension that surface when particularly complex sentences are presented (for instance, sentences with double negatives or dependent clauses).

3. An aphasic is alert to person and environment and enters the situation of being medically examined in appropriate fashion. He is intent on communicating thoughts regarding his own condition and surroundings. Again, there may be exceptions, particularly in the first few hours after an acute brain lesion, in which aphasic patients may appear inattentive and uninterested in communication. Or there may be patients, well into their chronic periods, in whom a depression will

not permit an appropriate relation with examiners and surroundings. The student of aphasia should develop a keen sensitivity to this important aspect of aphasia. As far as we can fathom, the view of the world from the point of view of the aphasic is impoverished by the lack of intact verbal processing but is NOT that of a confused, demented, or psychotic patient. Accordingly, the appearance of the aphasic patient is not that of an alienated individual. More often than not, beyond the barrier of handicapped communication, the examiner of an aphasic patient can empathize with his subject.

The Signs of Aphasia

Paraphasia

Paraphasia is the central sign of aphasia. It consists of a substitution of an incorrect and unintended word or sound for a correct one. If an entire word is substituted, the paraphasia is called GLOBAL or VERBAL. But the paraphasia may or may not be related to the type of word substitution. If the substitution belongs to the same semantic field (for instance, *chair* for *table*, or *jail* for *hospital*), it will be called SEMANTIC paraphasia. If not, it will be called RANDOM paraphasia. Words correctly used in a given sentence may reappear instants later, incorrectly used, in a new sentence. That is called PERSEVERATIVE or INTRUSION paraphasia. Finally, paraphasias can be substitutions of entirely novel words, NEOLOGISTIC paraphasias. If a single phoneme is substituted or added (if the word *table* becomes *trable* or *fable*), the paraphasia is designated PHONEMIC or LITERAL. Too many phonemic paraphasias may produce an unintelligible word. This is probably one of the mechanisms by which neologistic paraphasias are formed. Too many global paraphasias appearing in sentence after sentence give rise to JARGON SPEECH.

Paraphasias can appear in spontaneous speech or in dialogue, on repetition of spoken sentences or on reading aloud, and in writing as well. They can be noted also on naming tasks. But they are notably absent in automatic speech (emotional exclamations, series of numbers, calendar sequences).

Disturbance of Fluency

Although the general characteristics of speech in aphasic patients are not always easily classifiable, they tend to fall into one of two helpful categories: FLUENT or NONFLUENT. The designations can mean slightly different things to different authors, but for most aphasiologists, fluent speech is that which approximates normal speech in terms of the rate of word production, the length of each sentence, the melodic contour of the sentences, and the overall ease of the speaking act. In practical terms, it is usually measured by the longest continuous string of words that the patient produces in conversation. Fluent aphasic speech may actually be more abundant than normal speech. Nonfluent speech is the very opposite: The rate is low, sentence length is short, the melodic contour is lost, the production is effortful, there may be more pauses than actual words in a given time unit.

The matter of articulation is separate from the judgment of fluency or nonfluency. Most patients with fluent speech have perfect articulation, although some may have minor difficulties. Many patients with nonfluent speech have perfect articulation too, although some do not. But, as noted, the ability to articulate and the ability to formulate language are different. Even patients with severe nonfluent speech will be able to produce perfectly articulated automatized verbal sequences (as in counting or in emotional exclamations).

The measure of fluency has become one of the keys to the modern analysis of the aphasias, helping with classification and providing a powerful indication for the localization of lesion. Most patients with fluent aphasias have lesions located in the posterior aspect of the perisylvian region. Most patients with nonfluent aphasias have lesions located in the anterior aspect of the perisylvian region (Benson, 1967).

Disturbance of Repetition

A failure to repeat words or sentences is a hallmark of aphasia. The ability to repeat may be entirely lost or may be marred by phonemic paraphasias or by omissions of sounds and words. Repetition is impaired in most aphasic syndromes (see the section on syndromes later in this chapter), and in one of them, conduction aphasia, the impairment of repetition dominates the clinical presentation because of the lack of other pronounced defects. The impairment of repetition has localization value also. Its presence places the lesion firmly in the perisylvian region of the dominant hemisphere. Repetition defects are notably absent in the transcortical aphasias, in the so-called anomic aphasia, and in special syndromes such as pure alexia. In all of those entities, the responsible lesion is located outside the perisylvian ring. Patients with the transcortical aphasias may actually repeat only too well, echoing the examiner's words immediately after they are pronounced, often with little or no comprehension of what they are parroting. Such a defect is called ECHOLALIA.

Disturbances of Auditory Comprehension

Auditory comprehension can be impaired to variable degrees. Some patients may be able to participate in a colloquial conversation, giving appropriate verbal replies or indicating by nodding of the head, pointing responses, facial expression, or gesture that they understand the content of the messages they receive. Yet, confronted with laboratory tests, they may fail many items, particularly if specific details are included in the question or requested in the answer. Other patients may be quite impaired even in a simple conversation and will fail dramatically in the laboratory tests.

Disturbances of Reading and Writing

Reading can be disturbed in much the same way as auditory comprehension, although the two defects do not necessarily go together. For instance, patients with auditory comprehension defects usually have some reading impairment, but the proportion of those with both may be small in comparison with the proportion of those with auditory comprehension defects only. On the other hand, impairment of reading can appear in pure form without impairment of auditory comprehension or writing. In most cases of aphasia, however, impairments of reading, writing, and auditory comprehension appear together, although rarely to the same degree.

Apraxia

Many aphasic patients also present with apraxia, forms of which, from a practical and clinical standpoint, can be considered yet another sign of aphasia. APRAXIA may be defined as a disorder of the execution of learned movement that cannot be accounted for by either weakness, incoordination, sensory loss, or impaired comprehension or attention to commands. From a theoretical point of view, however, it should be clear that apraxia can appear in isolation, without aphasia, and that its many varieties and mechanisms justify a separate entity status. The presence of apraxia should be investigated in all aphasic patients, as it may interfere with the performance of acts requested through verbal command. Students of aphasia should be aware of the fact that patients do not "complain" of apraxia and that, except for the extreme forms of ideational apraxia, the phenomenon is neither immediately disruptive to the patient's life nor evident to the examiner. The reader is referred to Geschwind (1975) for a comprehensive view of the phenomenon.

Classification of Aphasia

Classifications are a necessary evil, but reviewing the classification systems of aphasia can be a discouraging task. The variety of criteria used over the past 100 years may disorient the reader at first. The diversity of the nomenclature will cause exasperation. The seeming conflict between systems that include as many as eight different varieties of aphasia and those that limit themselves to two or three will be a source of puzzlement. Yet, the student of aphasia should realize that the diversity and conflict reflect a historical evolution of the science of the aphasias and are more apparent than real. From the practical standpoint, few of the many available classification systems have survived. Current researchers and clinicians in leading aphasiological centers use but one or two of the more recent systems. Furthermore, some of the apparently discrepant systems are not really so, since they derive from different points of view in relation to the phenomena of aphasia. For instance, Weisenburg and McBride's (1935) classic designations of EXPRESSIVE, RECEPTIVE, and MIXED aphasia reflect a clinical vantage point. Luria's (1966) nomenclature—for example, EFFERENT and AFFERENT MOTOR, or DYNAMIC—reflects a physiological approach. On the other hand, Jakobson's (1964) description of CONTIGUITY (or combination) and SIMILARITY (or selection) defects is the product of a psycholinguistic point of view. It should be clear that the systems do not conflict but rather complement each other. Be that as it may, a modern researcher or clinician should have a working knowledge of the different classification systems, from Wernicke's (1874) to Geschwind's (1965). This should be complemented with a fully conversant use of one modern classification system: the proper definition of each of its categories, their anatomical and physiological significance, and their prognostic implications.

In our opinion, the system generally associated with the Boston school of aphasia is currently the most useful one. It can be used in conjunction with most forms of laboratory and bedside assessment and does not necessarily require the use of the Boston Diagnostic Aphasia Examination (BDAE). The Boston classification comprises all of the frequently encountered syndromes for which there is an established and accepted anatomical correlation. The nomenclature utilizes a combination of eponyms, clinically descriptive terms, and physiologically based terms and is quite evocative (see Goodglass & Kaplan, 1972). The following paragraphs contain a standard description of the major syndromes, in their acute phase. But the reader should be advised that some cases will only approximate the description and will fail to manifest all the characteristics detailed here.

The Syndromes of Aphasia

Wernicke's Aphasia

Wernicke's aphasia is the most fundamental and least controversial of aphasic syndromes. Speech is fluent and well articulated, with frequent paraphasias but preserved syntactic structure. Aural comprehension is defective. Repetition of words and sentences is defective also. In general, both reading and writing are disturbed.

Most patients present with language difficulties and may have no other evidence of neurological disease. (Right hemiparesis is infrequent and can be transient; right visual field defects are not the rule.) Thus, the diagnosis rests almost solely on the signs of aphasia, and the accuracy of the diagnosis is mandatory: For the unskilled examiner, a patient with acute Wernicke's aphasia may sound "confused," with the consequence that a psychiatric rather than neurological diagnostic approach may be taken. Even assuming that the mistake is corrected eventually, the delay can be disastrous.

In our experience, patients with Wernicke's aphasia are less easily frustrated than those with Broca's aphasia. Yet, the suspicious tendency of the Wernicke patients is more evident than in Broca's aphasia, and it should be recalled that these are among the few neurological patients who can develop a major paranoid syndrome and become homicidal.

This complex syndrome, which combines both output and input disturbances, is also known as RECEPTIVE aphasia, from Weisenburg and McBride's classification (1935), and as SENSORY aphasia, as Wernicke himself called it (1874), with appreciable modesty but little physiological sense. Kleist (1934) aptly called it WORD DEAFNESS, but the term is rarely used, while Brain (1961) named it PURE WORD DEAFNESS, an inaccurate designation, since patients with Wernicke's aphasia are indeed word deaf but clearly not in pure form. (Patients with pure word deafness do exist, however; they are unable to understand speech and to repeat words but speak fluently and WITHOUT paraphasias.) Head (1926) called it SYNTACTIC aphasia, which is an ambiguous designation.

Broca's Aphasia

The existence of Broca's syndrome is currently well established. Yet some of the major controversies in the history of aphasia have revolved around the nature and pathological correlation of Broca's aphasia. The first patient described by Broca in 1861 did not have what came to be known as Broca's aphasia, and it appears that the degree of involvement of Broca's area and of the surrounding frontal operculum produce considerably different degrees of aphasia (Mohr *et al.*, 1978). What currently is called Broca's aphasia can be defined as the opposition of Wernicke's aphasia. The speech is nonfluent. There are few words, short sentences, and many intervening pauses, and what words there appear are produced with labor and often with distorted sounds. The melodic contour is flat. The general appearance of speech is telegraphic, due to the rather selective deletion of many connective words. On the other hand, aural comprehension is relatively intact in colloquial conversation, although formal testing often discloses a defective performance. Repetition of words and sentences is impaired.

Unlike patients with Wernicke's aphasia, the patient with Broca's aphasia invariably presents with a right-sided motor defect (often a complete hemiparesis more marked in the upper extremity and face). As a consequence, patients with Brocas's aphasia are less vulnerable to misdiagnosis. Their presentation is clearly neurological. On the other hand, they are often depressed and respond to testing failures with "catastrophic" reactions (sudden weeping and refusal to proceed with examination) more frequently than do Wernicke's aphasics.

Broca's aphasia has also been known as EXPRESSIVE (Weisenburg & McBride, 1935) and MOTOR (Goldstein, 1948; Wernicke, 1874). For a time it was refused the status of aphasis and called ANARTHRIA (Marie, 1906), and, later, DYSARTHRIA (Bay, 1962). Head (1926) called it VERBAL aphasia.

Conduction Aphasia

The speech of conduction aphasics is fluent although usually less abundant than that of Wernicke's. There are commonly minor defects in aural comprehension, though comprehension of colloquial conversation is intact. But it is the impairment in repetition of words and sentences that dominates this syndrome. The defect takes many forms. Most commonly, patients repeat words with phonemic paraphasias, but often they will omit or substitute words, and they may fail to repeat anything at all if function words rather than nouns are requested. Comprehension of the defectively repeated sentences is good. Similarly, patients comprehend the sentences that they read aloud with numerous paraphasias. (This TRANSCODING performance from reading to oral expression is a form of repetition.)

Conduction aphasics often have some accompanying motor signs (paresis of the right side of the face and of the right upper extremity), but recovery is good. The syndrome has been known as CENTRAL aphasia, Goldstein's (1948) curious designation, and as AFFERENT MOTOR, Luria's term. Luria attempted to break down the syndrome, giving it a motor component (AFFERENT MOTOR) and an auditory one (ACOUSTIC AMNESIC). Kertesz (1979) proposed a comparable distinction (EFFERENT CONDUCTION and AFFERENT CONDUCTION).

Transcortical Sensory Aphasia (TSA)

Patients with TSA have fluent and paraphasic speech (global paraphasias predominate over phonemic ones) and a severe impairment in aural comprehension. Yet their repetition is intact (occasionally echolalic), setting them clearly apart from Wernicke's aphasics. The distinction of the syndromes is important since the localization of the lesion is different (see Chapter 2 on localization). This underscores the need to test repetition in every aphasic patient.

TRANSCORTICAL was the original designation of Goldstein, and it has held well through the years, both for TSA and for transcortical motor aphasia, some cases of which Luria preferred to call DYNAMIC aphasia (Luria & Tsevtkova, 1968).

Transcortical Motor Aphasia (TMA)

Patients with TMA have intact repetition, just as patients with TSA, and can have echolalia too. But the speech is nonfluent and troubled by phonemic and global paraphasias, perseveration, and loss of connective words. In our experience, auditory comprehension is impaired too when tested formally, although patients can often carry on a simple conversation at bedside.

Patients with TMA should be distinguished from those with mutism on several counts. Firstly, patients with TMA are inclined to communicate and do so, within their verbal limitations. Patients with mutism do not and are as impoverished in nonverbal as in verbal communication. Secondly, the speech of TMA is clearly aphasic; for example, there are unquestionable phonetic, lexical, and syntactical errors, whereas patients with mutism either produce no speech at all or utter a few short but linguistically correct sentences. Again, the distinction is important because the localization of the lesion is different.

Global Aphasia

As the name implies, global aphasics present with an almost complete loss of ability to comprehend or formulate verbal communication. Propositional speech may be reduced to a few words, the remainder of verbal communication consisting of emotional exclamations and serial utterances. Auditory comprehension is often reduced to a variable number of nouns and verbs, while the comprehension of functor words or of syntactically organized sentences is virtually negligible.

Anomic Aphasia

Patients with pure anomic aphasia are rare in our experience, but it is important to distinguish this syndrome from the SIGN of anomia. Anomia is present in practically all aphasic syndromes. Its significance by itself is limited. As a syndrome, anomic aphasia is characterized by a pervasive impairment of word finding, in any modality. But repetition is intact, and speech is fluent, well articulated, and grammatically correct. The terms AMNESIC aphasia and NOMINAL aphasia are synonymous.

Alexia with Agraphia

The pure syndrome of alexia with agraphia is rare if at all existent. More often than not, patients have signs of Wernicke's aphasia or of transcortical sensory aphasia. In the absence of aphasia, they generally have notable parietal lobe signs. But it is reasonable to make the diagnosis of alexia with agraphia when the disturbances of reading and writing predominate over the aphasic or parietal symptomatology. The fact that this syndrome can be associated with impaired as well as intact repetition, and with a greater or smaller extent of accompanying signs, suggests that a large segment of parietal and temporal lobe structures, cortical and subcortical, is engaged in the complex processes of reading and writing. Therefore, the anatomical significance of this entity is considerably smaller than that of most aphasic syndromes or of the syndrome of alexia WITHOUT agraphia (pure alexia).

Alexia without Agraphia (Pure Alexia)

As the designation implies, patients presenting alexia without agraphia become unable to read while they continue to be able to write, spontaneously or to dictation. (Many such patients can also copy writing, although they do so with difficulty.) Speech, auditory comprehension, and repetition are intact. Oral spelling of words (or its converse, the construction of words spelled orally) is normal. Reading in the tactile mode is normal, too. Whatever visual reading they can do is of single letters. (This often allows the patient to read aloud the letters of a word, one by one, and then reconstitute the word from this operation of spelling.)

Most patients have some form of accompanying visual function impairment. It can be a right homonymous hemianopia (the field of vision to the right of the vertical median is blind) or else a right hemiachromatopsia (loss of color perception without true blindness in the right hemifield). Most patients also have color anomia (a disturbance of naming colors with otherwise normal color perception). Some present with optic ataxia (a disturbance in the visual guidance of hand movements).

First described by Dejerine (1892), the syndrome was long forgotten and even denied but was revived by Geschwind (1965), who used it as a cornerstone for his theory of disconnection syndromes.

Pure Word Deafness

Pure word deafness is a rare syndrome. Patients have a profound loss of auditory comprehension and a complete impairment of repetition. Yet they produce normal fluent speech, mostly without paraphasias. It could be argued that pure word deafness, just as pure alexia, is not a true aphasia, since language formulation itself is not affected. From a physiopathological standpoint, both syndromes reflect the inability of appropriate verbal information to reach structures capable of decoding it, while those structures remain intact and permit regular inner language operations as well as normal exteriorization of well-formulated language. Yet there are many reasons why the two conditions should be discussed along with the aphasias. For one thing, they resemble aphasias from the standpoint of the communication impairment they produce. For another, anatomical and physiological knowledge derived from studying these two pure "input" disorders has contributed importantly to the understanding of the aphasias.

Atypical Aphasias

A considerable number of cases of aphasia fail to conform to any of the syndromes described here. This happens for several reasons. In some instances, although CT scan or postmortem examination confirm the presence of a typical cortical site of damage, the aphasia is milder or transient. The major cause of this is an unusual cerebral dominance disposition, whereby a left hander or more rarely a right hander may have either CROSSED DOMINANCE or AMBIDOMINANCE. But in other instances, it has been found, a noncortical locus of lesion is encountered in association with atypical aphasia syndromes. The lesion can be located in the deep nuclear masses of the brain or in both nuclear masses and the anterior limb of the internal capsule. Examples of the former have been reported in connection with thalamic and putaminal hemorrhage (Alexander & Lo Verme, 1980; Hier & Mohr, 1975). Examples of the latter have been found in connection with nonhemorrhagic infarction in the territory of the lenticular arteries (Damasio & Damasio, 1981; Naeser, 1979).

References

Alexander, M. P., & Lo Verme, S. R. 1980. Aphasia after left hemispheric intracerebral hemorrhage. *Neurology, 30*, 1193–1202.

Bay, E. 1964. Principles of classification and their influence on our concepts of aphasia. In A. V. S. De Reuck & M. O'Connor (Eds.), *Disorders of language.* London: Churchill.

Benson, D. F. 1967. Fluency in aphasia: Correlation with radioactive scan localization. *Cortex, 3*, 373–394.

Brain, W. R. 1961. *Speech disorders.* London: Butterworths.

Broca, P. 1861. Remarques sur le siège de la faculté du langage articulé, suivies d'une observation d'aphemie (perte de la parole). *Bulletin de la Société d'Anatomie* (Paris), *36*, 330–357.

Damasio, A., & Damasio, H. 1981. Aphasia with nonhemorrhagic lesions in the basal ganglia and internal capsule. *Archives of Neurology* (in press).

Dejerine, J. 1892. Des differentes variétés de cécité verbale. *Mémoires de la Société de Biologie,* Series 9, Vol. 4 (February 27), 61–90.

Geschwind, N. 1965. Disconnexion syndromes in animals and man. *Brain, 88*, 237–294, 585–644.

Geschwind, H. 1975. The apraxias: Neurological mechanisms of disorders of learned movement. *American Scientist, 63*, 188–195.

Goldstein, K. 1948. *Language and language disturbances.* New York: Grune & Stratton.

Goodglass, H., & Kaplan, E. 1972. *Assessment of aphasia and related disorders.* Philadelphia: Lea & Febiger.

Head, H. 1926. *Aphasia and kindred disorders of speech.* Cambridge: Cambridge Univ. Press.

Hier, D. B., & Mohr, J. P. 1977. Incongruous oral and written naming. Evidence for a subdivision of the syndrome of Wernicke's aphasia. *Brain and Language, 4,* 115–126.

Jakobson, R. 1964. Towards a linguistic typology of aphasic impairments. In A. V. S. De Reuck & M. O'Connor (Eds.), *Disorders of language.* London: Churchill.

Kertesz, A. 1979. *Aphasia and associated disorders.* New York: Grune & Stratton.

Kleist, K. 1934. *Gehirnpathologie.* Leipzig: Barth.

Luria, A. R. 1966. *Higher cortical functions in man.* New York: Basic Books.

Luria, A. R., & Tsevtkova, L. 1968. The mechanisms of dynamic aphasia. *Foundations of Language, 4,* 296–307.

Marie, P. 1906. Révision de la question de l'aphasie: La troisième circonvolution frontale gauche ne joue aucun rôle special dans la fonction du langage. *Semaine Médicale, 21,* 241–247.

Naeser, M. A. 1979. Putaminal aphasia. Paper delivered at the meeting of the Academy of Aphasia, San Diego.

Weisenburg, T., & McBride, K. 1935. *Aphasia.* New York: Commonwealth Fund.

Wernicke, C. 1874. *Der aphasische symptomencomplex.* Breslau: Cohn and Weigert.

4

Assessment of Aphasia

OTFRIED SPREEN and ANTHONY RISSER

This chapter will focus on the currently available methods of the assessment of aphasia. In order to view the development of assessment methods in context, a brief historical introduction will be necessary. In addition, we will attempt to establish a frame of reference for reviewing available methods by describing what would appear to us to be key requirements for an acceptable method in general and for the examination of brain-damaged populations in particular. We will then proceed to review the strengths and weaknesses of each of the currently available methods and finish with a discussion of the choice of methods in clinical work, with special reference to the widely differing problems, ranging from purely research-oriented questions to questions of measuring day-to-day improvement during therapy and assessing daily communicative ability in the home or occupational setting.

Historical Introduction

Even the earliest records of medical knowledge make reference to language disorders after brain damage (Benton, 1964). Accounts of simple clinical examinations were often included in such reports, but it was not until the second half of the nineteenth century (specifically since the publications of Broca; Joynt, 1964) that aphasia was explored more systematically. Case reports by Wernicke (1874/1908) and contemporaries contain detailed descriptions of examination procedures for individual patients, often extending over three or more printed pages. While some of these examinations were probably standard procedure in certain hos-

ACQUIRED APHASIA

Copyright © 1981 by Academic Press, Inc.
All rights of reproduction in any form reserved.
ISBN 0-12-619320-7

pitals, others were invented on the spot to explore individual features of a specific syndrome of aphasia. Understandably, the reports focused on the patient's specific disorder rather than on the examination procedure.

The clinical examination as developed in the late nineteenth century has been modified and augmented, but it has remained the essential tool of the clinical neurologist. Such examinations are exemplified in the writings of Jackson (1915) and Pick (1913) and in the more recent reports by Luria (1970) and Geschwind and Kaplan (1962). Some manuals document this approach (e.g., Strub & Black, 1977).

The clinical examination has a number of disadvantages, which gradually led to the development of more generally applicable and standardized assessment instruments. Clinical examinations tend to vary from one place to another, both in content and in the way in which they are administered; what is considered abnormal remains the subjective judgment of the clinician; and the examinations are difficult to replicate and compare. Early attempts to produce a more standardized examination were published by Head (1926), who insisted on a detailed "clinical protocol." Another examination procedure was published by Froeschels, Dittrich, and Wilheim (1932).

The first comprehensive battery of psychological and educational achievement tests for aphasic patients was used by Weisenburg and McBride (1935) in a 5-year study of 60 aphasic patients. Schuell (Schuell, Jenkins, & Jiménez-Pabón, 1964) calls this study a landmark because it was the first to use control subjects, to compare aphasic with nonaphasic brain-damaged subjects, and to use standardized methodology. Several other batteries were developed in the 1950s by Wepman (1951), Eisenson (1954), Wepman and Jones (1961), and Schuell (1955), partly as a result of intensive treatment efforts with World War II veterans. Benton (1964) reviewed the development of assessment procedures at that time and noted the work done in various centers, critizing that none of the procedures had been published in "usable form." The descriptions of procedures were insufficient, no standardization information was presented, nor were exact criteria for scoring or detailed guides for interpretation included. He compared the state of the art with the "pre-Binet stage" in intelligence testing: "We are today where intelligence testing was in 1900 [p. 263]."

Since Benton's review, several instruments have been published that present detailed administration and scoring criteria and that, at least in part, provide information on standardization and interpretation procedures. Our review will deal primarily with these more recently developed assessment techniques. Other reviews have been presented by Darley (1964, 1979) and Kertesz (1979).

Purposes of Assessment and Testing

Assessment procedures vary greatly, depending on the goal that the examiner hopes to accomplish. It is important to consider this point in evaluating and choosing specific procedures. Obviously, little is gained by administering a lengthy and difficult test battery designed for patients with mild language deficits to a bedfast patient with severe or global aphasia or for the purpose of evaluating short-term progress during therapy aimed at a specific problem (e.g., distinctiveness of articulation). In some patients, a clinical examination in the tradition of classical neurology (see Benson, 1979b) may be preferable as a brief evaluation of language disorders in the acute stage. Even for assessing specific training programs for a given patient, an individualized evaluation might be preferable to a standardized test for establishing a baseline and for measuring day-to-day progress.

Four general types of assessments may be distinguished: (*a*) screening procedures; (*b*) diagnostic assessment; (*c*) assessment for counseling and rehabilitation; and (*d*) progress evaluation.

SCREENING refers to a relatively brief and cursory examination for the purpose of detecting the presence or absence of a disorder. One popular application arising out of clinical psychology in the 1950s was screening for the presence or absence of ORGANICITY (a loose term referring to any form of damage to the nervous system affecting psychological functions), particularly in high-risk age groups and in conjunction with psychiatric evaluations. In relation to aphasia, screening would involve a brief examination with a highly sensitive instrument to detect the presence or absence of aphasia. Although some relatively brief, highly sensitive tests are available—either as part of detailed batteries or as separate instruments (Wheeler & Reitan, 1962)—testing for the purpose of screening has lost its attractiveness and usefulness since the 1950s. One reason for this is that the accuracy of screening devices is limited, usually around 80% (Spreen & Benton, 1965); another reason is that in clinical practice such "detective" work is hardly necessary, since most patients are referred with an established diagnosis of aphasia. Finally, the information obtained with such instruments reveals little to indicate how severe a problem the detected aphasia is in the daily life of the patient. As a result, screening tests have been all but abandoned. Reitan's test remains useful only in the context of a larger neuropsychological evaluation extending far beyond the language area. Of the existing tests, the Token Test and word fluency tests (to be described later) have in our experience been shown to be highly sensitive to even mild residual language disorders of an aphasic nature.

DIAGNOSTIC ASSESSMENT refers to an overall assessment of a patient's language performance for the purpose of arriving at a detailed description of areas of strength and weakness. Because of the comprehensive nature of this examination, it is suitable for intake examinations and/or reevaluations of patients with new or persisting complaints of language disorders. Diagnostic assessment tends to take very brief samplings of many different areas and may not necessarily be of use to the speech clinician interested in a detailed exploration of a particular problem. The diagnostic assessment also often attempts to arrive at a "diagnostic statement." Such a statement may either refer to the type of aphasia present or go beyond the description of the functional deficit and attempt to arrive at speculative conclusions about the nature and location of the underlying brain disorder itself. Most test authors advocate a particular "package" or battery of tests that, in their view, produces a comprehensive overview of all aspects of language behavior in the aphasic patient. As a result, fixed batteries are the almost inevitable choice of the clinician looking for a comprehensive instrument. Unfortunately, such batteries also reflect the particular school of thought as well as bias of the test author. For this reason, it becomes imperative to be fully familiar with the theoretical position of the author. Another disadvantage of the fixed battery approach is that it is difficult to include additional examination procedures and interpret them in relation to the battery itself because each instrument has been standardized and validated on somewhat differing populations. Nevertheless, such a flexible approach (i.e., adding and elaborating in certain areas, especially if weaknesses are found) may be the best choice for a speech clinician looking for additional information.

For the purpose of COUNSELING AND REHABILITATION, the approach of choosing a variety of assessment procedures, including a fixed battery, may be the most sensible choice. In particular, it would seem useful to gain as much information as possible on areas of strength, since this allows better-reasoned advice on what activities to pursue, what vocational options remain open to the patient, and how to structure a rehabilitation program. Counseling and rehabilitation also pose somewhat different questions than the diagnostic assessment can answer. Often it is not the ability of patients to name words or construct sentences from the materials presented in the laboratory situation that is most important, but rather their ability to make themselves understood and to communicate in day-to-day living. For this reason, the assessment shifts in emphasis from a strict testing situation to the observation (often expressed in terms of ratings, ranging from excellent to very poor) of communicative behavior. Another aspect of assessment in the rehabilitation setting concerns predictions of response to treatment and of recovery. While these questions have been poorly researched up to this time, they would seem crucial for decisions about the meaningful and economical planning for a given patient. Studies of predictive accuracy in a rehabilitation setting are only just beginning, and accuracy rates tend to be disappointing.

PROGRESS EVALUATION is closely related to assessment for rehabilitation. The clinician working with a patient would like to be able to chart day-to-day or week-to-week progress accurately rather than rely on subjective judgments or enthusiastic endorsements of the usefulness of therapy made by the patient or relatives. No formal tests have been developed specifically for this purpose, mainly because such progress assessments have to be tailor-made for each individual and his or her current level and range of deficit. For this reason, therapists may prefer to "lift" whole sections of an existing test in the appropriate area of deficit and range of difficulty and amplify such tests with additional material of their own choosing in order to establish a baseline of performance at the beginning of therapy. Repeat examinations after specified periods of training will then allow a plotting of progress over time. The methodology for the development of progress assessment techniques during therapy has been well established by authors in the behavior modification field (e.g., Lahey, 1973). The test–teach–test approach in education as well as in speech therapy has the advantage of being directly relevant to the material being taught or the language problem under training; no inferences from a general sampling of language behavior in test batteries is necessary. It has the disadvantage of not allowing observations about the broader, more general progress of the patient. For this purpose, the occasional diagnostic assessment will still be of benefit.

Construction Principles of Aphasia Tests

As pointed out earlier, a distinction can be made between the relatively informal (though frequently well structured and systematically executed) clinical examination for aphasia and more formal tests. While there will continue to be need for the clinical examination, more emphasis has been placed in recent years on the development of tests. Both clinical examination and tests may examine the same areas of difficulty; the distinction lies in the quantification of the test examination and in the opportunity to compare quantitative scores with reference norms. Hence, a test could be defined as a clinical examination that meets a number of psychometric requirements.

Rating Scales

Rating scales take a position somewhat in between the clinical assessment and psychometric tests. The clinician, who assigns a label of "mild," "moderate," or "severe" to the symptoms of a patient, is actually involved in a basic rating of severity. Ratings are frequently used (a) as a summary judgment of severity of any given symptom or syndrome and (b) as a specific judgment of aspects of a patient's behavior that cannot be readily measured. The first application refers to a complex process that weighs all the information on a given patient. A specific example is a professional's judgment in an indemnity suit in court; the professional may even be asked to specify whether the impairment affects 20% or 50% of the patient's ability before the onset of illness. The second application is of more specific interest in the context of this discussion. In this case, some aspect of the patient's speech behavior— for example, fluency of expression or ability to communicate in the home setting—is rated on a scale of levels or points. Usually, a rating scale does not exceed 7 points (from normal to very severe), since it has been demonstrated that rating scales with more than 7 points do not enhance the accuracy of the ratings but merely provide a false impression of greater accuracy. Rating scales should be subjected to careful interjudge reliability studies. Such reliability improves with very careful description of each rating point. For example, instead of marking the lowest point as "normal" and the highest as "very severe," each point should be illustrated in as much detail as possible with examples and descriptions. Rating scales are no substitute for psychometric testing, but they are extremely valuable if the information being rated cannot be readily tested or is too complex to be documented in test item scores. Ratings of communicative ability in the home or in a conversational setting are often made by an informant (e.g., a relative or a member of the nursing staff) rather than by the clinician who sees the patient only in a highly structured, isolated, and somewhat artificial examining or therapy situation.

The following section will describe the psychometric requirements for a well-constructed test. Some of these requirements also apply to rating scales. This description of psychometric requirements is given to establish the information that should be critically evaluated before a test or rating method is put to use in daily practice. It should, however, be stated beforehand that hardly any test or rating scale in the area of aphasia assessment fully meets the stringent psychometric requirements often demanded by the psychometric specialist and by associations concerned with standards of testing (APA, 1974). The reason for this is that most tests in the field of aphasia have been developed in individual laboratories in the context of clinical work and are not generally adopted by a large number of services and institutions. At the same time, the demand for such tests remains small (as compared for example to tests of general intelligence). Hence, the collection of norms and the conduct of validity and reliability studies proceeds slowly and is almost entirely dependent on the resources of the test authors and their collaborators. In other words, test development is demanding in terms of both time and money. Aphasia tests are not best-sellers; as a result, development has been less than optimal in most instances and completely neglected in others.

General Requirements for Tests

The most frequently stated requirements for tests of any kind are demonstrated validity, reliability, and standardization (Anastasi, 1976; Nunnally, 1967). Without going into detail, we will point out briefly the importance of each of these in general and then with specific reference to the field of aphasia.

STANDARDIZATION

Standardization refers to the test administration itself, which should be constant from patient to patient and from one examiner to another. If test administration and the conditions under which the test is administered are kept as controlled as possible, measurement error can be kept to a minimum. Any deviation from a standard administration procedure (e.g., prompting if the patient cannot respond readily, extending the time limits for answering) will inevitably produce more variability in test scores and hence undesirable variance when the scores of patients or groups of patients are compared. It may be tempting for the clinician to use the test material to explore how much a patient may improve as a result of simple aids given during the testing; however justified such a procedure, it should be understood that test results achieved under such modified conditions are no longer comparable to the published norms; that is, they contain an undesirable degree of measurement error.

The other aspect of standardization refers to the establishment of norms against which the performance of an individual patient can be compared. Norms essentially are a range of scores obtained from a refer-

ence group, including the mean score as well as the distribution of
scores from the highest to the lowest scoring subject in that group.
These are often expressed in percentile ranks or in relation to a normal
distribution score in terms of z scores, t scores, etc. Such converted
scores indicate a given patient's score in relation to the distribution. For
example, a score at the 90th percentile indicates a performance better
than 90% of the reference population. If the test is constructed for a
variety of populations, separate standardization procedures will have to
be conducted. For example, if scores tend to vary greatly with age, sex,
or socioeconomic status, separate norms will have to be established.
Occasionally, additional norms can be avoided by using correction
scores for these factors, but this may be impractical if two or more of
these factors interact with each other. Norms are usually produced for a
group of healthy men and women without neurological impairment or
aphasia. This allows the examiner to see how much a given patient's
score deviates from "normal." Norms developed for normal subjects
may not be sufficient for the evaluation of the aphasic patient; this question will be discussed later in the context of specific requirements for
tests of aphasia.

RELIABILITY

Reliability refers to the demonstration that on repeat administration
after a reasonable time interval and under the same conditions similar
results will be obtained for the same subject. Reliability is often demonstrated by giving an alternate form of the test during the same or at a
subsequent session, by comparing alternate (odd-numbered and even-
numbered) items of the test, by subdividing the test, or by measuring
item interrelationships by other means. Generally, reliability is best
demonstrated with normal, healthy subjects, since the measurement
error in patient populations and the likelihood of change in performance
due to changes in the patient's condition are high. Test scoring often
involves a certain amount of judgment on the part of the test administra-
tor. For example, if the patient is asked to describe the use of a
hairbrush, the response *for hair* may be judged to be unsatisfactory by
one scorer and satisfactory by another. In practice, interscorer differences can be reduced to a minimum if the test manual contains a
sufficient amount of scoring instructions and samples of how a given
item can be scored. One form of expressing scoring reliability is to give
test records to two or more independent scorers and compute a correlation coefficient between scorers. Such interscorer reliability is highly
desirable, since poor reliability of this type will obviously not only affect

the general reliability of the test but also introduce measurement error into studies of validity and other psychometric properties.

VALIDITY

Validity is probably the most crucial requirement for any test. It refers to the demonstration that a test measures what it claims to. Validity can be demonstrated in a variety of ways; typically, a distinction between predictive (or criterion-related), content, and construct validity is made. Of the three forms, the demonstration that a test is a valid "predictor" of whether or not a patient is aphasic is the most popular, though of limited value in several ways. The demonstration of validity relies entirely on the fact that the aphasic patient's performance can be discriminated from that of normal subjects on the basis of test results; in other words, the demonstration of validity comes close to the screening problem described earlier. Such a demonstration relies on the clinical judgment made for the aphasic group but neglects the fact that the discrimination between aphasics and normals could result from entirely irrelevant (for aphasia) or trivial test items. In the ideal case, other contrast groups in addition to healthy, normal subjects should be used (i.e., brain-damaged patients without aphasia). The question of validity for predicting membership in a specific subgroup of aphasics—for example, Broca's aphasia—will be addressed later.

Construct validity is often demonstrated by investigating the correlation of a new test with another test of known validity. However, since few tests in the aphasia field have such known validity, an alternative form of validity examination—the demonstration of factorial construct validity—is frequently used. In this case, factor analytic statistical techniques are used to show whether the tests in a given battery all contribute to a major factor of common variance that represents language functions.

Content validity refers to the adequacy of sampling from the domain of behaviors to be measured. In the case of testing for aphasia, for example, measuring verbal fluency alone would not be sufficient, because it does not appear to sample language behavior adequately (unless, of course, it could be shown that other expressive and receptive language functions all correlate highly and uniformly with word fluency). In other words, test items should be based on sound reasoning and should not be trivial or selectively biased. The content should also agree with the content area as defined by other researchers. The range and diversity of the content of a test can also be explored by factor analysis.

Specific Requirements for Tests with Brain-Damaged and Aphasic Patients

In addition to the general requirements for the construction of tests described in the previous section, several specific problems frequently occur in tests that are designed primarily for use with brain-damaged patients and specifically with aphasics. These questions arise in relation to the range of item difficulty, the need to clarify the nature of specific deficits revealed by the tests, the overlap of examinations for aphasia with measures of intelligence, the usefulness of a test in conjunction with recovery and therapy, and the overall conceptualization of the nature of aphasia.

Range of Item Difficulty

Range of item difficulty is usually determined by selecting from a range of "very easy" to "very difficult" items. In a well-constructed test, items should be homogeneously distributed; that is, the difficulty range (expressed in percentage of subjects passing each item) should rise in a linear fashion from the first to the last item. This principle of homogeneity of item distributions is relatively easy to follow if we are dealing with a test for a normal population that is reasonably well defined (e.g., all first grade children in selected, representative parts of the country). The principle can also be followed fairly well for a language test constructed to test normal adults. However, if aphasic subjects are used, most items would be far too difficult for a majority of the patients. As a result, most aphasic subjects would have scores in the bottom range of the distribution or even at a percentile of zero. Consequently, aphasia tests must shift the difficulty of item distribution toward the lower or "easy" end to make it possible to discriminate between mild, moderate, and severe aphasia. In other words, the range of item difficulty will have to be determined by the target population of aphasics, not by the general, healthy population. This shift inevitably produces a "ceiling" effect if the test is applied to normal subjects; normal subjects will usually score at or near the 100% correct range. It is, of course, possible to include items that are easy enough to discriminate between different degrees of aphasia as well as items difficult enough for a normal population; such a test, however, would be extremely lengthy and impractical. In short, for a test to be adequate in discriminating aphasics of different degrees, we will have to abandon the notion that this test can generally be useful for other populations with reasonably normal language behavior.

Clarification of Defects

Clarification of specific defects found in aphasics is necessary in many cases, especially if multiple handicaps (e.g., aphasia and motor disorder, aphasia and sensory disorder) are present. For example, if a patient cannot find the name of an object, we cannot automatically ascribe this deficit to an aphasic disorder. It is possible that the patient has difficulty recognizing the object visually or that some form of agnosia is present. If the patient cannot name an object placed in his hand, it is possible that sensory loss, inadequate motoric ability to handle the object, or inadequate stereognostic or kinesthetic recognition is responsible. Similarly, reading tasks, which are frequently part of an aphasia assessment, can be influenced by inadequate form discrimination and other factors. In a clinical examination, such alternative explanations are frequently obvious and quickly excluded by appropriate informal tests. It is important, however, to systematically check for such associated deficits, since the "test profile" produced at the end of testing with many standard batteries may easily be misinterpreted if used in a "blind evaluation" or by an inexperienced examiner. Some test batteries have included supplementary tests for associated deficits and developed clear rules as to when a supplementary test should be used. Such supplementary tests should also follow standard psychometric principles if they are to be used routinely. The inclusion of supplementary tests (see, e.g., Benton, 1967, 1972, p. 269) may expand the field of examination far beyond the area of aphasia.

Overlap with Intelligence Tests

The overlap of assessment of aphasia with measures of intelligence has often gone unnoticed, but it deserves special consideration in the context of item selection and in the context of our discussion of other defects found in association with aphasia. We do not intend to enter into the discussion of whether language-mediated behavior does or does not form an integral part of the cognitive ability of the individual or whether the presence of aphasia must of necessity affect the intellectual ability of the patient. Rather, it should be stressed that in the examination of aphasia the demands on the general intellectual abilities of the patient should be kept to a minimum; in addition, previously acquired knowledge of specific concepts and terms should influence the assessment of aphasia as little as possible.

The problem does not generally arise with the "easy" items used in aphasia tests; but when items for the "difficult" level are constructed, the separation of what is strictly language and what is intelligence becomes blurred. For example, naming tasks can be advanced to any level of difficulty by adding rare words and concepts that are likely to be found only in the vocabulary of the college-educated person of superior intelligence. Tasks requiring definitions invariably tend to place higher value on abstract, elegant wording and penalize the uneducated, less intelligent subject. Tasks requiring mathematical operations and the finding of superordinate concepts and similarities are, in fact, part of most recognized standard intelligence tests presently in use. For this reason, tests must be carefully scrutinized for content that exceeds the basic examination of language abilities. If such content cannot be avoided because of the range of item difficulties, the test must contain separate norms for patients of different ranges of intellectual and educational background or must apply adequate corrections for such factors. Although the premorbid intelligence of a patient is difficult to measure, it is usually possible to arrive at some basic judgment by considering the number of years of education, the level of occupational sophistication, and such ancillary information as may be available from nonverbal intelligence tests, estimates of the intellectual level of other family members, etc.

Use in Measuring Recovery

The use of tests in the context of recovery and therapy poses two problems. The first is essentially an additional validity problem—that is, whether or not a test is suitable for the measurement of recovery with or without therapy. Tests adequate for the measurement of recovery may be slightly different in content from tests that merely indicate the presence or type of aphasia and may require more items in certain difficulty ranges to allow the measurement of even small steps in recovery. A related question may be the ability of a test to predict recovery, which must be established independently of or in addition to other validation procedures.

The second related problem deals with the ability of patients to relearn what they have lost. This is a very neglected aspect of aphasia assessment. Most tests merely measure the status quo but deliberately exclude any practice or learning during the testing procedure. As pointed out earlier, providing cues to a patient during testing usually is seen as contributing to measurement error and hence must be avoided at all costs. If a test were to be designed to provide information on the relearning capacity of the patient, an entirely different approach to item construction would have to be taken. This approach would systematically include a variety of short learning trials with different kinds of cues in order to investigate whether the patient's language performance benefits, at least within the immediate testing situation. It should be obvious that the inclusion of such procedures in the assessment of aphasia would dramatically change the usual form of testing, affect retest reliability, and presumably add to the length of the test. Yet it is our impression that the benefits of such tests will outweigh the additional problems of test construction and validation and that such tests will be a major concern of test development in the future. Informal assessment of a patient's relearning capacity has, of course, been available for quite some time, and specific rules for such procedures have been developed in detail. This question will be addressed further in the last part of this chapter.

Conceptualization of the Nature of Aphasia

The conceptualization of the nature of aphasia is one recurrent theme underlying many of the considerations outlined in this section. The selection of tests is directly influenced by whether we see aphasia as a specific disorder of selected abilities or as a pervasive disturbance of communication, by whether we conceive of aphasia as unitary in nature or as consisting of many "subtypes." Benton (1967) in his discussion of this problem pointed out that the choice of a model of language functioning determines what kind of test we construct or use. He indicated that the problem is similar to the one posed by the conceptualization of intelligence; it is similar also in the sense that no common agreement exists. While Benton at that time still expressed some hope for the possibility of achieving a consensus, the development of research in aphasia (and in test construction) would seem to suggest that we have reached an impasse similar to that reached in the conceptualization (and testing) of intelligence. As a result, two approaches to test construction should be recognized as equally reasonable at this time:

1. To construct tests on the basis of one of the currently accepted conceptions of aphasia. This approach insures that the test measures all aspects viewed as important in a specific theoretical approach but makes it probable that the test will not be widely used as long as different conceptualizations of aphasia are held by other workers in the field.

2. To approach the problem pragmatically, avoid specific conceptualizations, and construct a test that contains a wide variety of probes of all abilities usually described by researchers of widely differing theoretical viewpoints. This pragmatic approach, also described by Benton and

quite commonly used in the field of intelligence testing, will not be fully satisfactory to any of the prevailing schools but may gain wider acceptance if the test instrument is otherwise well constructed and of demonstrated use in clinical practice. One drawback of this shotgun approach to test construction is the possibility of including redundant and/or highly specific material that may be irrelevant to the assessment of aphasia. This problem can be solved by future factor analytic investigations as long as the range of material is sufficiently wide to allow such conclusions.

Both approaches have been applied in the construction of currently used tests. In the following description of individual tests, we will make specific reference to the conceptual framework used in each for the information of the reader unfamiliar with a given instrument.

Current Methods for the Assessment of Aphasia

The following review of assessment procedures is given in an attempt to survey current and readily available methods and to provide sufficient introductory information for readers unfamiliar with some of the procedures to choose those methods most likely to meet their needs. Information on the test procedure itself, the choice and range of assessment, the psychometric properties of the test, the theoretical position of the test authors, and the most likely areas of use of each will be described. A documentation of test and reference sources is provided in the bibliography (see also Darley, 1979; Kertesz, 1979). We begin with descriptions of published clinical assessment procedures then discuss brief tests that may address only specific aspects of aphasia. Rating procedures and other measures of actual conversational speech in a communication setting will be considered next, and finally, comprehensive tests will be described. A short section on tests specifically designed for children is added.

Clinical Assessment

As mentioned in the introductory section of this chapter, not only is the clinical examination historically the primary method of assessing aphasia, but it also remains the standard tool of the clinical examiner, especially the neurologist as well as many speech clinicians. The advantage of the clinical examination lies in its flexibility, brevity, and suitability for even severely physically impaired patients, since the examiner can conduct a cursory examination at the bedside and follow up any errors made by the patient by further exploration with additional tasks, while at the same time skipping quickly across areas of strength where there is no obvious impairment.

Numerous versions of the clinical examination have been recorded, in formal descriptions within the contexts of a mental status examination in neurology (Strub & Black, 1977), a general neurological examination (Poeck, 1974), and specifically designed clinical examinations (Benson, 1979b), as well as in individual case descriptions (e.g., Geschwind & Kaplan, 1962). Some routine procedures—such as the "Paper Test" of Pierre Marie (1883), the "Hand–Eye–Ear Test" of Henry Head (1926), and Geschwind's (1971) "no ifs ands or buts" repetition as a simple task with high multiple demands on the patient's understanding, processing, and repetition ability—have become the standard repertoire of many clinical examinations. A detailed examination usually includes:

1. An evaluation of spontaneous or conversational speech, observing specifically the fluency of output, effort, articulation, phrase length, indications of dysprosody, paraphasias, and tendencies to omit words.
2. Repetition, including the standard repetition of digits and building to the repetition of multisyllabic words, complex sentences, or verbal sequences.
3. Comprehension of spoken language (e.g., Marie's test used the following instruction: "Here are three papers: a big one, a middle-sized one, and a little one. Take the biggest one, rumple it up and throw it on the ground. Give me the middle-sized one. Put the smallest one in your pocket."). For the patient with major motor impairment, it is necessary to restrict the examination to questions that can be answered with yes or no or, if speaking is impaired, by pointing.
4. Word finding, usually by asking for the names of common objects (e.g., the patient's clothes, body parts) both with and without prompting. Frequently the initial phoneme is offered as a cue, or an open-ended statement is provided to allow the word to be produced in appropriate embedding.
5. Reading, usually from newspaper or magazine material.
6. Writing, starting with the patient's own name and proceeding to dictated and spontaneous writing (e.g., "Describe your job.").

Luria (1966) provides an excellent detailed description of the clinical examination.

Since the clinical examination varies greatly in form as well as detail from one setting to another, no comparative evaluation of different examination methods will be attempted. Clinical examination skills must be acquired under close supervision in a clinical setting.

Schuell (1957) published a "short examination for aphasia" that presents a systematic clinical examination based on the model of the author's test (to be discussed later). This clinical examination provides a detailed check of auditory discrimination, recognition, and retention; visual discrimination, recognition, and recall; spatial orientation; involvement of speech musculature; sensorimotor involvement; word finding; and functional speech and writing. In a 1966 revision, Schuell recommends the use of 4-point rating scales for each of these functions and of 7-point severity ratings for the five major areas of impairment in aphasia. Schuell's revised examination represents an extension of the clinical examination by means of rating scale techniques that remain easy to use for clinicans without making demands of a formal test nature. Another attempt to establish a more systematic clinical examination by means of "behavioral analysis" was described by Sidman (1971).

In a reevaluation of her brief examination, Schuell (1966) carefully debates the merits of the clinical examination in comparison to the comprehensive test. She stresses that only a comprehensive test can assess all aspects of "aphasia, [which] deals with one of the most complex and perhaps the only unique function of the human brain [Schuell, 1966, p. 138]." For this reason, she recommends the use of a detailed test (i.e., the MTDDA[1]) and states that the use of the clinical examination does not replace the need for a full test examination.

Tests of Specific Aspects of Language Behavior

Several tests have been constructed for the detailed assessment of a specific function (e.g., language comprehension only; see also the detailed review of auditory comprehension tests by Boller, Kim, & Mack, 1977). Such tests usually make no claim to cover all aspects of aphasia but provide a relatively thorough assessment of the function in question. Since such functions are usually central to the aphasic disorder, however, these tests may also provide a reasonable discrimination between aphasic and nonaphasic patients in general. Some of these tests have been used as screening devices because of their good discrimination, although this was not necessarily the intent of the authors.

---

1. For full names of tests, see appendix to this chapter.

TOKEN TEST

The Token Test was introduced as a brief test designed by De Renzi and Vignolo in 1962 to examine subtle auditory comprehension deficits in aphasic patients. Since then, the original Token Test has been widely used and has spawned many variants—for example, short forms (Boller & Vignolo, 1966; Spellacy & Spreen, 1969; Van Harskamp & Van Dongen, 1977); alternate versions, including a concrete-objects version (Martino, Pizzamiglio, & Razzano, 1976); and a Token Test battery (Brookshire, 1978). The latest version of the original 1962 Token Test is found in De Renzi and Faglioni (1978) and De Renzi (1980).

The Token Test is a short and portable test that, in most versions, is composed of 20 plastic or cardboard token stimuli of two sizes (large and small), two shapes (square and round), and five colors. The tokens are laid out in front of the patient in a standard predetermined order; the patient must respond gesturally to the tester's oral command. The test is composed of a number of sections (six in the latest De Renzi version), ranging in increasing difficulty from such simple commands as "Show me a square," to "Show me a yellow circle," to "Show me a small green square," to more complex commands, such as "Pick up all squares except the yellow one."

There are no reported adult age differences on test performance; however, years of education has been found to influence performance and can be corrected for (De Renzi, 1980; De Renzi & Faglioni, 1978). Gallaher (1979) reports day-to-day retest reliabilities for the Token Test and its individual subsections to be greater than .90. Validation studies have shown the Token Test to be a strong and accurate discriminator between the performance of aphasic patients and that of normal adult hospitalized controls (De Renzi, 1980), nonaphasic right brain damaged controls (Boller & Vignolo, 1966; Swisher & Sarno, 1969), and nonaphasic diffuse and focal brain-damaged controls (Orgass & Poeck, 1966). Morley, Lundgren, and Haxby (1979) found that the Token Test discriminated particularly well between normals and aphasics with high levels of ability in comparison to the comprehension subtest of the BDAE and the PICA. Poeck, Kerschensteiner, and Hartje (1972) also demonstrated independence of the Token Test performance from the fluency–nonfluency dimension in aphasic patients. Cohen, Kelter, and Shaefer (1977) and Cohen, Lutzweiler, and Woll (1980) examined construct validity and other aspects of validity. The memory component of the Token Test was examined by Lesser (1976).

The Token Test has gained a good deal of popularity as both a clinical and an investigative test instrument. Two studies have also concentrated on specific training programs designed to improve comprehension ability on the Token Test (Holland & Sonderman, 1974; West, 1973). The many versions of the Token Test have led to some confusion about what a "Token Test" performance actually represents. Unfortunately, a test manual with a complete and organized discussion of the test and its usefulness as well as test normative values and reliability and validity statements, has yet to become available. However, two compilations of the work with the Token Test have been published (Boller & Dennis, 1979; McNeal & Prescott, 1978), and two English-language versions are commercially available (McNeal & Prescott, 1978=S; University of Victoria, 1969=S).[2] The test's advantages lie in sound discriminative validity, easy portability, and short administration times (less than half an hour). Brookshire (1975) advises the clinician to remember that, although the Token Test is a sensitive indicator of comprehension deficits, it is a measure of comprehension employing a limited stimulus array that, in itself, may not be highly generalizable to other stimulus arrays. For this reason, the clinician might wish to employ the Token Test along with other tests of auditory comprehension (e.g., the ACTS).

REPORTER'S TEST

De Renzi has employed the stimuli and most of the commands from the Token Test (De Renzi & Faglioni, 1978) to construct the Reporter's Test, a screening test for expressive deficits in aphasic patients (De Renzi, 1980; De Renzi & Ferrari, 1979). The Reporter's Test was designed to meet two specific goals: (a) to elicit organized speech; and (b) to limit the range of what the patient is expected to say. Whereas picture description tasks (e.g., BDAE or WAB) adequately fulfill the first goal, they fail on the second. Using the commands and stimuli from the Token Test is an attempt to satisfy both goals. The patient is required to act as a "reporter" on this task; that is, the patient must report the actions of the tester to an imaginary third person. For example, if the tester were to touch the large red circle stimulus, the patient must verbalize the relevant information necessary for a third person to reproduce the tester's action ("Touch the large red circle."). The Reporter's Test begins with several sample items to acquaint the patient with the task. The test is composed of five sections; the first four sections are taken from parts 2–5 of the Token Test.

De Renzi (1980) reports initial findings for the Reporter's Test in discriminating 24 aphasic patients from 40 hospitalized, nonaphasic, nonbrain-damaged controls. In this study, an actual third person sat next to the aphasic patient and performed as the aphasic instructed. Scoring

2. S refers to the source from which the exam can be obtained.

was on a pass–fail basis; partial credit was given for correct performances after repetition. Years of education, but not age, were significantly related to performance; for this reason, scores were corrected to account for education. Using a cutting score expected to produce 5% false positives, a 97% overall hit rate was obtained. One control and one aphasic patient were misclassified. Classification accuracy was higher for the Reporter's Test than for four other tests of verbal expression: visual naming, oral fluency, sentence repetition, and story telling.

De Renzi and Ferrari (1979) described aphasic performance employing both pass–fail scoring and weighted scoring (1 point for each bit of information on a trial but without particular credit for repetition). Aphasic patients, nonaphasic left brain-damaged patients, and nonaphasic right brain-damaged patients were described. Using the pass–fail scoring system, a cutting score of 18.35 resulted in a 92% hit rate, yielding 10% false positives in the sample of nonaphasic left brain damaged patients and 15% false positives in the right brain damaged sample. Sample classification on the Reporter's Test again proved superior to that of tests of visual naming, word fluency, sentence repetition, and story telling. Score corrections for eduational level are provided. Using the weighted scoring system, a cutting score of 54 resulted in an 82% hit rate, while yielding 15% false positives in the nonaphasic left brain-damaged group. The authors recommend the use of both scoring systems to offset the weaknesses of each: low classification for the weighted system and overly severe evaluation using pass–fail scoring.

A critical assessment of the utility of the Reporter's Test in a clinical setting must await detailed normative data as well as data indicating test reliability and validity. De Renzi (1980) reports low correlations between the Reporter's Test and tests of oral fluency (.17) and sentence repetition (.32) and significant, though moderate, correlations with visual naming (.41) and story telling (.49). The test correlates .66 with the Token Test.

In its current form, the Reporter's Test complements the Token Test in structure, brevity, and use as a screening device and certainly merits future psychometric evaluation. At the moment, De Renzi recommends that it be used following the Token Test, so that the patient is acquainted with the stimuli and the required commands.

AUDITORY COMPREHENSION TEST FOR SENTENCES (ACTS)

The ACTS (Shewan, 1980=S) is a recent addition to specific examinations of auditory comprehension. The current version is a revision of an earlier experimental version (Shewan & Canter, 1971). The ACTS format provides that sentences are spoken by the tester; the aphasic patient must point to one of four visual displays to indicate which display is correct for the stated sentence. Four preliminary trials are permitted. These trials also serve as a screening device to determine which patients are too impaired to perform the task. The preliminary trials are followed by 21 test items that vary along parameters of sentence length, vocabulary difficulty, and syntactic complexity. Both pass–fail and qualitative error-analysis scoring are possible; the use of each system is made easy by the clear and concise ACTS protocol sheet. The test manual states that an average of 10–15 min is required to complete the ACTS.

Shewan reports an ACTS internal consistency correlation coefficient of .82, as well as a test–retest reliability coefficient of .87. Two statements of validity are provided in the manual: (*a*) a correlation of .80 with an 8-point clinical rating of functional auditory–verbal comprehension; and (*b*) correlations of .52 with the auditory comprehension section of the BDAE and .89 with the WAB comprehension section. The low ACTS–BDAE correlation is attributed to the wide range of abilities assessed in the BDAE relative to the ACTS.

Information regarding the ACTS standardization sample of 150 aphasics of various etiologies and 30 normal adult controls is provided in the test manual. Means and standard deviations of the performance of various aphasic syndrome groups as well as typical profiles are included. Relevant qualitative group differences are also reviewed.

The revised ACTS test is brief, easy to administer and score, and requires simple nonverbal responses by the patient. It is reliable and a valid test instrument. It shows a good deal of promise as a test of comprehension for sentences that systematically vary in length, difficulty, and complexity. Cautions in evaluating ACTS performance, such as differences between the standardization sample and the clinician's expected referral base and educational and cultural influences on test performance, are carefully considered in the ACTS manual.

WORD FLUENCY TESTS

Word fluency tests are fast and efficient methods to assess verbal fluency in aphasic patients. The task involved is one of controlled association. The patient is required to produce as many words as possible that begin with a specific letter within a given time period. Two standardized tests of word fluency are available. The first word fluency test is part of the Spreen and Benton NCCEA examination (1977=S); The second is described by Wertz (1979).

The Spreen and Benton version requires the patient to say as many words as possible that begin with the letters *F*, *A*, and *S* within 1-min time periods. Proper names and words that differ only in suffix are excluded; performance is gauged in terms of the sum of admissible words in all three trials. Normative data, as well as corrections for age and level of education, are available in the NCCEA test manual (Spreen & Benton, 1977).

The letters employed in this version are all of the "easy" difficulty level, as defined by Borkowski, Benton, and Spreen (1967). Borkowski *et al.* examined the number of associations of normal adult females for 24 of the 26 letters of the alphabet. The number of associations was related with the difficulty level, as defined by both the Thorndike–Lorge count ($r = .80$) and the number of words per letter in *Webster's New Collegiate Dictionary* ($r = .74$). The authors also report that a heterogeneous sample of brain-damaged patients performed less well than normal adults at all levels of letter difficulty, lending validity to the testing method. Patients with low IQ were better differentiated with easy-level letters, whereas high IQ patients were better distinguished with more difficult letters.

Wertz (1979) describes a second word fluency test that employs the letters *S, T, P,* and *C* (all easy-level letters). In this version, proper names are permitted, and age and level of education corrections are not employed. Normative data are provided in Wertz and Lemme (1974) and Wertz, Keith, and Custer (1971). Standardized instructions for this version of the test are available in the protocol manual of the Veteran's Administration Cooperative Study on Aphasia (1973=S). This version of the task has also been employed to successfully discriminate brain-damaged and normal samples. Further, Wertz *et al.* report correlations between word fluency and PICA overall and verbal performance and the last section of the Token Test.

Tests of word fluency are quick and simple. Both versions described have proven discriminative validity. Reliability data, however, are lacking. Word fluency tasks may not be very sensitive in distinguishing at lower levels of ability, but they are capable of screening for the presence of less severe disability.

Short Screening Tests

The following tests have been deliberately designed to screen for the presence or absence of aphasia within a limited period of time. They are described here as short screening tests since they do not claim to provide a detailed description of the aphasic disorder but to check for and focus the direction on the problem if aphasia is present. Some of these tests are actually part of a larger neuropsychological test battery.

HALSTEAD–WEPMAN SCREENING TEST

The Wheeler and Reitan (1962; Heimburger & Reitan, n.d.=S) version of this screening device is designed to determine whether or not the patient can perform such simple tasks as spelling a word or naming an object. The test procedures are such that the clinician should elicit the patient's best possible performance. A large array of language function is briefly assessed by one or two items each. For example, the patient is required to draw a shape, name it, and spell it; to read (e.g., "See the black dog"); to do a single pencil-and-paper and a single "in-head" arithmetic problem; and to demonstrate object use and picture drawing.

The test takes approximately 20 min to complete. The test manual provides many illustrative examples of performances. As stated in the introduction of this chapter, screening tests of this type have seen little use recently because they provide very limited information and tend to show only limited accuracy. The test is usually given within the context of a complete neuropsychological test battery (Meier, 1974) intended to assess the full range of psychological deficits after brain damage. The screening efficiency of the test as a single measure (discrimination between aphasic and nonaphasic brain-damaged patients) has been reported as 80% correct (Krug, 1971).

APHASIA LANGUAGE PERFORMANCE SCALES (ALPS)

The ALPS (Keenen & Brassell, 1975=S) is designed to address the following questions: "What is the patient's best level of performance in each language modality, and how can we best use this information to plan effective therapy? [p. 3]." The authors consider the ALPS to be a "significant departure" from the trend toward psychometric objectivity in aphasia assessment as seen in such instruments as the MTDDA and the PICA. The endpoint of this psychometric trend, according to the authors, is such that the examiners "are encouraged, in short, to divest themselves in their own personality, to supress their individual responses to each change in their environments, and to behave rather like machines [p. 31]."

The ALPS is composed of four 10-item scales: listening, talking, reading, and writing. Item arrangement in each scale is in terms of difficulty. For each scale, a correct response is defined as that which the tester might expect from a normal adult. A correct or self-corrected response is given full credit (1 point); a correct response that requires prompting is given half credit (½ point). The tester is free to begin each scale at whichever level he or she feels the patient will be competent. A scale is terminated upon two consecutive failures. Criteria for determining normal performance, the need for prompting and the point in the subscale at which the patient will be competent are at the discretion of the tester. The number of correctly completed items is used as a score for each section and is directly translated into a scale of impairment. The authors provide an arbitrarily determined descriptive scale of impairment for each section, ranging from "profoundly impaired" for a scale score of 0–1 to "insignificant impairment" for a scale score from 9.5–10.

Normative data are not provided. Given the subjective nature of the ALPS administration, however, normative data would be, for all intents and purposes, of little value.

The authors report high test–retest reliabilities for each scale. Reliability coefficients from .83 to .94 are reported from a sample of 22 aphasics tested twice over a 3- to 5-week period. Split-half reliabilities for all scales of at least .86 are also reported from another sample of aphasic patients. In a sample of 23 aphasics, seven judges showed a high degree of concordance in scoring videotaped performances on the ALPS. The scales have also been statistically shown to increase in general difficulty. The validity of the ALPS has been examined relative to the PICA in one sample of 12 aphasic patients and a second sample of 50 aphasic patients: Overall and scale score were significantly correlated between the two tests.

To summarize, the ALPS would seem to fall into the gray area between clinical and psychometric assessment: While being systematized to a greater degree than many personal clinical examinations, the ALPS falls short of being a standard and comprehensive test instrument. The authors disclaim any psychometric intentions in creating the ALPS. Hence, the interested clinician would do well by weighing the positive and negative aspects of the ALPS against his or her own personal, informal clinical assessment rather than attempting, as the authors do, to contrast the ALPS with psychometrically established comprehensive aphasia examinations. The clinician looking for a brief and informal aphasia screening test might well consider the ALPS.

SKLAR APHASIA SCALE (SAS)

The SAS (revised SAS; Sklar, 1973=S) provides a brief assessment of the aphasic patient's residual abilities along four dimensions: auditory decoding, visual decoding, oral encoding, and graphic encoding. The four subtests are each represented by five areas that are each composed of five items. The SAS is constructed within the framework of a decode (input), transcode (process), and encode (output) model of language communication and its disabilities. Items on the SAS were chosen solely for their ability to sample verbal behavior; other items were omitted in deference to neuropsychological and neurological assessments of the patient.

Each response on the SAS is scored on a 5-point scale: a "correct" response (0), a correct though "retarded" response (1), a correct though "assisted" response (2), a "distorted" response (3), and an "erased" response (i.e., no response) (4). An impairment score for each subtest is obtained by finding the mean value of the four subtest impairment scores (0 = no impairment to 100 = full impairment). Five categories of the severity of total impairment are provided. The test author states that the total impairment index may be used prognostically in terms of potential benefit of therapy if modified by both the recency of the impairment and the patient's overall state of health.

SAS items were standardized on a sample of 20 adults ranging in age from 29 to 78 years. The test author reports high correlations between SAS performance and performance on Eisenson's aphasia examination, Schuell's short version based upon the MTDDA, and the Halstead–Wepman aphasia screening test in a sample of 12 aphasic patients. A second study found significant correlations between SAS performance and performance on the Wechsler–Bellevue, the Bender Visual–Motor Gestalt Test, and the Goldstein–Scheerer Cube Test. A third study (Sklar, 1963) found a significant correlation between SAS performance and autopsy findings of cerebral deterioration. Finally, findings from two factor analytic studies ($N = 65$ and $N = 111$) are provided in the test manual. Both are reported to have produced dimensions similar to the four subtest dimensions employed in the SAS.

In sum, the SAS is a brief aphasic examination designed to elicit relevant information on a patient's abilities along four dimensions of decoding and encoding. Although reliability data are not presented, the test author presents five studies examining the validity of the SAS as an instrument to assess language ability in aphasics. The test author states that the impairment index derived from SAS performance has prognostic significance; however, such prognostication is based on only a very simple index score (e.g., an aphasic performing with a score of 70 having a better prognosis than an aphasic scoring 15), and psychometric evaluations of SAS prognostic significance have not been presented so far.

Communication Profiles

The introduction of Sarno's Functional Communication Profile (FCP; Sarno, 1969; Taylor, 1965) marked the first psychometric attempt to assess language ability in its functional usefulness for everyday life. The newly available scale for Communicative Abilities in Daily Living (CADL) (Holland, 1980) is a further attempt to index the degree of disability faced by the patient in attempting to communicate in daily life. Rather than obtain pure, isolated samples of specific language behaviors, as tests of aphasia usually do, both the FCP and the CADL deal with such complex behaviors as the ability to make change, to communicate on the telephone, to read newspaper headlines and consumer-product labels, and to ask for, correct, and impart significant information to and from others. Hence, the type of information gauged on these profiles is a unique contribution to the overall assessment of the aphasic patient, providing the clinician with additional information, not usually available from formal testing procedures, regarding the communicative status of the patient.

FUNCTIONAL COMMUNICATION PROFILE (FCP)

The FCP (Sarno, 1969=S; Taylor, 1965) is designed as a measure of natural language use (such as that seen in everyday communication). Taylor (1965) distinguishes natural language use from the language elicited in the typically artificial and formal test setting. The FCP has been a germinal and important contribution to the assessment of the aphasic patient's communicative ability. The FCP attempts to index the aphasic patient's ability to employ language in common everyday situations, relative to the patient's estimated premorbid level of ability. "Normal" functioning on the profile is defined by the clinician's skilled estimation of the patient's previous language ability based upon available evidence. The effectiveness of a subjective rating scale of this type is directly related to the experience and skill of the user; therefore, it is *not recommended* for the clinically inexperienced or for those working in settings where few adult aphasics are likely to be seen (Sarno, 1969). It also may not be very useful in situations where little premorbid information is available.

A primary role of the clinician is to create an informal rapport with the patient wherein he or she can observe the patient's natural communicative behavior without resorting to formal testing. Forty-five behaviors (e.g., the ability to indicate yes and no, to read newspaper headlines, and to handle money) are rated on a 9-point scale of current ability as a proportion of estimated former ability. The scales range from "normal" (100%) to "absent" (0%) ability. The 45 behaviors are clustered into five categories: movement, speaking, understanding, reading, and miscellaneous (including calculation and writing). Overall cluster scores are obtained by determining the mean rating of the items in a cluster.

Despite the subjective nature of the scoring system, Sarno (1969) reports interrater reliability coefficients larger than .87 for each of the five subsections of the FCP. Reliability was determined for three judges using a sample of 20 right-hemiplegic patients with language symptoms of at least 2 months' duration.

The distinction between functional and psychometrically measured language functioning was examined by Sarno, Sarno, and Levita (1971).

Measurements of improvement were determined using original and follow-up performances on the NCCEA visual naming and identification by sentence (i.e., the Token Test) subtests and the speech and understanding subscales of the FCP. There was only a moderate relationship between the first and the second score on each of the two speech subtests (i.e., NCCEA visual naming and FCP speech) and no correlation between score changes on the two comprehension subtests (i.e., NCCEA identification by sentence and FCP understanding). The authors conclude that psychometric test improvement (as seen on the NCCEA subtests) need not be accompanied by functional, useful improvements in language ability.

The information obtained on the FCP is not designed to replace a comprehensive examination of the aphasic patient's language abilities and disabilities. Rather, its goal is to provide information not readily tapped by a standard examination: natural language capacity. The information yielded by a properly administered FCP may well be more easily translatable into a description of the patient's everyday capabilities than the information provided by a standard comprehensive examination. When properly used, the FCP may provide information on the functional consequences of the patient's aphasic condition that is not otherwise (except anecdotally) available. Repeated FCP administration may provide information on the recovery process of this functionally relevant communicative ability (Sands, Sarno, & Shankweiler, 1969; Sarno & Levita, 1979).

COMMUNICATIVE ABILITIES IN DAILY LIVING (CADL)

The CADL (Holland, 1980=S) is also designed to measure the communicative ability of the aphasic patient. Its purpose, like that of the FCP, is to provide supplementary nonredundant information, in the context of a full assessment of the aphasic patient, regarding functional language communicative ability. A good part of the test involves patient performance during simulated, cued-context, daily activities, such as dealing with a receptionist, communicating with a doctor, driving, shopping, and making telephone calls. Given the emphasis on communicative ability rather than on language ability per se, communication via oral, written, gestural, or any other method of transmission is acknowledged as significant.

The CADL is composed of 68 items, which are scored either "correct" (2 points), "adequate" (1 point), or "wrong" (0 points) on the basis of the success of the patient's attempt to communicate. For example, at one point the tester asks the patient, "Your first name is _____, right?" (filling in a fictitious name). If the patient's communicative act includes both a negative response ("No," headshake, written response, etc.) and his or her correct name, 2 points are alloted. If the patient simply replies with a negative response without further elaboration, the act is considered adequate but not fully appropriate. If the patient responds affirmatively, perseverates, echoes the question, or simply does not respond or responds incoherently, no points are given. Requests for repetition are considered to be legitimate communicative statements and are not penalized. However, if the patient fails to respond within 5 seconds, only partial credit (1 point for a correct response) is allowed.

Test standardization, reliability, and validity information from two principal studies are provided in the CADL test manual. In the initial study, 80 aphasic patients were assessed on an earlier 73-item version of the CADL, the BDAE, the FCP, and the PICA, as well as being observed during a 4-hour period to examine the frequency, appropriateness, and type of communicative behavior employed by the patient in everyday life. The internal consistency of the CADL in this sample was .97; 68 of the 73 test items showed item–total correlations of at least .40, indicating a high degree of test consistency. An interexaminer reliability coefficient of .99 was obtained for two scorers testing a subsample of 20 patients. The CADL manifests concurrent validity. The test correlated .87 with the FCP, .93 with PICA performance, and .84 with BDAE performance. The criterion validity of the CADL was assessed by determining the relationship between the CADL test score and behavior during a 4-hr observation period. Significant correlations between .60 and .64 were determined. The CADL also has demonstrated construct validity; test performance distinguished BDAE-determined types of aphasic patients. Global aphasics showed the poorest CADL performance. Wernicke's aphasics performed more satisfactorily than global aphasics but less well than Broca's aphasics, who in turn were inferior in performance to anomic aphasics.

In the second study, normative data were collected on 130 aphasic patients and 130 normal adults who varied in age, sex, and living situation (i.e., institution versus home). The manual reports better CADL performances for nonaphasics than for aphasics; for noninstitutionalized than for institutionalized groups; and for younger than for older groups; there was also a slight tendency for females to perform better than males. The aphasic patients showed a greater degree of heterogeneity in CADL performance than did normal adults. CADL performance was not influenced by either education or occupation. Again, global aphasics showed the worst performance, while anomic aphasics showed the best performance. Intermediate scores by mixed aphasic and Wernicke's aphasia groups and higher intermediate scores by Broca's aphasia and conduction aphasic groups were observed. Normative data in the form of sample means, standard deviation, cutoff scores, and item analyses are presented in the manual.

The CADL score is simply the sum of points earned on the 68 items. The manual describes 10 interrelated performance categories and presents error profiles for each type of diagnosed aphasia. The manual states that the CADL requires 35–45 minutes to complete. Two test protocols as well as a cassette tape recording of a third protocol are provided in the manual for training purposes.

The CADL, like the FCP, should provide a useful assessment tool for examining the functional consequences of aphasia. One study examines the usefulness of the test during functional communication focused therapy and in relation to the PICA (Aten, Caligiure, & Holland, in press). The clinician now has a choice of instruments for this type of assessment: the FCP and the CADL. Future work should indicate in which situations each test would be maximally efficient and useful.

Psycholinguistic Evaluation of Aphasic Language

While the assessment of communicative abilities in daily living discussed in the previous section makes use of conversational speech in a natural setting with limited structure, some studies have attempted to analyze conversational speech of aphasic patients in a setting that makes no specific demands on the patient at all. Ideally, one could monitor and record a patient's utterances on audio- or videotape in the course of a day in hospital or at home. The main goal of such studies is not, however, an assessment of communicative abilities but a more detailed study from a psycholinguistic point of view. Studies of use and abuse of syntax; grammar; word choice; frequency of word usage, pauses, and hesitations; speed of utterance; etc. can be conducted with such "free-speech" samples. The alternative approach is to focus on each aspect of psycholinguistic analysis individually and construct an experimental setting that allows an analysis of the types of errors produced by an aphasic patient.

Both the open-ended free-speech and the experimental approach have been used extensively in research with aphasia (Goodglass & Blumstein, 1973; Spreen, 1968). Insofar as these studies represent experiments rather than attempts to assess the aphasic patient's deficit, such studies will not be reviewed here. However, some of these studies have led to conclusions about the nature of the deficit in specific types of aphasia and can be translated into suitable methods of assessment.

These studies will be briefly described, and their potential application in the development of assessment techniques will be pointed out.

The first comprehensive studies of a psycholinguistic nature were conducted by Wepman and collaborators (Fillenbaum, Jones, & Wepman, 1961; Jones, Goodman, & Wepman, 1963; Spiegel, Jones, & Wepman, 1965; Wepman, Bock, Jones, & Van Pelt, 1956; Wepman & Jones, 1964). Part of this work is based on conversational speech by 50 aphasic speakers in response to the task of making up stories for the Thematic Apperception Test. Various linguistic paremeters were calculated, including grammatical form class usage, grammatical correctness, intelligibility, and word-finding problems (the latter three problems correspond to the syntactic, semantic, and pragmatic types of aphasia in Wepman's terminology). The studies involved complex calculations as well as judgments by linguistically trained researchers; they cannot be readily translated into more directly accessible forms of assessment.

The second major project was conducted by Howes and collaborators (Howes, 1964, 1966, 1967; Howes & Geschwind, 1964) and involved a detailed analysis of conversational speech of 5000 words of each of more than 80 aphasic and nonaphasic speakers. The analysis concentrated on lexical diversity (i.e., the frequency of word usage in aphasic versus nonaphasic speakers) and also distinguished between "fluent" and "nonfluent" speakers, who were viewed as similar to Wernicke's and anomic aphasics and to classical Broca's aphasics, respectively. Benson (1967) attempted to develop a simplified and clinically useful rating scale system based on the information of Howes's study and adding some additional rating dimensions. The ratings used a 3-point scale and involved the following aspects: rate of speaking, prosody, pronunciation, phrase length, effort, pauses, press of speech, perseveration, word choice, paraphasia, and verbal stereotypes. These 11 characteristics were related to radioactive brain scan localization. It was found that anterior lesions tended to produce speech with low verbal output, dysprosody, dysarthria, considerable effort, and predominant use of substantive nouns, whereas posterior lesions produced speech that was normal or near normal on all these features but showed paraphasia, press of speech, and a lack of substantive words.

A third study with a comprehensive analysis of conversational speech of a minimum of 1000 words from 50 aphasic and 50 normal speakers was conducted by Spreen and Wachal (1973; Wachal & Spreen, 1973) using a computer–scorer interaction analysis of various psycholinguistic aspects of spoken language. Crockett (1972, 1976) designed 5-point rating scales for 17 characteristics of speech—including rate of speech, prosody, pronunciation, hesitation, phrase length, effort, pauses, press of speech, perseveration, word choice, paraphasia, communication, naming, grammar, use of interstitial connectives, understanding of spoken language, and use of inflection, tense or gender, and neologisms— in an attempt to translate psycholinguistic speech characteristics into basic rating scale dimensions. Interrater agreement among five judges was satisfactory after some training and a carefully worded description of each characteristic was given.

Although both Benson's and Crockett's translation of psycholinguistic aspects of aphasic speech appeared to be quite successful within the limited scope of the research problem under investigation, further use of this approach has been limited up to this time. Some of the ratings have been incorporated into the Boston Diagnostic Aphasia Examination. Kerschensteiner, Poeck, and Brunner (1972) used a similar rating system for the study of conversational speech. Yet all three studies demonstrate clearly that it is possible to translate the somewhat elusive aspects of speaking style into rating scales that are readily understood and usable. Perhaps one reason for the infrequent use of such ratings has been that these attempts were made within the context of a relatively complex research project rather than in the context of an assessment-oriented project. Another reason may be that psycholinguistic aspects of aphasic speech are rather complex in themselves and not readily understood without prior training; hence, the clinically oriented examiner tends to shy away from the psycholinguistic evaluations and use the relatively more concrete standard testing and assessment methods instead.

Comprehensive Examinations

Unlike short screening tests or tests concerned with particular aspects of language functioning, comprehensive examinations of the aphasic patient's language ability seek to obtain a diverse sampling of performance at different levels of task difficulty along all dimensions of function that the test author deems relevant to language disability. Examples of dimensions common to most of these tests include oral expression, auditory comprehension, repetition, reading ability, and writing ability. Other dimensions vary according to the theoretical orientation of the authors.

Comprehensive examinations show a wide diversity of purpose, structure, utility, and adequacy as test instruments. For example, some tests are constructed to examine the localization of the lesion and to provide prognostic information regarding standard anatomically based aphasic syndromes. Others are concerned with eliciting behavior that will provide relevant information for the planning and initiation of re-habilitative intervention.

The tests chosen for this review are those in current use that are readily accessible to the clinician: the Appraisal of Language Disturbance (ALD) (Emerick, 1971), the Boston Diagnostic Aphasia Examination (BDAE) (Goodglass & Kaplan, 1972), the Minnesota Test for Differential Diagnosis of Aphasia (MTDDA) (Schuell, 1965), the Multilingual Aphasia Examination (MAE) (Benton & Hamsher, 1978), the Neurosensory Center Comprehensive Examination for Aphasia (NCCEA) (Spreen & Benton, 1977), the Porch Index of Communicative Ability (PICA) (Porch, 1967, 1973), and the Western Aphasia Battery (WAB) (Kertesz, 1979, 1980). Comprehensive tests that are no longer in widespread use, but are of historic value in the area of aphasia assessment, have been described in the introduction.

A common denominator of these test instruments is the need for adequate training and practice before the examination can be effectively employed. The choice of an assessment instrument is a serious decision for the clinician that not only involves personal preferences but also takes into consideration the clinical setting, the type of referrals that the clinician can expect, the stated intentions of the test instrument, as well as the adequacy of the examination as an at least minimally reliable, valid, and useful test instrument.

APPRAISAL OF LANGUAGE DISTURBANCE (ALD)

The author of the ALD (Emerick, 1971=S) views aphasia as an impairment of symbol functioning subsequent to cortical damage and characterized by one or more of the following symptoms: input disturbances via the modal channels, central processing disturbances, and output disturbances via modal channels. The stated purpose of this examination is to provide a systematic inventory of the patient's communicative abilities by examining input modalities, central processing, and output modalities to allow the clinician to determine the best avenues of reception and expression to initiate therapy.

The ALD is structured into three primary sections: (*a*) eight input–output pathways (e.g., aural to oral, aural to visual, aural to gesture, visual to oral, and visual to graphic); (*b*) a central language comprehension section in which matching, sorting and arranging, and manding (a Skinnerian term referring to requesting or demanding) are examined; and (*c*) a section on related factors, including tactile recognition, arithmetic, and an oral examination for signs of paralysis or other abnormality. The structure of the test follows closely the input–processing–output language model developed by Osgood and Sebeok (1965) and used in the Illinois Test of Psycholinguistic Abilities (ITPA) (McCarthy & Kirk, 1961) further modified by Wepman and collaborators (Wepman, Jones, Bock, & Van Pelt, 1960). The model is used in other tests as well (e.g., the SAS).

Normative data for the test are not reported nor are formal validity studies available. The test manual is very brief and frequently lacking in detail. According to the manual, material and procedures were developed on the basis of "intensive scrutiny of 75 aphasic patients." Fifty-six of these patients were retested after an interval of 2 weeks to 5 months, resulting in a reliability coefficient of .74 (.81 for a subsample of 39 neurologically stable patients). Interscorer reliability for 39 neurologically stable patients was .86.

There are several limitations to the usefulness of the ALD. First, a good many items considered as part of the assessment of central language processing are of questionable value. For example, two of the three matching tasks, given the author's conception of aphasia, might well be more parsimoniously labeled "visual-gesture" avenue tasks rather than "central language comprehension." Second, many tasks in this section and the related-function section are more adequately covered in other examinations. For example, the single object assembly and the single verbal arithmetic problem are more adequately assessed on such common test instruments as the Wechsler tests of intelligence. Third, the Peabody Picture Vocabulary Test (PPVT) (Dunn, 1965) is to be completed as part of the central language comprehension section; however, no instructions for incorporating PPVT test results into the ALD are provided. No decision rules are provided that would guide the reader in identifying types of aphasia. The author (Emerick, 1971) states this explicitly, stressing that "it is far more useful clinically to simply identify what the patient can and cannot do [p. 5]."

At present, the paucity of adequate psychometric studies, the brief and often uninformative test manual, and questionable test construction (i.e., "central language comprehension" section and the rather rigid adherence to a schematic model of language) offset any positive value that the ALD might possess relative to the other comprehensive examinations reviewed in this chapter.

BOSTON DIAGNOSTIC APHASIA EXAMINATION (BDAE)

The BDAE (Goodglass & Kaplan, 1972=S) is one of the most extensive aphasia examinations in popular use today. The primary focus of the BDAE is the diagnosis of classic anatomically based aphasic syndromes. This diagnostic goal is attained by comprehensive sampling of language components (e.g., speech fluency) that have previously proven themselves valuable in the identification of aphasic syndromes.

Goodglass and Kaplan state that the design of their instrument is based upon the observation that various components of language function may be selectively damaged by CNS lesions; this selectivity being an indication of: (a) the anatomical neural organization of language; (b) the localization of the lesion causing the observed deficit; and (c) the functional interactions of various parts of the language system. Several studies have been published to validate the stated purpose (Naeser & Hayward, 1978). Benson (1979a) states that knowledge of the classification system employed by the BDAE authors and their colleagues is necessary to adequately interpret the BDAE.

The BDAE is divided into five language-area sections (several areas were structured from a set of factor analyses described in the manual): (a) conversational and expository speech; (b) auditory comprehension; (c) oral expression; (d) understanding written language; and (e) writing. Each section is composed of a wide variety of diverse subtests. Each subtest attempts to measure a specific function in as purely isolated a fashion as possible. Supplementary language and nonlanguage tests that may or may not be of use in a given clinical setting are appended in the test manual.

The detailed examination of conversational and expository speech in the BDAE is an important and relatively unique aspect of this test. A "profile of speech characteristics," indexing verbal prosody, fluency, articulation, grammatical level, paraphasias, and word-finding difficulty, is derived from both a sample of free conversation and a sample of narrative speech. An overall rating of symptom severity is determined from these speech samples as well.

The profile and the severity rating are central to diagnostic decision making in the BDAE; particularly important is the fluency–nonfluency dimension. More detailed diagnoses incorporate information from the z-score profile sheet indicating subtest performance. The reliability of the speech characteristics profile was examined employing three judges who rated 99 patients' tape-recorded speech samples. The lowest correlation coefficients of .78 and .79 were obtained for word-finding difficulties and paraphasias, respectively. The other four scales had coefficients of at least .85.

Auditory comprehension is examined in the BDAE by word recognition in six distinct semantic categories, body-part identification, commands, and complex ideational material requiring yes–no responding. Expression is gauged on 12 subtests that include agility, naming, recitation, automatized sequences, and repetition. Articulation and the frequency of various types of paraphasias are recorded.

Understanding written language is assessed by four subtests, as is writing. Associative skills that either underlie reading or are by-products of the reading process (e.g., phonetic associations) are examined in the assessment of reading comprehension. Writing is assessed through mechanics, recall of written symbols, and word finding.

The BDAE is standardized on a sample of 207 aphasic patients with relatively distinct lesions and isolated, well-defined symptoms. Although standardization on such a large sample of patients is psychometrically useful, the clinician whose referrals do not reflect this select sample (i.e., referrals who may have lesions with a different bias in symptomology, severity, or socioeconomic background) may not be able to reference his or her patients directly to the BDAE sample. The z-score conversions for the various BDAE subtests are based upon data from varying numbers of these 207 aphasic patients. Converting a patient's performance to z scores allows an examination of patient strengths and weaknesses relative to this large group of aphasic patients.

The BDAE manual describes good internal consistency for all the test measures that contain a series of scorable items. Test–retest reliability has yet to be reported.

As with all other aphasia test instruments, the BDAE has both strong and weak points. Points in favor of the BDAE include its comprehensive sampling of behavior, its standardization based on a large sample of aphasic patients, and its attempt at a qualitative analysis of speech. Unfortunately, these strengths also reflect negative aspects of the test—namely, the time-consuming nature of BDAE administration, the select nature of the standardization sample, and the fact that the utility of a qualitative analysis is most likely directly related to the skill and experience of the professional performing the rating. The inclusion of a further standardization sample that is more randomly selected might well alleviate the second weakness described. A practical advantage of the BDAE is its portability relative to other assessment instruments. A Norwegian version of the test is available (Reinvang & Graves, 1975). Reinvang and Graves also attempt to clarify decision rules regarding the classification of the aphasias.

The ultimate usefulness of the BDAE must be determined by the needs of the individual clinician. The ability to operationally define classic aphasia syndromes, such as Broca's and Wernicke's aphasias, with this diagnostic instrument may be of importance to certain clinicians in certain settings. Other clinicians who may be looking for a comprehensive evaluation of aphasic performance that has prognostic value and that can be used to develop an intervention program for the patient might have to look elsewhere for a test instrument. The BDAE authors delineate clearly the primary goal of the test to facilitate such decisions.

MINNESOTA TEST FOR DIFFERENTIAL DIAGNOSIS OF
APHASIA (MTDDA)

The MTDDA (Schuell, 1965, 1973=S) is a comprehensive examination designed to observe the level at which language performance breaks down in each of the principal language modalities by examining the dimensions of impairment within each specific modality. The MTDDA systematically samples a very wide variety of language behavior in different modalities at different levels of task difficulty. To Schuell, the goal of a careful and comprehensive description of impairment in the aphasic patient is to provide a guide for effective therapeutic intervention. The construction of the MTDDA has represented a major breakthrough in the development of comprehensive aphasia test instruments that also meet requirements of standardization and objectivity. The current version of the MTDDA is the result of numerous systematic revisions of the original experimental version of the late 1940s. The author employed empirical factor analytic techniques (Schuell, Jenkins, & Carroll, 1962) as well as clinical experience to revise the structure of the test. The construction of the MTDDA reflects Schuell's theoretical consideration of aphasia as a unitary reduction of available language that crosses all language modalities and that may or may not be complicated by perceptual or sensorimotor involvement, by various forms of dysarthria, or by other sequelae of brain damage (Schuell & Jenkins, 1959, 1974b; Schuell *et al.*, 1964).

The MTDDA is composed of five sections: (*a*) auditory disturbances (represented by 9 subtests); (*b*) visual and reading disturbances (9 subtests); (*c*) speech and language disturbances (15 subtests); (*d*) visuomotor and writing disturbances (10 subtests); and (*e*) numerical relations and arithmetic processes (4 subtests). Within each section, subtest order is arranged from the least to the most difficult, with one minor discontinuity of order in the visual and reading disturbances section. Each section may be started at an estimated level of difficulty corresponding to the patient's ability (the "Binet method") and then continued to a point where the patient fails 90% or more of the items. Most items are scored either "correct" or "incorrect." Both the test manual (1965) and the companion monograph (1973) describe supplementary tests that should be considered for each section as well as the factor and intercorrelation structure for the sections of the test.

The auditory disturbance subtests include examinations of discrimination, retention span, and comprehension for vocabulary, sentences,
and paragraphs. The visual and reading subtests include examinations
of form and letter matching, matching printed words to pictures, matching printed to spoken words, reading comprehension for sentences and
paragraphs, and oral reading of words and sentences. The speech and
language subtests include 4 subtests that deal with speech movements
and articulation and 11 that deal with language, ranging from overlearned serial tasks to retelling a paragraph. Tasks of intermediate difficulty in this section include sentence completion, responding to questions, naming, and providing sentences. The visual and writing subtests
include 5 dealing with the reproduction and recall of visual forms and 5
dealing with written language, including spelling, producing sentences,
writing sentences to dictation, and writing a paragraph. The 4 numerical
and arithmetic subtests deal with functional arithmetic ability, minimizing the influence of education on performance. These tasks include coin
values, clock setting, and simple computations in the four basic arithmetic operations: addition, subtraction, multiplication, and division.

In terms of differential diagnosis, the author of the test has employed
the MTDDA to distinguish the following five aphasic syndromes: (a)
simple aphasia; (b) aphasia with visual involvement; (c) aphasia with
sensorimotor involvement; (d) aphasia with scattered findings compatible with generalized brain damage; (e) an irreversible aphasic syndrome (Schuell, 1974a). Schuell (1966, 1973) also added two additional
"minor syndromes": mild aphasia with persistent dysfluency (dysarthria) and aphasia with intermittent auditory imperception. Definitions,
signs, and MTDDA discriminations are provided in the monograph
(Schuell, 1973). However, as Zubrick and Smith (1979) point out, the
MTDDA was not designed to deal with broader issues of aphasic differential diagnosis: distinguishing aphasia from nonaphasic disorders
that may manifest language disturbance (e.g., memory loss, dementia,
severe hearing loss, and confusional state).

The length of the MTDDA is one feature that may or may not present
a problem for the user of the test. The large number of subtests include
many functions that exceed what some authors would consider the assessment of speech and language functions and range into material that
has been a traditional component of many standard intelligence tests.
Schuell's factor analysis may on closer inspection seem to reflect a major
first "general" factor that is closely related to the g obtained in factor
analyses of intelligence tests. Schuell and Jenkins (1959), however, consider this factor a general language factor, supporting their assumptions
about the unitary nature of language. Detailed information regarding

interpretation of the factor analytic findings are presented in Schuell, Jenkins, and Jiménez-Pabón (1964), as well as a careful analysis of the neurological, psychological, and social attributes of the aphasic and nonaphasic standardization samples. Schuell (1973) provides an examination of the differential neurological status of MTDDA-derived patient groups.

In sum, the MTDDA is an extensive examination of many facets of speech and language functioning. Great care has been taken in its construction, employing both clinical expertise and empirical technique. Potential users of the MTDDA should consider whether or not its length will be prohibitive in their clinical settings.[3] Potential users need also examine the congruence of the theoretical bases of the MTDDA relative to their own conceptions of the nature of aphasic deficits.

MULTILINGUAL APHASIA EXAMINATION (MAE)

The benefits to aphasiologists of having equivalent versions of a single aphasia examination for several language communities has been well stated by Benton (1967, 1968). The MAE (for English version, see Benton & Hamsher, 1978=S) has developed through the efforts of Benton and his North American and European collaborators to construct such an examination. English, French, German, Italian, and Spanish versions of the test are being prepared. The different language versions of the MAE are functionally equivalent in content rather than simply translations of an identical test. For example, the test of word fluency, rather than employing identical letters, uses letters that have corresponding levels of difficulty in each language (e.g., all letters are at an easy level of difficulty across language communities). Hence, performance on the task in each language is functionally equivalent.

The Benton and Hamsher version of the MAE is composed of eight areas of assessment: visual naming, sentence repetition, digit repetition, word fluency, spelling (oral spelling, writing to dictation, block-letter spelling), a version of the Token Test, aural comprehension of words and phrases, and reading comprehension of words and phrases. A rating scale of speech articulation based on verbal performance throughout the test session is also included. It ranges from 0 (speechless or usually unintelligible speech) to 8 (normal speech). Alternate versions of sentence repetition, word fluency, Token Test, and spelling are available if repeat assessments of the patient are necessary.

An MAE test manual citing reliability and validity data was not yet available at the time of this writing. The available documentation (i.e.,

---

3. A "very short form" was recently presented by Powell, Bailey, and Clark (1980).

Benton and Hamsher, 1978) in addition to providing standard test instructions, also provides normative information (in the form of percentiles) from a sample of normal adults without history or evidence of
neurological disability. Score adjustments for age and level of education
are also provided. It is hoped that the successful deployment of the MAE
in five language communities will facilitate direct comparisons of
individual–community case and sample data.

NEUROSENSORY CENTER COMPREHENSIVE EXAMINATION
FOR APHASIA (NCCEA)

The NCCEA (Spreen & Benton, 1977=S) is designed to provide a
comprehensive assessment of the following functions: language comprehension, language production, reading, and writing. The stated
goals of the NCCEA also include: to provide subtests that are sufficiently
complex that the clinician can obtain a relatively exact measure of performance level; to standardize and score performances such that necessary corrections for age, sex, and education can be made; to include
nonlinguistic subtests to insure valid intepretation of performance deficits on language tests as either linguistic in nature or due to other
dysfunction; and to include specific subtests that could be employed to
investigate current research questions in aphasiology (Benton, 1967).

The NCCEA is composed of 20 subtests that focus on the language
functions stated above and 4 "control" subtests of visual and tactile
functioning. Use of the control subtests is indicated when performance
deficits on certain subtests need to be differentiated as either language
related or visual or tactile in nature. Two of the NCCEA subtests—
identification by sentence (a version of the Token Test) and word
fluency—are viable screening tests in and of themselves, as previously
described. Digit repetition forward and backward with a modified administration and scoring system form 2 further subtests. Eight of the 20
language subtests and 3 of the 4 control subtests require the use of four
arrays of eight common objects. These objects are arranged in order of
difficulty from least to most difficult. The four sets are matched for item
difficulty. NCCEA subtests include stimulus presentations in either the
visual, auditory, or tactile modality. The remaining subtests include:
visual object naming, description of object use, tactile object naming for
each hand, sentence repetition, sentence construction, object identification by name, oral reading of names and sentences, oral reading of
names and sentences for meaning, object name writing, writing to dictation, copying sentences, and articulation. Unlike other aphasia test instruments, provisions for collapsing performance on several subtests

into category or modality performances are not provided in the test manual.

Several subtests provide a set of items for initial testing as well as a second set of items for use only if errors occurred in the first set. This feature tends to shorten administration time for the examination of areas in which a patient has no difficulties. The second set of items then provides more detailed quantitative information on problem areas. Single errors due to poor attention or other irrelevant causes will be reduced in their importance if the second set of items is passed correctly.

The range of item difficulty is limited. In an attempt to avoid highly specialized or low-frequency words, the authors used only very common objects for their object naming, identification, and similar tasks. As a result, the test has a rather low ceiling on some of the subtests, with the effect that very mild aphasic symptoms in highly educated patients may be missed. Other subtests, however, are "open-ceiling" tests for which this limitation does not apply.

Scores on the NCCEA are determined by response correctness. Incorrect responses and mispronounced correct responses are recorded verbatim, as are unusual features of the patient's performance, to yield qualitative performance information. An individual's performance on the NCCEA, when corrected for the influences of age and educational level as instructed, can be converted into percentile scores to yield relative levels of performance on each subtest and can be ranked on several profile sheets. These profile sheets allow the clinician to compare the patient's performance to that of samples of normal adults, aphasic patients, and nonaphasic brain-damaged patients. The aphasic and the nonaphasic brain-damaged samples consist of consecutive referrals for neuropsychological evaluation in an acute-care hospital setting. The norms are less appropriate if the clinician deals with a population of a different selective bias.

Reliability data are not provided in the test manual. The predictive validity of the NCCEA is reported by Lawriw (1976). The NCCEA as well as its individual constituent subtests differentiated aphasic from nonaphasic brain-damaged patients with a high degree of classification accuracy. Multiple discriminant analyses revealed between 76% and 90% correct classification. Discriminant weights were successfully cross-validated, with little loss of predictive validity within similar geographic and clinical settings. Concurrent validity with the WAB was demonstrated by Kertesz (1979). Concurrent validity for changes in language functions during therapy was reported by Kenin and Swisher (1972) for the overall FCP score; the authors noted the limited sampling on subtests other than auditory comprehension mentioned earlier. Another study reporting on the use of the test in the context of recovery during the first 3 months after onset of aphasia was presented by Ludlow (1977). She found significant differences in pattern of improvement between "Broca's" and "fluent" aphasics. Crockett (1976) demonstrated validity by examining the relationship between 17 rating scales of verbal behavior (including rate of speech, prosody, pronunciation, hesitation, phrase length, effort, pauses, press of speech, perseveration, word choice, etc.) and the corresponding NCCEA subtests and found high correlations. Crockett (1977) also demonstrated significant discriminant validity between four groups of patients.

The test has also been adapted into Italian, Japanese, and Spanish. A detailed description of the rationale and the details of test construction are not yet available, although the manual provides some of this information.

In summary, the NCCEA provides a comprehensive assessment of language functions for aphasic patients without the use of a specific model of language and without specifying a specific approach to delineating diagnostic types of aphasias. Psychometric development of the test since its original version in 1969 has been slow, but a fair amount of validation studies has accumulated. The development of three different profile sheets for score evaluation provides a distinct asset. On the other hand, the low ceiling of some of the subtests suggests that some aspects of language function in mildly or borderline aphasic patients cannot be adequately measured.

PORCH INDEX OF COMMUNICATIVE ABILITY (PICA)

The PICA (Porch, 1967, 1973=S) is designed to assess verbal, gestural, and graphic responsiveness subsequent to brain damage. A prime use of the PICA has been in assessing patient performance on multiple occasions postonset to determine the recovery of language ability. The PICA is composed of 18 subtests: 4 verbal, 8 gestural, and 6 graphic. A high degree of homogeneity among the subtests is established through the repeated use of 10 common, everyday objects of equal difficulty (e.g., a key, a cigarette) for a majority of the subtests. Subtest order is arranged so as to introduce minimal information during the earlier subtests that would be needed to perform later subtests. The use of many items of equal difficulty was employed to examine fluctuations in patient subtest performance over time. Similar to other aphasia tests, subtests were created to conform with a model of language functioning involving several possible input modalities, a central processor for incoming information and outgoing responses, and several possible output modalities (see ALD).

The PICA stresses the need to have a well-trained examiner in order for the test to have full usefulness. The potential user (in addition to being provided with an explicit and detailed description of the test, the standard testing environment, and proper test administration) is required to undertake a 40-hr workshop that emphasizes development of familiarity with the PICA scoring system and includes 10 PICA administrations under the supervision of a PICA-trained clinician. Because the PICA scoring system is considered to be the most difficult aspect of administering and evaluating the test, scoring is the primary focus of the requisite workshop traineeship. A persistent problem in recording responses to test items involves assessing and quantifying the given response as one of a wide variety of potential responses. As a compromise between two possible extremes (i.e., longhand notation of the characteristics of the response and simple pass–fail or normal–subnormal dichotomous scoring), the PICA uses a 16-point multidimensional scoring system, an attempt by the author to integrate the strengths of the two approaches while minimizing their weaknesses.

A given response to a PICA test item is evaluated along five relevant and basic dimensions: accuracy, responsiveness, completeness, promptness, and efficiency. A scoring system that considers all possible permutations of these five dimensions is, for all practical purposes, impossible and meaningless. Hence, 16 categories have been identified that represent various relevant combinations of these five dimensions, resulting in a 16-point ranked scale from "no response" (a score of 1) to "complex response" (a score of 16). For example, any attempt by the patient to perform at all on the task is scored at least a 6; all accurate responses are scored at least an 8. Additional points are given for a correct response after repeated instructions, for self-corrected responses, responsive ease, completeness, promptness, and efficiency. Porch (1967) reports the viability of the rank ordering of the 16 categories by providing empirical evidence available in the clinical literature as well as by pointing out the high agreement between PICA category ordering and the ranking of categories by 12 speech pathologists.

The individual item scores (180 possible) are transformed into an overall performance score, several modality scores, and individual subtest scores, for evaluative purposes. The overall performance score is considered as the best SINGLE index of the patient's general communicative ability. Modality scores yield information of the relative capacity of verbal, gestural, and graphic communicative ability. Subtest means provide further information on specific performances. Use of mean values require that statistical and conceptual assumptions of equal intervals between category levels be met. Whether this assumption is legitimate for the PICA has been the subject of a good deal of debate (e.g., see Martin, 1977; McNeil, 1979). While single item responses can be categorized on the 16-point scale (i.e., a score of 12 represents an incomplete response), mean values cannot be so categorized. Hence, mean scores cannot categorize the method by which the patient generally communicates but can only represent a performance level relative to either normative values or to the patient's other derived scores.

Data indicating that the PICA shows high interrater reliability as well as high test–retest reliability are provided in volume 1 of the test manual (Porch, 1967). The construct validity of the PICA is addressed logically, but not statistically, in this volume: Both the model of language functioning upon which the PICA is structured and the behaviors categorized in the scoring system have been noted in aphasiological literature. Holland (1980) reports concurrent validity of the PICA as .93 with the CADL scale, .86 with the FCP, and .88 with the BDAE.

Percentile data from normative samples of 280 left hemisphere damaged patients and 100 bilaterally damaged patients are presented in Volume 2 of the test manual (Porch, 1973). Percentiles for all principal transformed scores are provided. In addition to providing relative information for these transformed scores, percentiles are also utilized to determine a given patient's "aphasia recovery curve," employing the overall test percentile, the mean percentile of the nine highest-scored subtests, and the mean percentile of the nine lowest-scored subtests. Predictions on the scope of recovery can be attempted from this curve; a recovery ceiling is assumed when the three percentiles coincide (Porch, Collins, Wertz & Friden, 1980).

The underlying factor structure of the PICA has been addressed by Clark, Crockett, and Klonoff (1979a, 1979b). Three definable factors emerged from a factor analysis of Porch's original standardization sample ($N = 150$). The first factor was formed by the four verbal subtests, representing a pure dimension of verbal competence. Factor two represented five of the six graphic subtests. Factor three represented the eight gestural and the other graphic subtest; however, only four of the eight gestural subtests were principally defined by this factor. A higher-order factor analysis of the factor intercorrelation matrix indicated the presence of a general language impairment factor. PICA subtests showed loadings on this general factor as a function of task difficulty. A factor analysis of a second sample revealed five distinct factors: verbal competence, graphic expression, gestural demonstration of verbal and reading competency, basic gestural function, and graphic copying of geometric forms. The first four of these factors were highly intercorrelated, suggesting the presence of a general language impairment factor. These two studies suggest the presence of a basic general impairment factor for language; they also suggest a needed revision in the PICA subtest structure (3 or 5 distinct areas of interest rather than 18) and provide empirical evidence for the diversity of subtests subsumed under the gestural modality (Martin, 1977). DiSimoni, Keith, Holt, and Darley (1975) also found a high degree of redundancy among PICA subtests and conclude that a shortened form of the test may be more useful. A paper by DiSimoni, Keith, and Darley (1980) describes such a short version.

In sum, the PICA is a very well-developed and standardized test instrument that has been extensively employed in rehabilitative settings to track recovery postonset (a topic discussed in detail in the test manual). The two-volume test manual is exemplary compared to other descriptions of test construction in the field of aphasia assessment. The multidimensional scoring system has become, perhaps, the most criticized aspect of the test. Both rank order of the categorized behaviors (McNeil, Prescott, & Chang, 1975) as well as assumptions of equal interval scaling made by Porch (Martin, 1977) have been criticized. A well-written comprehensive critique of the PICA is provided by Martin (1977). Two further shortcomings of the PICA include the paucity of sampling auditory comprehension and the misleading labeling of several subtests as gestural when they entail other specific behaviors. McNeil (1979) suggests that such criticisms should not turn clinicians away from considering the PICA as a test instrument but rather should make them more cautious interpreters of PICA findings.

WESTERN APHASIA BATTERY (WAB)

The WAB (Kertesz, 1979, 1980=S; Kertesz & Poole, 1974) is a recent addition to the comprehensive assessment instruments for language functioning in aphasics. The primary goals of the WAB are to classify various aphasic syndromes (e.g., Broca's, Wernicke's, anomic, conduction) and to evaluate the severity of the aphasic impairment. The examination, designed for both clinical and research use, is composed of four language subtests and three performance subtests. Syndrome classification is determined by the pattern of performance on the four language subtests; the summed, overall performance on these subtests, yields a rating of performance severity (i.e., the APHASIA QUOTIENT). The four language subtests assess spontaneous speech, comprehension, repetition, and naming. The three performance subtests encompass reading and writing, praxis, and construction. Test items were selected to provide a wide enough range of difficulty for all grades of severity to be assessed.

Spontaneous speech is assessed in terms of the patient's speech both in response to questioning (e.g., "How are you today?") and in a description of a line drawing, much as in the BDAE. Speech is rated on two 10-point rating scales: an information content scale and a fluency scale that incorporates grammatical competence and the presence of paraphasias. Comprehension is assessed by yes–no questions that may be responded to verbally or nonverbally, depending on the capability of the patient, and by word recognition and sequential commands. Repetition is composed of 15 items that are scored either correct, phonemic error (partial credit), or error. This particular subtest does not appear to be as encompassing or as well structured as other repetition tasks (e.g., NCCEA sentence repetition). Naming is composed of object naming (without cuing or, if necessary, with tactile and/or phonemic cuing), word fluency, sentence completion, and responsive speech. An uncommon aspect of this test's construction is its dissociation of reading and writing ability (part of the PERFORMANCE QUOTIENT) from the other language subtests.

Standardization information is provided by Kertesz and Poole (1974) and updated by Kertesz (1979). These references include criteria for classification of aphasic syndromes based on the language subtest performances of a sample of 150 aphasic patients with various etiologies. Reliability and validity data are also provided. The WAB manifests high interrater reliability, good internal consistency, and high test–retest reliability. Successful criterion validity has been described by the author: Aphasics were differentiated from non-brain-damaged adults in their WAB performance. The use of the aphasia quotient distinguished aphasics from nonaphasic brain-damaged controls. Construct validity was assessed on a sample of 15 patients who were examined on both the WAB and the NCCEA. There were high correlations between corresponding subtests in the two examinations that ranged from .82 for spontaneous speech subtests to .95 for comprehension subtests.

A WAB test manual is just becoming available at the time of writing, although experimental and developmental work with the test has been carried out for several years. The most current WAB information source is Kertesz (1979). Response booklets and two-dimensional visual stimuli have just recently become commercially available (Kertesz, 1980). Actual objects, Raven's Coloured Progressive Matrices and WAIS blocks, are required for the battery and need to be purchased by the user. The author states that the language subtests can be administered in approximately 1 hr but that the full WAB would require at least two test sessions to complete.

In sum, the WAB is a recent addition to the assessment armamentarium. Like that of the BDAE, its primary usefulness would appear to be diagnostic: the classification of aphasic performances into traditional aphasic syndrome types. Explicit decision rules about which classification applies in an individual case are provided, although the test appears to operate with the assumption that all cases can clearly be classified as one of eight basic types. Such clear-cut classification is, of course, implicit in cluster analytic research but has little meaning for the "mixed" aphasias that occur much more often in clinical practice than this classification system suggests. Also, like the BDAE, the WAB offers a method of assessing spontaneous speech, though the WAB would appear to be less comprehensive than the BDAE in this regard. For example, fluency, grammatical competence, and the extent of paraphasias are combined into a single WAB scale, whereas they are assessed independently on the BDAE. The usefulness of the WAB as a research tool is well covered by Kertesz (1979); included in this reference is a review of a series of novel cluster analytic studies taxonomically examining aphasic syndromes of different etiologies over time (see also Kertesz & Phipps, 1980). Specific research has also dealt with the relationship between aphasia and nonverbal intelligence (Kertesz & McCabe, 1975).

Assessment of Aphasia in Children

The complex topic of aphasia in children is addressed in another chapter of this book. In the context of this chapter, we can deal with the assessment of aphasia only briefly, since a full discussion of the specific assessment problems in childhood would not fit within the space limitations and, more importantly, would deal with a topic that has found only limited attention in the aphasia assessment field.

The major obstacle encountered in designing assessment methods for children is that language ability increases with chronological age in the normal child and there is relatively high variability from child to child within a given age level. Full language competency is not reached until age 12–14 years (depending on definition of competency); after this age, further development takes place in terms of increased vocabulary, grammatical complexity, awareness of rules of generative grammar, etc. For these reasons, any assessment method for children requires the establishment of normative data for each year (or half-year) of age; because of the somewhat different rate of growth of language abilities in girls and boys, separate norms for each sex are also required. Obviously, the construction of suitable tests for children requires a much more extensive amount of psychometric work, especially for standardization, than does the construction of tests for adults; however, validity and reliability must also be fully established for each age level and cannot be taken for granted on the basis of studies involving children from all age levels.

Several tests of normal language development in children are available, such as the Illinois Test of Psycholinguistic Abilities (ITPA) (Kirk, McCarthy, & Kirk, 1968=S), but very few assessment techniques have been constructed or restandardized for children for the specific purpose of aphasia assessment (see review by Eisenson, 1972).

Among the brief or specific-purpose assessment methods, several adaptations of the sentence repetition method have been attempted. One report, which deals with 24 sentences that vary according to grammatical complexity in congenitally aphasic children, was reported by Bliss and Peterson (1975). Adaptations of the word fluency examination usually change from words starting with a given letter to animal names or similar groups for children who cannot be expected to have sufficient knowledge of spelling. DiSimoni (1978=S) published an adaptation of the Token Test for Children, standardized with 1304 children from preschool age 3 to grade 6 (age 12:6) from a mixed suburban population. The test manual also reviews several other studies investigating the scoring criteria as well as aspects of concurrent validity with other tests of auditory comprehension, including the ITPA and the PPVT (a test widely used with normal children). The Token Test has also been investigated in relation to socioeconomic status of the home, an important aspect of language development in children. Other tests of auditory comprehension not specifically designed for the assessment of aphasia but potentially useful are the Assessment of Children's Language Comprehension (Foster, Giddon, & Stark, 1973) and Carrow's (1972) Test for Auditory Comprehension of Language.

Comprehensive examinations for children available at this time include the already mentioned ITPA (which has been used for aphasia assessment in some studies), the Reynell Developmental Language Scales (Reynell & Huntley, 1971), the Northwestern Syntax Screening Test (Arndt, 1977; Lee, 1970), and the Utah Test of Language Development (Mecham, Jex, & Jones, 1967); no specific studies for children with acquired aphasia are available for these tests. Adaptations for children of comprehensive examinations for aphasia in adults have been presented for the NCCEA and the PICA. The NCCEA adaptation (Gaddes & Crockett, 1975) merely provides norms for children between ages 6 and 13 for each of the NCCEA subtests, but it has not been used in research studies with aphasic children. The norms presented show an acceptable gradual increase of scores with age for some subtests, whereas other subtests show a rapid increase within a limited age span, after which the test scores remain at ceiling level. The Porch Index of Communicative Ability in Children (PICAC) (Porch, 1979=S) contains a "basic battery" for 3-6 year olds and an "advanced battery" for 6-12 year olds. With the exception of some floor effects, score progression with age is satisfactory and reliability data are provided, but so far no validity studies with aphasic children have been reported. As with the PICA, the multidimensional scoring system poses some problems and requires extensive training.

Numerous other assessment procedures aimed at the general intellectual development of the child, but including one or more measures of language development, are available. They will not, however, be reviewed in this context, nor can the numerous available tests of articulation for children be considered here.

Assessment of Aphasia in Clinical Practice

This final section will present some general concepts and considerations regarding the assessment of aphasia in clinical practice. In particular, we will discuss the decision-making process before, during, and after the clinical assessment of questions of diagnosis, treatment planning, and prediction of recovery. Such decisions cannot be replaced by any assessment procedure—no matter how well constructed and "comprehensive" a test battery may be—but remain the responsibility of the clinician in consultation with related professionals involved with the individual patient.

Brookshire (1973) raises three major questions usually posed in aphasia assessment:

1. Does the patient have a speech or language disorder?
2. Are these speech or language defects treatable?
3. Can recovery of speech and language ability realistically be expected?

We would add to the first question the more basic supplementary question: What is the nature of the speech or language deficit? All four questions overlap with the various purposes of assessment described in the introductory section of this chapter: screening, diagnostic assessment, assessment for counseling and rehabilitation, and progress evaluation.

Decisions about the Presence or Absence of Aphasia

In clinical practice, this question may not arise if the patient is referred with an obvious diagnosis of aphasia of a moderate or severe degree. However, in a fair number of patients with mild or atpyical language disorders, such a decision must be made before we can proceed to other questions. On the surface, it would seem that well-validated tests of a more comprehensive or even of a screening type would be sufficient to provide an answer to this question. It should be remembered, however, that no test has a discrimination accuracy of 100% and that the gray area of false positive and false negative decisions encountered by any given test lies of necessity in the borderline area between mild aphasia and normal language function. Relying solely on cut-off points provided by test authors in patients with borderline impairment would, in effect, not be much better than random guessing. The clinician will have to use informed judgment to arrive at his or her own conclusion.

Premorbid Language Function and Intelligence

One major consideration for such an informed judgment is the evaluation of a given patient's language ability and intelligence before the onset of illness. The two factors, intelligence and language, are closely though not perfectly related. Since test results before the onset of illness are rarely available, a careful evaluation of the patient's educational history, professional or occupational background, language, and reading and writing habits must be made; relatives may be consulted with regard to this information and, at the same time, their judgment may be invited as to whether any language impairment is noticeable to them or not.

Another source of information may be provided by concurrently administered tests of general intelligence. Gross discrepancies between IQ tests and aphasia tests usually suggest selective language impairment. However, it must be remembered that many IQ tests rely heavily on tests involving verbal functions; only the so-called nonverbal component of IQ tests is useful in this regard. Once this information has been collected, an expected level of language function may be decided upon. Some tests allow a score correction based on the premorbid educational level to be added before interpretation; many other tests leave this consideration open.

A related but more difficult consideration concerns the sociocultural habits of the normal home and job environment of the patient. The need for verbal expression varies greatly from one sociological setting to another, and ethnic influences particularly tend to affect such factors as verbal fluency, general fund of information, vocabulary, articulation (and intelligibility), and prosody.

Bilingualism

Patients whose first language is not English pose a special problem in the assessment of aphasia. For such patients, the judgment of pre-morbid language ability in English becomes a difficult question. More-over, the question of a differential impairment in the two languages requires investigation. Various theories have proposed that the "older," the "more affectively favored," the "most frequently used" language is less affected by aphasia, whereas other studies point out either that little difference actually exists between languages (Obler & Albert, 1978) or that the language environment during recovery from brain damage is the crucial factor. It is usually sensible to refrain from any such generali-zation and to establish premorbid language competence and assess im-pairment for both languages.

Frequently, the examination in the second language is carried out by using the same assessment methods with or without the use of an in-terpreter. While this provides apparent close comparability of the as-sessment in the two languages, such comparability may be tenuous at best. Frequently, an "instant" translation of this type only poorly ap-proximates the difficulty level of vocabulary and grammar because of basic differences in the frequency of word use and grammatical structure in the two languages. The MAE described earlier addresses these prob-lems and attempts to provide fully equivalent forms in several lan-guages. Until this test is generally available, it is far more preferable to use foreign-language adaptations of assessment methods as far as they are available or even tests that were originally constructed in the second language. A review of foreign-language tests and adaptations does, however, exceed the scope of this chapter.

Motivational and Affective Considerations

Language does not exist in isolation. Patients who still show the acute aftereffects of brain damage are frequently apathetic, drowsy, and un-cooperative. Patients may also show considerable emotional reaction to their general neurological impairments; depression is frequent and most common during the phase of neurological "stabilization," when patients begin to realize the full extent of their disabilities. For these reasons, it is quite common that willingness to communicate is drastically reduced and test results are poor because of lack of motivation, inattention, or changes in consciousness. Again, this calls on the judgment of the clinician rather than for blind reliance on test results.

The Nature of the Speech and Language Deficit

Having arrived at a general diagnosis of aphasia, the description of the exact nature of the deficit becomes of paramount importance. What exactly is it that the patient can or cannot do? What degree of impairment is present in each of the areas under examination? A description of areas of strength is as important as the description of the areas of deficit, since the approach to treatment relies on both types of information.

Information about the nature of the deficit continually influences the process of assessment. As we find out about a specific area of weakness, a more detailed description of that area and related deficits will be required. Special testing procedures may be added to gather this information. Occasionally, it is necessary to continue the examination in this fashion after the initial assessment results have been reviewed.

The stress on diagnostic types of aphasia has led many test authors to develop a test pattern for each type either empirically or descriptively. As was pointed out earlier, the range of types of aphasia described varies from test to test, depending on the theoretical orientation of the authors. It is perhaps obvious from the preceding paragraphs that fitting a patient into a particular type on the basis of test results is of only limited preliminary diagnostic value. Types of aphasia have been related to location of lesion as well as to rate and stage of recovery, but—as with the borderline between aphasic and normal language function—the gray area between types presents serious problems. Perfect fit for individual patients into such types is rare, and general impairment defying any typology is the norm rather than the exception. For these reasons, the description of the nature of the language deficit must proceed beyond typology and produce an individual language profile for each patient.

Ancillary Assessment

The focus in this chapter, has been on an assessment of aphasia rather than on a general evaluation of a patient's deficit. The need to refer to results from general intelligence tests has already been mentioned. Similarly, the results of other cognitive, perceptual, and motor tests will be necessary (see also Spreen & Tuokko, 1981). Most importantly, the ancillary evaluation of basic motor and sensory functions is required. Certain language functions are likely to show severe deficits if the patient experiences impairment or distortions of visual perception or hearing. Patients are not likely to produce valid responses on tactile naming if impairment of motor functions or stereognosis is present. Some test authors have built in supplementary tests for such functions that are automatically administered if the patient fails on specific language tasks; in other tests, the clinician must ascertain the patient's basic abilities without such guidance. Either way, the description of the aphasic deficit will be strongly moderated if ancillary deficits are considered. Considerable training and experience is prerequisite to a full exploration of the results of such ancillary assessment.

Treatment of the Aphasic Disorder

Another chapter in this volume is devoted to a discussion of the treatment of aphasia. However, since many patients are referred mainly for an exploration of treatment options, the question should be considered briefly in relation to assessment. Obviously, if exploring treatment options is the primary purpose of assessment, the choice of assessment instruments will differ from the choice made for purely diagnostic purposes. Another major difference will be in the choice of additional procedures. Since it is well known that the presence of severe sensory or perceptual impairment or of severe memory impairment can invalidate treatment efforts, these ancillary factors should be carefully considered. Additional attention needs to be paid to the motivational state and the attentional capacities of the patient, both of which may interfere with the potential for treatment. Situational circumstances, family support, and other outside factors may have to be assessed. Most important in this context is an actual assessment of the relearning capacity of the patient. None of the existing assessment procedures provide a fully adequate opportunity to judge this capacity. For this reason, the clinician may resort to self-made tasks carefully calibrated in difficulty to the capacity of the patient. It is not necessary to construct entirely new material. Rather, much of the existing test material can be used as training material. For a simple, informal assessment of relearning, a brief series of items (e.g., word finding to pictures or objects; description of use; comprehension of words or sentences) can be used and repeated until all items are fully learned; the measure in this case would be the number of trials needed to reach criterion (e.g., full comprehension of five items). A repetition of the same procedure on the following day will indicate the "gain"—that is, how many fewer trials are needed for relearning of the same items.

Can Recovery Be Expected?

Increasing numbers of research studies are addressing the question of recovery. Some general rules (e.g., better recovery in younger, in female, and in left-handed patients with relatively recent onset) have been recognized, which are discussed elsewhere in this book. From an assessment point of view, some predictions of recovery can also be made (e.g., better recovery in patients with less severe aphasia, with comprehension deficits). It is important that assessment methods be chosen that provide as much information as possible on these points. It should be noted, though, that current knowledge about the prediction of the recovery process relies mainly on general and medical information about the patient rather than on test results.

Choice of Tests for Description of Language Deficit

No formal battery of tests can be recommended as sufficiently comprehensive to arrive at an optimal description of the nature of the speech and language deficit for an individual patient. In clinical practice, we, as well as many other clinicians, tend to use a flexible approach for which a comprehensive test battery is only the beginning. Complete reliance on a given test battery tends to introduce an element of rigidity that may result in failure to fully explore the patient's problem.

An optimal description may be gained by using one of the more comprehensive, well-validated instruments described in the preceding pages. This choice will depend on the purpose of the assessment as well as on individual preference and theoretical orientation. The comprehensive test chosen should be supplemented with other test procedures— specific-purpose tests (or parts of another comprehensive battery), a functional communication assessment, a clinical examination of specific problems and, if possible, specifically constructed tasks suitable for retraining, as discussed earlier.

The approach advocated here requires full knowledge of all available instruments as well as clinical skills and judgment. While parts of the examination may be conducted by a trained psychometrist, the full involvement of the clinician remains necessary. The approach does not lend itself to computerized test scoring and evaluation, advocated by some workers in the field of neuropsychology, since computer evaluation remains dependent on a fixed battery of tests.

Other considerations in the choice of assessment methods that need to be mentioned are (*a*) psychometric adequacy of a test; (*b*) portability of the test material; and (*c*) time requirements. In the first part of this chapter, psychometric requirements for a well-constructed test were stated explicitly. Obviously, the more a test meets the ideals of a psychometrically well-developed test, the more likely it is that valid and reliable results are obtained. Attention should also be paid to research conducted with a given instrument, since this provides additional information useful for making specific decisions about the nature of aphasia or about treatment and prognosis. Portability tends to be of no specific concern in a hospital-based laboratory but becomes a problem if bedside examination or examinations in other locations are frequently carried out. In this latter case, one would prefer a handy portfolio of pictures rather than a suitcase full of objects, even though any pictured item tends to lose some value on a "reality" dimension. Time is a crucial consideration in many facilities with heavy patient loads. However, the time requirements should be carefully weighed against the amount of information gleaned from a given test. Brevity is no virtue if crucial information is not collected. In fact, the approach advocated in this chapter suggests that time requirements should be of secondary importance and that experimental variants and additional procedures that may be of benefit to the patient in the long run should be used. If, on the other hand, brief screening is the only goal of assessment, then many of the short forms or screening devices deserve consideration.

A last point should be mentioned: Assessment is not an end in itself but must be considered in relation to the potential value to the patient. As Messick (1980) points out, the adequacy of a test is not dictated solely by psychometric soundness. Rather, the concept of construct validity must include the "ethics" of assessment; that is, it must provide a rational foundation for predictiveness and relevance as well as take into account the value implications of test interpretations per se.

Interpretation of Assessment Results

A few comments on the interpretation of test and other assessment results may be appropriate. Every clinician in the field of aphasia has his or her own model of how best to survey a summary sheet of assessment results—with and without frequent glances at the actual test records and notes on the behavior of the patient during testing. Many of the comprehensive tests provide, of course, their own grouping of the test information and hence a suggested approach to interpretation (e.g., summary scores for auditory comprehension, verbal retention, verbal expression). Other authors leave the approach to interpretation open to the test user. Our own approach (and that of many other clinicians) tends to be "syndromatic" in the sense that we tend to focus on the most seriously deviant score in the assessment record and scan for related information or test results. For example, if the patient's most serious

problem is on a test of word finding, we scan all related test results as
well as information about the patient's ability to find words in a conversational setting, in practical daily-life situations; for higher performance
on verbal and nonverbal short-term memory tests; etc. This allows a
better description of the deficit, that is, of whether the deficit is
generalized or specific to the testing situation, whether it is related to
"laboratory conditions" or a specific sensory modality, etc. Additional
assessment procedures may be necessary to fully evaluate this first
"syndrome." We then proceed to the next syndrome that would appear
to be reasonably independent of the first and again search for associated
deficits. In this fashion, one can move on to the least deviant score of the
assessment record, keeping in mind the estimated premorbid intelligence of the individual. Such syndromes may or may not be related to
each other; they may or may not reflect a "classical type" of aphasia with
localizing significance. The primary purpose is to gain a detailed picture
of the patients deficits in order of severity and in the context of other
related deficits. One can then proceed in the opposite direction, search-
ing for the highest score in the test record or the best preserved function
until the information in the assessment record is exhausted. Finally, a
reexploration of the syndromes is made by evaluating the actual behavior of the patient on individual tests or other assessment procedures
as well as on supplementary procedures given after a first, rough interpretation of the record. This will usually allow a description of the
patient in more detailed terms; for instance, we will no longer be describing "anomia for visually presented real objects" but can now include
details of how this deficit affects the patient and how rehabilitative
treatment may approach the deficit, building on strength but working
on weaknesses.

The approach described here is highly idiosyncratic in a deliberate
attempt to avoid preconceived models of language and/or brain
functions. However, until we have developed a more generally accepted
model of the language disorders and generally accepted standards of
procedure for generally accepted standard questions—and little progress
in that direction has been made so far—this outline of interpretation
procedures may provide the fullest utilization of assessment results at
the present state of development.

Appendix: Abbreviations for Aphasia Assessments

ACTS   Auditory Comprehension Test for Sentences
ALD   Appraisal of Language Disturbance

ALPS   Aphasia Language Performance Scales
BDAE   Boston Diagnostic Aphasia Examination
CADL   Communicative Abilities in Daily Living
FCP   Functional Communication Profile
ITPA   Illinois Test of Psycholinguistic Abilities
MAE   Multilingual Aphasia Examination
MTDDA   Minnesota Test for Differential Diagnosis of Aphasia
NCCEA   Neurosensory Center Comprehensive Examination for Aphasia
PIAT   Peabody Individual Achievement Test
PICA   Porch Index of Communicative Ability
PICAC   Porch Index of Communicative Ability in Children
PPVT   Peabody Picture Vocabulary Test
SAS   Sklar Aphasia Scale
WAB   Western Aphasia Battery
WAIS   Wechsler Adult Intelligence Scale

References

American Psychological Association. 1974. *Standards for educational and psychological tests.* Washington, D.C.: American Psychological Association.

Anastasi, A. 1976. *Psychological testing* (4th ed.). New York: Macmillan.

Arndt, W. B. 1977. A psychometric evaluation of the Northwestern Syntax Screening Test. *Journal of Speech and Hearing Disorders.* 42, 316–319.

Aten, J. L., Caligiure, M. P., & Holland, A. Efficacy of communication therapy for aphasic patients. *Journal of Speech and Hearing Disorders,* in press.

Benson, D. F. 1967. Fluency in aphasia: Correlation with radioactive scan localization. *Cortex, 3,* 373–394.

Benson, D. F. 1979. Aphasia. In K. M. Heilman & E. Valenstein (Eds.), *Clinical neuropsychology.* New York: Oxford Univ. Press. (a)

Benson, D. F. 1979. *Aphasia, alexia and agraphia.* New York: Churchill Livingstone. (b)

Benton, A. L. 1964. Contributions to aphasia before Broca. *Cortex, 1,* 314–327.

Benton, A. L. 1967. Problems of test construction in the field of aphasia. *Cortex, 3,* 32–53.

Benton, A. L. 1968. *Development of a multilingual aphasia battery: Progress and problems.* Paper presented at a meeting of the Research Group on Aphasiology of the World Federation of Neurology, Philadelphia, October 3.

Benton, A. L., & Hamsher, K. 1978. *Multilingual Aphasia Examination.* Iowa City: Benton Laboratory of Neuropsychology.

Bliss, L. S., & Peterson, D. M. 1975. Performance of aphasic and nonaphasic children on a sentence repetition task. *Journal of Communication Disorders, 8,* 207–212.

Boller, F., & Dennis, M. 1979. *Auditory comprehension: Clinical and experimental studies with the Token Test.* New York: Academic Press.

Boller, F., Kim, Y., & Mack, J. L. 1977. Auditory comprehension in aphasia. In H. Whittaker & H. A. Whittaker (Eds.), *Studies in neurolinguistics* (Vol. 3). New York: Academic Press.

Boller, F., & Vignolo, L. A. 1966. Latent sensory aphasia in hemisphere-damaged patients: An experimental study with the Token Test. *Brain, 89*(Pt. 4), 815–830.

Borkowski, J. G., Benton, A. L., & Spreen, O. 1967. Word fluency and brain damage. *Neuropsychologia, 5,* 135–140.

Brookshire, R. H. 1973. *An introduction to aphasia.* Minneapolis: BRK Publishers.

Brookshire, R. H. 1978. A Token Test battery for testing auditory comprehension in brain-injured adults. *Brain and Language, 6,* 149–157.

Carrow, E. 1972. Auditory comprehension of English by monolingual and bilingual preschool children. *Journal of Speech and Hearing Research, 15*(2), 407–412.

Clark, C., Crockett, D. J., & Klonoff, H. 1979. Empirically derived groups in the assessment of recovery from aphasia. *Brain and Language, 7,* 240–251. (a)

Clark, C., Crockett, D. J., & Klonoff, H. 1979. Factor analysis of the Porch Index of Communication Ability. *Brain and Language, 7,* 1–7. (b)

Cohen, R., Kelter, S., & Shaefer, B. 1977. Zum Einfluss des Sprachverstaendnisses auf die Leistungen im Token Test. *Zeitschrift fuer Klinische Psychologie, 6,* 1–14.

Cohen, R., Lutzweiler, W., & Woll, G. 1980. Zur Konstruktvaliditaet des Token Tests. *Nervenarzt, 51,* 30–35.

Crockett, D. J. 1972. *A multivariate comparison of Schuell's, Howes', Weisenburg and McBride's, and Wepman's types of aphasia.* Unpublished doctoral dissertation, University of Victoria.

Crockett, D. J. 1976. Multivariate comparison of Howes' and Weisenburg and McBride's models of aphasia on the Neurosensory Center Comprehensive Examination for Aphasia. *Perceptual and Motor Skills, 43,* 795–806.

Crockett, D. J. 1977. A comparison of empirically derived groups of aphasic patients on the Neurosensory Center Comprehensive Examination for Aphasia. *Journal of Clinical Psychology, 33,* 194–198.

Darley, F. L. 1964. *Diagnosis and appraisal of communication disorders.* Englewood Cliffs, N.J.: Prentice-Hall.

Darley, F. L. 1979. (Ed.) *Evaluation of appraisal techniques in speech and language pathology.* Reading, Mass.: Addison-Wesley.

De Renzi, E. 1980. The Token Test and the Reporter's Test: A measure of verbal input and a measure of verbal output. In M. T. Sarno & O. Hook (Eds.), *Aphasia: Assessment and treatment.* New York: Masson Publishers; and Stockholm: Almquist & Wiksell.

De Renzi, E., & Faglioni, P. 1978. Normative data and screening power of a shortened version of the Token Test. *Cortex, 14,* 41–49.

De Renzi, E., & Ferrari, C. 1979. The Reporter's Test: A sensitive test to detect expressive disturbances in aphasics. *Cortex, 15,* 279–291.

De Renzi, E., & Vignolo, L. A. 1962. The Token Test: A sensitive test to detect receptive disturbances in aphasics. *Brain, 85,* 665–678.

DiSimoni, F. 1978. *The Token Test for Children, Manual.* Hingham, Mass.: Teaching Resources Corporation.

DiSimoni, F. G., Keith, R. L., & Darley, F. L. 1980. Prediction of PICA overall score by short versions of the test. *Journal of Speech and Hearing Research, 23,* 511–516.

DiSimoni, F. G., Keith, R. L., Holt, D. L., & Darley, F. L. 1975. Practicality of shortening the Porch Index of Communicative Ability. *Journal of Speech and Hearing Research, 18,* 491–497.

Dunn, L. 1965. *Peabody Picture Vocabulary Test, manual.* Circle Pines, Minn.: American Guidance Service.

Eisenson, J. 1954. *Examining for Aphasia: A manual for the examination of aphasia and related disturbances.* New York: The Psychological Corporation.

Eisenson, J. 1972. *Aphasia in children.* New York: Harper.

Emerick, L. L. 1971. *The Appraisal of Language Disturbance, manual.* Marquette: Northern Michigan Univ.

Fillenbaum, S., Jones, L. V., & Wepman, J. M. 1961. Some linguistic features of speech from aphasic patients. *Language and Speech. 4,* 92–108.

Foster, R., Giddon, J., & Stark, J. 1973. *Assessment of children's language comprehension* (1973 Revision). Palo Alto, Calif.: Consulting Psychologists Press.

Froeschels, E., Dittrich, O., & Wilheim, I. 1932. [*Psychological elements in speech*] (E. Ferre, Trans.). Boston: Expression.

Gaddes, W. H., & Crockett, D. J. 1975. The Spreen–Benton aphasia tests, normative data as a measure of normal language development. *Brain and Language, 2,* 257–280.

Gallaher, A. J. 1979. Temporal reliability of aphasic performance on the Token Test. *Brain and Language, 7,* 34–41.

Geschwind, N. 1971. Current concepts: Aphasia. *New England Journal of Medicine, 284,* 654–656.

Geschwind, N., & Kaplan, E. 1962. A human cerebral deconnection syndrome. *Neurology, 12,* 675–685.

Goodglass, H., & Blumstein, S. 1973. *Psycholinguistics and aphasia.* Baltimore: Johns Hopkins Press.

Goodglass, H., & Kaplan, E. 1972. *The assessment of aphasia and related disorders.* Philadelphia: Lea & Febiger.

Head, H. 1926. *Aphasia and kindred disorders of speech.* New York: Macmillan.

Heimburger, R. F., & Reitan, R. M. n.d. *Testing for aphasia and related disorders.* Indiana University Medical Center.

Holland, A. L. 1980. *Communicative Abilities in Daily Living; manual.* Baltimore: Univ. Park Press.

Holland, A. L., & Sonderman, J. C. 1974. Effects of a program based on the Token Test for teaching comprehension skills to aphasics. *Journal of Speech and Hearing Research, 17,* 589–598.

Howes, D. 1964. Application of the word-frequency concept to aphasia. In A. V. S. de Reuck & M. O'Connor (Eds.), *Disorders of language.* London: Churchill.

Howes, D. 1966. A word count of spoken English. *Journal of Verbal Learning and Verbal Behavior. 5,* 572–606.

Howes, D. 1967. Some experimental investigations of language in aphasia. In K. Salzinger & S. Salzinger (Eds.), *Research in verbal behavior and some neurophysiological implications.* New York: Academic Press.

Howes, D., & Geschwind, N. 1964. Quantitative studies of aphasic language. In D. M. K. Rioch & E. A. Weinstein (Eds.), *Disorders of communication.* Baltimore: Williams & Wilkins.

Jackson, J. H. 1915. On the physiology of language. *Medical Times and Gazette, 2,* 275. (Reprinted in *Brain*, 1968, *38*, 59–64.)

Jones, L. V., Goodman, M. F., & Wepman, J. M. 1963. The classification of parts of speech for the characterization of aphasia. *Language and Speech, 6,* 94–777.

Joynt, R. J. 1964. Paul Pierre Broca: His contribution to the knowledge of aphasia. *Cortex, 1,* 206–213.

Keenan, J. S., & Brassell, E. G. 1975. *Aphasia Language Performance Scales.* Murfressboro, Tenn.: Pinnacle Press.

Kenin, M., & Swisher, L. P. 1972. A study of patterns of recovery in aphasia. *Cortex, 8,* 56–68.

Kerschensteiner, M., Poeck, K., & Brunner, E. 1972. The fluency–nonfluency dimension in the classification of aphasic speech. *Cortex, 8,* 233–247.

Kertesz, A. 1979. *Aphasia and associated disorders: Taxonomy, localization, and recovery.* New York: Grune & Stratton.

Kertesz, A. 1980. *Western Aphasia Battery.* London, Ont.: Univ. of Western Ontario.

Kertesz, A., & McCabe, P. 1975. Intelligence and aphasia: Performance of aphasics on Raven's Coloured Progressive Matrices (RCPM). *Brain and Language, 2,* 387–395.

Kertesz, A., & Phipps, J. 1980. The numerical taxonomy of acute and chronic aphasic syndromes. *Psychological Research, 41,* 179–198.

Kertesz, A., & Poole, E. 1974. The aphasia quotient: The taxonomic approach to measurement of aphasic disability. *Canadian Journal of Neurological Science, 1,* 7–16.

Kirk, S. A., McCarthy, J., & Kirk, W. 1968. *The Illinois Test of Psycholinguistic Abilities* (Rev. ed.). Urbana: Illinois Univ. Press.

Krug, R. S. 1971. Antecedent probabilities, cost efficiency, and differential prediction of patients with cerebral organic conditions or psychiatric disturbance by means of a short test for aphasia. *Journal of Clinical Psychology, 27,* 468–471.

Lahey, B. B. 1973. (Ed.). *The modification of language behavior.* Springfield, Ill.: Thomas.

Lawriw, I. 1976. A test of the predictive validity and a cross-validation of the Neurosensory Center Comprehensive Examination for Aphasia. Unpublished Master's thesis, University of Victoria.

Lee, L. L. 1970. A screening test for syntax development. *Journal of Speech and Hearing Disorders, 35,* 103–112.

Lesser, R. 1976. Verbal and non-verbal memory components in the Token Test. *Neuropsychologia, 14,* 79–85.

Ludlow, C. L. 1977. Recovery from aphasia: A foundation for treatment. In M. Sullivan & M. S. Kommers (Eds.), *Rationale for adult aphasia therapy.* Omaha: Univ. of Nebraska Medical Center.

Luria, A. R. 1966. *Higher cortical functions in man.* New York: Basic Books.

Luria, A. R. 1970. *Traumatic aphasia, its syndromes, psychology, and treatment.* The Hague: Mouton.

Marie, P. 1883. De l'aphasie, cecite verbale, surdite verbale, aphasie motire, agraphie. *Revue Medicale, 3,* 693–702.

Martin, A. D. 1977. Aphasia testing: A second look at the Porch Index of Communicative Ability. *Journal of Speech and Hearing Disorders, 42,* 547–561.

Martino, A. A., Pizzamiglio, L., & Razzano, C. 1976. A new version of the Token Test for aphasics: A concrete objects form. *Journal of Communication Disorders, 9,* 1–5.

McCarthy, J. J., & Kirk, S. A. 1961. *Illinois Test of Psycholinguistic Abilities* (Experimental ed.), Urbana, Ill: Institute for Research on Exceptional Children.

McNeil, M. R. 1979. Porch Index of Communicative Ability. In F. L. Darley (Ed.), *Evaluation of appraisal techniques in speech and language pathology.* Reading, Mass.: Addison-Wesley.

McNeil, M. R., & Prescott, T. E. 1978. *Revised Token Test.* Baltimore: University Park Press.

McNeil, M. R., Prescott, T. E., & Chang, E. C. 1975. A measure of PICA ordinality. In R. H. Brookshire (Ed.), *Clinical aphasiology, conference proceedings.* Minneapolis: BRK Publishers.

Mecham, M. J., Jex, J. L., & Jones, J. D. 1967. *Utah test of Language development.* (rev. ed.). Salt Lake City: Communication Research Associates.

Meier, M. J. 1974. Some challenges for clinical neuropsychology. In R. M. Reitan & L. A. Davison (Eds.), *Clinical neuropsychology: Current status and applications.* New York: Wiley.

Messick, S. 1980. The validity and ethics of assessment. *American Psychologist, 35,* 1012–1027.

Morley, G. K., Lundgren, S., & Haxby, J. 1979. Comparison and clinical applicability of auditory comprehension scores on the behavioral neurology deficit evaluation, Boston Diagnostic Aphasia Evaluation, Porch Index of Communicative Ability and Token Test. *Journal of Clinical Neuropsychology, 1* (3), 249–258.

Naeser, M. A., & Hayward, R. W. 1978. Lesion localization in aphasia with cranial computed tomography and the Boston Diagnostic Aphasia Examination. *Neurology, 28,* 545–551.

Nunnally, J. 1967. *Psychometric theory.* New York: McGraw-Hill.

Obler, L. K., & Albert, M. L. 1978. *The bilingual brain: Neuropsychological and neurolinguistic aspects of bilingualism.* New York: Academic Press.

Orgass, B., & Poeck, K. 1966. Clinical validation of a new test for aphasia: An experimental study of the Token Test. *Cortex, 2,* 222–243.

Osgood, C. E., & Sebeok, T. A. 1965. (Eds.). *Psycholinguistics: A survey of theory and research problems.* Bloomington: Indiana Univ. Press.

Pick, A. 1913. Die agrammatischen Sprachstoerungen. Studien zur psychologischen Grundlegung der Aphasielehre. Part 1. In (A. Alzheimer & M. Lewandowsky (Eds.), *Monographien aus dem Gesamtgebiet der Neurologie und Psychiatrie* (Vol. 7). Berlin: Springer.

Poeck, K. 1974. *Neurologie* (3rd ed.). Berlin: Springer.

Poeck, K., Kerschensteiner, M., & Hartje, W. 1972. A quantitative study on language understanding in fluent and nonfluent aphasia. *Cortex, 8,* 299–304.

Porch, B. E. 1967. *Porch Index of Communicative Ability: Theory and development* (Vol. 1). Palo Alto, Calif.: Consulting Psychologists Press.

Porch, B. E. 1973. *Porch Index of Communicative Ability: Administration, scoring, and interpretation* (Vol. 2). Palo Alto, Calif.: Consulting Psychologists Press.

Porch, B. E. 1979. *Porch Index of Communicative Ability in Children.* Vol. 1: *Theory and Development.* Palo Alto: Consulting Psychologists Press.

Porch, B. E., Collins, M., Wertz, R. T., & Friden, T. P. 1980. Statistical prediction of change in aphasia. *Journal of Speech and Hearing Research, 23,* 312–321.

Powell, G. E., Bailey, S., & Clark, E. 1980. A very short form of the Minnesota Aphasia Test. *British Journal of Social and Clinical Psychology, 19,* 189–194.

Reinvang, I., & Graves, R. 1975. A basic aphasia examination: Description with discussion of first results. *Scandinavian Journal of Rehabilitation Medicine, 7,* 129–135.

Reynell, J., & Huntley, R. M. 1971. New scales for the assessment of language development in young children. *Journal of Learning Disabilities, 4,* 549–557.

Sands, E., Sarno, M. T., & Shankweiler, D. 1969. Long-term assessment of language function in aphasia due to stroke. *Archives of Physical Medicine and Rehabilitation, 50,* 202–222.

Sarno, J. E., Sarno, M. T., & Levita, E. 1971. Evaluating language improvement after completed stroke. *Archives of Physical Medicine and Rehabilitation.* 52, 73–78.

Sarno, M. T. 1969. *The Functional Communication Profile: Manual of directions.* New York: New York University Medical Center–The Institute of Rehabilitation Medicine.

Sarno, M. T., & Levita, E. 1979. Recovery in treated aphasia in the first year post-stroke. *Stroke, 10,* 663–670.

Schuell, H. 1955. *Minnesota test for differential diagnosis of aphasia* (research ed.). Minneapolis: Univ. of Minnesota.

Schuell, H. 1957. A short examination for aphasia. *Neurology, 7,* 625–634.

Schuell, H. 1965. *Differential diagnosis of aphasia with the Minnesota Test.* Minneapolis: Univ. of Minnesota Press.

Schuell, H. 1966. A re-evaluation of the short examination for aphasia. *Journal of Speech and Hearing Disorders, 31,* 137–147.

Schuell, H. 1973. *Differential diagnosis of aphasia with the Minnesota Test* (2nd ed.). Minneapolis: Univ. of Minnesota Press.

Schuell, H. 1974. Diagnosis and prognosis in aphasia. In L. F. Sies (Ed.), *Aphasia, theory and therapy.* Baltimore: Univ. Park Press. (a)

Schuell, H. 1974. A theoretical framework for aphasia. In L. F. Sies (Ed.), *Aphasia, theory and therapy.* Baltimore: Univ. Park Press. (b)

Schuell, H., & Jenkins, J. J. 1959. The nature of language deficit in aphasia. *Psychological Review, 66,* 45–67.

Schuell, H., Jenkins, J. J., & Carroll, J. B. 1962. A factor analysis of the Minnesota Test for Differential Diagnosis of Aphasia. *Journal of Speech and Hearing Research, 5,* 350–369.

Schuell, H., Jenkins, J. J., & Jiménez-Pabón, E. 1964. *Aphasia in adults, diagnosis, prognosis, and treatment.* New York: Harper.

Shewan, C. M. 1980. *Auditory Comprehension Test for Sentences.* Chicago: Biolinguistics Clinical Institutes.

Shewan, C. M., & Canter, G. L. 1971. Effects of vocabulary, syntax, and sentence length on auditory comprehension in aphasic patients. *Cortex, 7,* 209–225.

Sidman, M. 1971. The behavioral analysis of aphasia. *Journal of Psychiatric Research, 8,* 413–422.

Sklar, M. 1963. Relation of psychological and language test scores and autopsy findings in aphasia. *Journal of Speech and Hearing Research, 6*(1), 84–90.

Sklar, M. 1973. *Sklar Aphasia Scale* (Rev. ed.). Los Angeles: Western Psychological Services.

Spellacy, F., & Spreen, O. 1969. A short form of the Token Test. *Cortex, 5,* 390–397.

Spiegel, D. K., Jones, L. V., & Wepman, J. M. 1965. Test responses as predictors of free-speech characteristics in aphasia patients. *Journal of Speech and Hearing Research, 8*(4), 349–362.

Spreen, O. 1968. Psycholinguistic aspects of aphasia. *Journal of Speech and Hearing Research, 11,* 467–477.

Spreen, O., & Benton, A. L. 1965. Comparative studies of some psychological tests for cerebral damage. *Journal of Nervous and Mental Disease, 140,* 323–333.

Spreen, O., & Benton, A. L. 1977. *Neurosensory Center Comprehensive Examination for Aphasia* (1977 revision). Victoria, B.C.: Neuropsychology Laboratory, Univ. of Victoria.

Spreen, O., & Tuokko, A. T. 1981. The neuropsychological assessment of normal and disordered cognition. In R. N. Malatesha & L. N. Hartlage (Eds.), *The neuropsychology of cognition.* Groningen: Sitjhoff and Nordoff, forthcoming.

Spreen, O., & Wachal, R. S. 1973. Psycholinguistic analysis of aphasic language: Theoretical formulations and procedures. *Language and Speech, 16,* 130–146.

Strub, R. L., & Black, F. W. 1977. *The mental status examination in neurology.* Philadelphia: Davis.

Swisher, L. P., & Sarno, M. T. 1969. Token Test scores of three matched patient groups: Left brain-damaged with aphasia; right brain-damaged without aphasia; non-brain-damaged. *Cortex, 5,* 264–273.

Taylor, M. L. 1965. A measurement of functional communication in aphasia. *Archives of Physical Medicine and Rehabilitation, 46,* 101–107.

Van Harskamp, F., & Van Dongen, H. R. 1977. Construction and validation of different short forms of the Token Test. *Neuropsychologia, 15,* 467–470.

Veteran's Administration Cooperative Study on Aphasia. Protocol manual, 1973.

Wachal, R. S., & Spreen, O. 1973. Some measures of lexical diversity in aphasic and normal language performance. *Language and Speech, 16,* 169–181.

Weisenburg, T. H., & McBride, K. E. 1935. *Aphasia.* New York: Commonwealth Fund.

Wepman, J. M. 1951. *Recovery from aphasia.* New York: Ronald.

Wepman, J. M., Bock, R. D., Jones, L. V., & Van Pelt, D. 1956. Psycholinguistic study of aphasia: A revision of the concept of anomia. *Journal of Speech and Hearing Disorders, 21,* 468–477.

Wepman, J. M., & Jones, L. V. 1961. *Studies in aphasia: An approach to testing.* Chicago: Education-Industry Service.

Wepman, J. M., & Jones, L. V. 1964. Five aphasias: A commentary on aphasia as a regressive linguistic phenomenon. In D. M. Rioch & E. A. Weinstein (Eds.), *Disorders of communication*. Baltimore: Williams & Wilkins.

Wepman, J. M., Jones, L. V., Bock, R. D., & Van Pelt, D. 1960. Studies in aphasia: Background and theoretical formulations. *Journal of Speech and Hearing Disorders, 25,* 323–332.

Wernicke, C. 1908. The symptom complex of aphasia. In A. Church (Ed.), *Diseases of the nervous system.* New York: Appleton. (Originally published, 1874.)

Wertz, R. T. 1979. Word fluency measure. In F. L. Darley (Ed.), *Evaluation of appraisal techniques in speech and language pathology.* Reading, Mass.: Addison-Wesley.

Wertz, R. T., Keith, R. L., & Custer, D. D. 1971. Normal and aphasic behavior on a measure of auditory input and a measure of verbal output. Paper presented at the American Speech and Hearing Association Convention, Chicago, November.

Wertz, R. T., & Lemme, M. L. 1974. *Input and output measures with adult aphasics.* Research and Training Center 10, Final report, Social Rehabilitation Services, Washington, D.C.

West, J. A. 1973. Auditory comprehension in aphasic adults: Improvement through training. *Archives of Physical Medicine and Rehabilitation, 54,* 78–86.

Wheeler, L., & Reitan, R. M. 1962. The presence and laterality of brain damage predicted from responses to a short aphasia screening test. *Perceptual and Motor Skills, 15,* 783–799.

Zubrick, A., & Smith, A. 1979. Minnesota Test for Differential Diagnosis of Aphasia. In F. C. Darley (Ed.) *Evaluation of appraisal techniques in speech and language pathology.* Reading, Massachusetts: Addison-Wesley.

5

Phonological Aspects of Aphasia

SHEILA E. BLUMSTEIN

The theory of language divides the linguistic system into components or levels. These levels include phonology, syntax, and semantics. Within each level, there are linguistic primitives that define the basic elements of the system. The nature of these elements, their organization, and the interaction of the levels constitute the theory of grammar. Implicit in the theory is the notion that the levels of language are in effect semiautonomous; that is, these levels are independent of each other and yet have to be inextricably linked during the communication process. As an example, the sounds of language can be studied independently of meaning, and yet they gain their linguistic significance ONLY because they convey meaning.

In this chapter, we will focus on the phonological component of the linguistic system in relation to adult aphasia. It is a useful heuristic to study aphasia in relation to each of the components of the grammar. And yet, as indicated here, it is important to emphasize that the components of the grammar are never entirely isolable. Perhaps more importantly, aphasia rarely evidences a deficit selective to only one linguistic component. Thus, studying phonology in aphasia does not imply that the patient is normal in other linguistic abilities. In fact, as we will note in the course of this chapter, the language behavior of aphasics shows clearly how the components of the grammar do interact in language processing.

The study of the phonological component affords in many ways a view of the effects of brain damage on language that other components cannot. In particular, phonology is embedded in physical reality—speech. Both at the level of production and perception, speech is the

129

primary interface with the linguistic code. In production, an idea is ultimately realized as a set of physiological events, and in perception, meaning is extracted from the acoustic waveform. Thus, unlike the other linguistic levels, which by their very nature are abstract, phonology relates to a physical reality. Moreover, the phonological component is the only linguistic level that can be studied in isolation from the others. For example, the perception of phonemic contrasts as /pa/ versus /ba/ can be examined independent of word meaning. Thus, it is possible to determine the extent to which a speech perception deficit may be selectively impaired independent of its relation to the semantic content of a word.

In this chapter, we will focus on three areas that relate to phonological processing in aphasia. We will first investigate speech production in order to characterize the nature of the speech deficits found in aphasia and to attempt to provide some insight into the underlying mechanisms responsible for these deficits. We will then turn to speech perception and explore the nature of the input deficits found in aphasia and suggest their possible underlying bases. Finally, we will discuss the relation between speech production and perception abilities in aphasia. Such study should help determine the extent to which production and perception deficits are either dissociated or linked and, as a result, will speak to the issue of the nature of the underlying organization of the phonological component in language processing.

The Phonological Component: A Model

Before considering these three areas, it may be useful to briefly elaborate a model of the phonological component of a grammar and review its primitives and their theoretical organization. The sounds of speech can be divided into two types of representation. The first is the phonemic level, which characterizes the minimal sound units that contrast meaning. For example, in English, the sounds /p/ and /b/ are each phonemes because they can be used to differentiate words in the language, for instance, *pear* versus *bear*. Phonology not only is concerned with the study of the individual phonemes of the language but also attempts to characterize how they combine in the language system. One can determine a grammar of phonology that specifies the combination of speech sounds for a particular language. It is the case in English, for example, that some combinations of sounds are allowable sequences, for instance, *brick* or the nonsense syllable *blick*, whereas others are not, **bnick*.

Although the phonemes are the minimal meaningful sound units of language, they are further divisible into smaller components or distinctive features (Chomsky & Halle, 1968; Jakobson, Fant, & Halle, 1962). These features describe the phonemes in terms of either the articulatory or acoustic characteristics that contribute to the phonemic identity of the segment. Figure 5.1 shows the bundle of distinctive features that characterize the phonemic segments /p/, /b/, and /d/. The phoneme /p/ is a consonant (in contrast to a vowel), [+consonantal]; it is produced with a complete closure of the vocal tract followed by an abrupt release, [+stop]; the closure occurs at the lips, [+bilabial]; and the vocal cords do not begin to vibrate until after the release of the stop closure, [−voice]. The phoneme /b/ shares all of the distinctive feature characteristics as /p/, with the exception of the voicing feature. For /b/, the vocal cords vibrate at the release of the stop consonant, and thus it is described as [+voice]. In contrast to both /p/ and/b/, /d/ is produced with a closure at the alveolar ridge, [−bilabial], and, as a result, is different from /b/ in place of articulation. Note also that /d/ is different from /p/ not only in place of articulation but also in voicing. Implicit in distinctive feature theory is the notion that sounds that are contrasted by a single feature are more alike articulatorily, acoustically, and psychologically than are sounds contrasting by several distinctive features. Thus, /p/ and/b/, distinguished by one distinctive feature, are more "similar" than are /p/ and /d/, distinguished by two distinctive features.

The phonological component of a grammar then consists of a characterization of the phonemes, rules for their combination, and distinctive feature specifications for the individual phonemes. Up to this point, the grammar has specified only the segments of speech. However, segments are embedded in a larger framework comprising stress and intonation patterns. Both stress and intonation form a part of what linguists call speech prosody or suprasegmentals, as they are melodic features of speech that span the domain of individual speech segments. The intonation or melody pattern of a sentence indicates to the listener, among

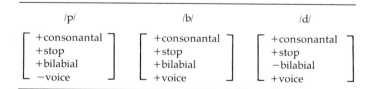

FIGURE 5.1 *Distinctive feature attributes of several phonemes in English.*

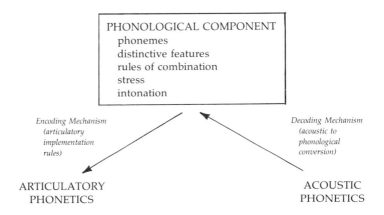

FIGURE 5.2. *A phonological model.*

other things, whether the sentence is a statement, question, or imperative.

From a theoretical point of view, linguists consider the phonological grammar to represent a central mechanism that subserves both speech production and speech perception. That is, the phonemes, features, organizational properties of segments, and suprasegmentals form the abstract grammar ultimately encoded in articulatory terms for speech production and decoded from the acoustic waveform for language comprehension. Figure 5.2 shows a schematic of the organization of such a model. Note that for production, the abstract phonological entities must be realized PHONETICALLY by means of articulatory implementation rules and that the acoustic signal must be encoded in terms of these abstract properties for comprehension. By phonetic is meant all of the detail required to realize the abstract phonological properties in terms of their actual production or perception. For example, the phoneme /p/ can occur in a number of phonological environments—in initial position as in *pill* and in a consonant cluster after /s/ in *spill*. The actual PHONETIC realization of the phoneme /p/ is different depending upon its environment. In initial position, the /p/ is aspirated, whereas after /s-/, it is not; that is, *pill*, /pɪl/ → [pʰɪl]; *spill*, /spɪl/ → [spɪl]. Thus, the study of phonology includes an analysis of the abstract properties of speech sounds, and phonetics includes the detailed physical characteristics of these speech sounds specified in terms of their articulatory parameters for production or in terms of their acoustic properties for perception.

Speech Production

Phonological Patterns of Dissolution

It has been observed clinically that nearly all aphasic patients produce phonological errors in their speech output. It was Paul Broca who first focused on the loss of articulatory capacity due to impairment of "la mémoire des moyens de co-ordination que l'on emploie pour articuler les mots [cited in Taylor, 1958, p. 126]."[1] In the ensuing 60 years, such aphasiologists as Hughlings Jackson (see Taylor, 1958), E. Froschels (1915), H. Head (1926), and M. Critchley (1952) noted that patients of nearly all clinical types make phonemic errors in their speech. These errors can be characterized according to four main types:

1. Phoneme substitution errors, in which a target phoneme is substituted for a different phoneme of the language, for example, *teams* → /kimz/.
2. Simplification errors, in which a target phoneme or syllable is lost, thus simplifying the phonological structure of the word, for example, *brown* → /bawn/.
3. Addition errors, in which a target phoneme or syllable is added to the word, for example, *papa* → /paprə/.
4. Environment errors, in which a target phoneme is replaced by or transposed with neighboring sounds, for example, *Crete* → /trit/, *degree* → /gədriz/.

It is interesting that, despite the clinical diversity of aphasic patients, all of these error types can be found across aphasic groups. Thus, the presence of such errors does not serve as a clinical diagnostic tool. Nevertheless, it is the PATTERN of errors rather than simply their presence that provides a means of characterizing and hopefully understanding the nature and bases of speech production deficits in aphasia.

For the most part, phonological studies have focused on the patterns of speech obtained for a particular diagnostic group. The groups studied have included primarily anterior and posterior patients. The reasons for the particular dichotomy made between these groups of patients corresponds largely to their remarkably different clinical characteristics. Anterior aphasics and especially a subgroup of these, Broca's aphasics, show a profound expressive deficit in the face of relatively preserved auditory language comprehension. Speech output is nonfluent in

---

1. "the memory of the means of coordination that one uses to pronounce words."

that it is slow, labored, and often dysarthric, and the melody pattern seems flat. Further, speech output is agrammatic. This agrammatism is characterized by the loss of grammatical words, such as *the* and *is* as well as grammatical inflectional endings marking number, tense, etc. Naming to confrontation is generally fair to good, and repetition is as good as or better than spontaneous speech output.

In contrast to the nonfluent speech output of the anterior patient, the posterior patient's speech output is fluent. Among the posterior aphasias, Wernicke's and conduction aphasias are perhaps the most studied in relation to phonology. The characteristic features of the language abilities of Wernicke's aphasia include well-articulated but paraphasic speech in the context of severe auditory language comprehension deficits. Paraphasias include literal paraphasias (sound substitutions), verbal paraphasias (word substitutions), or neologisms (productions that are phonologically possible but have no meaning associated with them). Speech output, although grammatically full, is often empty of semantic content and is marked with the overuse of high-frequency "contentless" nouns and verbs, such as *thing* and *be*. The patient also has a moderate to severe naming deficit, and repetition is also severely impaired. Another frequent characteristic of this disorder is LOGORRHEA or a press for speech.

Conduction aphasia refers to the syndrome in which there is a disproportionately severe repetition deficit in relation to the relative fluency and ease of spontaneous speech production and to the generally good auditory language comprehension of the patient. Speech output contains many literal paraphasias and some naming errors. In addition, these patients often evidence a moderate confrontation naming deficit.

As might be expected, because of the clinical observation that anterior aphasics have a severe output deficit, most studies have focused on this group. It is important to note that in this discussion results from studies concerning apraxia of speech and the speech output of Broca's aphasics are considered together. There has been an active dialogue in the literature between those who see apraxia of speech as a nonaphasic and selective articulatory deficit (Aten, Darley, Deal, & Johns, 1975; Johns & LaPointe, 1976) and those who consider apraxia of speech as part of a larger language or aphasic disorder (Buckingham, 1979; Martin, 1974, 1975; see also Chapter 9 of this volume). Whether apraxia of speech is a linguistically based disorder (i.e., affecting the phonological and consequently the linguistic system) or simply an articulatory disorder is difficult to determine from the obtained data. In order to dissociate these two possibilities, it is necessary to demonstrate that the patterns of articulatory errors are different from those of phonological errors, and, as we will see, similar patterns are derived regardless of whether the patient is labeled apraxic or aphasic. In reality, it would not be surprising to find similar patterns of phonological disintegration whether the errors are articulatory or linguistically based, primarily because theoretical linguistic assumptions are derived from the intrinsic nature or organization of the PHONETIC properties of speech in relation to their linguistic function. Thus, what is articulatorily simple is phonologically or linguistically simple, and what is articulatorily complex is also linguistically complex.

Turning to the patterns of speech output in anterior aphasics, common patterns of deficits are found. In particular, there are many more consonant than vowel errors (Keller, 1978; Trost & Canter, 1974). With regard to consonant errors, a greater number of substitution errors occur than any other type of error (Blumstein, 1973; Dunlop & Marquardt, 1977; Klich, Ireland, & Weidner, 1979; Trost & Canter, 1974). Further, patients have greater difficulty with consonants produced in initial than in final position, for example, *pete* versus *beep*. Moreover, simplification errors occur most commonly in the environment of consonant clusters and thus reflect an overall reduction in the complexity of the syllable structure.

The patterns of substitution errors can be studied in two ways. First, a phonemic analysis can be done in which the particular phoneme targets and their substitutions are listed. Such analyses have generally shown tremendous variability and inconsistency across patients (Trost & Canter, 1974; Shankweiler & Harris, 1966). Namely, it is impossible to predict what particular phonemes the patients will produce incorrectly, when those errors will occur, and exactly what phonemes will be substituted. As a result, several researchers have considered the errors to be unsystematic and random.

Nevertheless, further analysis reveals distinct patterns of dissolution. This analysis procedure considers the phonological RELATION between the target and substituted phoneme. Thus, the substitution of a /b/ for a /p/ represents, not the substitution of one whole sound unit for another, but rather the replacement of the voiced feature with the voiceless feature. As discussed earlier, linguistic theory makes implicit assumptions and predictions about the possible relations among the sounds of a language, and these have direct application to the types of speech production errors found in aphasia. Thus, phoneme substitutions should occur more commonly among sounds sharing a number of feature dimensions, for example, /p/–/b/ versus /t/–/w/. Moreover, sound substitutions should be characterized more commonly by single feature changes than by several feature changes. For example, /p/ → /b/ represents a single feature change of voicing, whereas /p/ → /z/ represents a change of the features of voicing, place of articulation (labial versus alveolar), and manner (stop versus fricative).

Roman Jakobson was the first researcher to suggest and ultimately to apply these theoretical principles to the study of aphasia and child language (Jakobson, 1968). Further studies have shown a remarkable uniformity in that, overall, many more single feature substitution errors are found than errors of several features (Blumstein, 1973; Martin & Rigrodsky, 1974; Trost & Canter, 1974). With regard to vowel errors, patterns of dissolution similar to those obtained for consonants can be found. Namely, substitution errors are the most common error type, and most errors reflect single feature substitutions (Keller, 1975, 1978; Trost & Canter, 1974).

Nevertheless, as already indicated, despite this systematicity and regularity, the particular occurrence of an error cannot be predicted (Blumstein, 1973; Hatfield & Walton, 1975). Moreover, substitution errors are not unidirectional; that is, voiced consonants can become voiceless and voiceless consonants can become voiced. Thus, the patterns of errors reflect statistical tendencies: When an error occurs, it will tend to be a single feature substitution, and the errors will more likely affect some features rather than others. In this sense, then, the performance of the patients is variable, but it is NOT random, as it follows specific phonological principles.

What these results suggest is that the patient has not "lost" the ability to produce either particular phonemes or to instantiate particular features. Rather, his speech output mechanism does not seem to be able consistently to encode the correct underlying phonemic (i.e., feature) representation of the word. As a consequence, the patient may produce an utterance that is articulatorily correct but that deviates phonologically from the target word; for example, for *team*, he produces /kim/. On other occasions, he may produce the same target correctly from both an articulatory and phonological point of view; for example, for *team*, he produces /tim/.

In general, the patterns of results obtained are stable across varying testing conditions. That is, in the studies described in the preceding discussion, a number of different procedures have been used to elicit the speech production data, including naming (Trost & Canter, 1974), repetition (Cohen, Dubois, Gauthier, Hécaen, & Angelergues, 1963; Kagan, 1977), reading (Bouman & Grünbaum, 1925; Dunlop & Marquardt, 1977), and spontaneous speech (Blumstein, 1973). However, it is important to emphasize that not all studies have reported similar results, and it may be that some of the differences obtained reflect the different testing procedures and stimulus sets used. For example, Trost and Canter (1974) found a different distribution of error types using a naming task compared to a repetition task. That is, subjects produced a greater proportion of responses that could not be judged phonemically in a naming task compared with repetition. Such differences are not at all surprising, considering the nature of these test paradigms. Failure to name reflects more than phonological output problems; rather, word-finding deficits can interact with the phonological disorder. In contrast, in repetition, an auditory model of the word is provided and therefore problems of word retrieval are controlled. However, a different variable is introduced in a repetition task; namely, the patient must be able to PERCEIVE correctly the auditory model. Thus, a repetition error could reflect a perceptual error, a production error, a memory deficit (the auditory model must be held in short-term store before it is repeated), or a combination of these three. It is important then in testing a patient that the nature of the task and its demands on the linguistic system be carefully considered and that the behavior of the patient be viewed in relation to the methodology used to elicit the stimuli.

Up to this point, we have reviewed only the behavior of anterior patients. However, a number of studies have investigated the phonological patterns of posterior aphasics as well. Clinically, of course, anterior and posterior patients represent contrasting speech output behaviors. The slow, labored, often dysarthric speech pattern of the anterior patient is opposed to the fluent, easily articulated, and facile output of the posterior patient. In fact, early researchers characterized the speech production patterns of anterior aphasics in terms of phonetic disintegration (Alajouanine, Ombredane, & Durand, 1939) and the patterns of posterior aphasics in terms of phonemic disintegration (Luria, 1966). Nevertheless, despite these differences, the speech production behavior of posterior patients breaks down into categories similar to the patterns of the anterior patients. In particular, more consonant than vowel errors are produced, substitution errors are among the most common error types, syllable structure of words is often simplified, and phonemic substitution errors involve single feature substitutions more often than substitutions of more than one feature (Blumstein, 1973; Burns & Canter, 1977; Degiovanni, Khomsi, Bosser, Souffront, Mollet, & Posson, 1977; Dubois, Hécaen, Angelergues, Chatelier, & Marcie, 1964; Green, 1969; Halpern, Keith, & Darley, 1976). Moreover, Wernicke's and conduction (both posterior) aphasics reveal similar patterns of production (Blumstein, 1973; Degiovanni *et al.*, 1977). That is, the patients can not be distinguished on the basis of the patterns of phonological disintegration.

In summary, phonological analysis of aphasic speech production indicates similar patterns of dissolution for both anterior and posterior aphasics. These errors can be characterized in terms of the frequency of phoneme substitution errors in which the relation between target word and actual production is distinguished primarily by single distinctive feature contrasts, simplification errors in which the complexity of a phonological form is reduced, the occurrence of intrusions of sounds or syllables, and also the influence of neighboring sounds on the final speech output. The stability of these patterns is evidenced by their occurrence across the different phonological systems in natural language—French (Bouman & Grünbaum, 1925; Lecours & Lhermitte, 1969), German (Bouman & Grünbaum, 1925; Goldstein, 1948), English (Blumstein, 1973; Green, 1969), Turkish (Peuser & Fittschen, 1977), and Russian (Luria, 1966), to name a few. Nevertheless, it is important to emphasize that different experimental tasks as well as differences in the type and complexity of the stimuli used (Martin, Wasserman, Gilden, & West, 1975) can contribute to variations among the basic patterns elucidated here.

Phonetic Patterns of Dissolution

As indicated in the previous section, an analysis of the phonological patterns of aphasic speech failed to differentiate among the various clinical types of aphasia. Taken as a whole, these results would suggest that similar mechanisms are responsible for the speech production patterns of aphasic patients. And yet, from a clinical point of view, such a conclusion does not seem warranted. Phonological analyses fail to capture what seems to be a quality distinction between the anterior and posterior aphasic. This distinction had been alluded to in the previous section under the rubric of phonetic versus phonemic disintegration. And it is just this distinction that the phonological analyses have ignored. In particular, the speech production characteristics of anterior aphasics are slow and labored and contain numerous PHONETIC distortions. These characteristics were not considered in the phonological investigations, where only errors that affected the PHONEMIC representation of the target word were considered. Thus, if a patient attempted to say *pear* and said [p^{hhh}ær], overly aspirating the initial consonant, this production would not be considered a phonological error, as the phonemic representation of the phonetic output was correct.

It has been a long-held observation that some patients, particularly anterior aphasics, produce phonetic errors. The implied basis for these errors is one of articulatory implementation; that is, the commands to the articulators to encode the word are inappropriate, poorly timed, etc. Perhaps the first researchers to investigate the nature of phonetic disintegration using instrumental measures were Alajouanine *et al.* (1939). Three principles were postulated to account for the patterns of consonant production they found in their patients: (*a*) paralytic, characterized by articulatory weakness; (*b*) dystonic, characterized by articulatory movements excessive in force and duration; and (*c*) apraxic, characterized by gross difficulty in forming articulatory movements to command and some difficulty upon imitation. More recent spectrographic analyses have supported the earlier findings (Lehiste, 1968). It is important to emphasize that in both of these studies patients classified either as having apraxia of speech or as anterior aphasics displayed similar patterns of behavior. These results suggest that anterior aphasics may have a speech production pattern qualitatively different from that of posterior aphasics when phonetic errors are also considered. Perhaps more importantly, it may be that the basis for many of the PHONOLOGICAL errors in anterior patients is actually phonetic in nature; that is, phonological errors, such as /p/ → /b/, may represent extreme phonetic distortions that are perceived by the listener in terms of a change in phonetic category from the target.

Several studies have attempted to address the nature of the phonetic productions in anterior aphasics. These studies have focused primarily on two phonetic dimensions, voicing and nasality, both requiring the integration of two articulators. In the case of the feature voicing, the dimension studied is voice-onset time—that is, the timing relation between the release of a stop consonant and the onset of glottal pulsing. For voiceless consonants, such as /p/, the vocal cords do not begin to vibrate until about 30 msec after the stop consonant is released, whereas for voiced consonants, such as /b/, vocal cord vibration begins either at the release of the consonant or some tens of msec after the release of the consonant. The production of nasal consonants also requires appropriate timing between two articulators—in this case, the release of the consonant and velum opening. For /m/, the velum must be open at the release of the consonant so that air may escape from both the oral and nasal cavities as the consonant is released. If the velum is not sufficiently open, air will be unable to escape through the nose and will consequently escape only through the oral cavity, resulting in the corresponding stop consonant /b/. Results of analyses of the production of both the voicing and nasal phonetic dimensions have shown that anterior patients evidence significant deficits (Blumstein, Cooper, Zurif, & Caramazza, 1977; Blumstein, Cooper, Goodglass, Statlender, & Gottlieb, 1980; Freeman, Sands, & Harris, 1978; Itoh, Sasanuma, Hirose,

Yoshioka, & Ushijima, 1980; Itoh, Sasanuma, & Ushijima, 1979). All of these studies have used acoustic measurements and have inferred that the basis for the deficit is phonetic and involves articulatory timing. More direct measures of articulatory timing using fiberoptics (Itoh, Sasanuma, Tatsumi, & Kobayashi, 1979; Itoh, Sasanuma, & Ushijima, 1979), computer-controlled X-ray microbeams (Itoh *et al.*, 1980), and electromyography (Shankweiler, Harris, & Taylor, 1968) have also shown that the timing relation among the articulators is impaired. Taken together, these results support the conclusion that motor programming for the synchronization of different articulators is impaired (Itoh, Sasanuma, & Ushijima, 1979) and, further, that there is a reduction in the capacity for independent movement of the articulators (Lehiste, 1968; Shankweiler *et al.*, 1968). Further, comparison of these patterns of speech with those of posterior patients has revealed that Broca's aphasics can be qualitatively distinguished from Wernicke's aphasics on the basis of their speech production. In particular, voice-onset time analyses have shown that Broca's aphasics display the timing deficits described here, whereas Wernicke's aphasics show minimal impairment (Blumstein, Cooper, Goodglass, Statlender, & Gottlieb, 1980). Anterior aphasics have evidenced phonetic deficits not only in consonant production but also in vowel production. A number of studies have shown that the formant frequencies for vowels (i.e., the frequencies corresponding to the resonant frequencies of the vocal tract) may be shifted and also display increased variability (Keller, 1975; Ryalls, 1981). Moreover, vowel duration is also increased compared to normal production (Ryalls, 1981). Taken together with the results for consonant production, it is clear that a characteristic of the speech production disorder of anterior aphasics is phonetic in nature and probably involves, at the very least, a deficit in articulatory programming and/or timing. What is of interest is that these phonetic distortions are present even in those utterances that are phonemically correct, that is, are categorized as belonging to the appropriate target phoneme (Blumstein, Cooper, Goodglass, Statlender, & Gottlieb, 1980; Ryalls, 1981). Thus, anterior aphasics seem to have a pervasive phonetic disorder that overlays their entire speech production.

Many of the phonological errors described in the preceding section probably reflected deficits of articulatory programming rather than planning. However, it is not clear whether the various types of errors and characteristics of segment production found in anterior aphasics can be attributed solely to articulatory deficits. Some of the voicing and nasal errors could well have reflected incorrect phoneme selection (i.e., inappropriate phoneme choice), as well as articulatory implementation problems. Moreover, it is difficult to attribute many of the error types—such as, errors of simplification, addition, and sequencing as well as consonant substitutions for place of articulation—to articulatory programming deficits. Thus, it may be the case that anterior aphasics evidence both a phonological deficit, implying a disorder in phoneme selection, as well as a phonetic deficit, implying a disorder in articulatory implementation. What is critical to emphasize is that, whatever the characteristics of the production deficits of anterior aphasics, they are similar in nature and kind to those found in anarthria, a disorder characterized by cortical or subcortical lesions producing severely impaired production with no paralysis of the speech musculature and no other associated aphasic symptoms (Lebrun, Buyssens, & Henneaux, 1973; Lecours & Lhermitte, 1976). Further, these patterns are different from those found in patients with dysarthria or with lesions in the lower motor neurons (Blumstein, Cooper, Goodglass, Statlender, & Gottlieb, 1980; Itoh *et al.*, 1980; Lebrun *et al.*, 1973).

The Production of Speech Prosody

Up to this point, the analysis of the speech production patterns in aphasia has focused on segmental features. Another important feature of speech production is its rhythm and melody, called speech prosody. The most common area of study in this regard is intonation, which is of interest for several reasons. On the one hand, intonation provides important clues concerning speech planning abilities. That is, several features characterize intonation patterns in declarative sentences in normal speech, and these features interact with syntactic complexity and sentence length. These features include:

1. Terminal falling fundamental frequency (or pitch) in utterance final position. That is, the pitch contour of the last word in a declarative sentence shows a sharp drop in frequency or pitch.
2. Fundamental frequency declination over the full sentence. That is, normally there is a higher fundamental frequency in the beginning and a lower fundamental frequency at the end of the sentence. This so-called declination effect usually occurs over the full range of a declarative sentence.
3. Lengthening of the final word in the sentence (Cooper & Sorenson, 1980).

In order for the speaker to produce the appropriate pitch contours and word duration, it is necessary for him to effectively preplan the sentence, taking into consideration its length and syntactic structure.

Besides studying planning behavior, the study of prosody is particularly important in understanding the nature of the speech production abilities of Broca's or anterior aphasics. As described earlier, one of the clinical features of anterior aphasia seems to be slow, labored speech in the context of a flattened intonation contour. It is useful then to see if acoustic investigations substantiate this clinical impression. To date, only a few studies have been conducted, and because only a few patients have been actually tested, the results should be considered preliminary. Nevertheless, they are extremely interesting. Analysis of two-word spontaneous speech utterances and reading in Broca's aphasics has shown that these patients have some rudimentary control over some features of prosody (Danley, deVilliers, & Cooper, 1979). There is a tendency for the patient to maintain a terminal falling fundamental frequency (although cf. Ryalls, 1980, for some conflicting data). This fall occurs even in utterances where the pauses between words may reach durations of as long as 7 sec. This suggests that Broca's aphasics do have a linguistic sense of an utterance and that even the very severe agrammatic patient is not simply stringing together lexical items, each one forming a holophrastic utterance.

Nevertheless, further analysis revealed a number of systematic problems in the production of prosody in these patients. In the first place, patients do not show utterance final lengthening. In fact, they show systematically longer durations in word initial than final position (Danley & Shapiro, 1980; Danley *et al.*, 1979). Interestingly, this finding does not correlate with the durations of utterances or the occurrence of pauses between words. These results are consistent with the findings of Goodglass and his colleagues that anterior aphasics need primary stress at the beginning of a sentence to initiate speech. Dubbed the stress-saliency hypothesis, it suggests that part of the production problem of the anterior aphasic is an increased threshold for initiating and maintaining the flow of speech (Goodglass, 1968; Goodglass, Quadfasel, & Timberlake, 1964). A second form of evidence of a prosodic deficit in Broca's aphasics is that these patients do not show normal declination patterns in longer utterances. Instead, the declination effect, usually occurring over the entire range of the sentence in normals, is found only in short phrases in Broca's aphasics. That is, the domain of the declination pattern seems to be limited to syntactic phrases, such as noun phrases or verb phrases and not the sentence as a whole. These are consistent with the findings of Goodglass and his colleagues, who showed that the utterances of Broca's aphasics are characterized syntactically by either noun phrases or verb phrases and rarely the concatenation of the two (Goodglass, Gleason, Bernholtz, & Hyde, 1972).

In sum, the patterns of phonetic disintegration clearly show that anterior aphasics have a different speech production pattern than do posterior aphasics. Phonetic disintegration can best be characterized in terms of a deficit in articulatory implementation of phonetic segments and especially in the timing of several articulatory maneuvers. In addition, the prosodic pattern of Broca's aphasics is also abnormal and reflects rudimentary melodic control over only a restricted syntactic domain.

Speech Perception

The Perception of Phonemic Contrasts

Like production studies, perception studies have focused mainly on the ability of aphasic patients to perceive phonemic or segmental contrasts, for example, *pear* versus *bear*. These studies have been motivated by two primary rationales. The first is to determine if segmental perception is impaired in aphasia. Such results should speak to the nature of the deficits of phonological processing at the receptive level. The second rationale is to ascertain the degree to which speech perception deficits form the basis for language comprehension deficits. It was Luria (1966) who elaborated this view in greatest detail with respect to Wernicke's aphasia. In particular, he argued that the severe comprehension deficit of these patients reflected the loss of "phonemic" hearing, that is, the ability to distinguish minimal phonological contrasts. He reasoned that if patients could not perceive phonological contrasts, then they would be unable to process words appropriately for meaning, resulting in a severe comprehension disorder. Such a view assumes that segmental perception underlies speech processing and further that language processing is hierarchically ordered, with speech analysis occurring before meaning is extracted from the signal itself.

Studies on segmental perception have indeed shown that aphasic patients do evidence deficits in processing segmental contrasts. Although such deficits are found in Wernicke's aphasics, they are by no means isolated to this particular group. Nearly all aphasics show some problems in discriminating phonological contrasts (Blumstein, Baker, & Goodglass, 1977; Jauhiainen & Nuutila, 1977; Miceli, Caltagirone, Gainotti, & Payer-Rego, 1978; Miceli, Gainotti, Caltagirone, & Masullo, 1980) or in labeling or identifying consonants presented in a consonant–vowel context (Basso, Casati, & Vignolo, 1977; Blumstein, Cooper, Zurif, & Caramazza, 1977). In terms of the feature relations of the consonants, the results are consistent with theoretical analyses of distinctive features. Namely, subjects are more likely to make discrimination errors when the test stimuli contrast by a single feature than when they contrast by two or more features (Baker, Blumstein, & Goodglass, 1981; Blumstein, Baker, & Goodglass, 1977; Miceli *et al.*, 1978; Sasanuma, Tatsumi, & Fujisaki, 1976). Further, discrimination errors on place contrasts—for example, /pa/ versus /ta/—are generally more common than are voicing contrasts—for example, /pa/ versus /ba/ (Baker *et al.*, 1981; Blumstein, Baker, & Goodglass, 1977; Miceli *et al.*, 1978).

The failure of patients to label or discriminate the sounds of speech has been explored for the most part in the context of natural speech. The use of natural speech in perception experiments has the advantage of providing all the cues necessary to signal a particular phonetic dimension. As a result, however, it is impossible to study the contribution of various components of the acoustic signal to the perception of the phonetic dimensions of speech. Studies of the speech perception abilities of normals have in fact attempted to chart out carefully those aspects of the acoustic signal critical to speech perception (Liberman, Cooper, Shankweiler, & Studdert-Kennedy, 1967). Using synthetic speech, acoustic parameters can be independently manipulated and controlled. A number of studies have explored the abilities of aphasic patients to perceive phonetic categories when presented with synthetic speech continua that vary in systematic steps along a particular acoustic dimension. Results have shown that patients have particular difficulties labeling these stimuli (Basso *et al.*, 1977; Blumstein, Cooper, Zurif, & Caramazza, 1977). To test labeling ability, subjects may be required to either repeat what they hear or point to a printed card containing the appropriate consonant or syllable. Interestingly, these patients may nonetheless be able to discriminate the same stimuli in a manner similar to normals (Blumstein, Cooper, Zurif, & Caramazza, 1977). This dissociation has been interpreted as reflecting the fact that the perception of the acoustic parameters defining the phonetic categories may be spared in aphasia, but the ability to use these dimensions to categorize the sounds of speech in a linguistically relevant way may be impaired. In fact, it was the Wernicke aphasics who seemed to demonstrate this dissociation more than the other aphasic groups tested, including Broca's, mixed anterior, and conduction aphasics (Blumstein, Cooper, Zurif, and Caramazza, 1977).

The Relation between Speech Perception and Auditory Language Comprehension

The dissociation of discrimination from labeling in speech perception begins to address the question of the relation between speech perception abilities and language comprehension. That is, the failure of Wernicke patients to maintain a stable category label might be the basis for their language comprehension deficits. Nevertheless, a number of studies that have compared speech perception abilities to auditory comprehension in aphasia have failed to show any systematic or strong correlations (Basso *et al.*, 1977; Blumstein, Baker, & Goodglass, 1977; Jauhiainen & Nuutila, 1977; Miceli *et al.*, 1980; for general discussion see Boller, 1978, and Lesser, 1978). That is, patients with good auditory language comprehension skills have shown impairments in speech processing; conversely, patients with severe auditory language comprehension deficits have shown minimal speech perception deficits. The failure to show a systematic relation between speech perception and language comprehension could be due to several factors. First, speech perception deficits may in fact underlie language comprehension deficits, but these deficits are revealed only in the context of larger streams of speech. Thus, focusing on the perception of segments in isolated words or syllables may not be a sensitive enough index. Second, the extraction of meaning from the auditory signal may require the perception NOT of segmental cues per se but rather of auditory patterns for individual words (Klatt, 1980). Thus, investigating segmental cues may not tap the primary perceptual deficit. Third, the underlying deficit in auditory comprehension may reflect an inability to relate sound representation to its appropriate meaning. Such a dissociation would be represented clinically by a deficit in word meaning as well as in speech perception. In this view, however, the word meaning deficit is not due to a speech perception impairment but rather due to an interaction of phonology and meaning (Baker *et al.*, 1981; Martin *et al.*, 1975).

Perhaps the only study that has shown a systematic relation between auditory perception ability and language comprehension in aphasia has been that of Tallal and Newcombe (1978). Interestingly, they focused on the auditory perception of rapidly changing acoustic information in both nonverbal and verbal stimuli. For nonverbal stimuli, they explored the ability of right brain-damaged and left brain-damaged aphasic patients to determine temporal order of two complex tones separated by various interstimulus intervals. For the speech stimuli, they focused on the perception of place of articulation, a phonetic dimension that seems particularly vulnerable in aphasia. One of the acoustic cues for place of articulation in stop consonants is the rapid motion of formant transitions. The rationale of Tallal and Newcombe's work was that aphasic patients may have a primary deficit in processing rapid acoustic events, and, as a result, the deficit is primarily auditory in nature. In this view, speech deficits are a secondary consequence of this disorder, and language comprehension deficits, as well, may be due to an inability to process normally auditory stimuli. Their results showed a dissociation between performance of left and right brain-damaged patients, with aphasics being selectively impaired in the nonverbal and language stimuli. Moreover, they found a correlation between performance on the nonverbal task and the Token Test, a test sensitive to auditory language comprehension deficits (DeRenzi & Vignolo, 1962). It is interesting to note that the Token Test requires, in the more complex parts of the test, the ability to sequence (i.e., order) a number of stimuli. The relation between this task and the sequencing deficit of auditory stimuli may be due to the nature of the two tasks (i.e., sequencing) rather than to an auditory impairment affecting language comprehension. In any case, on the basis of the obtained correlation, Tallal and Newcombe concluded that at least part of the comprehension deficit of aphasic patients reflects a disorder in auditory processing of rapid acoustic events. As to the place of articulation dimension, they demonstrated that lengthening the duration of formant transitions from 40 msec to 80 msec resulted in improved performance for only three out of six aphasic subjects. In fact, a more recent study has failed to show systematic improvement in either labeling or discrimination of place of articulation with extended formant transition durations (Blumstein, Tartter, & Nigro, 1981). Thus, although Tallal and Newcombe found a significant relation between processing of nonverbal auditory stimuli and language comprehension, it is not clear that the relation holds as strongly for speech stimuli.

Nevertheless, the hypothesis that auditory processing of rapid acoustic events underlies the language processing deficits of aphasics is an interesting one. A number of studies have shown that brain-damaged patients demonstrate increased thresholds for determining temporal order between two events in both the auditory and visual modalities (Efron, 1963; Swisher & Hirsh, 1972). Such findings are strongly correlated with aphasia (Bond, 1976; Efron, 1963; Swisher & Hirsh, 1972); however, they are not restricted to aphasic patients with left hemisphere lesions (Carmon & Nachson, 1971). In fact, it has been shown that both left and right anterior lobectomy patients with no aphasia show increased thresholds for temporal order judgments in the auditory modality (Sherwin & Efron, 1980). Thus, auditory deficits reflected in an inability to process rapidly presented acoustic events cannot be the primary basis for the language comprehension deficits of aphasic patients. If this were the case, all patients who evidence impairments in temporal order judgments should show an auditory language comprehension deficit. The presence of such deficits in nonaphasic patients mitigates against such an interpretation.

Nevertheless, the notion of time as a crucial variable in auditory language processing does have some support both in the clinical setting and in some subsequent experimental investigations. In particular, it has been reported that speaking slowly to an aphasic may enhance his language comprehension (Schuell, Jenkins, & Jiménez-Pabon, 1964). Several studies have shown that rate of stimulus presentation does enhance word retention (Cermak & Moreines, 1976) and overall language comprehension in aphasia (Albert & Bear, 1974; Bergman, Fiselson, Tze'elon, Mendelson, & Schechter, 1977; Lasky, Weidner, & Johnson, 1976; Weidner & Lasky, 1976). These findings seem to obtain for those patients who are not too severely impaired (Weidner & Lasky, 1976) and seems to interact with the syntactic complexity of the stimuli (Katz, 1979; Weidner & Lasky, 1976). Further, time alone does not seem to be the crucial variable—that is, comprehension performance is not necessarily enhanced with increased duration of the words themselves or of the pauses between words, but rather seems to hinge on increasing silent intervals at major syntactic breaks (Katz, 1979).

The Perception of Prosody

Prosodic cues serve a very important function in language processing. At the perceptual level, they provide an organizing framework for the different sentence types of language. For example, a rising intonation indicates a question, and a falling intonation, a statement. Both of these characteristics seem to be nearly universal properties of language (Lieberman, 1967). Stress is another suprasegmental component that is linguistically crucial, since it can serve to differentiate meaning in different lexical items. In English, for example, stress contrasts between *hótdog* and *hotdóg* or *cónvict* and *convíct* distinguish different syntactic classes or categories, that is, nouns and noun phrases versus nouns and verbs.

In contrast to the segmental features of language, the perception of prosodic cues (i.e., intonation and stress) seems to be remarkably well preserved in aphasia. Severely impaired aphasics have been shown to retain some ability to recognize and distinguish the syntactic forms of commands, yes–no questions, and information questions when marked by intonation cues (Green & Boller, 1974). This performance is superior to the determination of syntactic forms when marked by syntactic and lexical cues. Nevertheless, the perception of these intonation cues is far from normal, and patients still make many perceptual errors.

The perception of word accent in Japanese seems to be less impaired than the perception of segmental cues (Sasanuma *et al.*, 1976), and the perception of stress as a semantic cue distinguishing different lexical items in English is also relatively spared (Blumstein & Goodglass, 1972). Nonetheless, as with the intonation cues, the patient's performance is not completely normal.

What is of interest is that aphasic patient's performance seems to be relatively better preserved in the processing of prosodic cues compared to segmental cues. The reason for this dichotomy could reflect a hierarchical organization of phonological cues, with melody cues being simpler or perceptually more basic. Alternatively, it could reflect the participation of the nondominant hemisphere in the processing of these cues.

In sum, the perception of segmental cues in aphasia is clearly impaired. However, the patterns of disintegration are systematic and reflect the relation of the distinctive feature attributes of the phonemic contrasts. Nevertheless, all aphasic types evidence speech perception deficits, and further, such deficits do not seem to be the primary basis for the auditory language comprehension deficits found in these patients. Patients may show a dissociation between the ability to discriminate and label phonetic dimensions, suggesting that part of the so-called speech perception deficit reflects an inability to use the sounds of speech in a linguistically relevant way. In addition, aphasic patients show deficits in the processing of temporal order and rapidly changing acoustic events. It is not clear that this reflects an auditory rather than a linguistic basis to language processing problems. However, it does suggest that providing more time for the patient to process syntactically demarcated utterances does enhance their language comprehension. Finally, prosodic cues seem to show less impairment than segmental cues, perhaps reflecting the participation of the nondominant hemisphere in the processing of the suprasegmental dimensions of language.

The Relation between Production and Perception

Perhaps one of the most intriguing questions with regard to phonological deficits in aphasia is whether production and perception impairments are causally related. The implications of such a relation are that both production and perception are subsumed by a common underlying mechanism and that phonological deficits reflect a central disorder in which the internal phonological representation of sounds of language is affected (see Figure 5.2). The clinical consequence of this would be the presence of both production and perceptual deficits for speech in any particular aphasic patient. Dissociations between production and perception, on the other hand, suggest that there may be two independent phonological systems, one underlying production and the other underlying perception.

A number of studies have attempted to explore this issue, and the results are suggestive but far from conclusive. In particular, a general association of both production and perceptual deficits has been shown in anterior as well as posterior patients, and the severity of these deficits seems to be correlated (Basso *et al.*, 1977; Miceli *et al.*, 1980; Shewan, 1980). Nevertheless, the correlation is far from complete, since it has been shown that in all types of aphasics there can be dissociations between production and perception abilities. Some patients show no perceptual deficits in the face of poor production abilities (Miceli *et al.*, 1980; Shewan, 1980), whereas others with less severe phoneme output deficits are unable to make subtle phonemic discriminations (Miceli *et al.*, 1980).

Blumstein, Cooper, Zurif, and Caramazza (1977), comparing the production and perception of voice-onset time, concluded that there was no direct relation between the two abilities. In their study, only five out of nine subjects showed an association between production and perception. However, it is instructive to look in more detail at those patients who failed to show such a correlation, since some insight into the nature of the relation between these two abilities might be obtained. Of the four patients who showed a dissociation, three of them were anterior aphasics. Their performance was characterized by the presence of production errors in the context of normal perception. However, the production errors that these patients made were predominantly phonetic in nature and presumably reflected errors in articulatory programming rather than in phoneme planning. Of what significance is this observation? To help clarify this issue, let us consider what would be the clinical manifestation of a central phonological disorder. Presumably such a disorder would affect the internal representation of the sounds of speech. As a result, one would expect a disorder in phonemic output and input. The phonetic details of both production and perception should be intact. That is, discrimination of the acoustic attributes of the signal should be spared, despite perceptual impairment of the use of these sounds linguistically, and articulatory implementation of speech should be intact despite phoneme selection errors. Thus, the presence of phonetic errors in the context of normal perception suggests that there is a distinction between central disorders of phonology affecting both input and output modalities, and "peripheral" or phonetic disorders in which the central mechanism is spared but the phonetic properties of speech are affected. In this case, production and perception abilities may well be dissociated, affecting either output or input modalities.

Clearly, more research is needed to determine the relation between production and perception deficits in aphasia. It is critical that distinctions be made between central phonological disorders and those that affect phonetic manifestations. With a carefully defined distinction between phonetic and phonemic errors at both input and output levels, it may be possible to determine the extent to which speech production and perception are associated or dissociated. Such results may help determine the underlying bases for these disorders and more sharply differentiate phonological deficits in aphasia.

Conclusion

This chapter attempted to delineate the phonological patterns of aphasic speech and to provide some clues as to the nature of the mechanisms underlying such deficits. All clinical types of aphasia evidence some impairments in both speech production and speech perception. Nevertheless, careful analyses of the patterns of speech production indicated that the production process can be analyzed into at least two distinct stages, phonological planning and articulatory implementation. All patients show similar patterns of deficit at the first stage. However, the anterior patient is also impaired at the stage of articulatory implementation and, as a result, has both a phonetic and phonological impairment. Prosodic as well as segmental cues are affected in the production of anterior aphasics, suggesting that these patients have a general speech output deficit involving timing and fine motor control needed for speech output.

Analogous to speech production, at least two stages of perception are implicated in ongoing processing. The first involves the extraction of the acoustic properties of speech, and the second, the encoding of the attributes into linguistically significant dimensions. Dissociations between these two levels of perception are found in aphasia in the context of spared discrimination and impaired labeling. Nevertheless, the phonological patterns of perception involving the feature relations among segments is similar across aphasic patients.

Despite the presence of phonological disorders in nearly all aphasics, these impairments do not seem to correlate with the severity of language comprehension deficits. Consequently, speech perception deficits do not seem to form the basis for language comprehension deficits. Similarly, auditory deficits do not seem to underlie comprehension impairments.

What then is the relation between speech perception and language comprehension? It may be perceptual deficits underlie some language comprehension abilities; however, researchers to date have failed to focus on the appropriate dimensions. For example, ongoing speech processing requires the integration of acoustic events over a fairly long time interval, and current research has generally focused on short intervals, as, for example, the perception of speech segments. Some support for this view is that increasing the temporal parameters of the speech signal at crucial parts of the signal enhances language comprehension in some patients.

Finally, speech production and speech perception form part of a larger system, the phonological system, which presumably is central in nature. By central is meant that a common phonological system subserves both speech production and speech perception. The partial correlations obtained in studies comparing the relation between production and perception in aphasia would support this view. However, they also indicate that the so-called peripheral attributes of speech processing— that is, articulatory implementation in production and acoustic analysis in perception—may be impaired independently, thus affecting only one modality of speech and sparing the other. Such dissociations between production and perception emphasize the fact that despite a proposed common underlying mechanism subserving production and perception, the primary input and output characteristics of the phonological system are presumably independent of each other.

Acknowledgments

Many thanks to M. T. Sarno for her comments on an earlier draft of this paper. This work was supported in part by grant NS07615 to Clark University and NS06209 to the Boston University School of Medicine.

References

Alajouanine, T., Ombredane, A., & Durand, M. 1939. *Le syndrome de la désintégration phonétique dans l'aphasie.* Paris: Masson.
Albert, M., & Bear, D. 1974. Time to understand. *Brain, 97,* 373–384.
Aten, J. L., Darley, F. L., Deal, J. L., & Johns, D. F. 1975. Comments on A. D. Martin's "Some objections to the term apraxia of speech." *Journal of Speech and Hearing Disorders, 40,* 416–420.

Baker, E., Blumstein, S. E., & Goodglass, H. 1981. Interaction between phonological and semantic factors in auditory comprehension. *Neuropsychologia, 19,* 1–16.

Basso, A., Casati, G., & Vignolo, L. A. 1977. Phonemic identification defects in aphasia. *Cortex, 13,* 84–95.

Bergman, M., Fiselson, J., Tze'elon, R., Medelson, L., & Schechter, I. 1977. The effects of message speed on auditory comprehension in patients with cerebral cranial injury. *Scandinavian Journal of Rehabilitation Medicine, 9,* 169–171.

Blumstein, S. E. 1973. *A Phonological investigation of aphasic speech.* The Hague: Mouton.

Blumstein, S. E., Baker, E., & Goodglass, H. 1977. Phonological factors in auditory comprehension in aphasia. *Neuropsychologia, 15,* 19–30.

Blumstein, S. E., Cooper, W. E., Goodglass, H., Statlender, S., & Gottlieb, J. 1980. Production deficits in aphasia: A voice-onset time analysis. *Brain and Language, 9,* 153–170.

Blumstein, S. E., Cooper, W. E., Zurif, E., & Caramazza, A. 1977. The perception and production of voice-onset time in aphasia. *Neuropsychologia, 15,* 371–383.

Blumstein, S., & Goodglass, H. 1972. The perception of stress as a semantic cue in aphasia. *Journal of Speech and Hearing Research, 15,* 800–806.

Blumstein, S. E., Tartter, V., & Nigro, G. 1981. The perception of acoustic cues for place of articulation in aphasia. Manuscript in preparation.

Boller, F. 1978. Comprehension disorders in aphasia: A historical review. *Brain and Language, 5,* 149–165.

Bond, Z. S. 1976. On the specification of input units in speech perception. *Brain and Language, 3,* 72–87.

Bouman, L., & Grünbaum, A. 1925. Experimentell-psychologische Untersuchungen sur Aphasie und Paraphasie. *Zeitschrift fur die gesamte Neurologie und Psychiatrie, 96,* 481–538.

Buckingham, H. W., Jr. 1979. Explanation in apraxia with consequences for the concept of apraxia of speech. *Brain and Language, 8,* 202–226.

Burns, M. S., & Canter, G. C. 1977. Phonemic behavior of aphasic patients with posterior cerebral lesions. *Brain and Language, 4,* 492–507.

Carmon, A., & Nachson, I. 1971. Effect of unilateral brain damage on perception of temporal order. *Cortex, 7,* 410–418.

Cermak, L., & Moreines, J. 1976. Verbal retention deficits in aphasic and amnesic patients. *Brain and Language, 3,* 16–27.

Chomsky, N., & Halle, M. 1968. *The sound pattern of English.* New York: Harper.

Cohen, D., Dubois, J., Gauthier, M., Hécaen, H., & Angelergues, R. 1963. Aspects du fonctionnement du code linguistique chez les aphasiques moteurs. *Neuropsychologia, 1,* 165–177.

Cooper, W. E., & Sorenson, J. 1980. *Fundamental frequency in sentence production.* New York: Springer-Verlag.

Critchley, M. 1952. Articulatory defects in aphasia. *Journal of Laryngology and Otology, 66,* 1–17.

Danley, M., de Villiers, J. G., & Cooper, W. E. 1979. The control of speech prosody in Broca's aphasia. In J. J. Wolf and D. H. Klatt (Eds.), *Speech communication papers presented at the 97th meeting of the Acoustical Society of America.* New York: Acoustical Society of America.

Danley, M., & Shapiro, B. 1980. Speech prosody in Broca's aphasia. Unpublished manuscript.

Degiovanni, E., Khomsi, A., Bosser, E., Souffront, L., Moller, J. N., & Posson, J. 1977. Approche des troubles de l'integration phonémique chez les aphasiques interet d'analyses sonagraphiques. *Revue D'Oto-Neuro-Ophthamologie, 49,* 141–153.

DeRenzi, E., & Vignolo, L. A. 1962. The Token Test: A sensitive test to detect receptive disturbances in aphasia. *Brain, 85,* 665–678.

Dubois, J., Hécaen, H., Angelergues, R., Chatelier, M., & Marcie, P. 1964. Etude neurolinguistique de l'aphasie de conduction. *Neuropsychologia, 2,* 9–44.

Dunlop, J. M., & Marquardt, T. P. 1977. Linguistic and articulatory aspects of single word production in apraxia of speech. *Cortex, 8,* 17–29.

Efron, R. 1963. Temporal perception, aphasia, and déjà-vu. *Brain, 86,* 403–423.

Freeman, F. J., Sands, E. S., & Harris, K. S. 1978. Temporal coordination of phonation and articulation in a case of verbal apraxia: A voice-onset time study. *Brain and Language, 6,* 106–111.

Froschels, E. 1915. Zur Behandlung des motorischen Aphasie. *Archives Psychiatrist, 56,* 1–19.

Goldstein, K. 1948. *Language and language disturbances.* New York: Grune & Stratton.

Goodglass, H. 1968. Studies in the grammar of aphasics. In S. Rosenberg & J. Koplin (Eds.), *Developments in applied psycholinguistics.* New York: Macmillan.

Goodglass, H., Gleason, J. B., Bernholtz, N. A., & Hyde, M. R. 1972. Some linguistic structures in the speech of a Broca's aphasic. *Cortex, 8,* 191–212.

Goodglass, H., Quadfasel, F. A., & Timberlake, W. H. 1964. Phrase length and the type of severity of aphasia. *Cortex, 1,* 133–152.

Green, E. 1969. Phonological and grammatical aspects of jargon in an aphasic patient: A case study. *Language and Speech, 12,* 103–118.

Green, E., & Boller, F. 1974. Features of auditory comprehension in severely impaired aphasics. *Cortex, 10,* 133–145.

Halpern, H., Keith, R. L., & Darley, F. L. 1976. Phonemic behavior of aphasic subjects without dysarthria or apraxia of speech. *Cortex, 12,* 365–372.

Hatfield, F. M., & Walton, K. 1975. Phonological patterns in a case of aphasia. *Language and Speech, 18,* 341–357.

Head, H. 1926. *Aphasia and kindred disorders of speech* (2 vols.). New York: Hafner.

Itoh, M., Sasanuma, S., Hirose, H., Yoshioka, H., & Ushijima, T. 1980. Abnormal articulatory dynamics in a patient with apraxia of speech. *Brain and Language, 11,* 66–75.

Itoh, M., Sasanuma, S., Tatsumi, I., & Kobayashi, Y. 1979. Voice onset time characteristics of apraxia of speech. *Annual Bulletin of Logopedics and Phoniatrics, 13,* 123–132.

Itoh, M., Sasanuma, S., & Ushijima, T. 1979. Velar movements during speech in a patient with apraxia of speech. *Brain and Language, 7,* 227–239.

Jackson, J. H. 1958. *Selected writings of John Hughlings Jackson,* (Vol. 2) (J. Taylor, Ed.). New York: Basic Books.

Jakobson, R. 1968. [*Child language, aphasia, and phonological universals*] (A. R. Keiler, trans.). The Hague: Mouton.

Jakobson, R., Fant, G., & Halle, M. 1962. *Preliminaries to speech analysis.* Cambridge, Mass.: MIT Press.

Jauhiainen, T., & Nuutila, A. 1977. Auditory perception of speech and speech sounds in recent and recovered cases of aphasia. *Brain and Language, 4,* 572–579.

Johns, D. F., & LaPointe, L. L. 1976. Neurogenic disorders of output processing: Apraxia of speech. In H. Whitaker & H. A. Whitaker (Eds.), *Studies in neurolinguistics* (Vol. 1). New York: Academic Press.

Kagan, A. A. 1977. Articulatory difficulties of an aphasic with apraxia of speech. *South African Journal of Communication Disorders, 24,* 23–40.

Katz, B. 1979. The effects of slow speech on auditory comprehension in aphasia. Unpublished masters thesis, Brown University.

Keller, E. 1975. Vowel errors in aphasia. Unpublished doctoral dissertation, University of Toronto.

Keller, E. 1978. Parameters of vowel substitutions in Broca's aphasia. *Brain and Language, 5,* 265–285.

Klatt, D. 1980. Speech perception: a model of acoustic–phonetic analysis and lexical access. In R. A. Cole (Ed.), *Perception and production of fluent speech.* Hillsdale: Lawrence Erlbaum.

Klich, R. J., Ireland, J. V., & Weidner, W. B. 1979. Articulatory and phonological aspects of consonant substitution in apraxia of speech. *Cortex, 15,* 451–470.

Lasky, E. Z., Weidner, W. E., & Johnson, J. P., 1976. Influence of linguistic complexity, rate of presentation, and interphrase pause time on auditory-verbal comprehension of adult aphasic patients. *Brain and Language, 3,* 386–395.

Lebrun, Y., Buyssens, E., & Henneaux, J. 1973. Phonetic aspects of anarthria. *Cortex, 9,* 126–135.

Lecours, A. R., & Lhermitte, F. 1969. Phonemic paraphasias: Linguistic structures and tentative hypotheses. *Cortex, 5,* 193–228.

Lecours, A. R., & Lhermitte, F. 1976. The "pure form" of the phonetic disintegration syndrome (pure anarthria); Anatomo-clinical report of a historical case. *Brain and Language, 3,* 88–113.

Lehiste, I. 1968. *Some acoustic characteristics of dysarthria.* Switzerland: Biblioteca Phonetica.

Lesser, R. 1978. *Linguistic investigations of aphasia.* London: Arnold.

Liberman, A. M., Cooper, F. S., Shankweiler, D. P., & Studdert-Kennedy, M. 1967. Perception of the speech code. *Psychological Review, 74,* 431–461.

Lieberman, P. 1967. *Intonation, perception, and language.* Cambridge, Mass.: MIT Press.

Luria, A. R. 1966. *Higher cortical functions in man.* New York: Basic Books.

Martin, A. D. 1974. Some objections to the term apraxia of speech. *Journal of Speech and Hearing Disorders, 39,* 53–64.

Martin, A. D. 1975. Reply to Aten, Darley, Deal, and Johns. *Journal of Speech and Hearing Disorders, 40,* 420–422.

Martin, A. D., & Rigrodsky, S. 1974. An investigation of phonological impairment in aphasia: 2, Distinctive feature analysis of phonemic commutation errors in aphasia. *Cortex, 10,* 329–346.

Martin, A. D., Wasserman, N. H., Gilden, L., & West, J. 1975. A process model of repetition in aphasia: An investigation of phonological and morphological interactions in aphasic error performance. *Brain and Language, 2,* 434–450.

Miceli, G., Caltagirone, C., Gainotti, G., & Payer-Rigo, P. 1978. Discrimination of voice versus place contrasts in aphasia. *Brain and Language, 6,* 47–51.

Miceli, G., Gainotti, G., Caltagirone, C., & Masullo, C. 1980. Some aspects of phonological impairment in aphasia. *Brain and Language, 11,* 159–169.

Peuser, G., & Fittschen, M. 1977. On the universality of language dissolution: The case of a Turkish aphasic. *Brain and Language, 4,* 196–207.

Ryalls, J. 1980. Intonation and Broca's aphasia. Unpublished manuscript.

Ryalls, J. 1981. Motor aphasia: Acoustic correlates of phonetic disintegration in vowels. *Neuropsychologia,* in press.

Sasanuma, S., Tatsumi, I. F., & Fujisaki, H. 1976. Discrimination of phonemes and word accent types in Japanese aphasic patients. *XVIth International Congress of Logopedics and Phoniatrics,* 403–408.

Schuell, H. R., Jenkins, J. J., & Jiménez-Pabón, J. E. 1964. *Aphasia in adults.* New York: Harper.

Shankweiler, D. P., & Harris, K. S. 1966. An experimental approach to the problem of articulation in aphasia. *Cortex, 2,* 277–292.

Shankweiler, D. P., Harris, K. S., & Taylor, M. L. 1968. Electromyographic study of articulation in aphasia. *Archives of Physical Medicine and Rehabilitation, 49,* 1–8.

Sherwin, I., & Efron, R. 1980. Temporal ordering deficits following anterior temporal lobectomy. *Brain and Language, 11,* 195–203.

Shewan, C. M. 1980. Phonological processing in Broca's aphasics. *Brain and Language, 10,* 71–88.

Swisher, L., & Hirsh, I. J. 1972. Brain damage and the ordering of two temporally successive stimuli. *Neuropsychologia, 10,* 137–152.

Tallal, P., & Newcombe, F. 1978. Impairment of auditory perception and language comprehension in dysphasia. *Brain and Language, 5,* 13–24.

Taylor, J. (Ed.). 1958. *Selected writings of John Hughlings Jackson (Vol. 2)* New York: Basic Books.

Tikofsky, R. 1965. *Phonetic characteristics of dysarthria.* Michigan: Office of Research Administration.

Trost, J. E., & Canter, G. J. 1974. Apraxia of speech in patients with Broca's aphasia: A study of phoneme production accuracy and error patterns. *Brain and Language, 1,* 63–79.

Weidner, W., & Lasky, E. 1976. The interaction of rate and complexity of stimulus on the performance of adult aphasic subjects. *Brain and Language, 3,* 34–40.

6

Syntactic Aspects of Aphasia[1]

RITA SLOAN BERNDT and ALFONSO CARAMAZZA

The recent surge of interest in the phenomenon of aphasia is at least partly traceable to the notion that the theories and methods of linguistics and psychology, which have provided a framework for considering the structure and processes involved in language, might be useful in describing systematically the forms that language breakdown can take. Ultimately, the hope is that a detailed description of aphasic syndromes in terms of psycholinguistic components might result in a set of brain–function correlations that provides some information about how language is represented in the brain. In addition, the selective disturbance of linguistic components in aphasia might reasonably be expected to provide information about the functioning of those components in the normal system (Caramazza & Berndt, 1978).

The separate discussion of phonology, syntax, and semantics must not be taken, however, as an indication that these components function independently. The production and comprehension of language relies on a highly interactive system of linguistic structures and processes, and it is no simple matter to deal with them in isolation from one another. This is especially true for syntax—the component of the system that specifies the structural relations among words in sentences—since syntax cannot reasonably be separated from the other aspects of words that make up sentences. That is, while phonological investigations can proceed independently of syntax and semantics by presenting individual phonemes in isolation, syntactic structures necessarily involve the rela-

1. The preparation of this manuscript was supported by NIH research grant No. 16155 to the Johns Hopkins University.

157

tions among words and other morphemes that also have a specific phonological representation and encode a particular meaning. One implication of this lack of independence between syntactic structure and other aspects of language is that disruption at the level of phonological or lexical–semantic processing may appear to result in an impairment of syntax. Put differently, it is very difficult to uncover specifically syntactic impairments in patients who also show evidence of severe phonological or lexical–semantic disruption. For example, even if syntactic mechanisms were intact, patients would not be expected to perform a syntactic analysis in comprehension on a set of words they could not recognize for phonological or semantic reasons. These points will be developed in separate discussions of the syndromes of Broca's and Wernicke's aphasia.

Some additional introductory remarks must be made concerning the expected relationship between comprehension and production. The shift of emphasis away from the "expressive"–"receptive" distinction toward a view that aphasia impairs abstract linguistic components has encouraged the notion of the "central" linguistic deficit. That is, aphasia can be argued to result in a deficit that involves the actual form and content of the patient's knowledge about some aspect of language, rather than in impaired ability to use his or her (intact) knowledge in particular tasks (Whitaker, 1970). The argument that the aphasic patient suffers such a central deficit to a linguistic component predicts that the deficit will be manifested in all tasks that require the participation of the affected component, regardless of modality of input.

The theoretical assumption guiding these comments is that both comprehension and production involve the same linguistic structures; that is, the abstract syntactic rules that are necessary to guide the production of a successfully grammatical utterance are also needed to perform a syntactic analysis on a sentence in comprehension. The same applies to the auditory–verbal versus the visual channels of input and output. That is, the extraction of meaning from a written sentence is assumed to require the same syntactic information for correct comprehension as is the extraction of the same information from an aurally presented sentence. Planning the syntactic form of a sentence is assumed to involve similar syntactic structures regardless of whether the ultimate product is spoken or written. Although these generalizations are presumably true at an abstract structural level, they are not meant to imply that the same processing components are involved in comprehension and production (reading, listening, speaking, and writing). Clearly, the actual processes that are involved in planning and executing sentences and in listening to and understanding another's utterances are quite dissimilar, and ultimately they rely on different physiological systems altogether (see Garrett, 1980, for discussion). Similarly, the "real-time" processing demands of understanding a fleeting acoustic input in auditory comprehension are quite different from the requirements of extracting meaning from the static graphic input of a written sentence. The point is that, despite the differences in processing demands in these different tasks, they are all presumed to exploit the same structural information. If that information is disrupted, symptoms should be found in all of these performances, although they may not be manifested in the same way or to the same extent.

Syntactic Processing in the Normal System

Recent psycholinguistic approaches to the components of language have proceeded largely independently of current debates within linguistics concerning the proper characterization of the syntactic component. Instead, an effort has been made to provide linguistic descriptions that have psychological validity, but these may bear little relation to the formal rules of linguistic grammars.

In current psycholinguistic models, the rules of the syntactic component in language comprehension rely on surface structure parsing strategies that directly assign logical roles to major lexical items unless counterindicated by other syntactic and semantic information. This is essentially the approach of the Augmented Transition Network Models (Kimball, 1975), but it has also been adopted by an increasing number of psycholinguists working outside the framework of artificial intelligence (Clark & Clark, 1977).

A major portion of the syntactic processes within this framework is based on operations that specify co-occurrence relations among the category values of lexical items, such as the facts that a determiner can immediately precede a noun but not a verb, that a conjunction can conjoin two noun phrases or two verb phrases but not a noun phrase and a verb phrase, that within a clause a noun cannot immediately follow another noun, and so on. This set of co-occurrence relations serves to specify a surface structure parser that assigns grammatical roles to its constituents.

Within this type of model, the traditional distinction drawn by grammarians between the grammatical morphemes (both bound and free) and the class of "content" words (major lexical items) is especially important. The free grammatical morphemes (function words) play a crucial role in strategies for the segmentation of speech into constituents that are sufficient to determine logical roles, as in distinguishing between the following pairs of sentences:

> *The ball was hit to John.*
> *The ball was hit by John.*

Structural information in addition to that supplied by the grammatical morphemes—specifically information about the order in which noun phrases are arranged around the verb—is necessary to assign the logical roles in the following pair of sentences:

> *The boy chased the girl.*
> *The girl was chased by the boy.*

Therefore, a minimal description of the syntactic processing required to interpret an utterance consists in assigning category labels to lexical items, using the structure marking properties of the grammatical morphemes to parse the utterance into constituents, and attending to the order of constituents in the sentence sequence.

In general terms, the same basic elements are required for the production of syntactically correct sentences. From the initial formulation of a proposition to be expressed, the lexical items and a syntactic frame must be selected that encodes the grammatical morphemes and major lexical items of the sentence into the proper sequence (see Garrett, 1975, for a model of sentence production).

This very rudimentary description of syntactic processes constitutes only a limited part of what must be included in the syntactic component of a complete model of language processing, but it serves here as an adequate starting point for the consideration of syntactic disorders.

Syntactic Deficits in Aphasia

The productive deficits characterizing fluent and nonfluent aphasia types have for many years been described with reference to what are now considered to be syntactic descriptions (Goodglass, 1968). The speech production associated with damage to the anterior portions of the dominant hemisphere is described as AGRAMMATIC—largely devoid of the elements that provide syntactic structure. Speech produced by patients with damage in the posterior portions of the dominant hemisphere is described as PARAGRAMMATIC—characterized by an inappropriate use of syntactic elements. Although early descriptions suggested that both patient types showed evidence of disordered syntax, it is clear that these two syndromes involve very different types of disorders. Here we will assess work that investigates the extent to which each of these patient types suffers from what can be described as a syntactic deficit.

Broca's Aphasia

Agrammatic speech is one of the symptoms associated with Broca's aphasia, a symptom complex that is characterized by effortful, dysprosodic, short utterances composed largely of major lexical items (Goodglass & Kaplan, 1972). Clinically, the comprehension of the Broca's aphasic is said to be relatively spared. We have suggested elsewhere that the syndrome of Broca's aphasia involves a basic disruption of the syntactic component of the linguistic system (Berndt & Caramazza, 1980); here we will review the evidence, from production and from comprehension, that this is the case.

SPEECH PRODUCTION

The "telegraphic" appearance of the speech produced by Broca's aphasics results from a selective omission of the small "grammatical" words of the language—the articles, conjunctions, pronouns, auxiliary verbs, and prepositions that provide cues to the syntactic structure of sentences. The bound grammatical morphemes (e.g., plural and possessive markers on nouns; person, tense, and number inflections of verbs) tend also to be omitted in Broca speech. This qualitative description of agrammatic speech has been found to characterize the performance of these patients in spontaneous speech (de Villiers, 1974), in sentence completion tasks (Gleason, Goodglass, Green, Ackerman, & Hyde, 1975), in sentence repetition (Goodglass, Fodor &, Schulhoff, 1967), and in picture description (Gleason, Goodglass, Obler, Green, Hyde, & Weintraub, 1980). The omission of the structural, syntactic cues to sentence organization has been found in languages other than English, even though these elements may be represented in the surface structure in quite dissimilar ways. Descriptions of agrammatism are available for speakers of Russian (Luria, 1947/1970), Japanese (Panse & Shimoyama, 1973), Turkish (Peuser & Fittschen, 1977), and Ndebele (Traill, 1970).

The importance of the role of the grammatical morphemes in providing structural information about sentences has led to the interpretation of agrammatism as a disorder that affects the patient's ability to combine individual words into a unified sentence (Jakobson, 1956; Luria, 1947/ 1970). An alternative interpretation of agrammatism views the patient as omitting relatively inessential words in an effort to maximize the content of the message with the least amount of effort (Lenneberg, 1973; Pick, 1913). Within this view, the patient suffers no basic linguistic deficit; the fact that it is the grammatical elements that are lost is simply a function of their relatively low information value.

These two positions represent very different ideas about the nature of agrammatism in Broca's aphasia, and they should be evaluated within the context of the entire constellation of symptoms associated with the syndrome. In an attempt to characterize the productive aspects of agrammatism, researchers have exploited the fact that the omission of grammatical morphemes in Broca speech is rarely total. Some elements are always omitted or always produced, others will be retained in some contexts but not in others. Attempts to account for the pattern of omission in agrammatic speech have uncovered some regularities in the frequency of omission of various elements (de Villiers, 1974; Gleason *et al.*, 1975). The regular plural inflection (-*s*) and the present participle of the verb (-*ing*) are among the most frequent grammatical morphemes produced, while the markers required for other verb tenses (-*ed, will*) are among the least often produced. Although there is no obvious explanation for this ordering of probability of occurrence in Broca speech (see de Villiers, 1974, for discussion), several factors have been shown to be important.

Goodglass and Berko (1960) found that the syllabic form of a noun or verb inflection (*hors es*; *wait ed*) is more often produced by the agrammatic aphasic than is the nonsyllabic form (*dogs*; *play ed*). The added phonological salience of an additional syllable apparently facilitates production for the agrammatic patient, whereas it impairs production for Wernicke's aphasics and for small children.

Another factor that has been shown to affect the probability that a grammatical function word will be produced involves a combination of its phonological prominence (stress assignment) and position in a sentence. Goodglass (1968) has shown that the element most often omitted in Broca speech is an unstressed function word occurring in sentence initial position (Goodglass *et al.*, 1967). The same function word was shown to be much more subject to omission when occurring as the first element of an utterance (*Can birds fly*) than when occurring as the second element (*Birds can fly*), unless the initial functor was stressed (*Can't birds fly*). Goodglass (1968, 1976) argues that the agrammatic patient is most impaired in the ability to initiate speech and requires a "salient" (stressed) element to do so.

Although the importance of stress in function word production has been amply demonstrated, the value of stress as an explanation for the syndrome must be considered carefully. The utilization of stressed words by the agrammatic patient to initiate speech does not account entirely for the pattern of omission in Broca speech (Gleason *et al.*,

1975), nor does it explain the other structural characteristics of agramma- tic utterances discussed in the following pages. It may be that the regu- larities in patients' production of function words that can be attributed to stress are descriptions of mechanisms that the patient relies on to com- pensate for an inability to use standard linguistic means to structure utterances.

Nonetheless, the distinction between the grammatical morphemes and the substantive elements of a sentence can be formally described as involving a phonological distinction, and an explanation of Broca's aphasia based on the phonological properties of the elements omitted in agrammatic speech has been offered (Kean, 1978, 1980). This argument explicitly states that the deficit suffered by the Broca aphasic is phonological rather than syntactic. Agrammatic output results from a reduction of the phonological structure of a sentence to those elements (called phonological words) that function in the assignment of stress patterns in sentences. The grammatical morphemes are not phonologi- cal words—(that is, they don't play a part in the assignment of sentential stress)—and are therefore omitted. Although this hypothesis encounters some difficulties accounting for the data it was proposed to explain (see Kolk, 1978b), it is most deficient in its ability to deal with characteristics of agrammatic speech other than omissions. That is, there are structural features of the utterances produced by agrammatic speakers that are not easily explained as the result of phonological reduction.

The number and complexity of grammatical structures available to the agrammatic aphasic is severely reduced, and this reduction cannot be entirely explained as a by-product of a difficulty producing grammatical morphemes. That is, the correct production of certain syntactic construc- tions (e.g., questions) requires the production of a grammatical function word (i.e., an auxiliary verb). If the reduction of syntactic structure in Broca's aphasia were limited to loss of structures such as interrogatives that REQUIRE function word production, then this syntactic reduction might be viewed as a consequence of the loss of facility with function words. Then the simplification of syntactic structure in the Broca syn- drome might reasonably be thought to be a product of the patient's problems producing function words (which might be argued to result from "economy of effort" or phonological simplification), rather than as a reflection of a primarily syntactic disturbance.

The structural simplification appears to be far more profound in many cases than would be predicted by such an explanation, however. In the most severe cases, speech may consist of single words (primarily nouns) separated by pauses (Goodglass, 1976). Even less impaired patients, who may be capable of generating a simple "sentence" by juxtaposing a noun and a verb, may have difficulty producing other combinations involving substantives, such as two adjectives to modify a noun, or the expansion of a verb phrase to include an indirect object noun (Gleason *et al.*, 1975; Goodglass, Gleason, Bernholtz, & Hyde, 1972). That is, agrammatic constructions, such as *large white house* or *boy give mother book*, are rarely produced by Broca's aphasics, even though they require only major lexical items. More complex constructions—questions, negative sentences, relative clause constructions—are also rarely produced (Gleason *et al.*, 1980; Myerson & Goodglass, 1972).

It is important to note that agrammatic patients seem not to have lost the conceptual bases for these constructions and have no less need to convey complex information, despite their inability to use the linguistic means available to the normal speaker. Agrammatic patients often use alternative means to produce sentences equivalent to those constructions they do not produce (Gleason *et al.*, 1975, 1980), such as substitution of direct speech (e.g., *She said: Clean your room*) for a relative clause construction (*She told her to clean her room*).

The suggestion has been made that the structural abnormalities found in agrammatic speech include a basic inability to order syntactically the noun phrase and verb phrase elements to encode semantic information such as agent–action–object relations (Saffran, Schwartz, & Marin, 1980b). Although the production of correct word order has been assumed to be within the Broca patient's list of "spared" abilities (Goodglass & Kaplan, 1972), Saffran and colleagues argue that the frequent production of normal subject–verb–object (SVO) order by agrammatic patients results not from their utilization of syntactic ordering rules but from the application of a semantically based strategy of beginning utterances with animate nouns. In a picture description task, agrammatic patients ($N=5$) were considerably more likely to begin an utterance with an incorrect noun when the objects in the picture were alike in animacy (e.g., a dog chasing a cat; a pencil in a sink) than when the subject noun was animate and the object noun was inanimate (a boy pulling a wagon). The pictures eliciting the greatest number of ordering errors depicted an inanimate subject and an animate object (a ball hitting a boy).

Saffran, Schwartz, and Marin (1980b) argue that the agrammatic patient is unable to utilize the normal syntactic criteria for selection of the grammatical subject when generating a sentence but relies instead on the perceptual–conceptual salience of an animate constituent.

Speech Production: Summary and Interpretation. The results reviewed here demonstrate that the speech production characteristic of Broca's aphasia is deviant in ways that go beyond the frequent omission of the grammatical morphemes. Syntactic structure is greatly reduced, and abnormal constructions are produced that violate some of the most basic organizational principles of English syntax. Many of the structural characteristics of agrammatic speech cannot be interpreted as a by-product of the omission of grammatical morphemes and thus cannot be explained as a consequence of phonological simplification or economy of effort.

Several attempts have been made to provide an account of agrammatic production that is motivated by syntactic considerations. Marshall (1977) explicitly rejects the notion that agrammatism can be explained by hypotheses that focus on omission of the grammatical morphemes. Rather, Marshall offers an hypothesis that the structure of agrammatic speech results from the patient's failure to elaborate successfully the syntactic representation that underlies an utterance, so that the surface structure realization of the sentence contains only the major lexical items. That is, "elements are not 'deleted' before the articulatory program is run; they were never there in the first place [p. 141]." Although the precise mechanisms involved have not been spelled out, such a failure to elaborate a syntactic representation could presumably result in any and all of the structural deviations that characterize Broca speech.

Saffran, Schwartz, and Marin (1980a) argue that two separate deficits underlie agrammatic production: a syntactic deficit that results in the word order aberrations and other structural characteristics of agrammatic speech, and a phonological deficit that impairs the patient's ability to produce the grammatical morphemes. The reasons given for postulating dual impairments include the importance of phonological salience to the production of bound morphemes (as reported by Goodglass & Berko, 1960) and the occurrence of a patient who showed the characteristic structural deficits associated with Broca's aphasia but did not omit the grammatical morphemes. Saffran and co-workers argue that the two symptoms of agrammatism (structural abnormalities and omission of grammatical morphemes) reflect impairment to different stages in the production of sentences: the stage at which the syntactic frame is specified, and a stage of phonological realization. The validity of these separate stages is supported by data obtained on the production of speech errors by normals (Garrett, 1975).

We have argued that the omission of the grammatical morphemes, as well as the structural aspects of agrammatic speech, result from a disruption of syntactic processing abilities in Broca's aphasics that is reflected in all aspects of performance that requires syntactic analysis (Berndt & Caramazza, 1980; see also Caramazza & Berndt, 1978, Caramazza,

Berndt, Basili & Koller, in press; Zurif & Caramazza, 1976). That is, there is evidence that in tasks that do not require speech production, Broca patients are impaired in their ability to use the grammatical morphemes and other structural cues to arrive at a correct interpretation of sentences. This evidence, reviewed in the following section, can be combined with the production data to provide a comprehensive picture of the Broca syndrome.

COMPREHENSION AND OTHER "RECEPTIVE" ABILITIES

Clinical descriptions of Broca's aphasics have emphasized their relatively intact "receptive" abilities in contrast to their severe "expressive" problems (Goodglass & Kaplan, 1972; Wepman & Jones, 1964). In normal communicative situations, as well as in most clinical tests, Broca's aphasics appear to understand speech with little difficulty, although such tests as the Token Test (De Renzi & Vignolo, 1962), designed to find more subtle comprehension deficits, have shown that comprehension in these patients is less than intact (Poeck, Kerschensteiner, & Hartje, 1972).

The question of interest here is whether "subtle" comprehension deficits experienced by Broca's aphasics can be related to the types of problems they encounter in speech production. That is, do Broca's aphasics have relatively more difficulty with syntactic versus semantic aspects of sentences in comprehension? Several early attempts to demonstrate a syntactic comprehension deficit among Broca patients failed to find any qualitative differences in performance between Broca's and Wernicke's aphasics on sentence–picture matching tasks (Parisi & Pizzamiglio, 1970; Shewan, 1976; Shewan & Canter, 1971). The apparent similarity in the nature of comprehension errors produced by these disparate patient types supported the notion that comprehension is a "unitary" phenomenon that cannot be successfully decomposed into components that are subject to selective impairment (Boller, Kim, & Mack, 1977).

There are several reasons that this conclusion is not justified (see Berndt & Caramazza, 1980, for fuller discussion). First, in order to determine whether a patient is able to perform a syntactic analysis in sentence comprehension, the target sentences must be designed so that they REQUIRE syntactic analysis and cannot be successfully interpreted simply by understanding the individual meanings of the major lexical items. For example, Shewan and Canter's (1971) sentence materials included passive sentences, such as *The letter was mailed by the man*, which can be readily interpreted by anyone who knows the meanings of *letter*, *mail*, and *man* and who has an intact knowledge of the normal relations that obtain among these items in the world. Second, if a claim is to be evaluated that different patient types have different kinds of comprehension problems, then a means must be provided in the experimental situation for determining the cause of comprehension errors. For example, Parisi and Pizzamiglio (1970) included semantically reversible sentences, such as *The boy is pushed by the girl,* which requires syntactic analysis, but provided only one distractor type. Thus, all patients who failed to understand the sentence, either for syntactic or semantic reasons, could choose between the correct alternative and one other. Given this situation, it is not surprising that different "patterns" of performance failed to emerge.

During the last 5 years, several studies have been reported demonstrating that, when these factors are adequately controlled, Broca patients do indeed show evidence of a comprehension disorder that is qualitatively distinct from the comprehension disorder that is suffered by Wernicke's aphasics. The question that has not been completely resolved concerns the precise mechanisms that are responsible for this deficit. Again, the primary debate concerns whether or not the Broca patients' disorder can be wholly attributed to an inability to process the grammatical morphemes of the language. If so, explanations of agrammatism that hinge on the processing of grammatical morphemes might be extended to account for the comprehension deficits that have been demonstrated (Kean, 1980). On the other hand, if the Broca patients' comprehension problems can be shown to involve aspects of syntactic structure that are separate from the grammatical morphemes, then an explanation stressing a deficit that involves syntactic processing in general, including but not limited to processing of the grammatical morphemes, would be required.

There is considerable evidence that Broca's aphasics do not have complete control over the grammatical morphemes in comprehension. Heilman and Scholes (1976) demonstrated that Broca's aphasics failed to utilize a definite article to parse indirect object and direct object constituents. In a sentence–picture matching task, a group of nine Broca's aphasics responded to such sentences as

> *They showed her the horse shoes.*

> and

> *They showed her horse the shoes.*

as if the article were not there and the sentence were ambiguous:

> *They showed her horse shoes.*

Broca patients did not choose picture distractors that portrayed incorrect lexical items, although these were frequently chosen by a group of Wernicke's aphasics who were also tested.

Other investigations of Broca patients' abilities to process function words have shown that they are insensitive to the differential semantic value of the definite and indefinite articles (Goodenough, Zurif, & Weintraub, 1977) and that their memory for function words in the surface structure of sentences is significantly impaired relative to their memory for content words (Caramazza, Zurif, & Gardner, 1978). In an investigation of the role of sentential stress and word class on comprehension, Broca's aphasics responded more slowly to function words than to content words (independent of stress), unlike normal subjects (Swinney, Zurif, & Cutler, 1980).

In a series of metalinguistic studies that minimized the burdens imposed by the "real-time" processing constraints of auditory comprehension, aphasic patients and normal subjects were asked to make successive judgments of which two out of three words from a sentence "go best together" (Zurif, Caramazza, & Myerson, 1972; Zurif, Green, Caramazza, & Goodenough, 1976). Analysis is based on a matrix of the similarity judgments obtained from the patients' choices for all possible combinations of words from a target sentence. For normal subjects, this procedure has been shown to recover the hierarchical structure of sentence constituents (Levelt, 1970). The similarity judgments of Broca's aphasics yielded aberrant structures, in that content words tended to be grouped with each other rather than with function words. Normal noun phrases—articles plus nouns—did not result, although patients were somewhat more successful in producing tightly bound noun phrases when possessive pronouns (*my shoes*) rather than articles (*the shoes*) were the function word member of the constituent. The advantage of the pronouns relative to articles, which presumably resulted from their increased semantic information, was attenuated in semantically complex sentences (Zurif & Caramazza, 1976; Zurif et al., 1976).

In another type of metalinguistic task, German-speaking aphasics were required to rearrange the scrambled constituents of a sentence into the correct order (von Stockert & Bader, 1976). This sentence order task relied on the fact that the German language differentiates subject nouns from object nouns by a morphological variation of accompanying articles, while word order is relatively free. Some of the sentences, when arranged correctly syntactically on the basis of the article, were semantically anomalous (e.g., *The rabbit shoots the hunter*). Other sentences were grammatically structured nonsense, which also utilized the article variants to mark subjective and objective case. Broca's aphasics ($N=10$)

were virtually unable to order the nonsense strings using only morphological cues and produced very few correct orderings of the anomalous sentences. Instead, they most often produced syntactically deviant orders that expressed the nonanomalous semantic relation (e.g., *The hunter* [marked as object] *shoots the rabbit* [marked as subject]). Despite severely impaired reading comprehension, Wernicke's aphasics ($N=10$) produced syntactically well-formed sentences, presumably by relying on the morphological cues. These results are interpreted by von · Stockert and Bader as an indication of a double dissociation between syntactic and lexical–semantic abilities in these two patient types.

All of the results reviewed thus far can be interpreted as an indication that Broca's aphasics cannot process the grammatical morphemes. The argument has been made that it is precisely the elements that these patients omit in spontaneous speech that cause difficulties in comprehension tasks (Zurif & Blumstein, 1978). This problem with the grammatical morphemes could be said to result from a general disruption of syntactic processing abilities, or it could be attributed to some special characteristic of the class of grammatical morphemes, either phonological (Kean, 1980) or lexical (Bradley, Garrett, & Zurif, 1980), that renders them particularly susceptible to disruption.

The most important evidence available on this question involves further investigations of comprehension and metalinguistic abilities in Broca's aphasics. In a variation of Zurif and co-workers' metalinguistic task based on judgments of word relatedness within sentences, Kolk (1978b) demonstrated that some Broca's aphasics could not generate well-formed noun phrase constituents even when adjectives rather than articles were available as noun modifiers. Since adjectives do not share the "special" phonological or lexical properties of the class of function words, this result is interpreted as reflecting a basic disruption of the patients' ability to interpret sentence structure that was not linked in any obvious way to the grammatical morphemes.

Several comprehension tasks have been reported in which the interpretation of the sentence materials did not depend on any particular function word cue but required an interpretation of various surface structure cues, including word order. Caramazza and Zurif (1976) presented patients with center-embedded, object-relative constructions in a sentence–picture matching task. Some of the sentences employed strong semantic constraints (*The wagon that the horse is pulling is green*); others were semantically reversible (*The cat that the dog is biting is black*); and still others were semantically implausible (*The dog that the man is biting is black*). Picture distractors included foils showing a reversal of the actual agent–object relation (the "syntactic" distractor) and incorrect depictions of major lexical items (the "lexical" distractor). Broca's aphasics (N=5) performed well on the sentences with strong semantic constraints but performed at chance on reversible or implausible sentences when the pictured alternatives included a syntactic distractor.

Comprehension of the reversible center-embedded constructions requires syntactic processing that goes beyond a single function word marker and involves the ordering of the elements in the surface structure as well. No single functor provides a cue to the syntactic structure of these sentences, although the relative pronoun that introduces the clause has been shown to make processing somewhat easier (Fodor & Garrett, 1967).

Additional evidence that aspects of syntax in addition to the grammatical morphemes are disturbed in these patients was reported by Goodglass, Blumstein, Gleason, Hyde, Green, and Statlender (1979). Twelve Broca's aphasics were presented with subject-relative clause sentences, which did not employ a relative pronoun to mark the clause (e.g., *The man greeted by his wife was smoking a pipe*). Expanded versions of these sentences contained the same amount of linguistic information in a syntactically simpler construction (*The man was greeted by his wife and he was smoking a pipe*).

Broca's aphasics had significantly more difficulty understanding the syntactically complex versions of these sentences, providing strong evidence that the comprehension impairment in these patients involves a disruption of the ability to process syntactic information that is not limited to a failure to process the grammatical morphemes. Even in the most severe case that could be proposed—total inability to process ANY grammatical morphemes—the patient would be left with an identical residual string of substantives in both sentence types. The increased difficulty of the relative clause sentences must have resulted from factors other than (or in addition to) patients' difficulty processing the grammatical morphemes.

It should be pointed out that the results of these studies utilizing relative clause constructions have demonstrated a very high level of comprehension performance on the part of Broca's aphasics for sentences that do not require syntactic processing. It appears that these patients are quite capable of interpreting lengthy sentences when semantic cues are made available, a result that rules out a generalized comprehension problem or a short-term memory defect as possible explanations for their comprehension impairment. In addition, the good performance obtained from these patients in tasks with minimal syntactic demands supports the long-standing clinical description that comprehension is spared in Broca's aphasia.

Although it is the case that comprehension impairments are evident in these patients only under particular circumstances—when lexical–semantic information is not entirely sufficient for correct interpretation—it does not follow that the sentences that produce difficulty are necessarily long, infrequent, and/or complex constructions. Schwartz, Saffran, and Marin (1980) have demonstrated that Broca's (*N*=5) have great difficulty assigning agent–object roles to noun phrases in simple active and passive sentences when semantic cues are unavailable (*The robber was shot by the cop*). In addition, the same patients could not interpret simple locative constructions that were completely reversible (*The circle is behind the square*), even though they demonstrated good understanding of the prepositions themselves when word order was constrained (*The cow is in* [versus *beside*] *the barn*).

The primary syntactic cue to the underlying relations encoded by these simple reversible constructions is the order of the noun phrases around the verb or preposition. The Broca's aphasics who participated in this study appeared largely unable to use order information as a cue to determine the semantic relation in effect between the two nouns named in the sentence.

Summary. The evidence reviewed here indicates that the characterization of Broca's aphasia as an "expressive" deficit obscures a very systematic and now well-documented "receptive" deficit. In metalinguistic tasks, Broca's aphasics demonstrate a lack of understanding of the surface structure organization of sentences. In auditory comprehension, Broca's aphasics are deficient in their ability to use syntactic information about the structure of sentences to arrive at a correct interpretation of the meaning that the sentence encodes. There is considerable evidence that these impairments cannot be attributed solely to an inability to process the grammatical morphemes of the language, but involve other aspects of syntax, such as word order.

BROCA'S APHASIA: A SYNTACTIC DEFICIT

We have argued that the constellation of symptoms present in the production and comprehension of Broca's aphasics can be explained as a central disruption of the syntactic component of the language processing system, typically co-occurring with an independent disorder of articulation (Berndt & Caramazza, 1980). Such a disruption would have a predictable effect on the patient's ability to utilize the grammatical morphemes in production and in comprehension but should also produce additional aberrations in the syntactic structures produced and in the syntactic cues that can be utilized in comprehension. Since the deficit as proposed is assumed to involve a major component of the linguistic system that must be employed in all attempts to produce well-structured sentences or to extract meaning from sentences, it is expected that components of agrammatism will be found in the writing of Broca's aphasics and that the comprehension of written sentences should be impaired in the same way as it is in the auditory modality. There is some evidence that these predictions can be upheld both for writing (Goodglass & Hunter, 1970) and for reading (Samuels & Benson, 1979).

The hypothesis developed here is intended to provide the most parsimonious explanation possible for the constellation of symptoms that has been found in Broca's aphasia. It should be emphasized that the description of this syndrome as developed here is based on group studies that were focused on only one symptom at a time. There is little evidence with which to document the strong claim that all of these symptoms will be found to co-occur in all patients classed as Broca's aphasics. That is, we know little about whether patients can be found with agrammatism but without asyntactic comprehension, or vice versa. Until more data are available that document necessary cooccurrences of symptoms, it will be difficult to formulate stronger theories concerning the precise processing mechanisms that are compromised within particular syndromes.

For example, several of the metalinguistic studies reviewed in the preceding discussion divided the Broca patients into subgroups based on severity of productive deficits (Kolk, 1978a) or comprehension impairment (Zurif *et al.*, 1976) and subsequently reported differences in performance between the two subgroups. What is needed is enough information about the inabilities of the patients in the two subgroups that this heterogeneity within the syndrome can be elucidated. Another example is provided by Caplan, Matthei, and Gigley (in press), who report that 4 out of 10 Broca's aphasics were sensitive to syntactic distinctions in comprehending several types of gerundive constructions, while the remaining 6 were not. The authors explain this heterogeneity as a function of a difference in the ages of the patients who fell into the two groups, and no information is available concerning their performance on other tasks that might suggest an alternative explanation for the different types of performance obtained. In fact, the patients were classified as Broca's aphasics on the basis of dysprosody and utterance length, rather than on the basis of the presence of agrammatism, so it may be that some of the patients studied were cases of "pure anarthria" (Lecours & Lhermitte, 1976), who would not be expected to show a syntactic disturbance.

The importance of obtaining extensive information on patients' abilities in diverse language tasks cannot be overemphasized (see the discussion of conduction aphasia that follows). First, such information will provide a comprehensive picture of a patient's impairments and residual abilities that can be used in making decisions about clinical management. From a more theoretical perspective, accurate information about the co-occurrence of symptoms within a syndrome supplies the necessary basic information upon which theories of language impairment must be constructed. Without such information, we are reduced to providing accounts for individual isolated symptoms and may grossly misinterpret the locus of impairment.

Summary. The symptoms that characterize the syndrome of Broca's aphasia have been interpreted here as manifestations of a basic syntactic deficit, coupled with an independent deficit of articulation that affects speech production. The speech produced by these patients is typically composed of the simplest syntactic constructions, with frequent omission of the grammatical elements (the function words and bound grammatical morphemes) that provide structure to sentences. In tasks designed to constrain the production of words in a particular order, Broca patients have difficulty using the correct order of noun phrase elements to convey certain semantic relationships. In auditory comprehension and in metalinguistic judgments, Broca's aphasics are impaired in their ability to use syntactic cues, including grammatical morphemes and word order. The result is impaired comprehension of all sentences that cannot be interpreted solely on the basis of the major lexical items but require a syntactic analysis. All of these symptoms are interpreted as a manifestation of a syntactic impairment that should affect performance (in all modalities) in all tasks that require syntactic processing.

Conduction Aphasia

Perhaps the syndrome of conduction aphasia provides the most compelling evidence that our accounts of the mechanisms responsible for particular symptoms must be based on extensive information about the characteristics of the syndrome as a whole. Conduction aphasics produce relatively fluent and syntactically well-formed speech, exhibit good comprehension on clinical testing, and have inordinate difficulty repeating orally presented words and sentences.

Several of the tests of syntactic comprehension reported above found that conduction aphasics displayed the same "asyntactic" pattern that was displayed by the Broca patients (Caramazza & Zurif, 1976; Heilman & Scholes, 1976; see also Saffran & Marin, 1975). That is, comprehension was good only when semantic cues were available on which a correct interpretation could be based. Since the speech production of these patients is structurally well formed, this "syntactic" deficit seems to be limited to comprehension. It is not clear what specific mechanisms of syntactic processing could be responsible for such a deficit.

We have investigated some of the symptoms that co-occur with asyntactic comprehension in different patient types (Caramazza, Berndt, Basili, & Koller, in press). A conduction aphasic and two Broca patients were given a series of tests including sentence comprehension, story completion, oral reading, and sentence anagram. The two Broca patients displayed the total impairment in syntactic abilities described here: agrammatic speech, asyntactic comprehension, and asyntactic sentence construction in the anagram task. The conduction aphasic was impaired only in comprehension. The most important difference in performance between the two patient types was in the sentence anagram task. While the conduction aphasic rearranged the printed words of the anagram into a well-formed sentence without difficulty, both Broca patients were severely impaired in their ability to construct even normal noun phrase and verb phrase constituents.

We have argued that this pattern of performance in conduction aphasia can be explained by assuming that the syntactic processing mechanism is intact but is inaccessible during comprehension because of a severe limitation of the patient's short-term memory capacity (Caramazza, Basili, Koller, & Berndt, in press; see also Warrington & Shallice, 1969). This limitation of working memory prevents the elaboration of syntactic relations among lexical items during on-line processing, which results in an overreliance on the semantic information available in the major lexical items. These items are presumably better represented in the patient's long-term memory (assumed to be intact) than are the elements needed for syntactic analysis (i.e., the grammatical morphemes). Thus, the limitation of short-term memory capacity prevents adequate syntactic analysis in comprehension, because it interferes with the temporary storage of syntactic information during processing. The patient was able to construct sentence anagrams successfully by performing very simple local analyses—combining an article with a noun to form a noun phrase, for example—and then combining these small elements into a unified whole. The syntactic disruption present in Broca's aphasia prevented even these "local" syntactic analyses.

Summary. Patients classified as conduction aphasics have been shown to suffer from a syntactic comprehension deficit similar to the impairment found in Broca's aphasics. Unlike Broca patients, however, conduction aphasics show no sign of syntactic processing problems in speech production or in sentence anagram construction. It is argued that the asyntactic comprehension demonstrated in these patients results from a severely diminished capacity in auditory–verbal short-term memory, which interferes with their ability to store in working memory the output of an intact syntactic processing mechanism. The result is comprehension that relies on analysis of the major lexical items and thus appears to be intact for sentences that can be understood strictly by a semantic interpretation.

Wernicke's Aphasia

The investigation of syntactic abilities in Wernicke's aphasia is complicated by the severity of the lexical–semantic disturbances of these patients. As discussed in the chapter introduction, syntactic investigations cannot proceed independently of the words in a sentence. If a patient does not understand the words of a sentence or produces neologisms that the experimenter cannot identify, it is difficult to demonstrate that syntactic processing mechanisms are intact. Nonetheless, some claims have been made about the syntactic competence of Wernicke's aphasia that should be evaluated in light of the data.

The utterances produced by Wernicke's aphasics are often deviant syntactically, although these patients are said to produce a variety of grammatical constructions, including complex verb tenses and embedded subordinate clauses (Goodglass & Kaplan, 1972). The speech of Wernicke's aphasics is often quite devoid of informational content, but it usually gives the impression of being syntactically well formed. The suggestion has been made that the syntactic errors produced by these patients are a by-product of their pervasive word-finding problems, rather than a reflection of a disorder of syntax (Goodglass, 1968). That is, inappropriate selection of lexical items might result in serious grammatical violations, such as the use of a noun in a verb position or the use of an inanimate noun with a verb that requires an animate noun.

The strongest evidence available that syntax is spared in Wernicke's aphasia comes from the performance of German-speaking patients on the sentence order test (von Stockert & Bader, 1976). As discussed earlier, Wernicke patients were able to order sentence constituents correctly, despite severely impaired comprehension of the major lexical items, by using the morphological variant of the German article that

distinguishes subject nouns from object nouns. English does not provide an obvious analogue to this structural cue, and no studies have
been reported on which strong claims about preserved syntactic abilities
can be made about English-speaking Wernicke's aphasics. In all of the
studies reviewed here on Broca's aphasia that included Wernicke patients, the latter performed in general worse than the Broca patients but
did not limit their errors to the syntactic distractors.

The difficulty of separating lexical–semantic from syntactic factors in
the Wernicke patients' abnormal productions prevents definitive statements concerning the status of their syntactic abilities. Nonetheless,
several studies have been reported that undermine the assumption that
these patients produce utterances that are structurally normal. Gleason
et al. (1980) elicited narrative speech from groups of normal subjects as
well as from Broca's and Wernicke's aphasics ($N=5$ per group), using a
picture-story task. Although the Wernicke patients produced as many
words as did the normal group, their productions were much less syntactically diverse than the utterances produced by the normals. They
produced very few embedded constructions but tended to string a series
of clauses together with the conjunction *and*.

Another study that questions the syntactic "intactness" of Wernicke's
aphasics employs computer-aided acoustical analysis of the fundamental frequency (f_0) attributes of spoken sentences (see Chapter 5) (Cooper,
Danly, & Hamby, 1979). Several aspects of the fundamental frequency
contours of normal speakers have been shown to be affected in systematic ways by the syntactic structure of sentences (Cooper, 1980). This
technique thus offers the promise of providing a means for studying
patients' syntactic knowledge that does not necessarily rely on an intact
lexical–semantic system. Analysis was performed on the f_0 characteristics of sentences produced by five Wernicke's aphasics in a well-
practiced oral reading task. Several prosodic abnormalities were uncovered that indicated a failure of the patients to take into account overall
sentence length when programming an utterance. In addition, the Wernicke patients' f_0 functions were not influenced by major clause boundaries as are normal functions but seemed sensitive instead to phrase
boundaries within a clause. It appears that Wernicke's aphasics use
smaller-than-normal syntactic units in programming f_0 attributes, which
may indicate a disorder at the level of syntactic encoding.

Summary. The few studies reviewed here provide suggestions for future avenues of inquiry on the topic of the syntactic structure of the
utterances produced by Wernicke's aphasics. Although more research is
obviously required before the structural capabilities of Wernicke patients

are known, these studies indicate that their syntactic skills may be somewhat less than intact.

Summary and Conclusion

The syndrome of Broca's aphasia has been highlighted in this chapter, and evidence has been presented that the major symptoms associated with Broca's aphasia result from an impairment of the syntactic component of the linguistic system. It appears that the productive deficits associated with agrammatism may include such structural abnormalities as word order violations in addition to the frequent omission of the grammatical morphemes. The comprehension of Broca patients has been shown to be impaired for specific kinds of sentences, namely those that require syntactic (in addition to semantic) information for interpretation. This comprehension deficit appears to involve an impaired ability to use several types of syntactic cues, including word order and the grammatical morphemes. The syntactic deficit suffered by Broca's aphasics is assumed to involve a central component of the linguistic system and should be manifested in all modalities.

The syntactic capabilities of several other types of patients were also evaluated. Conduction aphasics demonstrate a comprehension deficit that is very similar to that of the Broca patients but show normal control over syntax in other tasks. The argument was presented that this appearance of asyntactic comprehension results from an impairment of short-term memory capacity in conduction aphasia that interferes with the patient's ability to perform ongoing syntactic analysis, even though the syntactic structures are intact.

The syntactic capabilities of Wernicke's aphasics are generally believed to be spared, although the severity of their other aphasic symptoms makes this claim difficult to evaluate. Several studies, using new techniques for evaluating aphasic performance, suggest that the fluent utterances produced by these patients are not syntactically normal.

Thus far in this chapter, there has been no discussion of the neuroanatomical correlates of the syndromes that have been discussed. The argument that Broca's aphasia represents a "pure" case in which one component of the system is disrupted while others are left intact suggests that it may be possible to "localize" syntax in the brain. Strong claims along these lines cannot be made, given the scarcity of localizing information for individual patients and our minimal understanding of the neurophysiological processes at work in the cerebral cortex (Caplan, in press). Nonetheless, Broca's aphasia may represent the best opportunity currently available to begin a search for specific neuroanatomical sites and neurophysiological processes that are involved in particular linguistic functions.

There is independent evidence that the syntactic component may be particularly suited to such an attempt. Several investigations of the language capacities of children and young adults who are functioning with only one cerebral hemisphere have demonstrated that a left hemisphere may be necessary for full syntactic competence (Dennis & Kohn, 1975; Dennis & Whitaker, 1976). The subjects of these studies were subjected to the surgical removal of the cortical portions of one cerebral hemisphere in order to control violent epileptic seizures. Subsequent language testing demonstrated that only those subjects with a remaining left hemisphere appear to have full control over syntax in comprehension. Subjects operating with only a right hemisphere demonstrate total phonological and semantic competence but are impaired in their ability to process complex syntactic constructions, such as passive negative sentences. The authors interpret these findings as evidence for the localization of syntax in the left hemisphere. Based on the data reviewed here on Broca's aphasia, it may be possible to further delimit the domain of syntax to the more anterior portions of the left hemisphere (Mohr, 1976). Although these suggestions must be approached with caution, they present the growing number of psychologists, linguists, neurologists, and speech pathologists who are interested in aphasia with exciting prospects for future research.

References

Berndt, R. S., & Caramazza, A. 1980. A redefinition of the syndrome of Broca's aphasia: Implications for a neuropsychological model of language. *Applied Psycholinguistics, 1*, 225–278.

Boller, F., Kim, Y., & Mack, J. 1977. Auditory comprehension in aphasia. In H. Whitaker & H. A. Whitaker (Eds.), *Studies in neurolinguistics* (Vol. 3). New York: Academic Press.

Bradley, D. C., Garrett, M. E., & Zurif, E. B. 1980. Syntactic deficits in Broca's aphasia. In D. Caplan (Ed.), *Biological studies of mental processes.* Cambridge, Mass.: MIT Press.

Caplan, D. On the cerebral localization of linguistic functions. *Brain and Language,* in press.

Caplan, D., Matthei, E., & Gigley, H. Comprehension of gerundive constructions by Broca's aphasics. *Brain and Language,* in press.

Caramazza, A., Basili, A. G., Koller, J. J., & Berndt, R. S. An investigation of repetition and language processing in a case of conduction aphasia. *Brain and Language,* in press.

Caramazza, A., & Berndt, R. S. 1978. Semantic and syntactic processes in aphasia: A review of the literature. *Psychological Bulletin, 85* (4), 898–918.

Caramazza, A., Berndt, R. S., Basili, A. G., & Koller, J. J. Syntactic processing deficits in aphasia. *Cortex,* in press.

Caramazza, A., & Zurif, E. B. 1976. Dissociation of algorithmic and heuristic processes in language comprehension: Evidence from aphasia. *Brain and Language, 3,* 572–582.

Caramazza, A., Zurif, E. B., & Gardner, H. 1978. Sentence memory in aphasia. *Neuropsychologia, 16,* 661–669.

Clark, H. H., & Clark, E. V. 1977. *Psychology and language.* New York: Harcourt Brace Jovanovich.

Cooper, W. E. 1980. Syntactic-to-phonetic coding. In B. Butterworth (Ed.), *Language production.* New York: Academic Press.

Cooper, W. E., Danly, M., & Hamby, S. 1979. Fundamental frequency (f_0) attributes in the speech of Wernicke's aphasics. In J. J. Wolf & D. H. Klatt (Eds.), *Speech communication papers presented at the 97th meeting of the Acoustical Society of America.* New York: Acoustical Society of America.

Dennis, M., & Kohn, B. 1975. Comprehension of syntax in infantile hemiplegics after cerebral hemidecortication: Left-hemisphere superiority. *Brain and Language, 2,* 472–482.

Dennis, M., & Whitaker, H. H. 1976. Language acquisition following hemidecortication. *Brain and Language, 3,* 404–433.

De Renzi, E., & Vignolo, L. A. 1962. The Token Test: A sensitive test to detect receptive disturbances in aphasics. *Brain, 85,* 665–678.

de Villiers, J. G. 1974. Quantitative aspects of agrammatism in aphasia. *Cortex, 10,* 36–54.

Fodor, J. A., & Garrett, M. F. 1967. Some syntactic determinants of sentential complexity. *Perception and Psychophysics, 2,* 289–296.

Garrett, M. F. 1975. The analysis of sentence production. In G. Bower (Ed.), *The psychology of learning and motivation advance in research and theory.* New York: Academic Press.

Garrett, M. F. 1980. Levels of processing in sentence production. In B. Butterworth (Ed.), *Language production.* New York: Academic Press.

Gleason, J. B., Goodglass, H., Green, E., Ackerman, N., & Hyde, M. R. 1975. The retrieval of syntax in Broca's aphasia. *Brain and Language, 2,* 451–471.

Gleason, J., Goodglass, H., Obler, L., Green, E., Hyde, M., & Weintraub, S. 1980. Narrative strategies of aphasic and normal-speaking subjects. *Journal of Speech and Hearing Research, 23,* 370–382.

Goodenough, C., Zurif, E., & Weintraub, S. 1977. Aphasics' attention to grammatical morphemes. *Language and Speech, 20,* 11–19.

Goodglass, H. 1968. Studies on the grammar of aphasics. In S. Rosenberg & K. Joplin (Eds.), *Developments in applied psycholinguistics research.* New York: Macmillan.

Goodglass, H. 1976. Agrammatism. In H. Whitaker & H. A. Whitaker (Eds.), *Studies in neurolinguistics* (Vol. 1). New York: Academic Press.

Goodglass, H., & Berko, J. 1960. Agrammatism and inflectional morphology in English. *Journal of Speech and Hearing Research, 3,* 257–267.

Goodglass, H., Blumstein, S. E., Gleason, J. B., Hyde, M. R., Green, E., & Statlender, S. 1979. The effect of syntactic encoding on sentence comprehension in aphasia. *Brain and Language, 7,* 201–209.

Goodglass, H., Fodor, I. G., & Schulhoff, C. 1967. Prosodic factors in grammar—evidence from aphasia. *Journal of Speech and Hearing Research, 10,* (1), 5–20.

Goodglass, H., Gleason, J. B., Bernholtz, N. A., & Hyde, M. R. 1972. Some linguistic structures in the speech of a Broca's aphasic. *Cortex, 8,* 191–212.

Goodglass, H., & Hunter, M. 1970. A linguistic comparison of speech and writing in two types of aphasia. *Journal of Communication Disorders, 3,* 28–35.

Goodglass, H., & Kaplan, E. 1972. *The assessment of aphasia and related disorders.* Philadelphia: Lea and Febiger.

Heilman, K. M., & Scholes, R. J. 1976. The nature of comprehension errors in Broca's, conduction and Wernicke's aphasics. Cortex, 12,(3), 258–265.

Jakobson, R. 1956. Two aspects of language and two types of aphasic disturbances. In R. Jakobson & M. Halle (Eds.), Fundamentals of language. The Hague: Mouton.

Kean, M. L. 1978. The linguistic interpretation of aphasic syndromes. In E. Walker (Ed.), Explorations in the biology of language. Montgomery, Vermont: Bradford Books.

Kean, M. L. 1980. Grammatical representations and the description of language processing. In D. Caplan (Ed.), Biological studies of mental processes. Cambridge, Mass.: MIT Press.

Kimball, J. 1975. Predictive analysis and over-the-top parsing. In J. Kimball (Ed.), Syntax and semantics, (Vol. 4). New York: Academic Press.

Kolk, H.H.J. 1978. Judgments of sentence structure in Broca's aphasia. Neuropsychologia, 16, 617–625. (a)

Kolk, H.H.J. 1978. The linguistic interpretation of Broca's aphasia. A reply to M. L. Kean. Cognition, 6, 353–361. (b)

Lecours, A. R., & Lhermitte, F. 1976. The pure form of phonetic disintegration syndrome (pure anarthria): Anatomo-clinical report of a historical case. Brain and Language, 3, 88–113.

Lenneberg, E. H. 1973. The neurology of language. Daedalus, 102, 115–133.

Levelt, W.J.M. 1970. A scaling approach to the study of syntactic relations. In G. B. Flores d'Arcais & W.J.M. Levelt (Eds.), Advances in psycholinguistics. Amsterdam: North-Holland Publ.

Luria, A. R. 1970. [Traumatic aphasia] (Douglas Bowden, trans.). The Hague: Mouton. (Originally published, 1947.)

Marshall, J. C. 1977. Disorders in the expression of language. In J. Morton & J. Marshall (Eds.), Psycholinguistics: Developmental and pathological. Ithaca: Cornell Univ. Press.

Mohr, J. R. 1976. Broca's area and Broca's aphasia. In H. Whitaker & H. A. Whitaker (Eds.), Studies in neurolinguistics (Vol. 1). New York: Academic Press.

Myerson, R., & Goodglass, H. 1972. Transformational grammars of three agrammatic patients. Language and Speech, 15, 40–50.

Panse, F., & Shimoyama, T. 1973. On the effects of aphasic disturbance in Japanese: Agrammatism and paragrammatism. In H. Goodglass & S. Blumstein (Eds.), Psycholinguistics and aphasia. Baltimore: Johns Hopkins Press.

Parisi, D., & Pizzamiglio, L. 1970. Syntactic comprehension in aphasia. Cortex, 6, 204–215.

Peuser, V., & Fittschen, M. 1977. On the universality of language dissolution: The case of a Turkish aphasia. Brain and Language, 4, 196–207.

Pick, A. 1913. Die agrammatischen sprachstonungen. Berlin: Springer-Verlag.

Poeck, K., Kerschensteiner, M., & Hartje, W. 1972. A quantitative study on language understanding in fluent and non-fluent aphasia. Cortex, 8, 299–304.

Saffran, E. M., & Marin, O.S.M. 1975. Immediate memory for word lists and sentences in a patient with deficient auditory short-term memory. Brain and Language, 2, 420–433.

Saffran, E. M., Schwartz, M. J., & Marin, O.S.M. 1980. Evidence from aphasia: Isolating the components of a production model. In B. Butterworth (Ed.), Language production. New York: Academic Press. (a)

Saffran, E. M., Schwartz, M. F., & Marin, O.S.M. 1980. The word order problem in agrammatism: II. Production. Brain and Language, 10, 263–280. (b)

Samuels, J. A., & Benson, D. F. 1979. Some aspects of language comprehension in anterior aphasia. Brain and Language, 8, 275–286.

Schwartz, M. F., Saffran, E. M., & Marin, O.S.M. 1980. The word order problem in agrammatism: I. Comprehension. Brain and Language, 10, 249–262.

Shallice, T., & Warrington, E. K. 1970. Independent functioning of verbal memory stores: A neuropsychological study. *Quarterly Journal of Experimental Psychology, 22,* 261–273.

Shewan, C. M. 1976. Error pattern in auditory comprehension of adult aphasics. *Cortex, 12,* 325–336.

Shewan, C. M., & Canter, C. J. 1971. Effects of vocabulary syntax and sentence length on auditory comprehension in aphasic patients. *Cortex, 7,* 209–226.

Swinney, D., Zurif, E., & Cutler, A. 1980. Effects of sentential stress and word class upon comprehension in Broca's aphasics. *Brain and Language, 10,* 132–144.

Traill, A. 1970. Transformational grammar and the case of an Ndebele speaking aphasic. *Journal of South African Logopedic Society, 17,* 48–66.

von Stockert, T. R., & Bader, L. 1976. Some relations of grammar and lexicon in aphasia. *Cortex, 12,* 49–60.

Warrington, E. K., & Shallice T. 1969. The selective impairment of auditory verbal short-term memory. *Brain, 92,* 885–896.

Wepman, J. J., & Jones, L. V. 1964. Five aphasias: A commentary on aphasia as a regressive linguistic phenomenon. In D. M. Rioch and E. A. Weinstein (Eds.), *Disorders in communication.* Baltimore, Md.: Williams & Wilkins.

Whitaker, H. A. 1970. Linguistic competence: Evidence from aphasia. *Glossa, 4,* 46–54.

Zurif, E., & Blumstein, S. 1978. Language and the brain. In M. Halle, J. Bresnan, & G. Miller (Eds.), *Linguistic theory and psychological reality.* Cambridge, Mass.: MIT Press.

Zurif, E., & Caramazza, A. 1976. Psycholinguistic structures in aphasia: Studies in syntax and semantics. In H. Whitaker & H. A. Whitaker (Eds.), *Studies in neurolinguistics* (Vol. 1). New York: Academic Press.

Zurif, E., Caramazza, A., & Myerson, R. 1972. Grammatical judgments of agrammatic aphasics. *Neuropsychologia, 10,* 405–417.

Zurif, E., Green, E., Caramazza, A., & Goodenough, C. 1976. Grammatical intuitions of aphasic patients: Sensitivity to functors. *Cortex, 12,* 183–186.

7

Lexical and Semantic Aspects of Aphasia

HUGH W. BUCKINGHAM, JR.

The present chapter treats the human lexicon—variously referred to as the mental dictionary, the dictionary, or simply the vocabulary. It will focus upon what happens to the lexicon, primarily located in the human cerebral cortex, as a consequence of damage to the nervous system. The studies referred to concern aphasia for the most part, but it will be necessary to draw from relevant findings on non-brain-damaged subjects as well as from certain linguistic studies of the lexicon. Lacking proper appreciation of the normal system, one cannot conceivably understand the disrupted system. The purpose of the chapter is to provide the reader with an outline of the many ways that lexical structure can be disturbed by brain damage. As a consequence, the reader will gain a deeper awareness of how words are represented in and manipulated by the brain and, more importantly, of how the system breaks down differently for different aphasics. Without such knowledge, one could not hope to understand, diagnose, or treat an aphasic with lexical disintegration.

Semantic Structure

I should mention at the outset that the dictionary is not the only domain of semantics, although aphasia studies have often limited inquiry to lexical semantics. Another extremely important area of semantics is concerned with truth values of propositions. To comprehend a sentence (or better yet, an ASSERTION of a speaker), the hearer must know that the speaker is claiming that the information conveyed by the sen-

ACQUIRED APHASIA

tence is, in fact, true. The hearer must also know what the speaker is claiming to be true. In addition, the hearer must understand the conditions under which the assertion would be considered true and under what circumstances it would not (Fodor, 1977, pp. 27–34). The study of meaning can involve reference, ideas, and behavior; meaning can be studied with regard to USE. Some have claimed that knowing what a sentence means is simply knowing the rules by which the sentence is to be used. By going through these rules, one, in effect, is verifying its truth (or falsifying it). However, truth value is limited to declarative sentences, since it makes no sense to speak of truth when considering promises, requests, warnings, threats, etc. Another domain of "use" semantics considers various of the "speech acts" under the rubric of pragmatics. The reader can consult Austin (1962), Searle (1971), Dillon (1977), Cole and Morgan (1975), Cole (1978), Sadock (1975), Fillmore and Langendoen (1971), and Katz (1972, 1977) for these and other traditional semantic issues. Before doing so, however, I would suggest reading Akmajian, Demers, and Harnish (1979, chaps. 11 and 12) and Fodor (1977). Little, if any, has beeen done in these areas as they might concern aphasia.

Semantic structure certainly must include what are known as selectional restriction rules, which subcategorize verbs on the basis of features for subjects and objects. For instance, an intransitive verb following a subject marked [+Human] will pick up the feature +[+Human__]. Accordingly, features are assigned to the nouns they occur with, so that, for example, the verb *roll* (for its intransitive reading) will be marked +[±Human__], since human and non human items may roll. The verb *laugh*, on the other hand, will be marked +[+Human__], since rocks do not laugh, nor do animals (see Newmeyer, 1980, chap. 3 for discussion of these issues as they relate to Chomsky's *Aspects* model of 1965). The notion of selectional restriction has clear syntactic implications and to an extent would explain why sentences such as *The rope shattered three clouds* are not grammatical. Issues such as these clearly rest at the boundaries between syntax and semantics, and nowhere would I want to imply that they are completely autonomous. Nevertheless, this chapter, to the extent possible, will not treat syntactic issues; those are dealt with in Chapter 6. As mentioned earlier, this chapter will treat aphasic disturbances of the mental dictionary.

The Structure of the Lexicon

The structure of the lexicon has been studied by anthropologists (Berlin & Kay, 1969), by psycholinguists (Deese, 1965; Miller & Johnson-

Laird, 1976), by aphasiologists (Lesser, 1978, chaps. 5 and 6), and by linguists (Gruber, 1976; Lehrer, 1974). Lexical information is indeed ubiquitous; it extends into practically every realm of the humanities and social sciences. Metaphor (Lakoff & Johnson, 1980; Ortony, 1979; Sacks, 1979), for example, can be studied with regard to brain damage (Winner & Gardner, 1977) or to artifical intelligence (Pylyshyn, 1979). Word meaning can provide clues to cultural differences (Whorf, 1956) as well. The importance of the mental lexicon can hardly be overestimated; I will now turn to a brief overview of what we know about how it is structured.

A study of the history of association psychology (such as Warren, 1921) will reveal that since the time of Aristotle it has been realized that words group into sets based upon the notion of "similarity". Eventually a taxonomy of "fields" (sets) was developed. Color terms have been studied extensively, both with respect to how they refer to distinct parcelings of the spectrum and with respect to the set of landmark or focal color terms (*black, white, red, green, yellow, blue,* and perhaps *gray*). These are TERMS, or labels, not colors in the physical sense, since, for instance, the label *red* (the landmark) may refer to different ranges (hues) along the spectrum. Colors may be intrinsic to some object (blood is intrinsically red) or simply accidental to some object (a telephone COULD BE red). Later we will see how color naming breaks down in brain damage. The reader should consult Miller and Johnson-Laird (1976, pp. 333–360) and Kay and McDaniel (1978) for extremely insightful treatments of color terminology. Semantic fields of kinship terminology have also been studied, most often by anthropologists such as Goodenough (1956, 1965). Again, Miller and Johnson-Laird (1976, pp. 360–373) provide a good outline of what is known about kinship terms. In addition, large sets of words are similar in that they relate to space. There is an extenisve set of labels for containers, pathways, and boundaries with relation to location and distance (Miller & Johnson-Laird, 1976, pp. 375–410). An equally interesting semantic sphere includes words having temporal relations. Practically all grammatical categories have words of a temporal nature. For instance, verb: *delay,* noun *year,* adjective: *late,* adverb: *subsequently,* preposition: *during,* and adverbial conjunction: *before* (Miller & Johnson-Laird, 1976, pp. 410–478). Even cooking terms have received serious linguistic study (Lehrer, 1969, 1974). Terms for body parts form a cohesive field, and later I will discuss how labeling versus locating body parts can be dissociated (Dennis, 1976). Room objects, food, and clothing represent additional semantic spheres of meaning, which, as we will see, have often been tested in aphasia. Finally, Miller and Johnson-Laird (1976, chap. 7) demonstrate that there exist quite pervasive semantic spheres for verbs relating to motion, possession, vision, and communication. This, then, is a brief statement of some of the relatively straight forward semantic bondings that comprise the lexicon.

Aside from bonding based upon semantic similarity, words can be related and grouped together through phonetic similarity, that is, by sound rather than by meaning. Acquisitional confusion in this realm can give rise to malapropisms. Often word association test responses will be words that are related to the stimulus by form alone.

To the extent that semantic and phonetic associations are based upon the metric of similarity, they may be considered paradigmatic; they exist along a vertical axis and can be said to be members of the same class.[1] At a very general level, we can claim that words of the same grammatical category are paradigmatically related. Paradigmatic errors in aphasia are selection errors where one form is substituted for another out of the same similarity class. We can also analyze paradigmatic relationships in terms of a hierarchy. For example (Buckingham, 1979,p. 274), consider the following words and categories: *property, household items, furniture, article for sitting, chair,* and *sofa. Property* is the highest superordinate, then *household item, furniture,* and so on. The last two words, *chair* and *sofa,* are referred to as CONTRAST COORDINATES by Goodglass and Baker (1976, p. 362) or as a MINIMAL CONTRASTIVE SET by Miller and Johnson-laird (1976, pp. 262–263). By MINIMAL is meant that each word in the set has EXACTLY the same superordinate terms. CONTRASTIVE implies that one and only one word in the set can apply to any given particular. For instance, a chair IS property, or IS a household item, or IS furniture, or IS an article for sitting, but it is NOT a sofa. *Sofa* has the same superordinate terms as a chair but is not a chair. As we will see, Goodglass and Baker's (1976) study of naming makes use of these concepts. The opposite of a superordinate is a hyponym; items beneath the superordinate are hyponyms. Most often, there will be some prototypical hyponym for a superordinate category—*Bird: robin* (but not *penguin* or *chicken*), *Fruit: banana* (but not *mango*), etc. It is not unreasonable to suggest that a prototype will be culturally determined in many cases. To an extent, categorical discreteness may be more clearly defined by prototypicality than by shared semantic features (Rosch, 1977). Nevertheless, characterizing precisely what constitutes some "normal member" of a category may prove to be more difficult than would be expected (Putnam, 1975). Prototypicality has also been studied in aphasias (Grossman, 1978, 1981). Words in these contrastive sets may also be synonyms or an-

---

1. I have found that this relational phenomenon is best explained with reference to "verb paradigms" usually found at the end of reference grammar books. Columns of verb forms are displayed showing tenses, aspectual forms, and their inflections. In each column, the verb forms are paradigmatically related—hence verb paradigms.

tonyms. Note that antonyms (considered to be polar opposites) are actually very much alike semantically. They must be if they share the same superordinate terms. The appreciation of antonymic contrasts in aphasia has also been investigated (Gardner, Silverman, Wapner, & Zurif, 1978). In addition, words may group into spheres in accordance with shape. Shape as an early distinguishing feature for children explains their "over extensions." For example, the use of the word *moon* for crescent-shaped objects is typical in initial stages of language acquisition (Clark & Clark, 1977, p. 492).

It goes without saying that the only way to quantify word relatedness is through the use of some sort of feature system. The problem, of course, is settling upon sufficient numbers and types. It is fairly well established that features such as [+Human], [+Abstract], [+Female] are of a high order of generality. But what of [+Married], [+Ferocious] for instance? The more specifically characteristic the features, the more residual in nature is that information. We might call the first type semantic, or defining, features and the second type characteristic, or residual, features. There is an interesting way to separate defining features from residual features (Akmajian *et al.*, 1979, p. 240; Miller, 1969). Take the features [+Male] and [+Married] and the noun *husband*.The sentence *That person is a husband* carries the information that the person is both male and married. The negation of that sentence *That person is not a husband*, in general circumstances, still carries the information that the person is male but no longer that he is married. The feature that is still "presupposed" under negation is usually the defining feature—not the residual feature. Take our previous example with the feature hierarchy for *chair*. Consider the sentence *That item is a chair. Item* carries with it both [+furniture] and [+for sitting in]. The negation *That item is not a chair*, in usual circumstances, still implies that it is a piece of furniture but certainly not necessarily that it is an item for sitting in. This is consistent with our hierarchy, since the defining feature [furniture] is higher on the scale than the characteristic feature [for sitting in]. We will need to appreciate this featural distinction when discussing Zurif, Caramazza, Myerson, and Galvin (1974) and Shanon (1978).

For the last serveral pages, we have been outlining paradigmatic relations between words. Let us now turn to another type of semantic relationship—syntagmatic. Whereas paradigmatic relations are vertical, syntagmatic relations are horizontal. These terms, it should be pointed out, were first developed by Ferdinand de Saussure (1959) and later brought to bear on the description and classification of the aphasias by Roman Jakobson (1964). As mentioned above, paradigmatic disturbances involve disordered selection of items. Syntagmatic disturbances, on the other hand, involve disordered combination of items in a string (i.e., along a horizontal axis). Lesser (1978, pp. 39–45) provides some further details concerning this important dichotomy. Syntagmatic lexical bonds, rather than being based upon similarity, are based upon contiguity. There are three principle types of syntagmatic relations: predication, coexistence, and synecdoche (part-for-whole).

Predication can involve adjective–noun sequences, such as *winter coat* or *kitchen chair*. The relationship between *cold* and *weather* is syntagmatic; *cold* is probably as closely bonded to *weather* as it is to *hot*. Object-description relations are most often expressed in copular sentences, such as *My uncle is a good wrestler*. Item-location relations exist between, for instance, *boat* and *water*, whereas instrument-function relations connect *watch* and *for telling time*. Words that are syntagmatically related through coexistence most often collocate, such as *needle* and *thread*, *peanut butter* and *jelly*, *bread* and *butter*, etc. Finally, part-for-whole relations involve referring to, for instance, a television by the word *tube* or a car by the word *wheels*.

The paradigmatic–syntagmatic dichotomy is of crucial importance for an understanding of the linguistic distinctions revealed in posterior aphasia versus anterior aphasia, since, in general, we can show that Wernicke's aphasics lose control of paradigmatic function, whereas Broca's aphasics lose control of syntagmatic function. The dichotomy captures the two most important ways in which lexical relatedness is structured in the mental dictionary. We will now turn our attention to the issue of accessing the vocabulary items.

Retrieval from the Lexicon

Theoretically, words must somehow be selected from the store and placed into certain positions of some preliminary linear structure. Just what this structure contains is not well understood, but most agree that it has a superimposed intonational pattern generated autonomously but in accordance with the syntactic, semantic, lexical, and pragmatic constraints of the message (Cutler & Isard, 1980). The structure presumably contains some minimal grammatical information (Clark & Clark, 1977, pp. 278–279) so that nouns will go into noun slots, verbs into verb slots, etc. Aphasic lexical errors as well as slips of the tongue in non-brain-damaged speakers (Buckingham, 1980; Söderpalm, 1979) reveal that selection processes take place AFTER grammatical category positions in sentences have been established, since the substituted word errors are always of the same grammatical category as the target forms. The psychological process of lexical retrieval must somehow work through the hierarchy to the level of the minimal contrastive set in most cases, since the errors are predominantly among the items in that set (i.e., *sofa→chair; apple→orange*).

Retrieval processes are invoked in natural settings during spontaneous speech or at confrontation naming. Psycholinguists, such as Goldman-Eisler (1964, 1968) and Butterworth (1979, 1980), have studied retrieval processes in ongoing speech by paying careful attention to pauses and hesitations, which I will discuss later. Much of our understanding concerning retrieval processes has come from confrontation testing of one form or another. Several investigators, such as Lesser (1978, p. 73), have warned of the "unnaturalness" of the task of requesting aphasics to name pictures and objects. It has been claimed that willfully producing labels for referents upon request taxes the volitional system, since the level at which the aphasic is forced to perform is metalinguistic. Accordingly, the naming disorder presumably indicates a failure to achieve the ABSTRACT ATTITUDE of which Kurt Goldstein (1948) continually spoke. To an extent, this could be said of all experimentation with aphasics, but most of the experimental studies with which I am familiar try to insure that the patient understands what is required of him or her and has the cognitive awareness at least to make intelligible attempts at performing what is required. This will often, however, give rise to the tendency of using much less severely involved patients, which may or may not be desirable.

Retrieval from the lexicon takes time, but before 1879 this fact was not appreciated. Warren (1921) details the history of association psychology and claims that through introspection the notion was derived that the more two items occurred together the tighter their bonding and the more likely one's presence would "call up" the other. This so-called law of contiguity was established hundreds of years ago. The act of naming came to be explained through this principle. A visual presentation of some object would evoke the spoken label for that object, since the two had been paired together often in the past. Items would also call up other items because of similarity. So essentially, association psychology had handed down two laws: contiguity and similarity. The reader should clearly recognize these as the historical roots of the dichotomy of syntagmatic and paradigmatic. Nevertheless, it was not until the psychology research laboratories started testing in the last quarter of the nineteenth century that quantification was made possible. The metaphor of "strength" for fixed associative bonding had been coined quite early in history, but it was not until Francis Galton's 1879 article in *Brain* (Warren, 1921, p. 215) that associative strength was correlated with the time it took a stimulus to call up its associate. Word association experimentation had come of age; now one could test to determine the relative strength of associative processes. Eventually, this experimental methodology using reaction time was extended to the testing of subjects whose associative function had been disturbed, thus providing a new way to examine aphasic disturbances of the lexicon.

Aphasic Disturbances of the Lexicon

D. Frank Benson (1979) has provided an excellent summary of the varieties of word-finding disturbances and an outline of their neurological correlates. The first he describes as WORD–PRODUCTION ANOMIA; here the errors are of two types—motor and paraphasic. The patient with articulatory disturbances usually has severe frontal lobe involvement and other motor difficulties; his disruption involves the articulatory manipulation of phonological forms, and the speech output is effortful and nonfluent. These are the word-finding problems of Broca's aphasia.

Paraphasic word-production anomia is a much more fluent disorder, and accordingly there is far less involvement of the motor cortex. Here, as with the motor patient, the problem is not with the retrieval of the phonological shape but with its execution. Unlike with the motor patients, the errors occur at the phonemic level. It is claimed that the phonemic disruption can be so severe as to render words completely unrecognizable. These patients will often fall into the category of conduction aphasia, and accordingly the cerebral involvement will include the left sylvian region between Broca's and Wernicke's area—or the area around the supramarginal gyrus.

Benson refers to the so-called pure anomic's access problems as WORD-SELECTION (WORD DICTIONARY) ANOMIA. This patient generally has no other production or comprehension problems. Benson noted that there has been much disagreement as to the anatomical localization of the syndrome except for the fact that "most researchers agree on a site posterior to the fissure of Rolando [p. 304]." Patients with SEMANTIC (NOMINAL) ANOMIA are like the "pure" cases, except they have difficulty comprehending the word, both printed and spoken. Theirs is perhaps a failure to appreciate the symbolic value of the word. It is generally felt that this syndrome results as a consequence of a more extensive lesion than that involved in the "pure" cases. The case Benson includes demonstrates a left frontoparietal lesion located in the cortical border zone, above and posterior to the sylvian fissure. A study of SEMANTIC APHASIA has appeared (Hier, Mogil, Rubin, & Komros, 1980) in which three cases are reported. Interestingly enough, these patients could partially understand isolated words but could not appreciate them in grammatical context. It was suggested that semantic aphasia involves the inability to grasp fully the meaning of words and grammatical constructions carrying syntagmatic relations, which are spatial in nature. It is significant that many of these patients have spatial disorders, which is likely due to the posterior parietal involvement. The patients in the Hier *et al.* study appeared to have more involvement than Benson's case. They had constructional apraxia, spatial agnosia, and some elements of Gerstmann's syndrome. One patient's tomogram revealed bilateral temporoparieto-occipital junction lesions. Benson's semantic anomia would then appear to be part of the full-blown syndrome of semantic aphasia.

Another anomic category discussed by Benson is CATEGORY-SPECIFIC ANOMIA, and the most commonly reported field affected comprises color terms (McKee & Damasio, 1979; Geschwind & Fusillo, 1966; Oxbury, Oxbury, & Humphrey, 1969). Quite often, this form of anomia is found as part of the syndrome of alexia without agraphia. The posterior cerebral artery is most often involved, and lesions often include the left occipital visual cortex and the posterior section of the corpus callosum (splenium). Interesting dissociations are often observed with color anomia. Recall that earlier we drew a distinction between objects that have intrinsic colors (grass is green) and those that have accidental colors (cup is green). Patients will often find it easier to name the color when it is pictured intrinsically than when it is not (Geschwind & Fusillo, 1966). Damasio, McKee, and Damasio (1979) discuss other determinants of variable performance in color anomia.

Body-part naming has been isolated as well. Dennis (1976) showed that the capacity to locate (by pointing to) body parts and to label them by their names can be dissociated. Dennis's patient was a 17-year-old girl who developed difficulties in naming body parts after resection of the left anterior temporal lobe. Yamadori and Albert (1973) have also described category-specific anomias. In addition, it has been demonstrated that different types of aphasics will reveal specific word category breakdowns. Goodglass, Klein, Carey, and Jones (1966; reprinted in Goodglass, 1978) showed that Wernicke's aphasics and anomics were significantly better at providing letter words than at providing object names. Broca's aphasics, on the other hand, showed no such significant difference.

The last type of aphasic anomia discussed by Benson is MODALITY-SPECIFIC. Here, for instance, the patient has difficulty naming visually presented objects, but not tactually presented objects. To name the object, the patient has to palpate it. This shows that the appreciation of perceptual attributes can be dissociated one from the other. A related finding has been provided by Gardner (1973). There he demonstrated the contribution of the tactile information in general to naming capacity. Gardner borrowed the Piagetian term OPERATIVE for describing those objects, parts of objects, or other entities that can be readily grasped, manipulated, or operated upon. Such items as mantle, ceiling, and floor are less manipulable than chair, vase, and telephone. When word frequency was controlled for, it could be shown that it was significantly easier to name operative objects as opposed to objects only knowable in a figurative way. The explanation for this is associationistic and has a history of hundreds of years (Warren, 1921). Naming depends upon the capacity to AROUSE (a key term in association psychology) a subset of actions of schemes of sensory experiences previously involved with the stimulus object. To the extent that there is a multiplicity of cross-modal associations built up, the visual stimulus object will be better matched with its associated articulate sign, the word. The operative object has a richer system of associates and can therefore be labeled more easily. Goodglass, Barton, and Kaplan (1968; reprinted in Goodglass, 1978) have suggested that most aphasics do not reveal discrete disconnecting lesions and thus will not as a rule present with such demarcated modality-specific deficits. These authors tested naming in aphasics across visual, tactile, olfactory, and auditory modes. Although there were differences in average raw scores, these were, save for a very few subjects, not significant. Goodglass *et al.* suggested that the various sense modalities could have different associative arousal capacities. This would explain the average raw score differences in naming across modalites.

The remaining types of anomia discussed by Benson are nonaphasic in nature and will therefore not be treated in this chapter. It will have been noted that many of these anomias arise from posterior cerebral damage; indeed it is generally felt that the semantic system is more dependent upon intact temporoparietal cortex. There is a fair amount of literature from experimental studies of nonaphasics that implicates the posterior regions of the cerebrum in semantic decoding.

Fedio and Van Buren (1974) demonstrated electrophysiologically that the left posterior temporoparietal cortex is important for proper retrieval of stored verbal information. Stimulation of this specific region produced anomic behavior. Such behavior was not induced by stimulating the left anterior temporal lobe or the right posterior temporoparietal cortex. Thatcher and April (1976) studied EEG-evoked potential correlates of semantic information processing and demonstrated large left–right asymmetries (left greater than right) from posterior cortical leads but not from anterior leads. Psychophysical studies of cognitive processing with EEG have often been criticized for not controlling for such variables as sensory differences in the stimuli, subjective states of subjects, different cognitive functions, sequence effects, and individual variation. Nevertheless, Chapman, McCrary, Chapman, and Bragdon (1978) controlled for many of these and still found that internal representations of meanings can be assessed by analyzing EEG responses. Molfese (1979) has, however, found not only that there is overlapping subcortical functioning during the processing of meaningful words but that the right hemisphere is operating as well. This does not mean that the two hemispheres are of equal functional importance for semantic processing, but rather that the right hemisphere is not dormant during dominate hemisphere cognitive functioning. One sees an increase in regional cerebral blood flow on the right side as well during language processing (Lassen, Ingvar, & Skinhøj, 1978). McKeever and Jackson (1979) have shown rather convincingly through a tachistoscopic reaction-time study that right visual field presentation of pictured objects gives rise to significantly faster naming rates for object naming and color naming. These studies, of course, simply discriminate left and right, not within the hemisphere. Wood, Taylor, Penny, and Stump (1980) studied regional cerebral blood flow increases in two groups of subjects. One group had to simply recognize words repeated from a previously presented list, while the second group had to decide if the words in the second list represented concrete objects that would fit into an area about the size of a living room. The authors found, among other things, significantly greater increases in left hemisphere blood flow in the semantic classification group than in the recognition memory group. Soh, Larsen, Skinhøj, and Lassen (1978) demonstrated decreased and abnormal blood flow to the crucial language centers in the cortex for specific aphasias. For example, when speaking, sensory aphasics showed at least marginal increases into Broca's area but no increase into the upper posterior temporal lobe region. Non-brain-damaged subjects always show increase in blood flow to Wernicke's area when speaking (Lassen *et al.* 1978). In sum, the combination of electrical stimulation, EEG, tachistoscopic, and blood flow studies in normals would seem to support the notion that left posterior cerebral zones are crucially involved in the lexical–semantic component of language.

Specific Linguistic Manifestations of Retrieval Disturbances

Brain lesions in the language areas will variously affect the patient's ability to find the lexical items necessary for one or another communicative purpose whether it is spontaneous speech, confrontation naming, or reading. In spontaneous speech, the objects are usually out of sight. This is the most natural setting in which providing spoken labels takes place. Some of what we know about the lexical–semantic difficulties in production comes from studying spontaneous speech samples, but most of what we know comes from confrontation testing. First, I would like to discuss the various manifestations of word blocks regardless of whether they are produced during a natural speech setting or as a response to directed testing. The first, in a sense, is the most obvious indicator of a word-finding block; it is the pause or hesitation (Butterworth, 1979, 1980; Goldman-Eisler, 1964, 1968). The speech output of the severely anomic is often characterized by pauses, usually directly after noun determiners, indicating a blocked noun. In the speech of a motor aphasic, it is obviously more problematic to determine if there is a true access deficit, because the hesitation could be occasioned by a motor initiation factor. Often this patient will produce audible groping in his attempts, and the first few segments may be on target. A true lexical block should show little evidence of "tip-of-the-tongue" behavior. Goldman-Eisler, referring to the doctrine of John Hughlings Jackson concerning automatic versus volitional processes in language production, noted that pauses in speech tended to occur before a high information load item was to appear. This is quite often where the aphasic hesitates, since anomic disturbances usually affect content words, which carry the lexical meaning for propositions. It should be cautioned that a great deal of hesitation due to word-finding problems will lead to disfluency in an otherwise fluent patient. Consequently, it is extremely important not to confuse an apraxic disfluency with an anomic disfluency. The pausing behavior that often precedes neologistic productions should not be taken as a claim that only severe jargonaphasics show hesitation behavior. In fact, Marshall (1976) has shown that delay is quite often a strategy for word finding in less severe or more fully recovered subjects. Furthermore, in these cases, the delay is more often followed by the production of the desired word than by a semantic or phonetic field error, a description, circumlocution, etc. Pausing behavior, therefore, seems to be used by aphasics who have differing degrees of severity with word finding.

Any type of field error is indicative of a word-finding block. With the field error, however, there is a lexical item incorrectly selected and substituted for the target rather than a pause in the stream of speech. Rinnert and Whitaker (1973) reported that the semantic confusions of the aphasic are often indistinguishable from word association responses of normals. Frequently the target and error are members of the minimal contrastive set. Antonymic forms as well may be substituted (Buckingham & Rekart, 1979). Gardner *et al.* (1978) demonstrated experimentally that Wernicke's aphasics, as opposed to Broca's, lose sensitivity to antonymic contrast on linguistic tasks. Asked to supply the "best opposite," Broca's aphasics more often supplied words indicating oppositions of qualities, whereas Wernicke's generally provided words that were syntagmatically related. Also, Wernicke's seemed to appreciate synonyms to a much greater extent than antonyms. This lack of sensitivity to antonymic contrast may underlie those cases where the lexical paraphasia is the antonym of the target. Another error type would be the substitution of a superordinate for one of its hyponyms. In fact, Goodglass and Baker (1976) noted that their patients with word finding problems maintained a surprising ability to appreciate superordinates. At this point, an important distinction needs to be drawn between hierarchically related superordinate structure and the minimal contrastive units. The former comprises the definitional structure for the items in the minimal set.

Definitions of objects, although in the superstructure, are often coded linguistically in sentential form, such as object description (*An oven is hot*) or instrument function (*A watch is for telling time*). Earlier I showed that these relations are predicative and therefore syntagmatic. Posterior aphasics, as mentioned, essentially control syntagmatic function and accordingly appreciate definitions and hence superordinate relationships expressed in sentences and phrases; this observation has been made repeatedly in the literature (Geschwind, 1967; Wepman, Bock, Jones, & Van Pelt, 1973).

At times, patients will substitute words that, given the sentential and conversational context, do not seem to be phonetically or semantically related to what would appear to be called for. The error is not a nonsense word and can be found in a dictionary of the speaker's language. Eugene Green (1969) refers to this as UNRELATED VERBAL PARAPHASIA. An example would be a sentence such as *It's kind of empty to mark these customers, too* (Buckingham, 1979, p. 278). *Empty* is certainly in the dictionary but does not appear to be at all appropriate in this context. Furthermore, it was not clear how the verb *mark* was to be understood.

Another very common substitute for an unretrievable word is the ANAPHOR. An anaphor is a word that has an antecedent, occuring either before or after it, to which it refers. Another general term is a PRO-FORM. The most common pro-forms are pro-sentences (*Jack's smart and he knows it*), pro-verbs (*Alice sings and I do, too*), and pronouns (*Al shaves after he brushes his teeth*). These are definite anaphors, since the referent is clear in all cases (*Jack is smart, sing, Al*). In addition, the referent (antecedent) appears somewhere in the lingusitic output. Indefinite anaphors, on the other hand, have a wide range of possible referents. Aphasics with access deficits will invariably use one or another type of indefinite anaphor. Where the retrieval involves a noun, the anaphor will be an indefinite pronoun. Such words as *thing, stuff,* and *guy* will stand for practically any object, as will the pronoun *one.* What is interesting in the anomic is that, despite the disrupted accessing ability, anaphoric processing remains intact. A significant distinction is still maintained in the linguistic system of the anomic—the distinction between sense and reference. This requires not only that the anaphoric elements be manipulated, but also that article usage be intact. Pronouns and articles are usually undisturbed (along with such other function words as conjunctions, prepositions, and forms of copula *be*) in posterior aphasics, but they carry a heavy semantic load. Indefiniteness usually relates to only the sense of the noun under consideration. For instance, *I want a ball* refers to any ball with no specific referent in mind, whereas *I want the ball* refers to a definite ball. In the first case, what is involved is sense; in the second, reference is involved. The anaphor *one* is normally pronominal under identity of sense, not reference. In the sentence *I don't know what you call it, but I have **one** at home,* the pronoun *one* is appreciated solely on the basis of the sense of the item involved, not the reference. For example, an anomic who cannot name *calendar* is very likely able to say *I saw one this morning* or *I have one at home.* As Miller and Johnson-Laird (1976) have shown, labeling objects at even the elemental indefinite pronoun level of *thing* requires a good deal of cognitive machinery. What it also indicates is that there is a word retrieval block and that the patient is compensating.

Circumlocution and confabulation are other linguistic compensations for access difficulty. This is often referred to as "empty speech" or LOGORRHEA and predictably will be comprised of indefinite terms and vague expressions. Mercer, Wapner, Gardner, & Benson (1977) published a study of confabulation in patients with severe memory loss and pointed out that confabulation is not necessarily in and of itself indicative of aphasia. Many jargonaphasics with demonstrable word finding difficulties, however, will confabulate a great deal (Kinsbourne & Warrington, 1963; Weinstein & Keller, 1963; Weinstein & Lyerly, 1976; Weinstein, Lyerly, Cole & Ozer, 1966), and their brain pathology often extends beyond the classical language zones to involve connections with the limbic-reticular system. Weinstein and Lyerly (1976) write that an extensive lesion in these regions "creates the milieu of brain dysfunction necessary for the maintenance of denial and hemi-inattention, mood changes, disorientation, reduplication and confabulation [p. 132]." Furthermore, the Mercer *et al.* patients had many of the same characteristics that jargonaphasics have—"pressured" speech output and an inability to self-monitor. In addition, nonsensical jargon will often resolve to analogues (Weinstein & Puig-Antich, 1974) of the jargon in later stages of recovery, where, in response to the same questions asked in the acute stage, the patient produces verbal stereotypes, officialese, cliches, malapropisms, and puns. All these productions were interpreted by Weinstein and Puig-Antich as verbal "gap fillers," most often lacking referential meaning. The point of all this is that at times lexical retrieval failures will manifest themselves through circumlocutory behavior.

Often a form of jargonaphasia will appear where many nouns or full noun phrases will be made up of isolatable words that do not exist in the dictionary of the aphasic's native language and that cannot be related to any conceivable target word on the basis of either sound or meaning. In the aphasia literature, these words are called neologisms. They can almost always be assigned to a grammatical category on the basis of their syntactic position or morphological inflection. They are articulated with fluency and ease, and their syllabic structure obeys all the phonological principles of the language in question. There appear to be four possible productive processes that could generate these nonrecognizable words. One could not logically involve a retrieval deficit; the other three could—and, in fact, do. Anyone working with neologistic jargonaphasics must understand the essential components of these error generating mechanisms, otherwise intervention may fail to affect the actual disorder.

I will first discuss the productive process that could result in a neologism but that does NOT imply a word block from the lexicon. The error mechanism is simply severe phonemic paraphasic distortion of the phonological shape of target words. The target word must be retrieved from the lexicon to make this theory work; the problem rests with phonemic execution and not lexical retrieval. Recall that Benson (1979) listed word-production anomia as a variety of word finding disturbance. I think we can safely say that word-production anomia cannot logically be a word finding disturbance, since how can you distort an item that you cannot retrieve? Benson's word-production anomia is of two types—motor and paraphasic. The paraphasic word production anomic will often produce so much phonemic paraphasia that words will be distorted beyond recognizability; the result is a neologistic form. Benson has published earlier accounts of neologisms presumably generated in this fashion (Benson, Sheremata, Bouchard, Segarra, Price, & Geschwind, 1973; Kertesz & Benson, 1970) and has shown that conduction aphasics with serious phonological impairment will produce neologisms. In any event, for this explanation to be logically consistent, the target word will have to be retrieved from the lexicon.

For the second possible error source, Butterworth (1979) and Buckingham (1981) have suggested that neologisms may arise under the conditions of a total word-finding block. Buckingham and Kertesz (1974, 1976) and Buckingham (1977a) argued that this is a reasonable alternative to a "phonemic distortion of target" theory. Butterworth (1979) has developed a random generating device that goes into operation, usually after a pause of .20 seconds or greater (Butterworth, 1980, p. 156). A mechanism of this nature can account for the production of the phonetic material of the neologism without claiming that the neologism was constructed by way of the patient's obliteration of the target word. It states that something totally different is going on in the subject's aphasia. The subject is, in a sense, producing strings of well-formed phonemes or syllables that fill in the gaps and compensate for words not retrievable from the lexicon. The fact that the device generates "randomly" accounts for the bizarre nature of neologistic expressions. Again, the only constraint under which this device must operate is that its output (i.e., the neologism) follow the syllabic patterns of the language.

A third possible source for a neologism comes from the perseveration of segments from a neologism produced earlier by the device. Buckingham, Whitaker, and Whitaker (1978, 1979) have demonstrated the pervasive effect of perseveration in neologistic jargonaphasia, and psycholinguistic studies (Buckingham, 1980; Shattuck-Hufnagel, 1979) have suggested speech production models for the linear ordering of phonological material, which, if disrupted, could account in interesting ways for perseveration. Note that the neologism generated through perseverative processes can be traced to an original target, but this target would have been produced by the random generating device and thus would have been neologistic itself.

Yet a fourth manner in which a neologistic word could reasonably arise has been suggested. Like the second and third alternatives, this, too, indicates a lexical retrieval deficit. This explanation involves a "two-stage" error, where initially there is a lexical selection error, which, before it reaches phonetic materialization, is distorted phonemically. Unlike the third neologistic process, the form that is subsequently distorted is a semantic field error and thus a real word in the language. This process has been proposed by several aphasia researchers (Brown, 1972, p. 62; Lecours & Lhermitte, 1972, pp. 304–305; Luria, 1970, p. 296). It should be clear to the reader at this point that in many instances, the production of neologisms indicates that the aphasic is having difficulty accessing the lexicon and that the forms being produced are in a sense "masking" this deficit. Up to now, I have been discussing the nature of semantic lexical associations, the selection of specific words from their associative fields or failure to do so. I have pointed to the many linguistic processes that aphasics can bring to bear in light of their retrieval deficits. But have I explained WHY they have these retrieval problems in the first place? I think not.

Explanations for Retrieval Disturbances

Much recent experimental work on aphasic lexicons has been carried out with the expressed purpose of demonstrating that brain damage will often loosen up the organization of the mental dictionary and thereby disrupt the system of verbal concepts. Once this is shown, it is then generally suggested that these disturbances in lexical structure are what underlie retrieval problems; thus, the explanation is shifted from access mechanisms alone to the atypical aphasic dictionary. Although there is a growing literature, some of it outlined in Lesser (1978, chap. 5), I will restrict my focus to Zurif *et al.* (1974); Goodglass and Baker (1976); Whitehouse, Caramazza, and Zurif (1978); and more recently Grober, Perecman, Kellar, and Brown (1980).

Zurif *et al.* used the "triadic comparison" procedure, where subjects (five Broca's, five Wernicke's as tested on the Boston Diagnostic Aphasia Examination, and five controls) were presented three words at a time and asked to choose the two felt to be most similar in meaning. The words used were 12 nouns, all marked [+concrete], but half (*mother, wife, cook, partner, knight,* and *husband*) marked [+Human] and half (*shark, trout, dog, tiger, turtle, crocodile*) marked [−human]. All were high-frequency words. Further semantic subdivision within the [+Human] set revealed three more distinguishing defining features [+Male], [+Female], and [+Person]. Recall that it is these higher-order superordinate features that keep their marking even under denial. If we are told that so-and-so is not a husband, we do not deny that the person referred to is [+Human] or [+Male] but simply that the feature for [Married] has changed from + to −. A similar breakdown into defining semantic features and characteristic residual features was done for the rest of the words so that, when interpreting the subjects' scores, the authors could tell whether the subjects were more sensitive to one type of feature or to another. The [−Human] group was divided into [+Fish] or [+Animal] (defining features), while several other residual features were arrived at—most importantly [±Ferocious]. Crucial for the analysis were characteristic features like [+Ferocious] and [+Married], because in their respective [±Human] sets they cut across semantic featural boundaries—[+Ferocious] across [Fish] (shark) and [Animal] (tiger, crocodile) and [+Married] across [Male] and [Female]. This provides a way to measure sensitivity to either defining features or characteristic features. If *wife* and *husband* are sorted together more than *wife* and *mother* or *husband* and *knight,* then presumably the subject is focusing his sensitivities upon the residual features and not upon the presupposed, higher superordinate, defining semantic features.

The analyses of the performances revealed several interesting distinctions between the controls and the aphasics and between the anterior and posterior aphasics. At the level of the [±Human] appreciation, both controls and anterior patients showed stability. The posterior group, even at this level, did not appear sensitive to the distinction. Instead, Zurif *et al.* found that the posterior aphasics would tend to group two words that could occur together syntagmatically. For instance, if the three words were *mother, husband,* and *cook,* the authors noted that the patient, as he placed the *mother* card with the *cook* card, would concurrently utter *My mother is a good cook.* Note that this accords with the fact that posterior aphasics still appreciate syntagmatic relations such as object description, here expressed in a copular proposition. Although the anteriors' lexical structure within [+Human] was rather like the controls, that within [−Human] was not. Interrelationships here were not as "tight" as they were for the controls, and the anteriors appeared to let the residual feature of [Ferocity] override the superordinates [Animal] and [Fish]. Shanon (1978) has found similar sensitivity to characteristic, residual features, but with a posterior patient. In general, the aphasics' lexical associative structure was weakened or loosened up so to speak—the posterior group more so than the anterior. The aphasics seemed more tied to the features of words relating to the immediate affective environment. I would note that the anteriors more often sorted *dog* with the [+Human] words in the triads. The posteriors, however, were clearly worse off than the anteriors in terms of organizational restructuring of the lexicon posttrauma. In the end, the authors suggest that "the data do indicate a relation between subjective lexical organization and word finding difficulties in aphasia [Zurif *et al.*, 1974, p. 185]". Further exploration of this claim is provided by a study by Goodglass and Baker (1976).

Under the assumption that labeling behavior depends on an intact lexicon and that retrieval processes depend upon a proper convergence of associations aroused (or revived) by the introduction of some sensory stimulus, Goodglass and Baker compared four groups of subjects: aphasics with low comprehension scores, aphasics with high comprehension scores, brain-damaged nonaphasics, and normal controls. The aphasics were grouped according to their performances on the Boston aphasia battery subtests of auditory comprehension. Words of high and low frequency were used; there were 8 high and 8 low for a total of 16. All were picturable. High-frequency words were *knife, cake, sheep, drum, bottle, desk, glove,* and *orange*. The low were *easel, cactus, flask, garter, accordian, awning, ostrich,* and *crowbar*. Initially all subjects were presented pictures of the items and asked to name them, so that comparisons could be made later between words labeled and not labeled. The general procedure was as follows. There were two testing sessions (8 pictures each—4 high and 4 low frequency). Each picture was placed in front of the subject one by one. While the subject was viewing a picture, a tape recording played 14 words, 7 with no relation to the pictured object and 7 with some form of association with it. The associative categories chosen by the authors were:

1. Superordinate, where the word names the class of which the target is a member (e.g., *plant* for *cactus*).
2. Attribute, which was an adjective describing a feature of the target (e.g., *sharp* for *knife*).
3. Contrast coordinate, another word that is a member of the same superordinate class as the target (e.g., *cow* for *sheep*). This category relation was discussed earlier in this chapter as the minimal contrastive set, and it was stressed that words in these sets are strongly paradigmatically related in that none appear in the definitional structures of the other. Note, on the other hand, that the superordinate *plant* will likely appear in the definition of *cactus* as will the attribute *sharp* for *knife*.
4. Functional associate, a verb depicting an action directed by or upon the target (e.g., *play* for *accordian*).
5. Functional context, the situation, general environment, or atmosphere in which the target occurs (e.g., *leg* for *garter*). Note that, like 1 and 2, functional associates and contexts also form part of definitional structure (e.g., *An accordian is something you play* or *A garter is worn on the leg*).
6. A phonetic associate (e.g., *Austria* for *ostrich*).
7. Identity, which was the spoken label for the object—a strong associate indeed!

Phonetic associates were simply not appreciated by the subjects and were consequently excluded from the analysis.

The subjects sat in front of a loudspeaker and held a rubber bulb in their left hand. The bulb was connected to a timer. They were instructed to squeeze the bulb if any of the words spoken from the recorder reminded them of the picture "even a little bit." The timing mechanism started at the last stressed syllable of the spoken stimulus word. Bulb pressure stopped it. As pointed out earlier, so-called strength of associate bonding can be measured in terms of the real-time delay for naming or recognizing associates. Zurif *et al.* (1974) did not, it will be recalled, use time as a measure.

Two response measures were studied: latency, when there was a response, and the number of trials, when the subject failed to respond to an associate (errors). In the first place, the high-comprehension group paralleled the two control groups in latency across associative categories—all were excellent on the identity associate. For that matter, so was the low-comprehension group. Notice however, that recognizing the identity associate was no more than recognizing a cue. Practically all aphasics who cannot find labels can recognize them if provided by the examiner. The high-comprehension and control groups all did very poorly on contrast coordinates and functional associates in terms of latency of response. The low-comprehension group was significantly different from all other in that it did surprisingly well with contrast coordinates but was remarkably impaired with functional associates. Error rates showed similar distinctions; again, the high-comprehension group paralleled the controls. The error rates (lack of response) for the contrast coordinates proved extremely interesting, since ALL groups failed to appreciate semantic connectivity among words in these minimal contrastive sets. Again, it is important to point out that the low-comprehension group did not differ from the other groups in detecting the identity category, but the error rate was extremely poor for all other associative detections. That is, the low-comprehension group knew enough to recognize the cue when provided but not enough to appreciate the normal range of associate bonds. Goodglass and Baker took this to mean that the low-comprehension aphasics "know WHAT an object is, but not ABOUT it [p. 367]." The semantic field is constricted. Note, however, that the words are not lost in any sense, rather their associative structures are narrowed or loosened up. Next, the authors examined the effect of the lexical disorganization on naming.

The low-comprehension group showed increased latencies across more categories than did the high-comprehension group for words they failed to label. Error rate for nonlabeled words was even more revealing. Although the high-comprehension group did not perform differentially to the associates of labeled versus nonlabeled words, the low-comprehension subjects had 50% greater error rates for associate appreciation of words they could not name. Analyses of variance demonstrated that word frequency was not significant for either comprehension group on latency of response or on success in naming. It is crucial to rule out word frequency as a significant factor for word finding problems, since frequency explanations are external to any one individual's lexical system. For this reason, deferring to word frequency counts is an uninteresting way to explain aphasic lexical behavior.

With respect to specific associative categories, it is significant that the superordinates were practically as intact as were the identity items, whereas the associates from within the minimal contrastive sets aroused little reaction. Also, somewhat surprising because of their essential syntagmatic relationships, functional contexts and functional associates were the most impaired in the low-comprehension subjects, who, in reality, were Wernicke's aphasics. The prediction would have been that the Wernicke's aphasics, with posterior lesions, should have shown better sensitivity to syntagmatic associates.

The basic findings from this study were, then, that both aphasic groups had shortened latency responses for recognizing associates of words they correctly named than of words they failed to name. The low-comprehension aphasics failed to respond to more associates in all categories for nonlabeled words than for labeled words. In fact, the difference was quite significant. There was a nonsignificant trend in this same direction for the high-comprehension group as well. The correlation between failure to name an object and failure to appreciate its semantic associates indicates that word finding deficits are related to disrupted associative structure.

In the same vein, Whitehouse *et al.* (1978) investigated how form and function interact in the labeling process. They looked at Broca's aphasics and anomic aphasics and asked whether one or both would show normal naming profiles (Labov, 1973) by altering labeling strategies in accordance with stipulated functions. Other research (Miller & Johnson-Laird, 1976) has shown that perceptual and functional information must be intact in order to decide whether a given object X is or is not labeled X. Whitehouse *et al.* realize that quite often aphasics will not be able to name an object on configuration test (or in general when they are asked the name of some item) but will be able to use the item in their patterns of ordinary daily use. What they did was study how aphasics (anterior versus posterior, roughly) utilize and integrate perceptual and functional attributes of objects "in order to find a verbal label [p. 65]."

The objects whose shapes and functional contexts were manipulated had to be labelable in their prototypical depictions; the objects on the manipulated continuum were bowl, cup, and glass. The functional phenomena were coffee poured from a pot into the container (cup function), cereal poured into the container (bowl function), and ice water poured from a pitcher into the container (glass function). Twenty-four drawings of containers were constructed so that, in a continuous scaling through gradual changes in shape, six drawings went from a prototypical cup to a bowl by adding to the width dimension. Similarly, six other drawings ranged from the prototypical cup, by increasing the height dimension, to a glasslike container. One group of 12 containers along the scale had handles; the other group did not have handles. The authors set these drawings up so that the three contextual (coffee, cereal, ice water) pictures could be fit to the container drawings such that they both appeared as one picture of some food substance being poured into some container. The situation was set up so that functional contexts and shapes could both be varied. Crucially, there were drawings of containers that had and did not have handles and whose shapes were at the border zones between cups and bowls and between cups and glasses. Each possible container was shown to the subjects in all possible contexts and once each with no context (neutral). While looking at each combined picture (container and context), subjects were offered a name (bowl, cup, or glass) presented orally and asked to indicate by raising their hands when the desired label was uttered.

For recognizing names with no context, the Broca's subjects behaved normally. They could name the prototypes and demonstrated sensitivity to the border zone areas. The posterior anomics appeared unable to integrate perceptual information. Regardless of the height or width, if it had a handle it was labeled *cup*. In addition, normals and Broca's invariably used context information in border zone cases to label; anomics, on the other hand, did not show effects of functional context. The anomics agreed with the examiner's utterance of *cup*, for instance, far more often than did the Broca's aphasics when the shape was glasslike AND when the context was pouring ice water from a pitcher.

In general, these findings accord with the previous two studies described. Broca's aphasics appear to have a much richer and better organized mental lexicon in terms of conceptual and functional information than do posterior aphasics. More recent support for this is provided by Grober *et al.* (1980), who found that the underlying representation of semantic categories is generally preserved in anterior aphasics but disrupted in posterior syndromes. The posterior group performs much worse at categorical boundaries and appears to selectively disregard defining features while placing complete reliance upon idiosyncratic characteristic features that tie the word more closely to personal situations and subjective experiences.

Aside from lexical associative disruption explanations for naming deficits, we should briefly mention two others—disconnection and neurodynamic breakdown. Disconnection-type explanations were inevitable once psychological associationism took hold in the study of human behavior. At first, of course, DISCONNECTION was used in a purely psychological (i.e., mental, nonphysical) sense, where one associate could be cut off, isolated, or disconnected from another. Benton and Joynt (1960, p. 214) claim that Johann Gesner (1738–1801), in his major work on aphasic descriptions (1770), was the first to introduce associative reasoning in explaining semantic–lexical deficits in patients with neologisms and lexical substitution errors. For Gesner, the patients' inability consisted in the failure to associate images or abstract ideas with their expressive verbal symbols.

Approximately 100 years later, anatomical structures such as the white fiber system were implicated in associative function. Once the general outline for this view was laid down in Wernicke (1977/1874), there was an increase in "diagram making," and disconnection of physical structures now became a plausible manner in which to explain disabilities in repetition, copying, reading aloud, comprehending, carrying out motor movements to command, and providing labels for objects presented in one stimulus mode or another. Not only did white fiber tracts connect areas within lobes and across lobes in one hemisphere, but there were interhemispheric (corpus callosum) fiber connections as well. Two important naming disconnections were then explainable. The first could arise from a lesion disconnecting Wernicke's area, where the acoustic–sound images were stored, from the angular gyrus, where the visual associates for objects were stored. As a consequence, when patients were shown an object or a picture of it and asked to name it, they could not. This type of explanation was so powerful that it remains today (Geschwind, 1974), despite arguments against it from Freud (1953/1891) to Brown (1977).

Benson (1979, p. 310) discusses another "anomia of disconnection," where the fibers involved form PART of the corpus callosum. Benson presents a case of "tactile" anomia following a lesion deep in the right frontal lobe lateral to the genu of the callosum (p. 311). When out of sight, an object placed in the left hand of the patient could not be labeled. The theory is that palpation with the left hand innervates right hemisphere tactile areas and that to name the palpated object the information from the tactile sensation region of the right hemisphere must travel through the anterior portion of the callosum to the language areas in the dominant left hemisphere. As long as the object remains out of sight, the patients cannot name it. Since the patients can later select the object from among a group, it does not appear that they did not know what the object was or somehow could not understand it. Another partial callosal disconnection anomia has been suggested for colors by Geschwind and Fusillo (1966). Here, visual color information is blocked from right to left transfer for naming. Unlike Benson's tactile anomia, which was secondary to anterior callosal lesions, the color anomia follows posterior callosal lesions in the splenium; the left visual cortex must also be damaged.

Note that the tactile anomia and the visual color anomia may occur with only PARTIAL hemispheric disconnections—anterior and posterior, respectively. For instance, the tactile anomia presumably would be corrected if visual information could reach the right visual cortex, since the information could cross the posterior callosum to the left side. There exist, however, patients who have had complete commissurotomy (total section of the corpus callosum) (Dimond, 1972; Gazzaniga, 1970; Sperry & Gazzaniga, 1967). These subjects will show the tactile anomia I have described, but they would NOT improve even were the right visual cortex to get information about the object. With tachistoscopic presentation of visual stimuli to one or the other visual field, naming experiments in the visual modality can be carried out with this "split-brain" population. For instance, visual stimuli presented exclusively to the right hemisphere (left visual field) of split-brain subjects cannot be named because the information received by the right visual cortex cannot traverse to the left language areas. In these cases, if the visual stimulus is not confined to the right hemisphere, the object will be named. Such is not the case with the color-specific anomia, since, for this syndrome to exist in the first place, there must be additional involvement in the left visual cortex. Some caution, however, should be maintained when interpreting the split-brain findings as they pertain to normal cortical function and capacity, since patients who undergo commissurotomy have usually had early brain insults bringing about abnormal functional rearrangement in the nervous system. Early lesions in the left hemisphere will force a functional shift to the would-be nondominant hemisphere, so that as adults, when they are tested postcommissurotomy, they will demonstrate more right hemisphere function than usual. This does not tell us what goes on in the normal right hemisphere, only what COULD go on.

In addition to semantic field disorganization and cerebral disconnection accounts of anomia, there is the neurodynamic theory of A. R. Luria (1972, 1973, 1974, 1975). The central physiological assumptions are Pavlovian in nature and focus upon characterizing normal and abnormal states of the cortex. When the brain is functioning as it should, physiological mechanisms operate under what are called "rules of force." When these rules of force are intact, strong or important stimuli evoke strong reactions, and weak or unimportant stimuli evoke weak reactions.[2] The "law of strength" in these cortical states is said to operate normally. Under these conditions, the subject is able to focus upon and attend to target behaviors as well as to select the most appropriate from among similar behaviors. The aftereffects of excitation as well as the similar but nonappropriate and unimportant stimuli are readily inhibited from rising to threshold in the undisturbed neurodynamic state.

An abnormal, or pathological, state of the cortex rearranges these neurodynamic forces; it is referred to as the "inhibitory phase." Under this condition, strong or important stimuli evoke reactions OF THE SAME STRENGTH as weak or unimportant stimuli. Since, here, all reactions are equally evoked, the cerebral state is also referred to as the "phase of equalization."

According to Luria, when the rule of force is functioning normally, and a word is needed, a multidimensional matrix of associated lexical items is evoked from which the proper word is to be selected. Subsequently, the subject attends to the task, directs his focus upon the appropriate word, and selects it, simultaneously inhibiting all other words in the matrix that have been subliminally aroused because of their similarity to the target word. If, however, the cortex has been damaged, and placed in the phase of equalization, word selection will be blocked because the whole matrix is aroused to equal strength so that NO form will be forthcoming. Anomia, then, for Luria (1974) is caused by "equal probability of the evocation of a whole complex of words which have some similarity [p. 9]." This briefly describes Luria's account of word-finding blocks. For sure, there is much more to his theories of cortical neurodynamics; I have restricted my comments to anomia only. The theory as a whole has some serious drawbacks (see Buckingham, 1977b), and it depends heavily on associative reasoning and terminology. Nevertheless, it represents an explanation of word-finding deficits quite different from the ones we have considered. The main stumbling block for the theory is that it is difficult to test. Consequently, it is impossible to know how one would go about disproving it, although if we follow the reasoning of Goodglass and Baker (1976) to its logical conclusion, we might have some cause to question it.

It would seem plausible to conclude from Luria's position that the more complex the matrix of lexical associates brought to mind by the aphasic, the more difficult it would be to inhibit all but the appropriate word from rising to threshold. A reduced semantic field with weakened

2. Warren (1921, pp. 144, 257) and Robinson (1976, p. 375) have both pointed to the associationist roots of Pavlovian neuropsychology, especially to the work of the eighteenth-century British association psychologist David Hartley (1959/1746, 1749).

associative strengths should, therefore, put LESS pressure on the inhibitory mechanism. Goodglass and Baker's (1976) study, however, leads to the conclusion that it is precisely BECAUSE of the reduced semantic fields that the patients have word-finding problems.

On the other hand, Luria's theory would predict that prompting the patient with some form of semantically associated cue, for example, would only cause further hindrance, since that cue would still need to be inhibited and possibly more so because its presence would have been greatly upgraded by the verbal stimulus. Marshall and Halvorson (1976), in a "point to" task with patients having word-finding difficulties, showed that providing the patients with several lexical associates only enhanced their confusion.

Since the term RETRIEVAL is a metaphorical and descriptive term, we cannot arrive at an ultimate account of word-finding problems in terms of it. That is, to claim that a patient has "retrieval" deficits is to describe the patient's behavior, but it does not account for or explain the behavior. One cannot explain X in terms of X. Therefore, since "retrieval" problems, "access" problems, or "word-finding" problems all describe the same behavioral abnormality, it makes no sense to use one term to explain the other. In this section, I have outlined three possible explanatory accounts for retrieval disturbances: (a) lexical structure disorganization; (b) cerebral disconnection; and (c) cortical neurodynamic irregularities.

The studies that propose (a) as an explanation do not claim that any words are lost from the lexicon. They claim that the boundaries between spheres are less distinct. This is not a reduction in the vocabulary in terms of number of lexical items. There has been great misunderstanding on this point, and it goes back in history to the original misconception that word-finding deficits result from "forgetting" the words.[3] In fact, everyone knows that the anachronistic term AMNESIC APHASIA does not really characterize anomia of any sort. Aphasics do not lose "memory for words." This is why such studies as Wiegel-Crump and Koenigsknecht (1973) although interesting in themselves, do not disprove any interesting accounts of word-finding problems.

These authors worked with four aphasics characterized as anomics. Out of a large corpus of words that the patients initially could not name, 40 were chosen for each patient in such a way that they could be equally distributed into five superordinate semantic categories: household items, clothing, foods, living things, and action words. In the 18 therapy sessions (2–3 per week, 1 hour sessions), 20 of these 40 words were

3. Benton and Joynt (1960, p. 211) quote from a case report written by Carl Linné in 1745, where the patient was said to have lost "the memory of all nouns."

drilled in all categories except foods. All patients were able to match pictures depicting distinct figural replicas having the same verbal referent; thus they presumably still had lexical conceptual structure intact. Nevertheless, this was not a labeling exercise and would seem to tap only that degree of functional information needed for the patients' patterns of everyday action and thought (Whitehouse *et al.,* 1978, p. 65). After therapy, the subjects made significant improvement in picture naming with *both* drilled and nondrilled test items. Not only were there far more correct responses, but there was also a significant reduction in response latency. Moreover, there was no significant difference in the improvement of nondrilled items within drilled categories versus improvement on items within the field of foods, which as a category had not been drilled. Thus, the therapy generalized not only to the nondrilled items in the drilled categories but also to the category of foods, which had not been drilled at all. The results are indeed interesting, especially as they demonstrate how clinical intervention may influence improved performance, and generalize to other behaviors. However, Wiegel-Crump and Koenigsknecht have disproved a theory that no one has held for a long time. The lexical structure disruption accounts of word-finding deficits are not that there is a reduction in the lexicon itself (Wiegel-Crump & Koenigsknecht, 1973, p. 411) or that there is an absolute loss of words (p. 417), but that the associative links within spheres of meaning are weakened. Consequently, Wiegel-Crump and Koenigsknecht's therapy sessions could have been somehow strengthening these bonds. By practicing the drilled items within a category, the patients were perhaps bringing the bonds into sharper focus; by fiat, this would serve better to delineate the nondrilled words in that category. This would account for the generalized improvement in the drilled categories. Practice with the four categories in therapy, by fiat, drew the fifth (foods) into sharper distinction from the rest. This could have aided labeling in that category and would account for the generalization to it. Therefore, this study, although significant in what it shows concerning therapy and its usefulness, does not necessarily contradict Zurif *et al.* (1974), Goodglass and Baker (1976), or Whitehouse *et al.* (1978). It only contradicts a trivial and anachronistic theory of word-finding problems that would claim, like Linné in 1745, that words had been lost from memory.

Concluding Remarks

In this chapter I have attempted to sketch an outline of psycholinguistic aspects of aphasic vocabularies, their structure, and their use. I focused my attention on the lexicon, since most of what we know about semantic systems in aphasia relates to it. At the outset I presented some basic concepts and theories of the structure of the lexicon as it presumably exists in the normal linguistic system. Without some notion of undisturbed patterns, descriptions of disturbed patterns would have no landmarks. The nature of retrieval from the lexicon in normals and the psychological accounts offered for selection and insertion were presented. The metaphoric nature of the term STRENGTH was pointed out, and it was suggested that the essential aspects of neuropsychological theories of the lexicon and retrieval from it have their roots firmly placed in a centuries-old association psychology. Aphasic disturbances of the lexicon were also addressed in terms of lesion location, and it was shown that localizing studies in normal populations often support findings from lesion studies. I outlined several distinct linguistic manifestations that indicate lexical access difficulties. This was followed by a presentation of various possible explanatory accounts for retrieval disturbances. It was stressed that word-finding (or naming) deficits can be DESCRIBED AS retrieval deficits but cannot be EXPLAINED BY retrieval deficits. There must always be a reason why the retrieval mechanism cannot function. Simply claiming it does not function says essentially nothing. Future work on the lexicon of aphasics and retrieval from it will have to be very insistent on this point.

References

Akmajian, A., Demers, R. A., & Harnish, R. M. 1979. *Linguistics: An introduction to language and communication.* Cambridge, Mass.: MIT Press.

Austin, J. L. 1962. *How to do things with words.* New York: Oxford Univ. Press.

Benson, D. F. 1979. Neurologic correlates of anomia. In H. Whitaker & H. A. Whitaker (Eds.), *Studies in neurolinguistics* (Vol. 4). New York: Academic Press.

Benson, D. F., Sheremata, W., Bouchard, R., Segarra, J., Price, R., & Geschwind, N. 1973. Conduction aphasia: A clinicopathological study. *Archives of Neurology, 28,* 339–346.

Benton, A., & Joynt, R. 1960. Early descriptions of aphasia. *Archives of Neurology, 3,* 205–222.

Berlin, B., & Kay, P. 1969. *Basic color terms: Their universality and evolution.* Berkeley & Los Angeles, Calif.: Univ. of California Press.

Brown, J. W. 1972. *Aphasia, apraxia and agnosia: Clinical and theoretical aspects.* Springfield, Ill.: Thomas.

Brown, J. W. 1977. *Mind, brain, and consciousness.* New York: Academic Press.

Buckingham, H. W. 1977. The conduction theory and neologistic jargon. *Language and Speech, 20.* 174–184. (a)

Buckingham, H. W. 1977. A critique of A. R. Luria's neurodynamic explanation of paraphasia. *Brain and Language, 4,* 580–587. (b)

Buckingham, H. W. 1979. Linguistic aspects of lexical retrieval disturbances in the posterior fluent aphasias. In H. Whitaker & H. A. Whitaker (Eds.), *Studies in neurolinguistics* (Vol. 4). New York: Academic Press.

Buckingham, H. W. 1980. On correlating aphasic errors with slips-of-the-tongue. *Applied Psycholinguistics, 1,* 199–220.

Buckingham, H. W. 1981. Where do neologisms come from? In J. W. Brown (Ed.), *Jargonaphasia.* New York: Academic Press.

Buckingham, H. W., & Kertesz, A. 1974. A linguistic analysis of fluent aphasia. *Brain and Language, 1,* 43–61.

Buckingham, H. W., & Kertesz, A. 1976. *Neologistic jargon aphasia.* Amsterdam: Swets & Zeitlinger.

Buckingham, H. W., & Rekart, D. M. 1979. Semantic paraphasia. *Journal of Communication Disorders, 12,* 197–209.

Buckingham, H. W., Whitaker, H., & Whitaker, H. A. 1978. Alliteration and assonance in neologistic jargon aphasia. *Cortex, 14,* 365–380.

Buckingham, H. W., Whitaker, H., & Whitaker, H. A. 1979. On linguistic perseveration. In H. Whitaker & H. A. Whitaker (Eds.), *Studies in neurolinguistics* (Vol. 4). New York: Academic Press.

Butterworth, B. 1979. Hesitation and the production of verbal paraphasias and neologisms in jargon aphasia. *Brain and Language, 8,* 133–161.

Butterworth, B. 1980. Evidence from pauses in speech. In B. Butterworth (Ed.), *Language production, Vol. 1: Speech and talk.* London: Academic Press.

Chapman, R. M., McCrary, J. W., Chapman, J. A., & Bragdon, H. R. 1978. Brain responses related to semantic meaning. *Brain and Language, 5,* 195–205.

Clark, H. H., & Clark, E. V. 1977. *Psychology and language: An introduction to psycholinguistics.* New York: Harcourt Brace Jovanovich.

Cole, P. (Ed.). 1978. *Syntax and semantics: Pragmatics* (Vol. 9). New York: Academic Press.

Cole, P., & Morgan, J. L. (Eds.). 1975. *Syntax and semantics: Speech acts* (Vol. 3). New York: Academic Press.

Cutler, A., & Isard, S. D. 1980. The production of prosody. In B. Butterworth (Ed.), *Language production, Vol. 1: Speech and talk.* London: Academic Press.

Damasio, A. R., McKee, J., & Damasio, H. 1979. Determinants of performance in color anomia. *Brain and Language, 7,* 74–85.

Deese, J. 1965. *Structure of associations in language and thought.* Baltimore, Md.: Johns Hopkins Press.

Dennis, M. 1976. Dissociated naming and locating of body parts after left anterior temporal lobe resection: An experimental case study. *Brain and Language, 3,* 147–163.

de Saussure, F. 1959. *Course in general linguistics.* New York: Philosophical Library.

Dillon, G. L. 1977. *Introduction to contemporary linguistic semantics.* Englewood Cliffs, N.J.: Prentice-Hall.

Dimond, S. 1972. *The double brain.* Edinburgh and London: Churchill Livingstone.

Fedio, P., & Van Buren, J. M. 1974. Memory deficits during electrical stimulation of the speech cortex in conscious man. *Brain and Language, 1,* 29–42.

Fillmore, C. J., & Langendoen, D. T. (Eds.). 1971. *Studies in linguistic semantics.* New York: Holt, Rinehart & Winston.

Fodor, J. D. 1977. *Semantics: Theories of meaning in generative grammar.* New York: Crowell.

Freud, S. 1953. [*On aphasia: A critical study*] (E. Stengel, trans.). London: Imago Publishing Co. (Originally published, 1891.)

Gardner, H. 1973. The contribution of operativity to naming capacity in aphasic patients. *Neuropsychologia, 11,* 213–230.

Gardner, H., Silverman, J., Wapner, W., & Zurif, E. 1978. The appreciation of antonymic contrasts in aphasia. *Brain and Language, 6,* 301–317.

Gazzaniga, M. S. 1970. *The bisected brain.* New York: Appleton.

Geschwind, N. 1967. The varieties of naming errors. *Cortex, 3,* 97–112.

Geschwind, N. 1974. *Selected papers on language and the brain.* Boston Studies in the Philosophy of Science, Vol. 16. R. S. Cohen & M. W. Wartofsky (Eds.). Dordrecht-Holland: D. Reidel Publ.

Geschwind, N., & Fusillo, M. 1966. Color naming defects in association with alexia. *Archives of Neurology, 15,* 137–146.

Goldman-Eisler, F. 1964. Hesitation, information, and levels of speech production. In A. DeReuck & M. O'Connor (Eds.), *Disorders of language.* Boston: Little, Brown.

Goldman-Eisler, F. 1968. *Psycholinguistics: Experiments in spontaneous speech.* London: Academic Press.

Goldstein, K. 1948. *Language and language disturbances.* New York: Grune & Stratton.

Goodenough, W. H. 1956. Componential analysis and the study of meaning. *Language, 32,* 195–216.

Goodenough, W. H. 1965. Yankee kinship terminology: A problem in componential analysis. *American Anthropologist, 67* (5, Pt. 2), 259–287.

Goodglass, H. 1978. *Selected papers in neurolinguistics.* Munich: Wilhelm Fink Verlag.

Goodglass, H., & Baker, E. 1976. Semantic field, naming, and auditory comprehension in aphasia. *Brain and Language, 3,* 359–374.

Goodglass, H., Barton, M. I., & Kaplan, E. F. 1968. Sensory modality and object-naming in aphasia. *Journal of Speech and Hearing Research, 11,* 488–496.

Goodglass, H., Klein, B., Carey, P., & Jones, K. 1966. Specific semantic word categories in aphasia. *Cortex, 2,* 74–89.

Green, E. 1969. Phonological and grammatical aspects of jargon in an aphasic patient. *Language and Speech, 12,* 103–118.

Grober, E., Perecman, E., Kellar, L., & Brown, J. W. 1980. Lexical knowledge in anterior and posterior aphasics. *Brain and Language, 10,* 318–330.

Grossman, M. 1978. The game of the name: An examination of linguistic reference after brain damage. *Brain and Language, 6,* 112–119.

Grossman, M. 1981. A bird is a bird is a bird: Making reference within and without superordinate categories. *Brain and Language, 12,* 313–331.

Gruber J. 1976. *Lexical structures in syntax and semantics.* New York: North-Holland Publ.

Hartley, D. 1959. [*Various conjectures on the perception, motion, and generation of ideas.*] (R. E. A. Palmer, trans., with introduction and notes by M. Kallich). The Augustan Reprint Society Publication No. 77–78. Los Angeles: William Andrews Clark Memorial Library. (Originally published, 1746.)

Hartley, D. 1749. *Observations on man, his frame, his duty, and his expectations* (2 vols.). London: Leake and Frederick.

Hier, D. B., Mogil, S. I., Rubin, N. P., & Komros, G. R. 1980. Semantic aphasia: A neglected entity. *Brain and Language, 10,* 120–131.

Jakobson, R. 1964. Towards a linguistic typology of aphasic impairments. In A. DeRuck & M. O'Connor (Eds.), *Disorders of Language.* Boston: Little, Brown.

Katz, J. J. 1972. *Semantic theory.* New York: Harper.

Katz, J. J. 1977. *Propositional structure and illocutionary forces: A study of the contribution of sentence meaning to speech acts.* New York: Crowell.

Kay, P., & McDaniel, C. K. 1978. The linguistic significance of the meanings of basic color terms. *Language, 54,* 610–646.

Kertesz, A., & Benson, D. F. 1970. Neologistic jargon: A clinico-pathological study. *Cortex,* 6, 362–386.
Kinsbourne, M., & Warrington, E. 1963. Jargon aphasia. *Neuropsychologia, 1,* 27–37.
Labov, W. 1973. The boundaries of words and their meanings. In C-J. Bailey & R. Shuy (Eds.), *New ways of analyzing variation in English.* Washington, D.C.: Georgetown Univ. Press.
Lakoff, G., & Johnson, M. 1980. *Metaphors we live by.* Chicago: Univ. of Chicago Press.
Lassen, N. A., Ingvar, D. H., & Skinhøj, E. 1978. Brain function and blood flow. *Scientific American, 239* (October), 62–71.
Lecours, A. R., & Lhermitte, F. 1972. Recherches sur le langage des aphasiques: 4. Analyse d'un corpus de néologismes; notion de paraphasie monémique. *L'Encephale, 61,* 295–315.
Lehrer, A. 1969. Semantic cuisine. *Journal of Linguistics, 5,* 39–55.
Lehrer, A. 1974. *Semantic fields and lexical structure.* Amsterdam: North-Holland Publ.
Lesser, R. 1978. *Linguistic investigations of aphasia.* London: Arnold.
Luria, A. R. 1970. *Traumatic aphasia.* The Hague: Mouton.
Luria, A. R. 1972. Aphasia reconsidered. *Cortex, 8,* 34–40.
Luria, A. R. 1973. *The working brain: An introduction to neuropsychology.* New York: Basic Books.
Luria, A. R. 1974. Language and brain. *Brain and Language, 1,* 1–14.
Luria, A. R. 1975. Basic problems of language in the light of psychology and neurolinguistics. In E. H. Lenneberg & E. Lenneberg (Eds.), *Foundations of language development* (Vol. 2). New York: Academic Press.
Marshall, R. C. 1976. Word retrieval of aphasic adults. *Journal of Speech and Hearing Disorders, 41,* 444–451.
Marshall, R. C., & Halvorson, K. A. 1976. Influence of semantic relatedness on the auditory comprehension of aphasic adults. Paper presented at the meeting of the American Speech and Hearing Association, Houston, Texas.
McKeever, W. F., & Jackson, T. L. 1979. Cerebral dominance assessed by object- and color-naming latencies: Sex and familial sinistrality effects. *Brain and Language, 7,* 175–190.
Mercer, B., Wapner, W., Gardner, H., & Benson, D. F. 1977. A study of confabulation. *Archives of Neurology, 34,* 346–348.
Miller, G. A. 1969. A psychological method to investigate verbal concepts. *Journal of Mathematical Psychology, 6,* 169–191.
Miller, G. A., & Johnson-Laird, P. N. 1976. *Language and perception.* Cambridge, Mass.: Belknap Press.
Molfese, D. L. 1979. Cortical involvement in the semantic processing of coarticulated speech cues. *Brain and Language, 7,* 86–100.
Newmeyer, F. J. 1980. *Linguistic theory in America: The first quarter-century of transformational generative grammar.* New York: Academic Press.
Ortony, A. (Ed.). 1979. *Metaphor and thought.* Cambridge: Cambridge Univ. Press.
Oxbury, J. M., Oxbury, S. M., & Humphrey, N. K. 1969. Varieties of color anomia. *Brain, 92,* 847–860.
Putnam, H. 1975. Is semantics possible? In H. Putnam (Ed.), *Mind, language, and reality: Philosophical papers* (Vol. 2.). Cambridge: Cambridge Univ. Press.
Pylyshyn, Z. W. 1979. Metaphorical imprecision and the "top-down" research strategy. In A. Ortony (Ed.), *Metaphor and thought.* Cambridge: Cambridge Univ. Press.
Rinnert, C., & Whitaker, H. A. 1973. Semantic confusions by aphasic patients. *Cortex, 9,* 56–81.

Robinson, D. N. 1976. *An intellectual history of psychology.* New York: Macmillan.

Rosch, E. 1977. Classification of real-world objects: Origins and representations in cognition. In P. N. Johnson-Laird & P. C. Watson (Eds.), *Thinking: Readings in cognitive science.* Cambridge: Cambridge Univ. Press.

Sacks, S. (Ed.). 1979. *On metaphor.* Chicago: Univ. of Chicago Press.

Sadock, J. M. 1975. *Toward a linguistic theory of speech acts.* New York: Academic Press.

Searle, J. R. (Ed.). 1971. *The philosophy of language.* London: Oxford Univ. Press.

Shanon, B. 1978. Classification and identification in an aphasic patient. *Brain and Language,* 5, 188–194.

Shattuck-Hufnagel, S. 1979. Speech errors as evidence for a serial order mechanism in sentence production. In W. E. Cooper & E. C. T. Walker (Eds.), *Sentence processing: Psycholinguistic studies presented to Merrill Garrett.* Hillsdale, N.J.: Erlbaum.

Söderpalm, E. 1979. *Speech errors in normal and pathological speech.* Lund: CWK Gleerup.

Soh, K., Larsen, B., Skinhøj, E., & Lassen, N. A. 1978. Regional cerebral blood flow in aphasia. *Archives of Neurology,* 35, 625–632.

Sperry, R. W., & Gazzaniga, M. S. 1967. Language following surgical disconnection of the hemispheres. In C. H. Millikan & F. L. Darley (Eds.), *Brain mechanisms underlying speech and language.* New York: Grune & Stratton.

Thatcher, R. W., & April, R. S. 1976. Evoked potential correlates of semantic information processing in normals and aphasics. In R. W. Rieber (Ed.), *The neuropsychology of language.* New York: Plenum.

Warren, H. C. 1921. *A history of the association psychology.* London: Constable Press.

Weinstein, E. A., & Keller, J. J. A. 1963. Linguistic patterns of misnaming in brain injury. *Neuropsychologia,* 1, 79–90.

Weinstein, E. A., & Lyerly, O. 1976. Personality factors in jargon aphasia. *Cortex,* 12, 122–133.

Weinstein, E. A., Lyerly, O., Cole, M., & Ozer, M. 1966. Meaning in jargon aphasia. *Cortex,* 2, 166–187.

Weinstein, E. A., & Puig-Antich, J. 1974. Jargon and its analogues. *Cortex,* 10, 75–83.

Wepman, D., Bock, R., Jones, L., & Van Pelt, D. 1973. Psycholinguistic study of aphasia: A revision of the concept of anomia. In H. Goodglass & S. Blumstein (Eds.), *Psycholinguistics and aphasia.* Baltimore, Md.: Johns Hopkins Press.

Wernicke, C. 1977. [The aphasia symptom complex: A psychological study on an anatomic basis.] In G. H. Eggert (Ed. and trans.), *Wernicke's works on aphasia: A sourcebook and review.* The Hague: Mouton. (Originally published, 1874.)

Whitehouse, P., Caramazza, A., & Zurif, E. 1978. Naming in aphasia: Interacting effects of form and function. *Brain and Language,* 6, 63–74.

Whorf, B. L. 1956. *Language, thought and reality.* Cambridge, Mass.: MIT Press.

Wiegel-Crump, C., & Koenigsknecht, R. A. 1973. Tapping the lexical store of the adult aphasic: Analysis of the improvement made in word retrieval skills. *Cortex,* 9, 410–417.

Winner, E., & Gardner, H. 1977. Sensitivity to metaphor in organic patients. *Brain,* 100, 719–727.

Wood, F., Taylor, B., Penny, R., & Stump, D. 1980. Regional cerebral blood flow response to recognition memory versus semantic classification tasks. *Brain and Language,* 9, 113–122.

Yamadori, A., & Albert, M. L. 1973. Word category aphasia. *Cortex,* 9, 83–89.

Zurif, E., Caramazza, A., Myerson, R., & Galvin, J. 1974. Semantic feature representations for normal and aphasic language. *Brain and Language,* 1, 167–187.

8

Auditory Comprehension in Aphasia

KAREN RIEDEL

Not so long ago, it was common practice to describe the aphasias according to the obvious differences in behavior in different language modalities. This framework assumed that speech and comprehension were diametrically opposed; the terminology used to describe this state of affairs reflected this conception. Aphasics were said to manifest either an "expressive" or "receptive" disorder, or a "motor" rather than "sensory" disorder.

Currently, the syndromes of aphasia are classified according to aberrations in verbal output—that is, the overall fluency of speech, the presence or absence of articulatory disorders, paraphasia, the content of vocabulary, and intactness of syntax. This is accomplished with a fair degree of certainty since the parameters of speech are readily observed, taped, transcribed, described, and analyzed. Identifying the dimensions of the defects in auditory comprehension of spoken language is quite another matter because they can only be inferred from an aphasic individual's response to what he hears.

It is, however, difficult to know whether the adequacy–inadequacy of an aphasic person's response to controlled spoken units reflects actual comprehension. Add to the fact that, in the real world, variables influencing comprehension are not precisely controlled. An aphasic with limited comprehension of individual linguistic units can frequently employ his understanding of known situations to infer from content what is expected of him, so that in many familiar situations responses to spoken language appear appropriate. On the other hand, the aphasic with fairly intact comprehension subjected to unfamiliar, unnatural, anxiety-

215

provoking situations often manifests considerable inconsistency in understanding relatively simple material.

It goes without saying, that one can assume very little about comprehension disorders in aphasia without an in-depth examination using a number of different techniques and careful observation of a patient's overall behavior in a variety of situations. Although the techniques of assessment have become more refined over the years, it is important to keep in mind that the fundamental problems of where, how, and what is examined persist without firm agreement as to which factors are the most relevant.

Recently, linguists have brought their tools and descriptive techniques to the study of aphasia, which has effected important changes in the direction of speech comprehension research. Linguistic parameters have been defined, and the variables are more systematically controlled so that the differences in dimensions of comprehension in the various syndromes of aphasia can be investigated. But intimately related to language disorders are a multiplicity of nonlinguistic factors that have implications for not only how the aphasic understands language in the real world but how he performs on tests designed to assess parameters of comprehension ability.

In this chapter, the following topics will be treated: the historical basis of fundamental issues, contemporary investigations, the problems of assessment, the implications of studies using the Token Test, and the evolution of auditory comprehension recovery.

Theoretical Issues

To put current investigations of comprehension into proper perspective, it is instructive to look at the manner in which basic theoretical issues have evolved. Boller (1978, 1979) and Boller, Kim, and Mack (1977) have reviewed the contributions of many early investigators in aphasia. For purposes of this chapter, only the major theoretical positions concerning auditory comprehension of spoken language will be discussed.

The major contribution of Carl Wernicke's discovery of sensory aphasia was his focus on the problem of language comprehension in aphasia and its localization to the left temporal area (Eggert, 1977, p. 47). This immediately spurred investigation into the nature of comprehension disorders, and over a period of years, Wernicke formulated a theoretical model to account for impaired auditory processing. The model associated the location of the brain lesion with different varieties

of comprehension disorders. Subcortical damage, he concluded, inter-
fered with the transmission of spoken language to the cortical sensory
speech area and resulted in "pure word deafness." Localized damage to
the sensory speech area resulted in impairment of the sensory imagery
necessary for comprehension of word concepts, producing sensory
aphasia. Nonlocalized cerebral damage resulted in impairment of the
higher mental processes of conceptualization. Damage at this level was
said to result in dementia.

Wernicke later revised his theory about the nature of the deficits in
sensory aphasia and interpreted the loss of comprehension as a result of
the loss of word sound perception, more precisely, an impairment of
that portion of the hearing scale within which the speech process takes
place (Eggert, 1977, p. 45).

Pierre Marie (translated by Cole & Cole, 1971) challenged nearly all of
Wernicke's assertions. In his opinion there were not several discrete
clinical syndromes, but only one "true" aphasia, the "aphasia of Wernicke" or sensory aphasia. Broca's aphasia was viewed as simply Wernicke's aphasia plus anarthria. He took issue with the concept of centers
for "sensory images," pointing out that aphasics understand individual
words but fail to understand words when combined in a sentence. Furthermore, he emphasized that aphasics manifest deficits that go beyond
the auditory–verbal modality and stated that the common unifying disorder was a "marked diminution of intellectual capacity in general [p.
54]."

Based on early experimental investigations (Marie & Vaschide, 1903a,
1903b, 1903c, 1903d) in which he compared aphasics' reaction times,
immediate memory for words, and word association to normal, Marie
found all aphasic patients markedly deficient. He concluded that the
intellectual impairment was both quantitative and qualitative in nature.
Pierre Marie departed from Wernicke and other of his contemporaries
who viewed intellectual disturbances as accessory to aphasia. To him,
they were THE central deficit.

Arnold Pick's theoretical model of aphasia is credited with laying the
groundwork for the study of language as a mental process, which is the
domain of contemporary psycholinguistics (Spreen, 1973). Pick conceived of language comprehension as a complex hierarchical process,
the stages of which were not additive but led to greater perceptual clarity
and increased refinement in understanding the utterance. He believed
the understanding of single words evoked the general concept of the
content of the utterance and preceded the stages of linguistic processing,
which led in turn to the correct specific concept. Pick was unique among
his contemporaries in emphasizing the primacy of the sentence, the role

of prosody, and the closeness of the spoken sentence to the grammar of thought. He valued aphasic's responses to language, since by observing the responses, he could identify and study the aborted stage of processing.

The application of linguistics to the investigation of comprehension disorders in aphasia was furthered by Roman Jakobson (1970). Linguistic analysis, he believed, provided both quantitative and qualitative evidence to differentiate the major forms of aphasia. He thought that each syndrome involved a disturbance in one of two fundamental operations, selection or combination.

Both encoding and decoding of speech involved these basic operations, but in reverse. He hypothesized that in encoding, the speaker begins with the selection of constituents before combining them into a whole. In decoding, however, the listener begins with context, the combinatory process, before analyzing the constituents. The "motor" aphasic, selectively impaired in the operation of combination—that is, in the use of contextual information—is forced to rely on analyzing constituent words. In "sensory" aphasia, the antecedent process of combination and contextual comprehension is preserved, but the selection or analysis of constituent lexical items is selectively impaired. He believed disturbances of selection have a greater impact than the disturbances of combination on comprehension of meaning.

The notion underlying Luria's model of aphasia (Luria, 1958, 1964; Luria & Hutton, 1977) is that brain lesions result in a fundamental defect in the neurodynamic operations of analysis and synthesis. The primary disturbance has repercussions on a whole complex of linguistic and nonlinguistic functions. The quality of the disturbance or symptom complex is dependent on the location of the lesion. Thus, qualitatively different auditory comprehension defects are produced by various lesions in the left hemisphere, and each disturbance can be traced to a single irreducible defect. Lesions of the temporal zone result in sensory aphasia, or acoustico-gnostic aphasia, due to a defect in the auditory analyzer responsible for the discrimination of speech sounds. A second type of temporal zone comprehension disorder, acoustico-mnesic aphasia, is due to difficulty in retention of word sound traces. The word heard subsequently interferes with the one heard before; that is, although individual words are comprehended adequately, failure is encountered when words are presented in a sentence or a series. Lesions of the zone where the temporal, parietal, and occipital lobes meet, results in semantic or pure amnesic aphasia, a linguistic disturbance due to failure in "simultaneous synthesis."

The aphasic individual afflicted with a lesion in this area has difficulty understanding the simplest logicogrammatical constructions. He is unable to comprehend units of words that require combining a number of elements into a single whole concept and therefore fails to understand such utterances as *father's brother* versus *brother's father*. He is also unable to transform word order to achieve an accurate interpretation of passives, for example, *A boy was bitten by a dog*, and he has difficulty with phrases involving spatial relations, for example *circle under the triangle*.

Luria implies that the comprehension disorder in frontal lesions (efferent motor aphasia) is a secondary disturbance reflecting the defects of inner language associated with the disintegration of dynamic schemes of expression.

Jason Brown's theory (1972), expanded in 1977, represents a departure from traditional formulations regarding the nature of aphasia. Following and expanding Arnold Pick in emphasis on hierarchical systems of cognition, Brown conceives of aphasia as the result of disturbances within the linguistic phase of the hierarchy but points out analogous patterns of breakdown in all functional systems: language, praxis, perception. The clinical forms of aphasia represent different stages in the formation of language in normal speech production. In each syndrome of aphasia, there is a conjoint reduction of the expressive–receptive unit to a given stage. He accepts the broad distinction between anterior and posterior aphasias, and classifies aphasia along traditional lines. However, Brown's interpretation of aphasic syndromes is unorthodox. The symptoms comprising each syndrome are analyzed in relation to the stage of regression in the cognitive hierarchy that they represent.

Brown asserts that the nonlinguistic (perceptual) changes found are not added to but are a part of the reduction and vary predictably according to the stage of language that is disturbed. Emotional changes, too, represent not reactions to the disturbance but subjective components attached to each level, a suggestion rather unique in contemporary literature.

The contemporary literature pertaining to speech comprehension in aphasia is dominated by discussions that allude to the basic controversies that were widely disputed at the beginning of this century. Are the speech symptom complexes of aphasia reflective of different central mechanisms underlying the comprehension of spoken language? If so, what is the evidence of these differences? If there is a unifying deficit underlying the comprehension disturbance, what is its nature? Are the differences in comprehension ability in aphasia only quantitative? What is the nature of auditory–verbal perception deficits? How does the perceptual function operate? How central and/or integral are the many non-linguistic deficits manifested by aphasics to their problem in comprehending language?

Contemporary Studies

Linguistic Factors in Comprehension

Lesser (1978) identified two major contributions of the linguistic approach to the study of language disorders in aphasia: (*a*) the recognition that language has structure, which is presumably hierarchical in nature, and from which can be derived the basic units of language to be studied (i.e., phonemes, morphemes, etc.); and (*b*) the provision of a framework that permits the analysis of the aphasias as a central disorder affecting the phonological, syntactic, and semantic levels of function. The linguistic approach deemphasizes the traditional dichotomies that referred to a disproportionate impairment in one avenue of input–output processing (e.g., motor–sensory, expressive–receptive, auditory–visual, decoding–encoding).

INVESTIGATIONS OF PHONOLOGICAL FACTORS

It seems reasonable to assume that at least part of the difficulty aphasics evidence in understanding spoken language might be due to or associated with an impairment in processing the sounds of the language. There are three major questions concerning phonological perception in aphasia:

1. Is the disturbance specific to or greater in Wernicke's aphasia than in other syndromes?
2. Is there a correlation between phonological disturbances and overall comprehension ability?
3. Is there a correlation between phonological disorders in speech and an impairment in phonological perception?

Luria (1958) hypothesized that lesions in the temporal lobe resulted in damage to an auditory analyzer responsible for the phonematic analysis of speech. The disorder resulted in the collapse of the phonemic structure of words, which affects the individual's comprehension of word meaning (spoken language) as well as other related abilities associated with the syndrome of sensory or Wernicke's aphasia.

The hypothesis that the severe comprehension disorder manifested in Wernicke's aphasia is due to an underlying deficit in phonemic processing has been tested in several investigations. Each involves a different method, and this may be of crucial significance. Investigators have usually used a discrimination or picture identification paradigm, both of which have inherent problems in validity. This can be controlled to some extent by the careful modification of presentation and scoring methods.

Blumstein, Baker, and Goodglass (1977) administered to aphasic patients an extensive phoneme discrimination test comprised of three parts: a test that compared word pairs differing in one or two distinctive features (voice–place), a task in which test syllables differed (*describe–prescribe*), and a test in which the sounds were reversed in order (*tax–task*). Though clearly the most impaired group in overall comprehension as assessed by the Boston Diagnostic Aphasia Examination, Wernicke's aphasics performed better on these phoneme discrimination tasks than did the two other groups, the mixed anteriors (nonfluent speech with comprehension deficits) and residual posteriors. All aphasic groups manifested phonological discrimination disturbances on all three tasks, and all groups performed significantly better when real-word stimuli were used rather than nonsense words. The authors concluded that the marked comprehension disorder found in Wernicke's aphasia could not be attributed to a low-level speech discrimination defect since they performed the discrimination tasks better than other aphasic subtypes, and their discrimination scores improved just as much as other groups' scores when meaningful words were added.

Gainotti, Caltagirone, and Ibba (1976) administered the Verbal Sound and Meaning Discrimination Test to a relatively large group of aphasics. The examination was designed to study both the phonemic and semantic levels of language processing. This test requires that the patient point to a picture named by the examiner in an array that includes, in addition to the correct identification, a phonemically similar, a semantically similar, and a nonrelated picture. On this task, phonemic confusions were not confined to Wernicke's aphasics, and all aphasic subgroups made fewer phonemic errors than semantic errors.

Given the pervasiveness of semantic disorders in aphasia, it seems crucial to examine the relationship between phonological and semantic factors. To specify the nature of this relationship, Baker, Blumstein, and Goodglass (1981) administered to Wernicke's and Broca's aphasics a series of phonological discrimination tests in which both phonological distinctions and semantic requirements were systematically controlled. Their results indicated that, although Wernicke's aphasics were more

impaired than Broca's on all tests, their performance was disproportionately impaired when the requirements for semantic processing were
increased. Phonological factors, however, played a role in discrimination, since in all cases, discriminations involving one distinctive feature
(voice or place) resulted in more errors than did two-feature contrasts
(voice + place).

It is also conceivable that sentence context might play a role in
phonological processing, though this area has not received much systematic investigation. Gardner, Albert, and Weintraub (1975) gave a
picture-choice test in which two of the six alternatives were phonemically related to a target word contained in a sentence. They found
phonemic confusions were a slightly more prevalent error type than
semantic confusions in posterior aphasics, a group composed of fluent
aphasics with and without significant comprehension difficulty.

Goldblum and Albert (1972) speculated that Wernicke's aphasia may
comprise a heterogeneous group with respect to the perception of
speech sounds. They identified two groups by the qualitatively different
responses obtained on a phoneme discrimination test. Specifically, for
one group of sensory aphasics in which a word deafness component was
evident, discrimination errors occurred primarily on items where the
phonemic difference between words was small. For a second group, in
which there was a marked disturbance for both written and spoken
language, discrimination errors occurred with equal frequency in
phonemically dissimilar and similar words. The investigators concluded
that there was no single factor underlying the speech perception deficit
in Wernicke's aphasia.

The distinction between Wernicke's aphasia and word deafness has
been discussed by Ziegler (1952) and M. N. Goldstein (1974). Word
deafness is a relatively rare disorder, the diagnosis of which is based on
a striking unimodal impairment of auditory comprehension. Patients
may disregard speech and behave as if they were deaf, but on hearing
testing, they respond to rather low-intensity nonspeech sounds. Unlike
Wernicke's aphasia, speech, writing, and reading are essentially intact,
though some patients present disproportionately milder symptoms of
aphasia in other language modalities. In many cases of pure word deafness, the disorder is said to have evolved from a Wernicke's-type syndrome (M. N. Goldstein, 1974). It is possible that the entity referred to as
Wernicke's or sensory aphasia actually comprises a range of disorders
in which the relationship between phonological and semantic factors
varies.

In contrast to Wernicke's aphasia, in which semantic processing is
disturbed, the impairment in pure word deafness is said to involve a

selective phonological processing disorder. This claim is given support in a study by Saffran, Marin, and Yeni-Komshian (1976). Specifically, the patient studied was given a variety of speech perception tests in which the perceptual phenomena under experimental conditions with normal subjects are well known (identification of natural stop consonants, judgments of voice-onset time, identification–discrimination of synthesized stop consonant–vowel combinations). Error patterns were systematic, and the patient discriminated and identified stop consonants very abnormally. For example, unlike normals, the patient's perception of stop consonants in consonant–vowel syllables varied according to the following vowel, an indication that perception had an acoustic rather than phonetic basis. In addition, dichotic listening tests indicated total suppression of right ear signals, suggesting that analysis of speech was accomplished by right hemisphere mechanisms and could be best characterized as "acoustic" rather than "phonetic" processing.

At this stage of investigation, it does not appear reasonable to conclude that the severe comprehension deficits found in the classical description of Wernicke's aphasia are solely or even significantly influenced by a purely phonological perceptual disorder. Rather, there is no simple relationship between phonological discrimination and auditory comprehension in Wernicke's aphasia. The phonlogical deficit is influenced by semantic processing factors, and semantic identification is affected by phonological factors. In addition, there is the possibility of different varieties of phonological disorders among the population of Wernicke's aphasics.

The notion that damage to the left hemisphere, whatever the locus of the lesion, impairs phonemic perception and that the degree of impairment has more to do with the overall severity of the comprehension deficit than with whether the lesion was posterior or anterior has also received only limited support in experimental studies.

Disturbances in phoneme discrimination coexisted with impaired sentence comprehension in less than half of the patients in a study reported by Carpenter and Rutherford (1973). Miceli, Gainotti, Caltagirone, and Masullo (1980) found a significant but only partial correspondence between disorders of phonological analysis and general comprehension. In the Blumstein, Baker, and Goodglass (1977) study, patients in the mixed anterior group, who consistently performed poorly on the three discrimination tasks, were not the most impaired in overall speech comprehension ability. Jauhianen and Nuutila (1977) also found no correlation between disturbances in feature discrimination in aphasia and Token Test score.

There is contradictory evidence as to the type of contrast most vulnerable in aphasia. Blumstein, Baker, and Goodglass (1977) and Miceli, Caltagirone, Gainotti, and Payer-Rigo (1978) found discrimination of place contrasts (e.g., *b–d*, *p–t*) more difficult than voicing contrasts (e.g., *p–b*, *t–d*) in aphasia. In Blumstein's study, place contrast errors were the predominant error type manifested by posteriorly damaged aphasics (Wernicke's, anomics, conduction, and transcortical sensory). No difference in errors on types of contrasts were found in anterior aphasics. In contrast, Carpenter and Rutherford (1973) found the voicing cue contrast (e.g., *staple–stable, base–bait, kit–kid*) significantly more difficult than place contrasts for all aphasic groups. Jauhianen and Nuutila (1977) found vowels and consonants with back place of articulation more easily discriminated than other phonemic contrasts in aphasics with left cerebrovascular accidents (CVA). Phonological discriminations involving two distinctive features, voice and place, are clearly easier for aphasics than discriminations involving the single feature of either voice or place. Greater phonological distance apparently facilitates discrimination (Blumstein, Baker, & Goodglass, 1977; Baker *et al.*, 1981).

Several studies have used synthesized speech to investigate phonemic discrimination or identification (Basso, Casati, & Vignolo, 1977; Blumstein, Cooper, Zurif, & Caramazza, 1977; Tallal & Newcombe, 1978). Using synthesized speech, it is possible to construct stimuli that vary in a given acoustic parameter along a continuum. The one most often used is the voice-onset-time (VOT) continuum. When normal listeners are asked to identify stimuli varying in VOT (from *da* to *ta*), they readily assign the stimuli to one or the other class, but fail to perceive the small steplike acoustic changes at any location except the perceived phonemic boundary. Moreover, when asked to discriminate between stimuli, they are unable to discriminate those stimuli they have assigned to the same class but are able to reliably discriminate those stimuli identified as belonging to two separate classes.

Basso *et al.* (1977) found that 70% of aphasics they tested did not exhibit a sharp boundary in the perception of *da* and *ta* stimuli, and in some cases no boundary occurred at all. The defect was more common among nonfluents (95%) than fluent aphasics (58%). Though there was a significant correlation between the phonemic identification defect and comprehension scores, there was also considerable individual variation. Some patients with poor comprehension performed well, whereas some with relatively preserved overall comprehension performed poorly.

Blumstein, Cooper, Zurif, and Caramazza (1977) using a similar paradigm asked patients not only to identify but also to discriminate sounds along a continuum. Three patterns of performance were identified: a group of patients who performed similar to normal subjects on both identification and discrimination tasks; a group who failed to reliably discriminate or identify stimuli along the VOT continuum; and a third group who performed the discrimination task normally but failed to identify reliably. The authors suggested that for this group, comprised primarily of Wernicke's aphasics, the problem was not an inability to discriminate phonological contrasts, but rather a defect in assigning a category label to the stimulus; in other words, these patients were unable to use phonological information in a "linguistically relevant" way. There was no relationship between severity of auditory comprehension and difficulty on the two tasks. In fact, some patients with good comprehension failed both tasks.

Using synthetic speech to investigate an auditory rather than linguistic basis for phonemic discrimination difficulty in aphasia, Tallal and Newcombe (1978) found that aphasics who were interval sensitive in the analysis of nonverbal sounds were also deficient in their ability to process the rapidly changing formant transitions that are required to distinguish between /ba/and/da/. When the duration of formant transitions cuing the distinction was increased from 40 to 80 msec, performance improved. The investigators suggested that the deficit in understanding speech is due to an underlying specific defect in processing rapidly changing acoustic events. Pertinent to this, Blumstein reports in Chapter 5 in this book that she found no difference in identification and discrimination function when formant transitions are extended.

Using an entirely different methodology, Mostofsky, Vanden-Bossche, Sheinkopf, and Noyes (1971) investigated whether aphasics perceived distances among the various distortions of spoken language and undistorted speech. A prose passage was presented in a clear version and four distorted versions (slowed, speeded, reversed, and computer-synthesized vocoded). Normal and aphasic subjects were asked to make judgments about the similarity of distorted to clear versions. Aphasics' judgments differed from those of the normal controls in that the aphasics appeared to judge clear speech more similar to distorted speech than normals did. The distance of the individual aphasic's judgments from the cluster of normal judgments had no relationship to the aphasic's performance on a standard test of auditory comprehension, but it did relate to a clinical ranking of comprehension; that is, the nearer the aphasic's judgments to the normals', the less auditory comprehension deficit he was judged to have.

Having derived only scattered and somewhat contradictory evidence to link phonological or discrimination disorders with either the comprehension deficit manifested in Wernicke's aphasia or with the overall comprehension ability in aphasia, research in phonological perceptions has turned to another dimension: the association of phonological perception deficits with disturbances in phonological production. A central integrating sensorimotor mechanism of phonological processing that affects both the production and analysis of speech has been hypothesized.

Two types of phonological disturbances can be identified in the speech of aphasics: a phonemic disorder without phonetic distortions, usually accompanied by verbal paraphasia found in Wernicke's aphasia; and a primarily though not exclusively phonetic disorder associated with agrammatism in Broca's aphasia. Studies have looked at the phonological problems of one or the other or both populations. Gainotti, Caltagirone, and Ibba (1976) found only "mild" correspondence between discrimination errors on the Verbal Sound and Meaning Discrimination Test and phonemic errors in the speech production of Wernicke's aphasics with both phonemic and mixed paraphasia and Broca's aphasics. Blumstein, Cooper, Zurif, and Caramazza (1977) reported that the ability to perceive the VOT categorically in no way relates to the ability to produce voice and voiceless stops. Studies of patients described as manifesting "speech apraxia" or "phonetic disintegration" have shown the correlation between the productive impairment and phonemic discrimination to be weak (Aten, Johns, & Darley, 1971; Johns & Darley, 1970) or nonexistent (Shankweiler & Harris, 1966).

In more recent and well-defined studies, Shewan (1980) found an association between phoneme sequence recognition and production deficits in some Broca's aphasics. Miceli *et al.* (1980) identified a group of patients comprised of members from fluent and nonfluent categories, in which patients with phonemic production deficits performed more poorly on a test of phonemic discrimination than did those without phonemic production defects. Both sets of findings, at least in part, support a central mechanism hypothesis. There were, however, patients in both studies whose phonological discrimination function was unrelated to the severity of phonological errors in speech.

One important area that has been almost totally overlooked in aphasia research is prosodic processing. As a result little is known about how much the aphasic relies on intonation for auditory comprehension. If prosody functions to maintain a coherent auditory signal, facilitate phrase groups, draw attention to lexical meaning, and enhance syntactic analysis by cuing sentence form, engaging the listener emotionally, and communicating affective information, one would suspect that prosody might play a role in aphasics' comprehension of speech. Since Boller and Green (1972) found that even very severely impaired patients retain an ability to distinguish between different types of sentences, prosody might be rather resilient in aphasia. Another possibility is that a defect in prosodic processing may be impaired in patients who manifest dys-prosody in speech. For example, Broca's aphasics have been shown to use prosody differently from normals in the processing of open (content) versus closed (function) class words under varying conditions of sentence stress (Swinney, Zurif, & Cutler, 1980).

Some studies have found prosodic processing to be impaired commensurate with impaired comprehension. For example, Feyereisen reports (in press) that ability to match prosodic information to a picture depicting emotional content is correlated with the severity of comprehension deficits in aphasia. Schlanger, Schlanger, and Gerstman (1976) found that both right and left hemisphere damaged patients are impaired in matching emotionally toned sentences to pictures depicting emotions. Bond (1976) also showed aphasics to be more impaired than other brain-damaged patients in their ability to profit from the imposition of rhythm to organize nonspeech sounds into patterns or phrases.

In summary, except in the case of the relatively rare disorder of pure word deafness, current studies have provided scant evidence to support the notion of a phonemic basis for the comprehension disorder found in aphasia. Regardless of the methodology used and in spite of the fact that aphasics generally perform more poorly than normals or other brain-damaged subjects on tasks designed to measure phonological discrimination and identification, performance deficits are not clearly linked to a particular variety of aphasia, nor do they seem directly related to the extent of the overall comprehension disorder. There is a partial correlation between scores on phonological discrimination tests and severity of comprehension, but there are always some subjects, who, despite poor discrimination, perform well on auditory comprehension tasks and others who manifest preserved comprehension but fail to reliably discriminate or identify phonological parameters. In addition, discrimination and identification are separable for some aphasics, tentatively Wernicke's aphasics, whose ability to discriminate phonological features is superior to their ability to label stimuli.

The lack of correspondence between performance on tests of phonological perception and comprehension of spoken language raises certain questions as to the nature of the language comprehension process. The hypothesis that perception of phonological parameters (place and voicing) are a prerequisite for understanding spoken language is not supported. Rather, there is a complex relationship between phonological and semantic factors involved in the aphasic's ability to discriminate words.

Some investigators (Lesser, 1978) have suggested that, given the benefit of prosody, semantics, and syntax, the listener may require little in the way of phonemic analysis, and phonological perception may be peripheral rather than basic to the process of understanding speech. This is in fact similar to Brown's theory of perceptual regression (1977, p. 93), in which he postulates that speech perception begins at the semantic level and proceeds through levels until the final abstract auditory level of phonemic or morphemic perception takes place.

Another possibility is that phonological discrimination is so basic a function of the left hemisphere that deficits are only manifested with very severe damage and the performance differences reflect other linguistic or nonlinguistic factors (i.e., inability to maintain a category label, short-term memory deficits, defective decision making, etc.). It is important to note in this regard that patients manifesting severe comprehension deficits retain some ability to analyze the phonology of their language, to distinguish their own language from a foreign tongue, and to differentiate between phonemic jargon and real words (Boller & Green, 1972). Phonological structure in this sense would appear rather resilient compared to the parameters of semantics and syntax investigated in aphasia.

Obviously, further research in phonological perception is required before it will be possible to define the relative importance of phonological factors in the various syndromes of aphasia.

DISORDERS OF SEMANTIC AND SYNTACTIC
PROCESSING IN APHASIA

Traditionally, the study of comprehension has treated individual words separately from sentences. In fact, aphasia batteries customarily include a word-identification task, in which a patient is instructed to point to a picture or object named by the examiner, and several types of sentence comprehension tasks. If comprehension proceeded in a unidimensional, additive fashion, then this format would be sufficient. The linguistic approach to aphasic disorders, however, assumes a multidimensional impairment in the comprehension of individual words and in the sensitivity to different sentence forms among the various types of aphasia. It follows that linguistic research has attempted to separate semantic from syntactic processing disorders in investigations of comprehension in aphasia. There appears to be a basic interrelationship between syntax and the lexicon that makes this an almost impossible task.

Disturbances in Comprehension of Single Words. This section will examine studies of single-word comprehension. The first objective is to discover the source of the variation in the understanding of isolated words, then to explore the differences among various types of aphasia and to see to what extent overall severity of comprehension is related to semantic comprehension.

Word frequency seems a significant factor in predicting word comprehension. Schuell, Jenkins, and Landis (1961), using the Ammons test, found an orderly and predictable reduction of vocabulary comprehension based on the relative frequency of word usage in the language.

Some writers have suggested that certain semantic category names (colors, body parts, furniture, etc.) are more difficult than others for aphasics. Goodglass, Klein, Carey, and Jones (1966) tested a large sample of aphasics manifesting Broca's, Wernicke's, and amnesic aphasia and found a similar rank order of difficulty for all types of aphasia. Comprehension of object names was followed by action names, color names, and number and letter names. Moreover, the order of difficulty in comprehending names of the five different semantic categories was dissociated from the aphasics' production of the name on visual confrontation. For example, object names, though easiest to comprehend, were the most difficult to name; letters, the most difficult to comprehend, were the easiest for most groups to encode. The most notable comprehension difficulty was the failure of Wernicke's aphasics to identify body-part names.

Poeck, Hartje, Kerschensteiner, and Orgass (1973) questioned the existence of a rank order of difficulty among semantic classes. Comparing comprehension of body-part names and object names, they found no differences associated with semantic category. Aphasics who were able to identify body parts, either by pointing to their own body or to pictures depicting the body part, were also able to identify object names, and aphasics with poor understanding of body-part names were equally poor at identifying object names.

Without more substantial evidence for a rank order of difficulty for different semantic categories, it seems premature to conclude that aphasics show consistently more difficulty with item names belonging to one category than another. One would predict that a task requiring identification of dissimilar object names is considerably easier than one requiring identification of letter names that are phonemically, visually, and semantically similar. Methodological factors must be carefully controlled in order that the differences among categories are not an artifact of the test design rather than inherent language factors. This is not intended to minimize the importance of the reported presumably rare cases of category-specific anomias in which naming and identification are selectively disturbed for color or body parts. Rather, the prevalence of differences among semantic categories in a general population of aphasics remains unclear.

Schuell and Jenkins (1961) emphasized the susceptibility to semantic association errors in word identification. Comparing the difference between three types of errors—semantic, acoustic, and random—they found that aphasics, regardless of the degree of comprehension impairment, made more semantic association errors than other types of errors. Random errors were prevalent in severely impaired patients, whereas in mild aphasia, semantic errors were the only error type.

Psycholinguistic investigations of semantic comprehension in aphasia have utilized a multiple-choice technique in which semantically controlled alternatives are presented to test the hypothesis that aphasics who show a prevalence of semantic paraphasia in speech (Wernicke's, anomics) are selectively impaired in semantic identification.

For example, to test whether semantic confusions in comprehension are more frequent in patients exhibiting semantic paraphasia in speech, Pizzamiglio and Appicciafuoco (1971) administered a multiple-choice test in which the semantic relatedness of the alternatives was controlled to four groups (Broca's, Wernicke's, amnesics, global). The patient was asked to point to the picture names from a group of four semantically similar choices (e.g., priest, God, church, Bible). Semantic errors were frequent among all aphasic subtypes, including Broca's aphasics. To some extent, the number of errors paralleled the overall severity of aphasia. When Wernicke's and Broca's aphasics were matched for severity, no difference was found between groups.

Similar findings were reported in a subsequent study by Gainotti *et al.* (1976) in which the link between production and comprehension in phonology and semantic processing was investigated. Using the Verbal Sound and Meaning Discrimination Test, the subjects were asked to identify from six alternatives including not only the correct one but also a semantically related, a phonemically related, and three nonrelated items. No differences between clinical types in either the type or frequency of comprehension disorders were evident. In each clinical syndrome, the incidence of pathological performance was related to the severity of aphasia. Though there were no differences in semantic error frequency between patients classified as Wernicke's or Broca's aphasics, there was a clear-cut difference within the Wernicke's (fluent) category associating semantic errors in production with semantic errors in comprehension. The bias toward semantic association errors in all forms of aphasia led Gainotti *et al.* (1976) to conclude that semantic disintegration is the most basic problem in all forms of aphasia.

Semantic association errors were also more prevalent than phonemic confusions in Gardner *et al.*'s (1975) investigation of the contribution of sentence context to word meaning. In this study, however, the

anterior-damaged (nonfluent, Broca's) aphasics evidenced more semantic errors than did the posterior-damaged (Wernicke's) aphasics.

There is evidence to suggest, however, that not only are aphasics
prone to semantic association errors when identifying from among
closely associated word choices but right brain damaged nonaphasics
also evidence a significant proportion of semantic errors (Lesser, 1974)
and a similar breakdown in semantic knowledge is found in dementia
(Swartz, Marin, & Saffran, 1979). Swartz *et al.* suggest that the lexical
processes, particularly those closely tied to the perceptual mechanism,
are more bilaterally represented than the phonological or syntactic processes. Brain damage regardless of the hemisphere involved affects performance of identification tasks involving choices that are closely related
semantically.

Bilateral representation of semantic knowledge may also account for
the unusual preservation of single-word identification on tasks involving unrelated word choices. Support for the notion of bilateral representation of semantic knowledge might be inferred from several sources.
For example, object identification is a frequent area of improvement over
time even in global aphasia (Sarno & Levita, 1981). Some aphasics score
in the adult range on such vocabulary identification tests as the Peabody
Picture Vocabulary Test (Goodglass, Gleason, & Hyde, 1970). Aphasic
subjects as a group performed slightly better than nonaphasic right brain
damaged subjects on the English Picture Vocabulary Test (Lesser, 1974).
Moreover, in studies of commissurotomized patients, the right hemisphere has demonstrated an extensive single-word vocabulary, though
its ability to handle syntactic analysis is limited (Zaidel, 1976).

In brief, performance on word identification tasks and overall severity
of comprehension correlate in aphasia. Although semantic confusions
are the most pervasive error type on picture choice tests, this task fails to
discriminate among diagnostic categories of aphasia, and it is questionable whether a word identification technique reliably discriminates
aphasics from other brain-damaged subjects. The semantic specifications of the objects or pictures presented is a factor in the accuracy of
responses.

To isolate differences in semantic processing, other methodology is
necessary. Using a reaction time task, Baker and Goodglass (1979) found
a significant difference between Broca's and Wernicke's aphasics in the
decoding of individual substantive words. The Wernicke's aphasics required significantly longer time to identify concrete object names (mean
response time 650 msec) than did Broca's, whose mean response time
(200 msec) compares with normal's reaction times, and all groups responded more quickly to high-frequency than low-frequency items. The

magnitude of the decoding time in Wernicke's aphasics correlated highly with comprehension scores on the Boston Diagnostic Aphasia Examination. They concluded that the Wernicke's aphasic's need for increased processing time to identify single words reflected their reduced ability to recognize a particular picture as representative of a concept, in other words, their conceptual deficit.

While this investigation dealt only with substantives, other studies have examined differences among aphasic subtypes in the handling of other parts of speech.

Goodglass *et al.* (1970) explored the multidimensionality of comprehension disorders and found that patients with traditional aphasia syndromes had different types of comprehension difficulty. Specifically, anomics performed significantly worse on the Peabody Picture Vocabulary Test (PPVT) compared to their other performances, supporting the assertion of a parallel between a disturbance in the comprehension of a specific feature of language (nouns, verbs) and the verbal production of that feature. Broca's aphasics performed well on the PPVT but were unusually impaired in pointing to objects named in series, sometimes failing with a series of only two items. The authors attribute this failure to difficulty in the performance of sequential actions, a variable possibly dissociated from comprehension of the actual words used. No parallel was found between Broca's aphasics' limited use of prepositions and an inability to understand them. In fact, using a picture verification task, Broca's aphasics understood prepositional relationships better than did Wernicke's aphasics, who use prepositions normally in speech.

Smith (1974) tested aphasics' ability to understand prepositional relationships and administered a test that required them to arrange objects in a specified location (e.g., *Put the coin in the cup*). Patients were then asked to describe the arrangement placed in front of them. The scoring system allowed for a comparison between lexical and prepositional errors. In contrast to Goodglass *et al.* (1970), Smith found that patients who produced no relational words were markedly impaired in understanding these words and one anomic patient made more errors on nouns than on relational words. Smith attributed the difference between the two studies to the increased sensitivity of this task. However, the sensitivity of the task may not be selective to the understanding of the particular prepositions included. She noted that instructions that called for the manipulation of only one object were more often followed than those calling for the manipulation of two, suggesting that this task may also have been tapping a disturbance in sequential actions rather than a disturbance in the comprehension of specific prepositions. Though

Smith's study has certain limitations, it suggests a correspondence between disturbances in production and comprehension.

Certain relational words appear unusually difficult for aphasics to
understand; specifically, prepositions of location (*between, next, by, beside*); reversible relationships (*over–under, right–left, before–after*) and
quantifiers (*more–less*). Lenneberg, Pogash, Cohlan, and Doolittle (1978),
having found a consistent rank order of difficulty among individual
words, suggested that the unusual difficulty in understanding words
signifying temporal–spatial relationships is a manifestation of a basic
cognitive, rather than purely linguistic, defect. They attribute the deficit
to a failure in SIMULTANEOUS SYNTHESIS, a term Luria introduced. It
refers to a basic inability to understand concepts in which a number of
temporal–spatial elements make up a whole. Sasanuma and Kamio's
(1976) study of forms expressing temporal order (before and after) identified three different patterns of performance equally distributed among
four different aphasic subtypes. Gardner, Strub, and Albert's (1975) case
report describes an individual who manifested a particular difficulty in
understanding words that expressed temporal arrangements in the auditory modality but had only minimal difficulty with the same concepts
when presented in written form. This report suggests that the impairment may, in certain cases, be selective to the modality of presentation.
Hier, Mogil, Rubin, and Komros (1980) reported on a study of three
"semantic" aphasics whose auditory comprehension deficit was characterized by extraordinary difficulty in grasping the meaning of words that
embody spatial significance (*beside, under, behind, before, right, left,* etc.),
though the comprehension of other single words as assessed by a vocabulary test was intact.

Psycholinguists have turned their attention to exploring the impairment in the abstract relationships between words as a means of studying
the nature of the semantic disturbance found in aphasia.

Goodglass and Baker (1976) divided an aphasic population into two
groups based on the severity of comprehension impairment to study the
impact of such deficits on semantic organization. Information about a
patient's semantic field was obtained by analyzing the error rate and
reaction time in identifying spoken words that related to a target word.
Association categories for each word included in addition to identity
(e.g., *orange*), a superordinate (*fruit*), attribute (*juicy*), coordinate (*apple*),
function associate (*eat*), and function context (*breakfast*). The patient was
shown a picture, asked to name it, and asked to indicate recognition of a
link between the words heard and the pictured item by pressing a rubber bulb. Low- and high-comprehension aphasics differed both quan-

titatively and qualitatively on this task. Although the high-comprehension group exhibited a somewhat greater spread of scores, their performance essentially paralleled that of the normal group. The low-comprehension group, however, demonstrated a different order of difficulty among the categories. For example, for low-comprehension aphasics, the contrast coordinate (e.g., *apple*) had the second fastest time rather than the slowest, as in the case of normal and high-comprehension aphasics. Functional context (e.g., *breakfast*), relatively easy for high-comprehension and normal groups, was among the most difficult for the low-comprehension group, and the functional associate stimuli (e.g., *eat*), which required the longest reaction times for all groups, were markedly slower for the low-comprehension group. Low-comprehension group error rates were exceptionally high for these last two categories, leading the investigators to conclude that a qualitative change in semantic organization occurs with seriously impaired com-prehension. Moreover, when error rate and reaction time data were compared with naming ability, the pictures that patients failed to name were those for which they had failed to respond to a number of as-sociates of the target word. Though this was most prevalent with low-comprehension aphasics, the trend was also evident in high-comprehension aphasics.

This study is important in two respects; first, it presents evidence for qualitative differences in semantic organization dependent on severity of comprehension, and second, it identifies a central (semantic) mechanism linking the comprehension of semantic associates with a specific production defect (i.e., object naming). Goodglass and Baker did not categorize their group into diagnostic classes, but only with respect to comprehension. It is unclear, therefore, whether the qualita-tive difference in semantic organization is selective to a particular sub-type of aphasia or whether it cuts across diagnostic category and is a function of the severity of the comprehension impairment.

In this connection, Zurif, Caramazza, Myerson, and Galvin (1974) investigated the disturbances in semantic representation in two sub-types of aphasia. Broca's aphasics, who by definition have relatively spared comprehension, grouped words with respect to semantic fea-tures in a manner resembling normal subjects. In contrast Wernicke's aphasics, who generally manifest significant comprehension distur-bances, were strikingly deviant in their clustering of words. The inves-tigators pointed out, however, that one Wernicke's aphasic with a mild comprehension disturbance actually clustered words in a manner similar to the Broca's group, suggesting that the pattern of semantic disorganization may be less related to diagnostic category than to the severity of comprehension impairment.

Affective meaning is another aspect of semantic organization that has been investigated in aphasia. Zurif and co-workers (Zurif *et al.*, 1974) noted that the clustering patterns of Broca's aphasics seemed governed more by affective and concrete relationships between words than by the abstract relationships upon which normal subjects base their semantic decisions. Mostofsky *et al.* (1971), in a preliminary study of connotative meaning, found that the ability to make connotative judgments was dissociated from type and severity of aphasia, leading them to assert that the affective and communicative systems are not equally impaired in aphasia.

Gardner and Denes (1973) administered a modified pictorial version of Osgood's Semantic Differential, a test designed to tap the affective or connotative component of word meaning, which requires a subject to rate a word on a number of qualitative dimensions. The accuracy or closeness of aphasics' judgments to normal was then compared with the ability to match words to the appropriate referent (i.e., denotative component). To test connotation, patients were asked to point to whichever abstract design went with a spoken word. Several other factors were explored, such as differences in connotation between concrete and abstract words and between noun and adjectives. The findings indicated that, although patients with mild comprehension disorders achieved high scores on a simple denotation test, aphasics were inferior to normal subjects in both connotation and denotation testing. The subject's performance on the test of connotative comprehension correlated highly with performance of denotative comprehension. Within the aphasic population, the results might have been predicted on the basis of a clinical assessment of comprehension deficits; global, Wernicke's, anomic, Broca's, transcortical motor, and conduction aphasics scored from low to high in that order. Surprisingly, there was no difference in error rates in connotation of performance between abstract and concrete nouns or adjectives and nouns. The most significant finding, however, was that connotation is not, at least on this measure, more preserved than denotation.

The investigation of disturbances in semantic organization in aphasia has really only just begun. Buckingham's Chapter 7 in this volume outlines the various ways semantic organization might be impaired in cerebral damage. At this point studies in which the severity of comprehension has been examined in relation to the qualitative changes in the semantic network are limited.

Undoubtedly, further probing will permit greater understanding of lexical comprehension than is possible at this time. So far, what is known about aphasics' comprehension of single words consists of an accumulation of observed phenomena for which there are only tentative explanations. Investigations using semantically related word choices have exposed the possibility that semantic knowledge is extremely vulnerable, not only in left-sided lesions producing aphasia, but in nonaphasic right brain damage and in generalized brain disease as well. It is also likely that semantic (word) discrimination errors are equally pervasive in all aphasic types and that the degree of impairment correlates with overall comprehension ability. On the other hand, word–picture identification in the case of unrelated choices indicates word recognition is quite preserved in aphasia. Goodglass and Baker's (1976) study also suggests that the mere pointing to an object name may indicate little with respect to limitations in the underlying semantic disturbance.

Many factors have been suggested as influencing the comprehension of individual words: word frequency, familiarity, affective aspects, semantic and grammatic category, and redundancy of semantic information in sentences in which the word appears. However, the degree to which these are important, and for which variety of patient, remains unclear. Diagnostic category, as it reflects presumed locus of lesion, has been identified as a variable in performance of different word comprehension tasks, though explanations of differences must be seen as tentative. Severity of the comprehension disturbance and the overall severity of the aphasic condition is interwoven with, and sometimes overrides, the specific type of aphasia. There is some indication that severity is not just a quantitative reduction in function, but that it is also qualitative in its impact on the semantic component of language.

Comprehension Disorders and Syntax. Contemporary researchers applying linguistic theory to the study of aphasia have sought evidence to support the notion that the agrammatism of Broca's aphasia is more than an economy of expression due to a purely motor encoding disorder. To them, it represents a disturbance in syntactic knowledge, "a conceptual agrammatism," affecting grammatical competence in both speech production and comprehension (Goodglass, 1973). Originally, researchers reasoned that certain grammatical forms would be expected to be more difficult for Broca's aphasics to understand than for Wernicke's aphasics, whose grammar in production appears nearly intact. Early studies, however, were relatively unsuccessful in isolating selective deficits among classical subtypes. Goodglass (1973) reported a study using a two-picture

choice technique in which aphasics' recognition of contrasting morphological forms (e.g., verb tense, subject–object order, active and passive,
singular and plural) were tested. All groups of aphasic patients demonstrated essentially the same rank order of difficulty in contrast discrimination.

A more elaborate picture choice test of syntactical structure was used
by Parisi and Pizzamiglio (1970) and in Lesser's (1974) English translation of their test. Twenty contrasts were tested, including tense, plural-
ity, negation, gender, prepositions, indirect–direct objects, passive–
active, etc., by having subjects identify which of two pictures matched a
spoken sentence. Both studies found the syntax test highly sensitive to
aphasia; however, neither study revealed any significant qualitative differences among aphasia subtypes. Parisi and Pizzamiglio found a high
correlation among syntax discrimination performance, degree of comprehension disturbance, and overall severity. The Italian study found
the direct–indirect object contrast the most difficult, whereas Lesser's
replication of the Italian study demonstrated that some aphasics have
disproportionate difficulty with sentences in which the sequencing of
words is critical to interpretation—that is, reversible active subject–
verb–object sentences (*The boy is chasing the dog; The dog is chasing the
boy*). Lesser felt that sentence length was not a factor, since long sentences with subordinate clauses proved easier for aphasics to understand than short reversible sentences. The minor role of sentence length
was also demonstrated in the study of sentence comprehension by Shewan (1969) and Shewan and Canter (1971), which also failed to find any
qualitative differences in performance among aphasic subtypes.

The picture verification method has several serious shortcomings. It is
very difficult to select distractor items (i.e., pictured alternatives) that
permit errors based on faulty syntactical analysis to be isolated from
errors due to lexical miscomprehension. The number of choices presented may also influence error rate. It is impossible to isolate from
impaired syntactic analysis other factors affecting decision making, such
as impulsivity and impaired short-term memory.

As the methodology for testing syntactic processing deficits has become more refined, some reliable differences among various subtypes of
aphasia have been uncovered. Interest in linguistic investigation continues to focus on the comprehension status of Broca's aphasics. Investigations have, therefore, examined the degree to which Broca's aphasics,
relative to other aphasic subtypes, are impaired in handling sentences
that depend on the comprehension of grammatical morphemes and syntactic relationships. For example, Goodenough, Zurif, and Weintraub
(1977) demonstrated that Broca's aphasics do not use the article to

modulate the meaning of the noun phrase. Given a black circle, a black square, and a white circle and asked to press the black one (i.e., the black one of the two circles), they fail to choose the black circle.

An abnormal pattern of morphological processing was demonstrated by Broca's aphasics on a word monitoring task designed by Swinney *et al.* (1980). They reported that Broca's aphasics respond more slowly and make more errors than normal subjects on close class (function) than on open class (content) words regardless of sentence stress. Heilman and Scholes (1976) found Broca's aphasics insensitive to the definite article *the* in parsing indirect–direct object constituents required to understand the difference between such sentences as *He showed her the baby pictures* and *He showed her baby pictures.* Conduction aphasics also failed to appreciate the indirect–direct object distinction and performed similar to Broca's aphasics. In contrast, Wernicke's aphasics not only made more errors than the other two groups but also more often than not chose lexical distractor items in the picture verification task.

Caramazza, Zurif, and Gardner (1978) presented sentences orally to anterior (Broca's) and posterior (Wernicke's) aphasics. After hearing the sentence, the subject was presented with one word from the sentence and asked to recall the word that followed it. If unable to say the word, a multiple-choice array was presented from which to choose the word. Both groups of aphasics had significantly more difficulty retrieving function words than content words, suggesting that neither group was able to use syntactic information embodied in function words in sentence processing or in the construction of memory representations.

Comprehension of syntactic relationships that depend on the word order of a sentence rather than on the function word cue was investigated by Caramazza and Zurif (1976). They presented Broca's, conduction, and Wernicke's aphasics with four types of center-embedded, object-relative sentences (e.g., *The cat that the dog is chasing is brown*) and asked subjects to point to the pictorial representation. Sentences included nonreversible, in which interpretation was determined by semantic constraints (*The apple that the boy is eating is red*); reversible, in which the correct interpretation was based on syntactical knowledge (*The boy that the girl is chasing is tall*); improbable (*The boy that the dog is patting is fat*); and control sentences (*The boy is eating a red apple*). The picture choice distractors were also systematically controlled. Results showed that both Broca's and conduction aphasics selected the correct picture for nonreversible sentences but misidentified pictures depicting reversible (syntactically constrained) sentences. These findings support the notion that Broca's comprehension is biased toward lexical knowledge and impaired when syntactic information (word order) cues interpretation. The conduction aphasics' performance paralleled that of Broca's aphasics, whereas Wernicke's aphasics were essentially insensitive to either the syntactic or semantic factors. Since several Wernicke's aphasics were eliminated on the basis of an inability to accomplish the task, the authors suggest the relatively high overall performance of this group was due to the fact that their population was not truly representative of Wernicke's aphasia.

To investigate whether it is the overgeneralization of conventional word order (active voice or subject–verb–object, SVO) or the insensitivity to functors that makes passive reversible sentences more difficult than active voice constructions, Swartz, Saffran, and Marin (1980) presented a picture verification task to a group of agrammatic patients. Subjects showed no tendency to overgeneralize word order from active to passive, but four out of five failed to interpret passive sentences. Three of the subjects even failed to apply a consistent SVO reading to active voice sentences. A similar task involving reversible locative prepositions (e.g., *The circle was under the square*) and transitive verbs (*The square shoots the circle*) was administered. In all cases, agrammatic patients were unable to decode the syntax of word order in a consistent manner. Individual patients adopted different strategies on different days, but they were unable to use a fixed principle to uncover the relational structure of sentences.

Further support for the notion of a selective impairment of syntactic comprehension in Broca's aphasia is demonstrated by the study reported by Goodglass, Blumstein, Gleason, Hyde, Green, and Statlender (1979). When expanded versions of center-embedded sentences are presented as two contiguous simple sentences (e.g., *The man greeted by his wife was smoking a pipe* versus *The man was greeted by his wife and he was smoking a pipe*), Broca's aphasics' comprehension improves. Expanded versions contain the same information but (*a*) are presented in less encoded or syntactically simpler manner; and (*b*) are longer than control sentences. Not all patient groups profited from expansion. Expansion aided Broca's aphasics with poor comprehension but made little difference to Wernicke's aphasics. It actually depressed the performance of conduction aphasics with significant comprehension deficits. Since comprehension improved with longer sentences in Broca's aphasics, as long as the grammatical relationships among words were clearly specified, short-term memory deficits were ruled out as an influence. The relatively poor performance of conduction aphasics on expanded versions, however, suggests that short-term memory deficits might account for their difficulty comprehending center-embedded sentences. This was in fact the conclusion reached by Saffran and Marin (1975), who reported findings on a conduction aphasic with a selective short-term memory deficit that affected his ability to understand syntactically complex sentences of increased length. Their results demonstrated that although short-term memory is markedly defective in conduction aphasia, long-term memory is preserved. They found that the patient's performance on a variety of immediate memory tasks was similar to normal subject's performance on delayed recall tasks.

Several tasks were administered, but the most relevant was the patient's performance on the immediate recall of sentences. The patient was permitted to paraphrase information, since his verbatim repetition was limited to four to six words. In general, the paraphrased sentences evidenced preserved sentence comprehension despite the obvious short-term memory limitations, but when surface structure was complex, as in center-embedded sentences, reversible passives, or passives preceded by introductory phrases, sentence meaning was misinterpreted.

The authors suggest that in the case of conduction aphasia, the patient relies on long-term storage for sentence comprehension and, in general, successfully interprets meaning. On sentences for which the subject and object are reversible, however, the patient is forced to assume the first noun of the utterance is the subject and the next is the object. Since the phonemic record is not available, so that the patient is unable to reconsider his reading of the sentence, more often than not the sentence paraphrase reveals a misinterpretation based on information presented at the beginning of the sentence.

Berndt and Caramazza (Chapter 6 of this volume) report on a study of Caramazza, Basili, Koller, and Berndt (in press) that investigated the differences in the syntactic abilities of conduction and Broca's aphasics. Conduction aphasics were clearly superior to Broca's aphasics in performing a sentence anagram task. This supports the suggestion of Saffran and Marin (1975) that in conduction aphasia the capacity to handle syntax is retained but the ability to make use of skills that put heavy demands on short-term memory is reduced.

In summary, studies of syntax consistently demonstrate that Broca's aphasics (anterior–nonfluent) are unable to process function words and grammatical morphemes efficiently, nor can they handle syntactically complex encoded utterances. It is reasoned that Broca's aphasia involves a specific kind of comprehension disturbance. Specifically, Broca's aphasics are limited in their ability to profit from the role of grammatical morphemes in assigning relationships among words and organizing sentence structure and are impaired in their ability to manipulate word order not dependent on any function word cue. They understand sentences to the degree that they are able to derive correct meaning from the lexical items, their preserved knowledge of the world, and the overall situation.

Posterior aphasics (Wernicke's—fluent), on the other hand, seem impaired both in their understanding of lexical information and in their ability to profit from syntactic information provided by grammatical morphemes. In general, studies show that they do as poorly as Broca's on tests of syntactic comprehension. Whether this is a by-product of the severe lexical impairment, a reflection of a specific syntactic disorder in addition to the lexical impairment, or a reflection of some nonspecific performance variable remains unclear. Equivocal findings with respect to syntactic abilities of fluent aphasics reflect both the inherent difficulties in attempting to isolate the semantic from syntactic level of language and difficulties in obtaining a truly representative population of this variety of aphasia that can cope with the task demands of these studies. As in studies of semantic disturbance, the severity of the disorder influences both the type and degree of syntactic comprehension.

Conduction aphasics perform very much like Broca's aphasics. The assertion that conduction aphasics, deprived of the specific phonemic record, must rely on lexical comprehension as do Broca's aphasics seems reasonable. Practically speaking, however, studies have shown that patients of all subtypes exhibit some degree of short-term memory impairment (Albert, 1976; Caramazza *et al.*, 1978). It is not clear if the deficit in short-term memory plays a different role in various subtypes or whether short-term memory is language specific or involves all input processing. It is also possible that a performance reduction in short-term memory may reflect a more global retrieval deficit.

SUMMARY OF LINGUISTIC STUDIES

At this point in time, some conclusions can be drawn from the extensive investigations of comprehension at each of the various linguistic levels. Using different experimental methods to investigate phonological, semantic, and syntactic abilities in aphasia, studies indicate that the large majority of patients have some degree of impairment at all levels, though impairment may not correlate with the overall severity of comprehension. It is fairly uncommon for one level to be selectively impaired, the one exception being the rare syndrome of pure word deafness, which involves a marked selective disturbance in phonological processing. However, partial correlations are found in studies that demonstrate a disproportionate impairment of phonological discrimination in a part of the population of aphasics who manifest phonological errors in speech. There is also a high correlation between semantic discrimination and identification in patients whose primary symptom is verbal (semantic) paraphasia, as well as a selective insensitivity to grammatical markers in patients presenting agrammatism. These findings support the existence of central mechanisms that affect both speech production and comprehension.

It is also clear that the degree of impairment at each level is unequally related to the overall comprehension ability. In most studies disturbances at the phonological level seem quite dissociated from overall comprehension ability (Lesser, 1978), and it may well be that the phonological level operates as a relatively peripheral part of the language system. Disturbances at the semantic level are pervasive among all aphasic subtypes and are also found in individuals suffering brain lesions outside the language areas. The degree of semantic deficit seems most closely associated with the severity of overall comprehension disturbance.

The results of a number of linguistic investigations suggest that syntactic deficits are common in all aphasic subtypes. Although syntactic tests do not adequately differentiate subgroups of aphasia, such tests reliably discriminate nonaphasic brain-damaged individuals from aphasics (Lesser, 1974; Mack & Boller, 1979; Parisi & Pizzamiglio, 1970). It is not difficult to understand that performance on syntactically weighted tests does not correlate with other measures of comprehension. Most clinical tests of comprehension rely heavily on the understanding of particular lexical items, which is relatively spared in some forms of aphasia. The impact of syntactic deficits on the overall comprehension ability of aphasics is, therefore, more superficial and may only be apparent when sentence interpretation is dependent on grammatical morphemes or on complex syntactic relationships among the words of a sentence.

Nonlinguistic Factors in Comprehension

Historically, the relationship between the linguistic and nonlinguistic factors that affect comprehension in aphasia has been a controversial issue. One notion is that comprehension impairment reflects an underlying conceptual deficit that affects both spoken language and many nonverbal abilities. Another line of reasoning postulates an underlying nonlinguistic auditory processing disorder that affects linguistic function. That is, the inability to understand spoken language is thought to be secondary to a defect in discriminating and analyzing the acoustic properties of the signal. Other investigators maintain that language and nonlanguage processes are distinct from each other. Still others have suggested that specific defects in cognition, perception, awareness, and affect are associated with each aphasic syndrome.

AUDITORY PERCEPTUAL FACTORS

Investigators are in reasonably good agreement that in the case of pure word deafness the sounds of speech are not perceived normally. Some studies indicate that patients with this condition also manifest AUDITORY AGNOSIA, a term that refers to the inability to match an environmental noise with its source. (For a review and discussion, see Vignolo, 1969.)

Nonverbal sound recognition is generally tested by presenting taped sounds (barking, gunshots, etc.) and asking the subject to identify the picture depicting the sound source (dog, pistol), In addition to the correct picture, the subject is presented alternatives, including one depicting an acoustically similar source, one with a semantically associated source, and one with no relationship to the test sound. Presumably, acoustic errors reflect a discriminative disorder and semantic errors an associative defect. Several studies have investigated aphasics' ability to perform this task, and their findings have revived the long-standing discussion as to whether the perceptual deficit in aphasia is best characterized as an associative–semantic or a purely auditory–discrimination defect.

Spinnler and Vignolo (1966) administered such a sound recognition test to unilaterally brain-damaged subjects. Although not all aphasics scored in the impaired range, poor performance was found only in the aphasic group. Sound recognition impairment was more frequent in Wernicke's aphasia than other aphasic syndromes, and test scores correlated significantly with a test of auditory verbal comprehension. Furthermore, the aphasic group was the only group in which "semantic" errors outnumbered "acoustic" errors. The investigators concluded that the impairment in sound recognition in aphasia was due not merely to a discriminative disorder but rather to a common associative–semantic disorder that transcends spoken language and is the basis for the nonverbal sound recognition impairment and the deficit in auditory comprehension. The argument for a central associative–semantic disturbance in aphasia was further elaborated by Faglioni, Spinnler, and Vignolo (1969). They found that the nonverbal sound recognition defect was associated with performance on other tests of conceptual abilities. In contrast, aphasics were found to be unimpaired in a test of basic sound recognition.

Strohner, Cohen, Kelter, and Woll (1978) demonstrated, however, that when pictured alternatives are controlled for acoustic and semantic properties subjects show no specific error type. Furthermore, they found no difference between Broca's and Wernicke's aphasics in their ability to match a sound with its source, though performance highly correlated with a test of comprehension. Strohner *et al.*, therefore, took issue with the notion of a common semantic basis for the connection between nonverbal sound recognition and comprehension disorders in aphasia. Instead they postulated that the primary difficulty in aphasia is an impairment in analyzing a characteristic feature of the stimulus regardless of the perceptual modality. They considered both "semantic" and "acoustic" disorders part of the cognitive disorder found in aphasia.

The major difference between the two sets of findings is in the interpretation of the root of the problem. All studies demonstrated that a portion of the aphasic population evidences a defect in nonverbal sound recognition that correlates with an impairment in the comprehension of spoken language. It remains unclear, however, which individual aphasics are likely to manifest such difficulty. Goldblum and Albert (1972) identified a subgroup of Wernicke's aphasics in whom an impairment on phonemic discrimination tasks was linked with an impairment on a test of nonverbal sound recognition and another group in whom phonemic discrimination deficits were mild and nonverbal recognition defects were rare. Varney (1980) emphasizes, furthermore, that there are some aphasics who, despite severe deficits in comprehension of spoken language, have no difficulty linking sounds with their sources. He suggests that, although in many aphasics nonverbal sound recognition deficits and auditory comprehension disorders are correlated and have a common basis, severe comprehension disorders are sometimes selectively linguistic and exist independently of a disturbance in nonverbal sound recognition. Obviously, it is necessary to specify further the comprehension profiles of aphasics with preserved and impaired nonverbal recognition to elucidate the interconnection of nonverbal sound recognition and language comprehension disorders.

NONVERBAL DISORDERS ASSOCIATED WITH
COMPREHENSION IMPAIRMENT

It is not within the scope of this chapter to discuss the extensive literature concerning the nonverbal intellectual deficits in aphasia (see Chapter 11 of this volume). However, it is appropriate to point out that many nonauditory abilities have been found to be highly associated with spoken language comprehension. Particularly notable are interpretations of symbolic gestures (Gainotti & Lemmo, 1976), associations of objects with their color and use (De Renzi, Faglioni, Scotti, & Spinnler, 1972), performance on the Raven's Progressive Matrices (Basso, De Renzi, Faglioni, Scotti, & Spinnler, 1973; Kertesz & McCabe, 1975), and the qualitatively different styles and abnormalities of visual stimulus exploration among various syndromes of aphasia (Tyler, 1969). These investigations have supported the notion that disorders of speech comprehension are associated with disturbances of higher mental function that transcend spoken language.

The assertion that the basic difficulty in aphasia is a failure at a very early stage of auditory analysis was proposed by Efron (1963), who found that aphasics require much greater intervals between stimuli to judge which of two sounds come first. Efron reasoned that aphasia might well be considered an epiphenomenon of a more fundamental nonlinguistic deficit in temporal analysis. The suggestion spurred a great deal of research activity examining the possible auditory–temporal basis for aphasia. This line of research demonstrated that, compared to other brain-damaged individuals, aphasics were impaired in analyzing the temporal properties of stimuli. Studies have shown that aphasics have difficulty discriminating and matching complex nonverbal sounds (Tallal & Newcombe, 1978), judging the presence of dichotically presented clicks at various temporal separations (Lachner & Teuber, 1973), and, for some patients, judging the order of both auditory and visual stimuli (Brookshire, 1978a; Swisher & Hirsh, 1972). However, the evidence to support the link between difficulty in temporal resolution and comprehension disorders in aphasia is weak. In fact, Efron (1963) found those aphasics most impaired in their temporal judgments were those with the most preserved comprehension of spoken language.

It is also important to note that Carmon and Nachson (1971) found that left-brain-damaged individuals without aphasia were impaired in their ability to sequence lights and sounds. The strongest evidence against a fundamental temporal ordering deficit in aphasia is provided by Sherwin and Efron's study (1980) of right and left temporal lobectomized individuals, which indicated that an elevated threshold for performing temporal order judgments was unrelated to aphasia or dominant hemisphere lesions.

The hypothesis that an impairment in basic auditory processing is implicated in comprehension disorders has, however, been supported by Tallal and Newcombe (1978), whose findings correlated with an impairment in processing nonverbal sounds at decreased interstimulus intervals, a failure to process rapidly changing acoustic information in synthetic speech syllables, and a reduction in spoken language comprehension. It is anticipated that further studies will attempt to specify the nature of the temporal defect and its connection with the language processing deficits in aphasia.

Although findings that support the notion of an auditory–temporal defect as the basis for the comprehension disorder in aphasia are equivocal, many investigations have indicated that aphasics profit from additional time to process speech. Ebbin and Edwards (1967) found performance on a speech sound discrimination task improved for some aphasics with increased interstimulus intervals. Reducing the rate of enunciation resulted in a significant improvement in aphasics' ability to identify common object names embedded in a sentence (Gardner *et al.*, 1975). In another study, decreasing the rate of speech improved the identification of objects named serially and sentence repetition in patients' manifesting mild comprehension disorders (Weidner & Lasky, 1976). Decreasing the rate of presentation aided aphasics' ability to make semantic but not phonemic comparisons on a word detection task (Cermak & Moreines, 1976).

In addition, Sheehan, Aseltine, and Edwards (1973) found that inserting silence around individual phonemes improved the younger aphasic individual's comprehension scores, though silences between words had no enhancing effect. Inserting pauses in Token Test commands has also been found to have a facilitating effect on performance, though increased processing time may not enhance comprehension when sentence structure is complex (Liles & Brookshire, 1975). Similarly, Poeck and Pietron (1981) found that "stretching" speech signals has a positive effect on Token Test performance. Investigations manipulating speech electromechanically have found that expansion improves performance for some aphasics, whereas speech compression has a detrimental effect (Parkhurst, 1970), and too much deviation from normal speech rate in either direction interferes with word comprehension (Di Carlo & Taub, 1972).

There is no question that aphasics often fail to understand speech at a normal rate and benefit from additional processing time. The effect of speed, though perhaps not universal, is potent and seems independent of the form of aphasia. This impairment need not be explained as a failure due to a defect in nonlinguistic temporal analysis. It is just as reasonable that, given the reduction in efficiency in aphasics' linguistic processing, more time is necessary to mobilize defective comprehension strategies. Merely increasing processing time does not seem to benefit all patients or improve performance on those operations that are not within a patient's linguistic capacity.

SHORT-TERM MEMORY DEFICITS

Despite the near universality of short-term memory deficits in aphasia, there may be little correlation between the severity of short-term memory deficits and the severity of the comprehension disorder.

For example, conduction aphasics, who manifest a striking reduction in verbatim repetition and other short-term memory tasks, show remarkably intact sentence comprehension (Saffran & Marin, 1975).

Short-term memory is tested in various ways: verbal repetition or pointing to objects serially named or visually presented. Tzortzis and Albert (1974) isolated two types of short-term memory deficits in aphasia: memory for items and memory for order. Albert (1976) demonstrated that, while the short-term memory deficit is more conspicious as information load is increased, aphasics have a marked reduction in recall of total items regardless of information load. Furthermore, memory deficits of items named was sometimes dissociated with memory for the order of the series. When memory performance was correlated with anatomical localization data, Albert found that every aphasic with a perisylvian lesion also showed defective short-term memory. Short-term memory was not, however, linked to any specific variety of aphasia.

EMOTIONAL FACTORS

Clinically, one is impressed by what appears to be markedly enhanced comprehension when aphasic patients are exposed to material relating to their feelings or other emotionally charged topics (illness, loss, personal life, etc.); by contrast, comprehension is not as good with the neutral material used in standardized assessment measures.

Boller, Cole, Vrtunski, Patterson, and Kim (1979) studied the effects of emotional content on comprehension of spoken language in severe aphasia. High emotional content commands (*Show me how to shoot a gun*), yes–no questions (*Are you going to a nursing home?*), and informational questions were matched with control sentences of low emotional content. The high emotional content sentences precipitated a significantly greater number of correct and appropriate responses than did those of low emotional content. However, high emotional content can sometimes work against effective processing. For example, Wechsler (1973) found aphasics recalled more details of a neutral story than of a story dealing with illness.

Greater responsiveness to topics of high personal relevance and selective forgetting of unpleasantness is certainly not selective to aphasia, but the impact of emotional content on comprehension function is clinically important, often contributing to the variability in aphasic performance. Variability in functional comprehension has also been related to the anxiety precipitated by stressful communicative situations (Schuell, 1953b). In clinical performance, anxiety may account for the detrimental effect of discouraging instructions (Stoicheff, 1960).

There is a general tendency for aphasic patients to overlook disorders of comprehension while readily acknowledging speech, writing, reading, and even subtle cognitive impairments. To some extent, acknowledgment of the inability to understand spoken language may be associated with an admission of intellectual dysfunction, a concept more threatening to some aphasics than difficulty speaking. This notion is partially supported by the fact that some patients admit to having experienced comprehension difficulty in the past, while denying present difficulty despite objective findings to the contrary.

GENERAL PSYCHOLOGICAL FACTORS

Some investigators have placed great emphasis on the role of more general effects of brain damage on language function. While the significance of these symptoms may be argued, no one will dispute the prevalence of a variety of behaviors that, though unrelated to the form and content of language, account for a substantial proportion of failure in linguistic performance. K. Goldstein (1948) particularly stressed the importance of general organic behaviors in explaining the reduction of function in aphasia. He maintained that there is a rise of threshold and retardation of excitation for all stimuli, resulting in slower reaction time; a lability of thresholds resulting in an inability to sustain a given performance; reduced equalization between excitation and inhibition that results in perseveration; increased dependency of performance on external factors resulting in distractibility; a blurring of the figure–ground boundaries; and loss of abstract attitude evident in difficulty initiating an activity, shifting voluntarily from one set to the next, or making a choice by keeping two aspects in mind while grasping a whole.

However one may interpret such symptoms, these general effects of brain damage have grave consequences for an aphasic's ability to follow and respond to spoken language, complicate formal assessment of language comprehension, and account for variability in performance from one situation to the next. In overall terms, they result in reduced efficiency for receiving and acting on input from the external world. Though there are few systematic studies of the influence of these general factors on speech comprehension, it is not difficult to demonstrate differences in accuracy of response to a given linguistic unit under different circumstances.

In a preliminary study, Lenneberg *et al.* (1978) were able to demonstrate marked differences in aphasics' ability to understand single words, by manipulating such external factors as order of presentation, number of choices, environmental and verbal content, length of utterance, and controlling for perseveration. Error scores were compared item by item and analyzed in each condition for every patient. This permitted quantification of the degree to which performance on a word comprehension test could be attributed to linguistic factors, nonlinguistic general factors (cognitive), or physiological variability. They found that nonlinguistic performance factors contributed as little as zero and as much as 95% of the errors made on the test. The more severely impaired patients showed a higher proportion of errors due to externally controlled factors than did less severely impaired patients.

As a result of their findings, Lenneberg and his co-workers suggested that, in studies of language function, only less severely affected aphasics be used as subjects, since if patients are ordered in terms of severity, the importance of these "nuisance factors" increases and makes it difficult to observe actual language dysfunction.

Valuable information has been obtained, however, from the investigation of preserved comprehension in severe aphasia. Boller and Green (1972) and Green and Boller (1974) studied the comprehension of global and Wernicke's aphasics and found certain regularities in the rudimentary comprehension processes of this group despite marked individual differences in some patients. When responses of severely impaired patients were scored for appropriateness of facial expression or other behavioral responses rather than for correctness, retention of some linguistic comprehension was demonstrated. As a group, although they had difficulty distinguishing between conventional English and semantic jargon, they were able to distinguish between their native language and a foreign language or phonemic jargon. Some preserved appreciation of sentence structure was also evident in the subjects' tendency to use more jargon in response to questions requiring information than in response to yes–no questions and verbal commands. They appropriately disregarded irrelevant introductory material, and the frequently observed superiority of responses to whole body and limb commands over responses to other commands was supported. The most unexpected finding was that patients responded far better when the examiner faced the patient and when natural speech, rather than tape-recorded messages, were used.

The external cues provided by a natural setting appear to improve language comprehension. Contextual information, whether it be verbal or situational, enhances an aphasic's comprehension of the general meaning of spoken language and the understanding of particular syntactic structures. The importance of context in comprehension was supported by Stachowiak, Huber, Poeck, and Kerschensteiner (1977), who found aphasics' comprehension of material presented in a literary context to be superior to performance on clinical comprehension tests. Wilcox, Davis, and Leonard (1978) demonstrated that the aphasics' responses to indirect requests referable to videotapes of naturalistic situations were far superior to their comprehension as measured by standard aphasia comprehension batteries. This held true regardless of clinical type or severity of aphasia, though in the more severely impaired patients' overall performance was somewhat poorer.

It is obvious that a variety of externally controlled nonlinguistic factors, such as rate of speech or presentation, emotional content of utterance, and verbal or situational context, affect aphasics' comprehension of speech; however, it is not obvious for which aphasics and for what reasons this should be so. Aphasics manifest a vast number of deviant behaviors not clearly related to their language disturbances, ranging from retarded reaction time to inability to sustain performance levels, perseveration, difficulty sorting irrelevant from relevant details, difficulty shifting from one set of response requirements to the next, inability to relate to concerns outside the immediate environment, deviant affectual display, and varying degrees of denial. With few exceptions to date, those interested in clinical classification have paid little attention to the regularity of various nonlinguistic factors that are possibly qualitatively different in the varieties of aphasia. Little is known about the evolution of these symptoms, which ones persist to what degree and for whom. That all of these factors interact with aphasics' comprehension of spoken language and must be considered in clinical assessment cannot be denied.

Clinical Assessment

There is a general consensus among clinical practitioners of the need for in-depth testing of spoken language comprehension in aphasic patients. There is, however, disagreement as to the direction it should take and what clinical diagnostic and practical requirements it should attempt to meet. (For further discussion of the issues surrounding assessment of aphasia, refer to Chapter 4 of this volume.) Test designs are never completely comprehensive and, from a practical point of view, need not be. Obviously, the judicious selection of a particular assessment instrument depends on the clinical and research needs one wants to satisfy as well as on sufficient familiarity with the limitations and advantages of the instrument. It is particularly important that the interpretation of comprehension deficits not be limited to information derived exclusively from the particular assessment instrument used.

With this in mind, it seems essential to specify clinical needs. A battery assessing comprehension should include instruments that (*a*) distinguish between aphasic and nonaphasic individuals; (*b*) identify mild disorders not obvious in an interview; (*c*) permit a reliable and valid inference to be made about the extent to which overall understanding of spoken language is impaired, along a complexity continuum; (*d*) permit identification of critical linguistic parameters; (*e*) contribute to diagnostic classification; (*f*) identify nonlinguistic but contributing factors, such as the perceptual, motor, cognitive, and affective aspects; (*g*) examine comprehension in a variety of situational settings; and (*h*) have a sufficient range of difficulty that improvement can be documented over time. Research needs are different from clinical needs, and the choice of instruments to assess comprehension must be carefully considered with respect to the purpose and design of the study. Not all of these needs are adequately satisfied by existing instruments.

Although assessment measures are described in Chapter 4, it seems important to consider the features of existing batteries of comprehension tests.

The Boston Diagnostic Aphasia Examination (BDAE) (Goodglass & Kaplan, 1972) contains an auditory comprehension section containing four subareas: word discrimination, which utilizes a picture choice format involving six semantic categories (objects, forms, letters, actions, numbers, and colors) and is scored for correctness, speed, and identification of category; body-part identification, in which the patient must point to body parts on himself and the examiner, and scoring reflects both speed and correctness; verbal commands, in which the amount of auditory information presented ranges from one to five units, and scoring reflects correctness only; and complex ideational material, which requires answers to paired yes–no questions concerning both factual material not related to the immediate environment and material read to the patient and is scored by the number of yes–no pairs that are correct.

Though not formally a part of the BDAE, several supplementary language tests are included to test patients' comprehension of prepositions of location; understanding of *before* or *after*; ability to follow commands that involve *Touch* _____ *with the* _____ *and With the* _____, *touch the* _____; understanding of subject–verb–object order in passive constructions; and understanding of possessive relationships.

The Minnesota Test for the Differential Diagnosis of Aphasia (MTDDA) (Schuell, 1965) contains seven subtests of auditory comprehension, all of which are scored for accuracy only. The subtests are recognizing common words (picture choice format), discrimination between paired words that are phonemically similar, recognizing letters (multiple-choice format in which a card containing several auditorily confusable letters is presented), identifying items serially named (patient is asked to point to items in a picture given a one to two unit series), understanding sentences (simple yes–no questions about common factual information), following directions (patient performs commands with the several common objects presented), understanding a paragraph (yes–no questions pertaining to a paragraph read to a patient). There is also a test of verbal memory span for digits and sentences.

The Neurosensory Center Comprehensive Examination for Aphasia (NCCEA) (Spreen & Benton, 1969) includes two auditory comprehension subtests: identification by name, in which the patient points to real objects named by the examiner, and identification by sentence (Token Test) (see Spreen and Risser, Chapter 4 of this volume). Twenty plastic tokens are presented in a prescribed array. The patient is asked to identify and follow a series of verbal commands that entail responding to words designating two sizes, two shapes, and five colors. The Benton–Spreen version comprises six progressively more complicated parts.

The Auditory Comprehension Test for Sentences (ACT) (Shewan, 1979) is a picture verification sentence comprehension test that requires the patient to select one of four pictures that matches the sentence spoken by the examiner. Vocabulary, sentence length, and syntactic complexity are systematically controlled. Scores reflect not only correctness but promptness and self-correction. Types of errors (lexical or syntactic) and position of error in a sentence can be reflected quantitatively in the score.

Porch Index of Communicative Ability (PICA) (Porch, 1967). This battery is divided into three subdivisions: gestural, verbal, and graphic. Stimuli are presented either gesturally or verbally. Two subtests assess specifically the patient's understanding of spoken language: ability to point to objects whose function is given verbally by the examiner, and ability to point to objects named. Subtests are presented in an hierarchical manner, progressing from the one that requires the least information to the one that requires the most. The scoring procedure is complicated and based on a 16-point binary-choice multidimensional scale. Accuracy, responsiveness, completeness, promptness, and efficiency are built into the scoring method.

The Functional Communication Profile (FCP) (Sarno, 1969; Taylor, 1965) is not a formal test but rather a rating scale. Aphasics' ability to understand spoken language is assessed in a situation that simulates as far as possible everyday conversation and real-life situations. The "understanding" subtest is one of five sections of the profile. The examiner rates 15 different behaviors on a 9-point scale from 0 to normal, taking into account a presumed premorbid proficiency. Behaviors include such varied responses as awareness of environmental sounds and emotional voice tone, recognition of one's own name and the names of family members, recognition of objects and action names, ability to follow simple, gestured, and complex commands, and understanding of simple one-to-one, group, and complex rapid conversation.

Some of the needs specified earlier are partially satisfied by the individual tests described. For example, the Token Test is a valuable aid in helping to discriminate aphasics from nonaphasics. There is a relatively small error rate, and depending on the study, between 84% and 91% of aphasics are so differentiated by Token Test score (Hartje, Kerschensteiner, Poeck, & Orgass, 1973; Orgass & Poeck, 1966; Spellacy & Spreen, 1969; Swisher & Sarno, 1969). One must keep in mind, however, that elderly brain-damaged individuals without clinical evidence of aphasia frequently show reduced scores on the Token Test, so that scores must be considered in the context of a patient's history and clinical state.

Left-brain-damaged patients who show no obvious speech production deficits may score more poorly than other brain-damaged individuals (Boller & Vignolo, 1966). The Token Test is useful in exposing the less apparent comprehension deficits of Broca's, conduction, and mild fluent varieties (De Renzi & Vignolo, 1962), though it is not very helpful in classifying subtypes (Poeck, Kerschensteiner, & Hartje, 1972). It is extremely useful in documenting changes in input processing over time (Prins, Snow, & Wagenaar, 1978; Sarno & Levita, 1979). The nonredundant highly artificial, linguistically and cognitively demanding features of the Token Test expose deficits and real changes not observable using other assessment procedures. It is extremely limited, however, in areas where other tests excel, namely, in tapping the lower end of the scale and the variations in severe comprehension deficits. Further discussion of the Token Test will follow this section.

The relatively new ACT (Shewan, 1979) provides the stimuli and format for more detailed linguistic analysis than is possible with the older batteries. The author reports that overall scores also help to differentiate among the comprehension abilities of Broca's, Wernicke's, and amnesic aphasics, though aphasics as a group show equal impairment across the parameters of vocabulary, sentence length, and syntax.

Though not intended to be used as the only measure of communication abilities, nor as a substitute for comprehensive and systematic investigation of aphasic behavior, the FCP (Sarno, 1969; Taylor, 1965) is a useful tool for quantifying the patient's responses to spoken language and for rating present proficiency. Such factors as patient's age, education, professional status, and estimated premorbid proficiency are considered in making the assessment. Its value is in encouraging a point of view that goes beyond the scores obtained on formal tests and in artificial settings, by focusing on a patient's actual use or behavior in a real communication event.

In summary, although there is always a certain amount of lag between knowledge obtained and its clinical application, the direction of aphasia testing has followed the trends of aphasia research. The recent emphasis on psycholinguistics has uncovered needs partially addressed by a test such as the ACT (Shewan, 1979). The very wide use of the Token Test has led investigators to questions and concerns that were only informally acknowledged. Pragmatic aspects of communication and issues of validity that address whether or not an instrument tests the patient's actual function in the course of everyday communication are more seriously considered, though no test is truly successful in this area. The very nature of the comprehension dimension plus the fact that there is controversy about all aspects of comprehension deficits in aphasia, makes demands on test design that are almost impossible to meet.

The Token Test: Research Findings

The Token Test seems to have initiated or at least contributed to the recent focus on auditory comprehension disturbances in aphasia. In the years since its original publication, the test has gained widespread use as both a clinical and a research tool. (For an in-depth account of Token Test research, refer to Boller and Dennis, 1979.)

On the surface, the test appears to be a relatively straightforward comprehension task, but it obviously embodies a variety of linguistic and cognitive requirements to which the left-hemisphere-damaged patient with aphasia is peculiarly sensitive. Although research has greatly increased our understanding of the factors that contribute to the test's difficulty, it remains impossible to ascertain the basis for errors on specific items and it is difficult to interpret the meaning of the overall score.

De Renzi and Vignolo (1962) designed the Token Test to uncover subtle comprehension deficits in patients whose disturbance appeared limited to expression and in mild sensory aphasics. Certain features were built into the test that added to its sensitivity but perhaps detracted from its clinical usefulness. The language of the commands is non-redundant, and the items used (i.e., shapes, sizes, colors) provide no inherent clues to enhance comprehension. The format is artificial without situational cues that might obscure comprehension loss. Cultural and intellectual factors are minimized by the selection of high-frequency common words. In the first four sections, commands are controlled for length and number of critical items presented, and the response mode is limited to pointing. In the final sections, the commands are more syntactically complex, require a more complicated motor response, and vary in length. Inherent in the test design is a lack of separation between the lexical and syntactic aspects of each command.

Following De Renzi and Vignolo's original study, the first research application verified the sensitivity of the instrument to receptive deficits in mild aphasia (Hartje *et al.*, 1973; Lesser, 1974; Orgass & Poeck, 1966, 1969; Spellacy & Spreen, 1969; Swisher & Sarno, 1969). These studies supported De Renzi and Vignolo's (1962) finding that any patient showing evidence of aphasia in speech production will likely have a reduced Token Test score. They directed attention to the fact that the disturbance manifested by motor or Broca's aphasia was not isolated to speech production and provided evidence for the pervasiveness of comprehension deficits in aphasia, or at least for those complex cognitive and linguistic abilities tested by the Token Test.

Many revisions have been proposed, and generally those Token Test versions most widely used are revisions of the original. Authors have reduced the number of items (De Renzi, 1979; Spellacy & Spreen, 1969) and varied the shape of the tokens (Spreen & Benton, 1969), their color (Scotti & Spinnler, 1970), and the scoring system (Orgass & Poeck, 1966), yet the instruments retain discriminative power. In fact, Part V is so highly discriminative that it has been used by itself (Poeck, Orgass, Kerschensteiner, & Hartje, 1974). In addition, the discriminating power is not limited to auditory language comprehension. A written version proves equally difficult for aphasics (Poeck & Hartje, 1979).

On the other hand, investigations have shown that the diagnostic usefulness of the Token Test is limited. Poeck and co-workers (Poeck *et al.* 1972; Poeck *et al.*, 1974) found no quantitative or qualitative difference in overall score or performance on any subtest among motor, sensory, and amnesic aphasics.

The range of Token Test application in aphasia research has been extensive. Experimental investigations have correlated Token Test performance with other measures of comprehension (Lesser, 1974; Needham & Swisher, 1972; Orgass & Poeck, 1969), with other nonverbal auditory abilities (Faglioni *et al.*, 1969; Tallal & Newcombe, 1978), and with visual abilities (Birchmeier, 1980). It has also been used to compare reduced performance in aphasia with the normal language acquisition in children (Poeck *et al.*, 1974; Whitaker & Noll, 1972), to experimentally train auditory comprehension (Holland & Whitney, 1979; Salvatore, 1976), to assess right hemisphere comprehension (Zaidel, 1976, 1977b), and to document recovery (Prins *et al.*, 1978; Sarno & Levita, 1979).

Most recently, Token Test performance has been used as an independent variable for clinicopathological correlation. By dividing the aphasic
population into low- and high-comprehension groups, the locus and
extent of lesions implicating degrees of performance reduction have
been studied (Vignolo, 1979).

Several studies have explored the microstructure of each command to
isolate linguistic factors contributing to command complexity (De Renzi
& Vignolo, 1962; Whitaker & Noll, 1972; Whitaker & Selnes, 1978;
Whitaker & Whitaker, 1979). Among the linguistic parameters identified
were the grammatical ambiguity of verbal expressions denoting shape,
the semantic dependence of the grammatical elements (prepositions,
articles, adverbs, and conjunctions), the ambiguity of reference for locative prepositions, the switch from implied to overt instrumental use of
the word *touch*, the processing demands of two verb commands, and
the unique role played by many of the verbs used.

Mack and Boller (1979) designed a Token Test that independently
varied the linguistic requirements of syntax, lexicon, and sentence
length; reduced the total size of the array from 20 to 8; minimized motor
demands; and revised scoring procedures in order to increase the test's
power to discriminate among clinical types. The most substantial revision was in the final section involving syntactically complex commands.
They divided this section into two parts: one testing understanding of
locative prepositions and the other testing words denoting sequential
order (e.g., *after, when, if . . . then*).

Consistent with other psycholinguistic studies, an analysis of items
discriminating aphasics from nonaphasics demonstrated that the commands that involved words indicating a temporal sequence and reversible center-embedded sentences were particularly problematic for
aphasics. The modified test resulted in a more definable separation between nonfluents with and without significant comprehension disorder,
and clear differences in both the number and type of errors made between the nonfluent and fluent categories. Specifically, nonfluent
aphasics with good comprehension evidenced only syntactic errors.
Nonfluents with comprehension loss and fluent aphasics made both
stimulus and syntactic errors. The mean number of stimulus errors was
obviously greater in the fluent group; nonfluents with good comprehension had a near normal stimulus error rate. The number of stimulus
errors for nonfluent aphasics with comprehension loss fell between the
numbers of the other aphasic groups.

Kreindler, Gheorghita, and Voinescu (1971) varied the concrete–
abstract nature of the items and the order of the wording of stimulus
elements in commands. In addition to the abstract shape (*square* and

circle), they added two concrete shapes (*house* and *flower*) and two words of presumed intermediate abstractness (*dwelling* and *plant*). The items were presented in two sizes and colors.

They found that shape words always yielded significantly more errors than did words denoting other attributes; these were followed by words denoting color and size. However, the difference in error rate between shape and color was significantly greater for the abstract shape words (*square, circle*) than for the concrete items (*house, flower*). The concrete versus abstract property of words affected the scores of aphasics with milder comprehension disorders. In those with severe impairment, the error rate was too high to yield a significant difference. Word order of elements was also a significant factor in performance. The third position was always better decoded for all variants, though the shape name was consistently more difficult than other attribute categories.

Lesser (1979) investigated whether the use of real object names and a change in the grammatical class of shape words would improve aphasics' performance. Predicting that inherent multisensory cues would enhance comprehension, she administered a version in which object names (e.g., **sponge** *square*) were substituted for the words denoting color. This task, however, proved more difficult than the standard version for aphasics.

In a version in which shape names were unambiguously modifying adjectives (e.g., **square** *sponge*), comprehension of the attribute improved, but this version was also no easier than the standard form. Lesser suggested that the real objects may have further increased the artificiality of the test and added to rather than decreased processing difficulty. One interesting sidelight of Lesser's study was the high correlation between aphasics' verbal descriptions of an item and their ability to identify the item when named, which suggests part of the difficulty handling Token Test commands may be attributed to a central semantic retrieval deficit.

Lesser (1976) also argued that because of the many nonlinguistic cognitive demands of the test, Token Test data are not suitable material for linguistic analysis. She particularly stressed short-term memory requirements, though she reported that memory demands are so interrelated with other linguistic, perceptual, and motor requirements that it is impossible to isolate short-term memory constrictions. She maintained that when input–output systems are overloaded, information about the nature of the aphasics' linguistic impairment is obscured by other performance errors.

Given the many possible reasons for failing to understand Token Test commands, it is likely that different aphasics perform poorly for entirely different reasons. To assess performance variables contributing to Token Test scores, Brookshire (1978b) expanded on the test design and administered a battery of Token Tests to right and left hemisphere damaged individuals. The battery presented three different forms: a standard test, a configurational test in which subjects select one of four pictured groupings to match a spoken sentence, and a visual test in which a pictured arrangement is matched to one of four pictures. Each form was presented in an immediate- and delayed-response mode. The results showed marked uniformity in rank order of performance in the various forms presented under the two conditions. Patient's showing atypical patterns in performance with respect to memory or visual search could be isolated from those showing the typical aphasic performance patterns.

In summary, the complexity of linguistic and cognitive demands the task places on the aphasic must not be underestimated. Many factors influence performance on the Token Test, including linguistic factors: analyzing items that are closely related semantically, the grammatical features of predication, location, subordination, temporal sequence, and adverbial phrases; difficulty with particles, implicit and overt verbs; and the extralinguistic factors: lack of redundancy in the message, difficulty managing a series of shifting but similar tasks, defects in attention and concentration, fatigue, visual spatial deficits, difficulty handling the abstractness of tokens, the artificiality of the task, impaired analysis of a whole into a series of elements, and reliance on volitional movements of the hand, to name only the most obvious.

The Token Test is often criticized for not contributing as much as it should to the diagnosis of aphasia. It was, however, constructed with a certain purpose in mind—to be a highly demanding task, free of cultural, intellectual, and situational factors, that could help separate the aphasic from the nonaphasic population. This the test does well. It is also one of the best overall indicators of severity, correlating highly with the size of the lesion on CT scans (Naeser, Hayward, Laughlin, Becker, Jernigan, & Zatz, 1981).

The wealth of data derived from the years of clinical and experimental use of the Token Test has resulted in a greater appreciation of the complexity of receptive disturbances in aphasia. Though it is impossible to know on what basis a patient fails to perform a particular command, the regularities and peculiarities of aphasics' overall performance have raised relevant questions regarding the nature of and dimensions involved in comprehension disorders. One expects that, in the future, investigations using the Token Test will attempt to isolate and control factors affecting performance in order to provide information defining patterns of performance in the various aphasic syndromes.

Evolution of Comprehension Disorders in Aphasia

Information about the recovery of comprehension is necessary for practical and theoretical reasons. It is essential for the clinical worker to appreciate the significance of a patient's comprehension status in a particular time frame and to be able to predict and interpret changes in the evolution of symptoms. Furthermore, the information gained from recovery data raises theoretical questions regarding neurological compensation and functional restitution.

There are at least two major reasons to examine the evolution of comprehension disorders: first, to discover to what extent in what respect, and for which diagnostic groups comprehension changes over time; and second, to examine the significance of comprehension disturbance relative to overall recovery.

Although recovery studies have tended to be less concerned with the evolution of a particular symptom than with the general trends of recovery, there is something to be learned from recovery findings. There have been a few systematic investigations of the evolution of aphasia in the post-CVA patient (Kenin & Swisher, 1972; Kertesz, 1979; Kertesz & McCabe, 1977; Lomas & Kertesz, 1978; Prins *et al.*, 1978; Sarno & Levita, 1979; Vignolo, 1964).

With few exceptions, recovery studies investigating language change have found that, at all levels of severity, comprehension precedes expression on nearly all clinical comprehension measures in the evolution toward normal function. All patient groups studied, including severe or global aphasia, show some degree of improvement in comprehension in the first few months (Lomas & Kertesz, 1978) and some severe (global) aphasics continue to improve substantially in their ability to understand sentences in the 6–12-month period (Sarno and Levita, in press). Both Prins *et al.* (1978) and Demeurisse, Demol, Derouck, de Beuckelaer, Coekaerts, and Capon (1980) found that, while all aphasic groups improved on tests of auditory comprehension, fluents or Wernicke's aphasics improved slightly more than other patient groups. Sarno and Levita (1979) found their fluent group improved slightly faster than their nonfluent group on the Token Test in the first 3 months postonset, but the nonfluent group had exceeded the fluent by 6 months postonset.

The initial status of comprehension impairment has long been considered a prognostic indicator for the extent of overall recovery in aphasia (Schuell, 1953a). This impression is supported by research findings. High-comprehension groups, whether fluent or nonfluent, made significant improvement at initial stages in overall test scores in Lomas and Kertesz's (1978) study of spontaneous evolution. Neuroradiologic studies also support the implication of this finding. Kertesz (1979) reports that the larger the lesion, the poorer the comprehension. There is a high significant negative correlation between lesion size and score on a measure of overall language function (the aphasia quotient). The CT scan studies of Yarnell, Monroe, and Sobel (1976) and Naeser, Hayward, Laughlin, and Zatz (1981) show similar results.

This major finding should, however, be considered with another very common finding of recovery studies. Improvement in comprehension is found without concomitant changes in speech (Prins *et al.*, 1978; Sarno & Levita, 1981; Vignolo, 1964). This is particularly true of patients with "mixed expressive" (Vignolo's group) and global aphasia (Sarno and Levita's group) as well as the perhaps similar "severe nonfluent" in Prins's study, though Prins *et al.* reported that a few individual cases showed sufficient improvement in speech to be reclassified on successive tests. The disparity between recovery in speech and comprehension led Vignolo (1964) to conclude that the factors limiting recovery in oral expression are found within expression itself, supporting the notion that separate mechanisms are involved in the act of speaking and in reception of spoken language.

Many general theories have been proposed to account for the phenomenon of recovery, including cortical equipotentiality, substitution of function, plasticity, individual variations in hemispheric specialization, and functional comprehension. Although the extent of recovery in the comprehension of language in chronic aphasia is sometimes considerable, few explanations exist as to why this should be so since lesion size does not alter.

Some investigators have suggested that the right hemisphere is responsible for the improvement in comprehension function, and there are data to support such a claim. For example, the split-brain research done by Zaidel (1976, 1977a, 1977b) demonstrates that the isolated right hemisphere is capable of a considerable degree of lexical and some limited syntactic comprehension. It should also be noted that Pieniadz, Naeser, and Koff (1979) report increased recovery in comprehension to be correlated with atypical increased right occipital width on CT scan findings. Dichotic listening study findings also support increased right hemisphere responsibility in recovery. Pettit and Noll (1979) found that, as language comprehension improves, there is a corresponding increase in left ear scores and a decrease in right ear performance. Johnson, Sommers, and Weidner (1977) discovered that the severity of aphasia correlates with the magnitude of left ear preference. Thus, the difference between speech and auditory comprehension in evolution may represent the inherent abilities and limitations of the right hemisphere.

Prins *et al.* (1978) offer a linguistic explanation of the disparity between speech and comprehension in recovery. They suggest that the apparent difference in vocal and auditory modes is at least partially a function of the differences in linguistic requirements of the two modalities. The task of the listener is relatively restricted. The process can be reasonably successful when forced to rely primarily on lexical processing, a minimal amount of syntactic analysis, heuristic strategies, and an understanding of the world. On the other hand, speaking is far more demanding.

Given the marked improvement in comprehension during evolution, one suspects that the aphasic becomes more effective at employing both nonlinguistic and linguistic strategies. Yet these factors have not been explored in any systematic way. In the only systematic study of the evolution of comprehension, Pizzamiglio, Appicciafuoco, and Razzano (1976) sampled the phonetic, semantic, and syntactic discrimination abilities of a group of aphasics over a 12-month period. In the first year postonset, they found that patients improved most on the linguistic levels in which they were most defective. That is, Broca's aphasics improved significantly on the phonetic and syntactic tests but not on the semantic tests. Wernicke's aphasics improved on the semantic discrimination test but not on the phonetic or syntactic measures.

The dynamic changes through which the syndromes evolve provide an untapped area of investigation. Research in linguistic recovery could expose the rank order of difficulty in parameters of phonology, semantics, and syntax and provide the quantitative analysis of qualitative features of comprehension impairment against a backdrop of degree of improvement.

Concluding Comments

It is becoming increasingly obvious as we accumulate more research data that the linguistic operations that are disturbed in aphasia are far more complex than ever imagined. It is also apparent that the comprehension of spoken language involves much more than the decoding of an acoustic signal and the understanding of the literal meaning of words. The very nature of comprehension poses tremendous methodological problems, for as we define dimensions and control variables to study the process, we must sacrifice the complexity of the interrelationships among linguistic parameters. Certainly, a simplistic model cannot account for the variety of preserved and impaired receptive language abilities observed in aphasic patients. In addition, given the intimate relationship of language comprehension with attention, perception, imagery, concept analysis, abstraction, and emotional factors, it could be argued that this aspect of communication defies our ability to study and know it. Yet if we dismiss comprehension disorders because of their complexity, we limit our understanding of the impact of the pathological process in language function.

Our clinical impressions suggest that diagnostic subtypes of aphasia categorized on the basis of shared speech characteristics do not represent homogeneous groups with respect to comprehension. This factor may contribute to the inconclusiveness of study findings. Although selective input deficits are evident in some cases, they are often not attached to any particular variety of aphasia. Rather, for each group there is a range of overall comprehension ability and a pattern of more or less impaired characteristics.

One other consideration is noteworthy. Given the inherent variability affecting performance of brain-damaged individuals, the results of even the most elegant experimental design must be considered tentative. While variability affects performance in all aspects of aphasia research, it is particularly important in the study of comprehension, since by its nature it cannot be directly observed. Complicating matters further is the fact that the population with the most complex and severe comprehension disturbance (i.e., sensory-Wernicke's) is the one least amenable to study. One might even question whether the Wernicke's aphasics selected for research are truly representative of that diagnostic group.

Whether or not the traditional methods using group statistics are applicable to a parameter of communication as complex as comprehension in a population as diverse as aphasia is also equivocal. Although it may be possible to isolate factors in comprehension, data derived from groups may also mask significant findings. One might question whether it is possible to generalize group findings to the individual patient.

Finally, it is important to point out that the bulk of research pertaining to comprehension disorders in aphasia has been accomplished in the past two decades. With the increased attention to this aspect of aphasia, we have become aware of a great many things, the most crucial of which is the enormity of the task before us.

References

Albert, M. 1976. Short-term memory and aphasia. *Brain and Language, 3,* 28–33.
Aten, J. L., Johns, D. F., & Darley, F. L. 1971. Auditory perception of sequenced words in apraxia of speech. *Journal of Speech and Hearing Research, 14,* 131–143.
Baker, E., Blumstein, S., & Goodglass, H. 1981. Interaction between phonological and semantic factors in auditory discrimination. *Neuropsychologia, 19,* 1–15.
Baker, E., & Goodglass, H. 1979. Time for auditory processing of object names by aphasics. *Brain and Language, 8,* 355–366.
Basso, A., Casati, G., & Vignolo, L. A. 1977. Phonemic identification defects in aphasia. *Cortex, 13,* 84–95.
Basso, A., De Renzi, E., Faglioni, P., Scotti, G., & Spinnler, H. 1973. Neuropsychological evidence for the existence of cerebral areas critical to the performance of intelligence tasks. *Brain, 96,* 715–728.
Birchmeier, A. 1980. Feature analysis and the Token Test. *Brain and Language, 10,* 98–110.
Blumstein, S., Baker, E., & Goodglass, H. 1977. Phonological factors in auditory comprehension in aphasia. *Neuropsychologia, 15,* 19–30.
Blumstein, S., Cooper, W., Zurif, E., & Caramazza, A. 1975. Levels of speech perception dissociated in aphasia. Paper presented at the Academy of Aphasia, Victoria, British Columbia, October.
Blumstein, S., Cooper, W., Zurif, E., & Caramazza, A. 1977. The perception and production of voice-onset time in aphasia. *Neuropsychologia, 15,* 371–383.
Boller, F. 1978. Comprehension disorders in aphasia: A historical review. *Brain and Language, 5,* 149–165.
Boller, F. 1979. Introduction: Testing for comprehension: A short history of comprehension tests up to the Token Test. In F. Boller & M. Dennis (Eds.), *Auditory comprehension: Clinical and experimental studies with the Token Test.* New York: Academic Press.
Boller, F., Cole, M., Vrtunski, B., Patterson, M., & Kim, Y. 1979. Paralinguistic aspects of auditory comprehension in aphasia. *Brain and Language, 7,* 164–174.
Boller, F., & Dennis, M. (Eds.) 1979. *Auditory comprehension: Clinical and experimental studies with the Token Test.* New York: Academic Press.
Boller, F., & Green, E. 1972. Comprehension in severe aphasia. *Cortex, 8,* 382–394.
Boller, F., Kim, Y., & Mack, J. 1977. Auditory comprehension in aphasia. In H. Whitaker & H. A. Whitaker (Eds.), *Studies in neurolinguistics* (Vol. 3). New York: Academic Press.
Boller, F., & Vignolo, L. A. 1966. Latent sensory aphasia in hemisphere-damaged patients: An experimental study with the Token Test. *Brain, 89,* 815–830.
Bond, Z. S. 1976. On specification of input units in speech perception. *Brain and Language, 3,* 72–87.
Brookshire, R. H. 1978. Auditory comprehension and aphasia. In D. F. Johns (Ed.), *Clinical management of neurogenic communication disorders.* Boston: Little, Brown. (a)
Brookshire, R. H. 1978. A Token Test battery for testing auditory comprehension in brain injured adults. *Brain and Language, 6,* 149–157. (b)
Brown, J. 1972. *Aphasia, apraxia and agnosia: Clinical and theoretical aspects.* Springfield, Ill.: Thomas.
Brown, J. 1977. *Mind, brain and consciousness: The neuropsychology of cognition.* New York: Academic Press.
Caramazza, A., Basili, A. G., Koller, J. S., & Berndt, R. S. An investigation of repetition and language processing in a case of conduction aphasia. *Brain and Language,* in press.
Caramazza, A., & Zurif, E. 1976. Dissociation of alogrithmic and heuristic processes in comprehension: Evidence from aphasia. *Brain and Language, 3,* 572–582.

Caramazza, A., Zurif, E. B., & Gardner, H. 1978. Sentence memory in aphasia. *Neuro-psychologia, 16,* 661–671.

Carmon, A., & Nachson, I. 1971. Effect of unilateral brain damage on perception of temporal order. *Cortex, 7,* 411–418.

Carpenter, R., & Rutherford, D. 1973. Acoustic cue discrimination in adult aphasia. *Journal of Speech and Hearing Research, 16,* 534–544.

Cermak, L., & Moreines, J. 1976. Verbal retention deficits in aphasic and amnesic patients. *Brain and Language, 3,* 16–27.

Cole, M. F., & Cole, M. 1971. *Pierre Marie's papers on speech disorders.* New York: Hafner.

Demeurisse, G., Demol, O., Derouck, M., de Beuckelaer, R., Coekaerts, M., & Capon, A. 1980. Quantitative study of the rate of recovery from aphasia due to ischemic stroke. *Stroke, 11,* 455–458.

De Renzi, E. 1979. A shortened version of the Token Test. In F. Boller & M. Dennis (Eds.), *Auditory comprehension: Clinical and experimental studies with the Token Test.* New York: Academic Press.

De Renzi, E., Faglioni, P., Scotti, G., & Spinnler, H. 1972. Impairment in associating colour to form, concomitant with aphasia. *Brain, 95,* 293–304.

De Renzi, E., & Vignolo, L. A. 1962. The Token Test: A sensitive test to detect receptive disturbances in aphasics. *Brain, 85,* 665–678.

Di Carlo, L., & Taub, H. 1972. The influence of compression and expansion on the intelligibility of speech by young and aged aphasic (demonstrated CVA) individuals. *Journal of Communication Disorders, 5,* 299–306.

Ebbin, J., & Edwards, A. 1967. Speech sound discrimination of aphasics when inter-sound interval is varied. *Journal of Speech and Hearing Research, 10,* 120–125.

Efron, R. 1963. Temporal perception, aphasia and déjà vu. *Brain, 86,* 403–424.

Eggert, G. H. 1977. *Wernicke's works on aphasia: A sourcebook and review.* The Hague: Mouton.

Faglioni, P., Spinnler, H., & Vignolo, L. A. 1969. Contrasting behavior of right and left hemisphere damaged patients on a discriminative and a semantic task of auditory recognition. *Cortex, 5,* 366–389.

Feyereisen, P. Decoding paralinguistic signals. *Journal of Communication Disorders,* in press.

Gainotti, G., Caltagirone, C., & Ibba, A. 1976. Semantic and phonemic aspects of auditory language comprehension in aphasia. *Linguistics, 154,* 15–28.

Gainotti, G., & Lemmo, M. A. 1976. Comprehension of symbolic gestures in aphasia. *Brain and Language, 3,* 451–460.

Gardner, H., Albert, M., & Weintraub, S. 1975. Comprehending a word: The influence of speed and redundancy on auditory comprehension in aphasia. *Cortex, 11,* 155–162.

Gardner, H., & Denes, G. 1973. Connotative judgments by aphasic patients on a pictorial adaptation of the semantic differential. *Cortex, 9,* 183–196.

Gardner, H., Strub, R., & Albert, M. 1975. A unimodal deficit in operational thinking. *Brain and Language, 2,* 333–344.

Goldblum, M., & Albert, M. 1972. Phonemic discrimination in sensory aphasia. *International Journal of Mental Health, 1,* 25–29.

Goldstein, K. 1948. *Language and language disturbances.* New York: Grune & Stratton.

Goldstein, M. N. 1974. Auditory agnosia for speech ("pure word deafness"). *Brain and Language, 1,* 195–204.

Goodenough, C., Zurif, E., & Weintraub, S. 1977. Aphasics' attention to grammatical morphemes. *Language and Speech, 20,* 11–19.

Goodglass, H. 1973. Studies on the grammar of aphasics. In H. Goodglass & S. Blumstein (Eds.), *Psycholinguistics in aphasia.* Baltimore: Johns Hopkins Press.

Goodglass, H., & Baker, E. 1976. Semantic field, naming, and auditory comprehension in aphasia. *Brain and Language, 3,* 359–374.

Goodglass, H., Blumstein, S., Gleason, J. B., Hyde, M., Green, E., & Statlender, S. 1979. The effect of syntactic encoding on sentence comprehension in aphasia. *Brain and Language, 7,* 201–209.

Goodglass, H., Gleason, J. B., & Hyde, M. 1970. Some dimensions of auditory language comprehension in aphasia. *Journal of Speech and Hearing Research, 13,* 595–606.

Goodglass, H., & Kaplan, E. 1972. *The assessment of aphasia and related disorders.* Philadelphia: Lea & Febiger.

Goodglass, H., Klein, B., Carey, P., & Jones, K. J. 1966. Specific semantic word categories in aphasia. *Cortex, 2,* 74–89.

Green, E., & Boller, F. 1974. Features of auditory comprehension in severely impaired aphasics. *Cortex, 10,* 133–145.

Hartje, W., Kerschensteiner, W., Poeck, K., & Orgass, B. 1973. Note: A cross-validation study on the Token Test. *Neuropsychologia, 11,* 119–121.

Heilman, K. M., & Scholes, R. J. 1976. The nature of comprehension errors in Broca's, Conduction, and Wernicke's aphasics. *Cortex, 12,* 258–265.

Hier, D., Mogil, S., Rubin, N., & Komros, G. 1980. Semantic aphasia: A neglected entity. *Brain and Language, 10,* 120–131.

Holland, A., & Whitney, J. 1979. Nondiagnostic uses of the Token Test. In F. Boller & M. Dennis (Eds.), *Auditory comprehension: Clinical and experimental studies with the Token Test.* New York: Academic Press.

Jakobson, R. 1970. *Selected writings* (Vol. 2) The Hague: Mouton.

Jauhianen, T., & Nuutila, A. 1977. Auditory perception of speech and speech sounds in recent and recovered cases of aphasia. *Brain and Language, 4,* 572–579.

Johns, D. F., & Darley, F. L. 1970. Phonemic variability in apraxia of speech. *Journal of Speech and Hearing Research, 13,* 556–583.

Johnson, J. P., Sommers, R. K., & Weidner, W. E. 1977. Dichotic ear preference in aphasia. *Journal of Speech and Hearing Disorders, 20,* 116–129.

Kenin, M., & Swisher, L. P. 1972. A study of pattern of recovery in aphasia. *Cortex, 8,* 52–68.

Kertesz, A. 1979. *Aphasia and associated disorders: Taxonomy, localization and recovery.* New York: Grune & Stratton.

Kertesz, A., & McCabe, P. 1975. Intelligence and aphasia: Performance of aphasics on Raven's Coloured Progressive Matrices (RCPM). *Brain and Language, 2,* 387–395.

Kertesz, A., & McCabe, P. 1977. Recovery patterns and prognosis in aphasia. *Brain, 100,* 1–18.

Kreindler, A., Gheorghita, N., & Voinescu, I. 1971. Analysis of verbal reception of a complex order with three elements in aphasics. *Brain, 94,* Part II, 375–386.

Lachner, J., & Teuber, H. L. 1973. Alteration in auditory fusion thresholds after cerebral injury in man. *Neuropsychologia, 11,* 409–415.

Lenneberg, E., Pogash, K., Cohlan, A., & Doolittle, J. 1978. Comprehension deficit in acquired aphasia and the question of its relationship to language acquisition. In A. Caramazza & E. Zurif (Eds.), *Language acquisition and language breakdown.* Baltimore: Johns Hopkins University Press.

Lesser, R. 1974. Verbal comprehension in aphasia: An English version of three Italian tests. *Cortex, 10,* 247–263.

Lesser, R. 1976. Verbal and non-verbal memory components of the Token Test. *Neuropsychologia, 14,* 79–85.

Lesser, R. 1978. *Linguistic investigations of aphasia: Studies in language disability and remediation.* New York: Elsevier.

Lesser, R. 1979. Turning tokens into things: Linguistic and mnestic aspects of the initial sections of the Token Test. In F. Boller & M. Dennis (Eds.), *Auditory comprehension: Clinical and experimental studies with the Token Test.* New York: Academic Press.

Liles, B. Z., & Brookshire, R. H. 1975. The effects of pause time on auditory comprehension of aphasic subjects. *Journal of Communication Disorders, 8,* 221–235.

Lomas, J., & Kertesz, A. 1978. Patterns of spontaneous recovery in aphasic groups: A study of adult stroke patients. *Brain and Language, 5,* 388–401.

Luria, A. R. 1958. Brain disorders and language analysis. *Language and Speech, 1,* 14–34.

Luria, A. R. 1964. Neuropsychology in the local diagnosis of brain damage. *Cortex, 1,* 3–18.

Luria, A. R., & Hutton, T. 1977. A modern assessment of the basic forms of aphasia. *Brain and Language, 4,* 129–151.

Mack, J. L., & Boller, F. 1979. Components of auditory comprehension: Analysis of errors in a revised Token Test. In F. Boller & M. Dennis (Eds.), *Auditory comprehension: Clinical and experimental studies with the Token Test.* New York: Academic Press.

Marie, P., & Vaschide, N. 1903. [Experimental research on the immediate memory of aphasics.] *Revue Neurologique, 11,* 322. (a)

Marie, P., & Vaschide, N. 1903. [Experimental research on the mental life of aphasics.] *Revue Neurologique, 11,* 228–231. (b)

Marie, P., & Vaschide, N. 1903. [Mental automatism of aphasics.] *Revue Neurologique, 11,* 1127–1128. (c)

Marie, P., & Vaschide, N. 1903. [Research on the association of ideas in aphasics.] *Revue Neurologique, 11,* 722–724. (d)

Miceli, G., Caltagirone, C., Gainotti, G., & Payer-Rigo, P. 1978. Discrimination of voice versus place contrasts in aphasia. *Brain and Language, 6,* 47–51.

Miceli, G., Gainotti, G., Caltagirone, C., & Masullo, C. 1980. Some aspects of phonological impairment in aphasia. *Brain and Language, 11,* 159–169.

Mostofsky, D., VandenBossche, R., Sheinkopf, S., & Noyes, M. 1971. Novel ways to study aphasia. *Rehabilitation Literature, 32,* 290–298.

Naeser, M. A., Hayward, R. W., Laughlin, S. A., Becker, J. M. T., Jernigan, T. L., & Zatz, L. M. 1981. Quantitative CT scan studies in aphasia. II. Comparison of the right and left hemispheres. *Brain and Language, 12,* 165–189.

Naeser, M., Hayward, R. W., Laughlin, S., & Zatz, L. M. 1981. Quantitative CT scan studies in aphasia. I. Infarct size and CT numbers. *Brain and Language, 12,* 140–164.

Needham, L., & Swisher, L. P. 1972. A comparison of three tests of auditory comprehension for adult aphasics. *Journal of Speech and Hearing Disorders, 37,* 123–131.

Orgass, B., & Poeck, K. 1966. Clinical validation of a new test for aphasia: An experimental study of the Token Test. *Cortex, 2,* 222–243.

Orgass, B., & Poeck, K. 1969. Assessment of aphasia by psychometric methods. *Cortex, 5,* 317–330.

Parkhurst, B. 1970. *The effect of time altered speech stimuli on performance of right hemiplegic adult aphasics.* Paper presented at the Annual Convention of the American Speech and Hearing Association, New York, New York.

Parisi, D., & Pizzamiglio, L. 1970. Syntactic comprehension in aphasia. *Cortex, 2,* 204–215.

Pettit, J. M., & Noll, J. D. 1979. Cerebral dominance in aphasia recovery. *Brain and Language, 7,* 191–200.

Pieniadz, J., Naeser, M., & Koff, E. 1979. CT scan reversed cerebral hemispheric asymmetries and improved recovery in aphasia. Paper presented at the Academy of Aphasia, San Diego, California, October. Manuscript submitted for publication.

Pizzamiglio, L., & Appicciafuoco, A. 1971. Semantic comprehension in aphasia. *Journal of Communication Disorders, 3,* 280–288.

Pizzamiglio, L., Appicciafuoco, A., & Razzano, C. 1976. Recovery of comprehension in aphasic patients. In Y. Lebrun & R. Hoops (Eds.), *Recovery in aphasics.* Neurolinguistics 4. Amsterdam: Swets & Zeitlinger, B. V.

Poeck, K., & Hartje, W. 1979. Performance of aphasic patients in visual versus auditory presentation of the Token Test: Demonstration of a supra-modal deficit. In F. Boller & M. Dennis (Eds.), *Auditory comprehension: Clinical and experimental studies with the Token Test.* New York: Academic Press.

Poeck, K., Hartje, W., Kerschensteiner, M., & Orgass, B. 1973. Sprachverständnisstörungen bei aphasischen und nicht-aphasischen Hirnkranken. *Deutsche Medizinische Wochenschrift, 98,* 139–147.

Poeck, K., Kerschensteiner, M., & Hartje, W. 1972. A quantitative study on language understanding in fluent and nonfluent aphasia. *Cortex, 8,* 299–304.

Poeck, K., Orgass, B., Kerschensteiner, M., & Hartje, W. 1974. A qualitative study on Token Test performance in aphasic and non aphasic brain damaged patients. *Neuropsychologia, 12,* 49–54.

Poeck, K., & Pietron, H-P. 1981. The influence of stretched speech presentation on Token Test performance of aphasic and right brain damaged patients. *Neuropsychologia, 19,* 133–136.

Porch, B. E. 1967. *Porch Index of Communicative Ability.* Palo Alto, Calif.: Consulting Psychologists Press.

Prins, R. S., Snow, C. E., & Wagenaar, E. 1978. Recovery from aphasia: Spontaneous speech versus language comprehension. *Brain and Language, 6,* 192–211.

Saffran, E. M., & Marin, O. S. 1975. Immediate memory for word lists and sentences in a patient with deficient auditory short-term memory. *Brain and Language, 2,* 420–433.

Saffran, E. M., Marin, O. S., & Yeni-Komshian, G. H. 1976. An analysis of speech perception in word-deafness. *Brain and Language, 3,* 209–228.

Salvatore, A. P. 1976. Training an aphasic adult to respond appropriately to spoken commands by fading pause time duration within commands. In R. H. Brookshire (Ed.), *Clinical aphasiology: Conference proceedings.* Minneapolis: Minn.: BRK Publishers.

Sarno, M. T. 1969. *The Functional Communication Profile: Manual of directions.* New York University Medical Center, Institute of Rehabilitation Medicine.

Sarno, M. T., & Levita, E. 1979. Recovery in treated aphasia in the first year post stroke. *Stroke, 10,* 663–669.

Sarno, M. T., & Levita, E. 1981. Some observations on the nature of recovery in global aphasia after stroke. *Brain and Language, 13,* 1–12.

Sasanuma, S., & Kamio, A. 1976. Aphasics' comprehension of sentences expressing temporal order of events. *Brain and Language, 3,* 495–506.

Schlanger, B., Schlanger, P., & Gerstman, L. 1976. The perception of emotionally toned sentences by right hemisphere-damaged and aphasic subjects. *Brain and Language, 3,* 396–403.

Schuell, H. 1953. Aphasic difficulties understanding spoken language. *Neurology, 3,* 176–183. (a)

Schuell, H. 1953. Auditory impairment in aphasia: Significance and retraining techniques. *Journal of Speech and Hearing Disorders, 18,* 14–21. (b)

Schuell, H. 1965. *Differential Diagnosis of Aphasia with the Minnesota Test.* Minneapolis, Minn.: Univ. of Minnesota Press.

Schuell, H. M., & Jenkins, J. J. 1961. Reduction of vocabulary in aphasia. *Brain, 84,* 243–261.

Schuell, H., Jenkins, J. J., & Landis, L. 1961. Relationship between auditory comprehension and word frequency in aphasia. *Journal of Speech and Hearing Research, 4,* 30–35.

Scotti, G., & Spinnler, H. 1970. Colour imperception in unilateral hemisphere-damaged patients. *Journal of Neurology, Neurosurgery, and Psychiatry, 33,* 22–28.

Shankweiler, D. P., & Harris, K. S. 1966. An experimental approach to the problem of articulation in aphasia. *Cortex, 2,* 277–292.

Sheehan, J., Aseltine, S., & Edwards, A. 1973. Aphasic comprehension of time spacing. *Journal of Speech and Hearing Research, 16,* 650–675.

Sherwin, I., & Efron, R. 1980. Temporal ordering defects following anterior temporal lobectomy. *Brain and Language, 11,* 195–203.

Shewan, C. M. 1969. An investigation of auditory comprehension in adult aphasic patients. Paper presented at the Annual Convention of the American Speech and Hearing Association, Chicago, Illinois, November.

Shewan, C. M. 1979. *Auditory Comprehension Test for Sentences.* Chicago: Biolinguistics Clinical Institutes.

Shewan, C. M. 1980. Phonological processing in Broca's aphasics. *Brain and Language, 10,* 71–88.

Shewan, C. M., & Canter, G. 1971. Effects of vocabulary, syntax and sentence length on auditory comprehension in aphasic patients. *Cortex, 7,* 209–226.

Smith, M. D. 1974. On the understanding of some relational words in aphasia. *Neuropsychologia, 12,* 377–384.

Spellacy, F. J., & Spreen, O. 1969. A short form of the Token Test. *Cortex, 5,* 390–397.

Spinnler, H., & Vignolo, L. A. 1966. Impaired recognition of meaningful sounds in aphasia. *Cortex, 2,* 337–348.

Spreen, O. 1973. Psycholinguistics and aphasia: The contribution of Arnold Pick. In H. Goodglass & S. Blumstein (Eds.), *Psycholinguistics and aphasia.* Baltimore: Johns Hopkins Press.

Spreen, O., & Benton, A. R. 1969. *Neurosensory Center Comprehensive Examination for Aphasia.* Victoria, B. C.: Neuropsychology Laboratory, University of Victoria.

Stachowiak, F. J., Huber, W., Poeck, K., & Kerschensteiner, M. 1977. Text comprehension in aphasia. *Brain and Language, 4,* 177–195.

Stoicheff, M. L. 1960. Motivating instructions and language performance of dysphasic subjects. *Journal of Speech and Hearing Research, 3,* 75–85.

Strohner, H., Cohen, R., Kelter, S., & Woll, G. 1978. "Semantic" and "acoustic" errors of aphasic and schizophrenic patients in a sound–picture matching task. *Cortex, 14,* 391–403.

Swartz, M., Marin, O. S., & Saffran, E. 1979. Dissociations of language function in dementia: A case study. *Brain and Language, 7,* 277–306.

Swartz, M., Saffran, E., & Marin, O. S. 1980. The word order problem in agrammatism: Comprehension. *Brain and Language, 10,* 249–262.

Swinney, D., Zurif, E., & Cutler, A. 1980. Effects of sentential stress and word class upon comprehension in Broca's aphasia. *Brain and Language, 10,* 132–145.

Swisher, L., & Hirsh, J. 1972. Brain damage and ordering of two temporally successive stimuli. *Neuropsychologia, 10,* 137–151.

Swisher, L. P., & Sarno, M. T. 1969. The Token Test scores of three matched patient groups: Left brain-damaged with aphasia, right brain-damaged without aphasia, non brain-damaged. *Cortex, 5,* 264–273.

Tallal, P., & Newcombe, F. 1978. Impairment of auditory perception and language comprehension in dysphasia. *Brain and Language, 5,* 13–24.

Taylor, M. L. 1965. A measurement of functional communication in aphasia. *Archives of Physical Medicine and Rehabilitation, 46,* 101–107.

Tyler, H. R. 1969. Defective stimulus exploration in aphasic patients. *Neurology, 19,* 105–111.

Tzortzis, C., & Albert, M. 1974. Impairment of memory for sequences in conduction aphasia. *Neuropsychologia, 12,* 355–366.

Varney, N. 1980. Sound recognition in relation to aural language comprehension in aphasic patients. *Journal of Neurology, Neurosurgery, and Psychiatry, 43,* 71–75.

Vignolo, L. A. 1964. Evolution of aphasia and language rehabilitation: A retrospective exploratory study. *Cortex, 1,* 344–367.

Vignolo, L. A. 1969. Auditory agnosia: A review and report of recent evidence. In A. L. Benton (Ed.), *Contributions to clinical neuropsychology.* Chicago: Aldine Press.

Vignolo, L. A. 1979. Lesions underlying defective performances on the Token Test: A CT scan study. In F. Boller & M. Dennis (Eds.), *Auditory comprehension: Clinical and experimental studies with the Token Test.* New York: Academic Press.

Wechsler, A. F. 1973. The effect of organic brain disease on recall of emotionally charged versus neutral narrative texts. *Neurology, 23,* 130–135.

Weidner, W. E., & Lasky, E. 1976. The interaction of rate and complexity of stimulus on the performance of adult aphasic subjects. *Brain and Language, 3,* 34–40.

Whitaker, H. A., & Noll, D. 1972. Some linguistic parameters of the Token Test. *Neuropsychologia, 10,* 395–404.

Whitaker, H. A., & Selnes, O. A. 1978. Token Test measures of language comprehension in normal children and aphasic patients. In A. Caramazza & E. B. Zurif (Eds.), *Language acquisition and language breakdown.* Baltimore: Johns Hopkins Press.

Whitaker, H. A., & Whitaker, H. 1979. Lexical, syntactic, and semantic aspects of the Token Test: A linguistic taxonomy. In F. Boller & M. Dennis (Eds.), *Auditory comprehension: Clinical and experimental studies with the Token Test.* New York: Academic Press.

Wilcox, J., Davis, A. G., & Leonard, L. B. 1978. Aphasics comprehension of contextually conveyed meaning. *Brain and Language, 6,* 362–377.

Yarnell, P., Monroe, P., & Sobel, L. 1976. Aphasia outcome in stroke: A clinical neurological correlation. *Stroke, 7,* 514–522.

Zaidel, E. 1976. Auditory vocabulary of the right hemisphere following brain bisection or hemidecortication. *Cortex, 12,* 191–212.

Zaidel, E. 1977. Auditory language comprehension in the right hemisphere following cerebral commissurotomy and hemispherectomy: A comparison with child language and aphasia. In A. Caramazza & E. Zurif (Eds.), *Language acquisition and language breakdown.* Baltimore: Johns Hopkins Press. (a)

Zaidel, E. 1977. Unilateral auditory language comprehension on the Token Test following cerebral commissurotomy and hemispherectomy. *Neuropsychologia, 15,* 1–18. (b)

Ziegler, D. K. 1952. Word deafness and Wernicke's aphasia: Report of cases and discussion of syndrome. *Archives of Neurology and Psychiatry, 67,* 323–333.

Zurif, E., Caramazza, A., Myerson, R., & Galvin, J. 1974. Semantic feature representations for normal and aphasic language. *Brain and Language, 1,* 167–187.

9

Explanations for the Concept of Apraxia of Speech

HUGH W. BUCKINGHAM, JR.

The term APRAXIA OF SPEECH has had an extremely variable history and has been used to describe different types of behaviors, in different types of patients, and under different stimulus conditions. It is a term used, often with qualifying modifiers, to describe syndromes or parts of syndromes. Since there is, and has been, so much variability in the way the term has been used, it becomes very confusing when it is simply incorporated to label a specific patient. Since there have been different conceptualizations of "apraxia," it stands to reason that apraxia of speech may also not be completely well defined throughout the literature on the topic. It is the purpose of this chapter to outline the various ways in which apraxia has been explained so that the reader will have a proper appreciation of the complexities involved. In this chapter I would like to propose that under certain interpretations there are additional forms of apraxia of speech that differ from the frontal speech apraxias. Frontal lobe apraxia of speech has been referred to as aphemia, Broca's aphasia, motor aphasia, anarthria, verbal aphasia, phonetic disintegration of speech, apraxia, apraxic dysarthria, cortical dysarthria, and oral verbal apraxia.

I would like to propose further that certain phonological functions as understood by linguists operate IN PARALLEL WITH and at a distinct level from the hierarchically organized sensorimotor practic functions of the brain. The phonological functions involve selecting and sequencing of phoneme-like units that speakers BELIEVE themselves to be uttering. In actuality, they are uttering sounds, or PHONES which may then be considered as being produced by nervous firings giving rise to complex and synchronous muscular contractions resulting in acoustic impingements

271

on the air. Practic brain function is involved at the neurological level throughout the whole process from ideation to production. However, these processes must be worded carefully so as not to imply that phonemes are articulated. The nature of the phoneme is such that it cannot be uttered. It is a "psychologically real" abstract unit for which no invariant factor, articulatory or acoustic, has yet been found. Consequently, an anomaly results when it is maintained that phonemes are uttered, produced, articulated, distorted, etc. Phonological functions of selecting and sequencing phonemes are much too abstract and ideational in nature to be considered "motoric."

Another claim to be made in this chapter is that the subphonemic errors made by Broca's aphasics typically involve disturbed limb–praxic function for the vocal tract musculature involving motor commands for outputting speech sounds (phones)—the units for which, together with their serial order, having been "fed forward" from the ideational level.[1] The result is an effortful, groping speech output, usually seen when the left frontal lobe is damaged in the region of the third convolution. This syndrome has also been referred to as an apraxia of speech, which leads to the principal thesis of this chapter. One can plausibly argue, given the historical development of the notion of apraxia, that the apraxias in general admit of alternate explanations: one that involves disconnection lesions and another that involves cortical lesions of centers. The explanatory mechanisms for both are different. This state of affairs has resulted in much confusion over the issue of apraxia and the consequent

1. I am aware that as this sentence reads I am dangerously close to the fallacy that John Hughlings Jackson (1931/1878a) warned against. He believed that a "psychical state" (an "idea of a word" or simply "a word") cannot produce an articulatory movement, which is clearly a physical phenomenon. Rather, it was "discharge of the cells and fibers of the anatomical substratum of a word [which] produces the articulatory movement [p. 156]." In general, Jackson states, "In our studies of diseases of the nervous system we must be on our guard against the fallacy that what are physical states in lower centers fine away into psychical states in higher centers; that, for example, vibrations of sensory nerves become sensations, or that somehow or another an idea produces a movement [p. 156]." Phonemes, like words, are abstractions and like the "psychical" elements of Jackson do not "fine away" into physical articulatory production. I believe that this dualism of Jackson is appropriate and should be carefully considered when dealing with phonemes and neurological theories of speech production. That is, the problems are precisely what Jackson was defining last century. Phonemes are mentalistic constructs of the mind; they have psychological not physical reality. Fromkin and Rodman (1978) write, "A phoneme is an abstract unit. We do not utter phonemes; we produce phones [p. 109]." That is, we produce phonetic segments. They quote the early twentieth-century linguist Edward Sapir: "In the physical world the naive speaker and hearer actualize and are sensitive to sounds, but what they feel themselves to be pronouncing and hearing are 'phonemes' [p. 102]."

notion of apraxia of speech. The problems have been recalcitrant principally because the arguments are at the level of explanation and not at the
level of data.

Historical Background

Prior to the work of John Hughlings Jackson and Hugo Liepmann,
who are usually credited with developing the notion of apraxia, Paul
Broca (1960/1861) considered two alternative views for explaining the
speech problem of his patient, Leborgne (Tan). The first, which he eventually adopted, was that the patient had lost his "faculty[2] of articulate
speech." This was an intellectual faculty and consisted of the "memory
for the procedure one has to follow in order to articulate the words [p.
54]." This was not a general faculty of speech, but rather one aspect
dealing with "the faculty to coordinate the movements which belong to
the articulate language [pp. 54–55]." Broca also considered the possibility that aphemia might "be a kind of locomotor ataxia, limited to the
articulation of sounds [p. 54]." Were this to be the case, Broca reasoned,
the disorder would not be the loss of an intellectual faculty "which
belongs to the thinking part of the brain [p. 54]," but rather "it would
only be a special case of the general coordination of actions, a faculty
which depends on the motor centers of the central nervous system [p.
54]." At the time of Broca's paper, the "Bell-Magendie" sensorimotor
dichotomy had not reached the cerebral cortex (Young, 1970); consequently, it was difficult to conceive of a CORTICAL motor (nonintellectual) system, and therefore damage to the cortex should only disrupt
"intellectual faculties"; motor organization and function were not considered to be intellectual. Broca states quite succinctly, "Everyone knows
that the cerebral convolutions are not motor organs [p. 70]." Subsequent
to Broca's presentation, the stage was set for the arguments as to
whether Broca's aphasia involves language or speech, although in 1861
the discussion was whether it was an intellectual impairment or a nonintellectual problem with locomotion. It certainly parallels the present-day
disputes over whether lesions in areas 44 and 45 of the dominant left

2. The preponderance of the word FACULTY is due to the development of the faculty
   psychology of the eighteenth-century Scottish philosophers Thomas Reid and Dugald
   Stewart. Franz Gall drew heavily from the Scottish school when developing his theories
   of phrenological faculties. These theories subsequently influenced Bouillaud, who
   passed them on to Auburtin and Broca. Thirty-five years before Broca, Bouillaud (1825)
   had argued (in support of Gall) that the "faculty of articulate language" is mediated in
   the anterior lobes of the brain (Young, 1970).

hemisphere cause an aphasia or an apraxia. It is claimed that the second option focuses on the motor system rather than on the language system.

Benton and Joynt (1960) showed that speech-specific lingual paralysis secondary to brain damage is a long-observed phenomenon, having been reported by Soranus of Ephesus (A.D. 98–135), Paracelsus (1493–1541), and Johann Schenck von Grafenberg (1530–1598). The same observation of speech-specific lingual paralysis was made by Auburtin and Bouillaud (Stookey, 1963), both of whom were precursors of Broca. In addition to noting simply that the patient could swallow, masticate, etc. but could not utter words normally, it was further observed by Baillarger (Alajouanine, 1960) and by Auburtin (as reported in Broca, 1960/1861, p. 52) that the patient could quite fluently produce speech automatisms. Still, a third observation of the Broca's aphasic was made. Broca wrote "that they can immediately WHEN BEING ASKED bring their tongue up, down, right, etc. But, however precise these movements may appear to us they are infinitely less so than the excessively delicate movements which the language demands [p. 54; emphasis added]." From this description provided by Broca, we have apraxia of speech without oral-facial apraxia (at least no involvement of the tongue).

A fourth description was also provided where there was a "nonpro-trusion" of the tongue upon VERBAL request. Jackson (1931/1866) wrote, "In some cases of defect of speech the patient seems to have lost much of his power to do anything HE IS TOLD TO DO, even with those muscles that are not paralyzed. Thus, a patient will be unable to put out his tongue when we ask him, although he will use it well in semi-involuntary actions, e.g., eating and swallowing [p. 121; emphasis added]." He goes on to add, "He will not make the particular grimace he is told to, even when we make one for him to imitate [p. 121]." Twelve years later, in an article appropriately entitled "Remarks on Non-Protrusion of the Tongue in Some Cases of Aphasia," Jackson (1931/1878b) again wrote, "It will have been noticed by every medical man that some patients who have loss or defect of speech do not put out the tongue WHEN THEY ARE ASKED [p. 153; emphasis added]." Jackson, unlike Broca, is describing an ap-raxia of speech WITH oral-facial apraxia. It was Jackson who first stressed that the disorder was one of volitional movement; he considered that encoding a propositional message was highly volitional as was the pro-trusion of the tongue upon verbal–acoustic command. Incorporating voli-tion as an explanatory device for certain movement disorders goes back at least to Jackson (1931/1874) where he describes the "three degrees of the use of the word 'no'." Uttering *no* when requested to do so was more volitional than uttering *no* in the normal course of conversation. Its production was considered most automatic (and consequently less volitional) when used emotionally as a negative command. It is important to point out that Jackson had to rule out any paralysis in order to account for the less volitional movements. In his explanations, it was also necessary for him to rule out comprehension loss. To note a failure to perform on verbal command is not a significant observation if it can be shown that the patient simply does not understand the command.

This historical development is well known now, especially with the publication of von Bonin (1960) and the selected writings of Jackson edited by J. Taylor (1932); several investigators of apraxia of speech have referred to the pioneering work of Jackson (De Renzi, Pieczuro, & Vignolo, 1966, p. 50; Head, 1926, p. 94; Johns & LaPointe, 1976, p. 185; Mateer & Kimura, 1977, p. 262).

It is necessary, however, to mention that at this point in history an unfortunate ambiguity was developing. The results of this ambiguity are evident today. The patient who, to the verbal command, was unable to grimace or to protrude the tongue for Jackson might have had a lesion disconnecting the area for comprehending language and the area for outputting the motor commands. He would not necessarily have had any lesions at all in the motor zones of the frontal lobes. On the other hand, the lesion could have been in the frontal cortical motor zones. In this case, disconnection would not serve as the crucial element of explanation, but rather the explanation would rest at the motor level. The disconnection hypothesis crucially involved LANGUAGE as a stimulus condition; the other did not. Therefore, the mechanisms would be quite distinct. The nondisconnection hypothesis would emphasize the mechanism as breakdown in motor planning and sequencing, whereas the other would emphasize disconnection of motor zones and language comprehension zones. Geschwind (1975) states, "The explanation . . . tries to account for all the apraxias on the basis of disconnection of the areas in which the command is comprehended from those areas where the command is carried out [p. 190]." The nondisconnection proponents require that their "apraxia" be caused by some lesion in an important cortical area. The disconnection position does not require this. Again, I am making the claim that once the phrase "when they are asked" comes up in the history of aphasia, the interpretive ambiguity arises. I further claim that the ambiguity has led to the two distinct views of apraxia; the issues became crystalized when aphasiologists began trying to characterize an "apraxia of speech."

The work of Hugo Liepmann shows that he utilized both types of explanation. His "limb-kinetic" apraxia was caused by lesions in the frontal motor association areas, and his "ideational" apraxia stemmed from damage to the sensory association zones in the posterior temporoparietal regions (Brown, 1972; Head, 1926). Liepmann felt that motor aphasia was a particular form of limb-kinetic apraxia of the "glossolabiopharyngeal" apparatus; subsequently, he added the larynx to this string of anatomical modifiers (Head, 1926, p. 99). According to Liepmann, a limb-kinetic apraxia was characterized by a "loss of kinaesthetic memories of a definite part of the body [Head, 1926, p. 97]." The patient had "lost the power to execute certain combinations of acquired movements" and "delicate movements" were impossible (Head, 1926, p. 98). Accordingly, Liepmann, when speaking of motor aphasia as a type of limb-kinetic apraxia, was extending the notion of "limb" to the speech articulators as well as to the arms. In a sense, this is not unreasonable. When Liepmann discussed this type of apraxia, he did not make reference to the stimulus-specific language command but rather invoked the Jacksonian notion of volition as the key explanatory device. That is, the patient could be said to be apraxic in his speech behavior, even though no one had provided a verbal command to behave linguistically, that is, to speak. Clearly, except for repetition, speakers articulate of their own accord—something quite different from performing some behavior upon verbal command from a second party. Again, disconnection apraxia principally involves motor isolation from auditory zones for language comprehension or from posterior visual zones. The historical oddity in all this is that Liepmann also introduced the first in-depth description of ideomotor types of apraxia, which were clearly connectionistic in nature.[3] Here, the ideational and motor-kinesthetic processes are separated from one another rather than lesioned themselves. By postulating an internal initiating ideational component, Liepmann could explain this type of apraxia without restricting the output disturbances to those elicited by linguistic verbal commands. Once again, the "will" was incorporated as the command generator, so to speak. These confusions have no doubt led Geschwind (1965) to state that "the designation 'apraxia' is an inadequate one unless the stimulus conditions are

---

3. A disconnection theory will, of course, admit of a lesion to some center if that center is anatomically connected to (and between) Wernicke's area and a primary motor area. Consequently, the ensuing explanation will still be connectionistic. I have in mind the lesions in the prefrontal motor association cortex, which still, according to Geschwind's model, disconnect the primary cortical motor area from Wernicke's area rather than destroy "programmed memories for movement," etc. In addition, there is Geschwind's (1969) description of lesions which simply disconnect the angular gyrus from Wernicke's area, and lesions that actually damage the gyrus itself. The resulting syndromes are different, but in both cases, the essential mechanism is disconnection of Wernicke's area from the occipital visual cortex. Certainly, Geschwind uses center explanations in dealing with certain failures to respond on imitation, but these failures are not apraxic-like, rather they are due to motor weakness. We will see later that Geschwind has another explanation for certain other failures on imitation.

specified [p. 606]." For this reason, it has always been strange to me, at least, that researchers who describe nonconnectionistic apraxias of speech elicit so much of their data by asking patients to REPEAT (Johns & Darley, 1970). Disconnection explanations are classic for repetition deficits (Kinsbourne, 1972; Wernicke, 1977/1874). Aside from a supramarginal gyrus ideokinetic apraxia, Liepmann (1900) also described the "sympathetic" ideokinetic apraxia of the left limbs arising from callosal disconnections in the anterior regions or from left prefrontal lesions, both of which disconnect the dominant language zones from the right hemisphere motor areas.

Before leaving the earlier studies of apraxia, it is instructive to look at how Henry Head's discussion of the issue served to extend the interpretive ambiguity. When writing about Liepmann and apraxia in his chapter entitled "Chaos," Head provides some more chaos by beginning the section with the clear implication that the apraxic behavior is secondary to a linguistic command, such as "told to protrude his tongue," "show his teeth to command," and "execute such movements to order" (Head, 1926, p. 93). Up to this point in Head's treatment, the label APRAXIA is directly linked with the language stimulus condition as an essential component. It would therefore be subject to a connectionistic explanation. However, by page 95 in Head's discussion, we are told that an apraxia of speech is a disorder with the "higher mechanics of verbal formulation [p. 95]." Since formulation is involved, it is now possible to consider the stimulus condition as self-induced on the part of the speaker. It is this point at which the "will" is usually invoked. Once the concept of volitional or purposive behavior comes to the foreground, the "will" may serve as the stimulus condition. Consequently, the disconnection explanation would no longer be necessary. As we shall see, this is exactly what happened in the further developments in apraxia of speech and the concomitant nonconnectionistic explanation.

It would appear, then, that there is ample historical precedent for two quite distinct explanations for movement disorders, which in both cases are referred to as "apraxia." One explanation leads to the acceptance of an apraxia of SPEECH, the other does not. Consequently, one's position as to what constitutes an apraxia in general has largely determined one's stand on whether or not it makes sense to talk about an apraxia of speech. Several current stands will now be discussed against this historical backdrop.[4]

---

4. Table I in Johns and LaPointe (1976) contains an illuminating collection of clinical descriptions of limb-kinetic speech deficits from Auburtin (1861) to Shankweiler, Harris, and Taylor (1968).

Current Stands

One current position regarding apraxia of speech is often referred to as the "Mayo School" position. The influence of F. L. Darley, Arnold Aronson, and J. R. Brown is obvious, and many researchers (with clinical and theoretical goals alike) have, in one way or another, been extending their views. The list of publications is long indeed, and much of the work has appeared since the late 1960s. The excellent summary provided by Johns and LaPointe (1976) is written from the point of view of the Mayo tradition of a center lesion apraxia of speech. Their claim is that this is what others have called Broca's aphasia. Furthermore, the apraxia of speech is caused by lesions in the frontal motor association areas, although this school, in the early stages of its formulations, seemed to feel that any articulatory disturbance was apraxic in nature, that is, essentially motoric. The further important claim of this school is that an apraxia of speech is not a language problem at all; therefore, the term Broca's APHASIA is somewhat anomalous for these investigators, since aphasia should refer only to language disturbances. Two clear historical points are made by this school. First, it adopts Broca's postulated (but ultimately not chosen) explanations that the disorder is primarily motoric, not a higher-level linguistic problem. Second, the Mayo School would agree with Liepmann that what is involved is a type of limb–kinetic apraxia of the glossolabiopharyngeal musculature. Consequently, the mechanism involved need not be connectionistic. In addition, the Mayo position separates apraxia of speech from oral–facial apraxia, although like most others (for instance, De Renzi *et al.*, 1966), the proponents are well aware that the two most often occur together.

Another proposal may be regarded as the result of a reaction to the early positions of the Mayo School that every nondysarthric articulation problem was an apraxia of speech. To the extent that the Mayo position now equates apraxia of speech with only Broca's aphasia, this second proposal will not represent a problem for its position. This second proposal makes a clear distinction between frontal articulatory disorders and posterior articulatory disorders. The work reported in Canter (1973), Trost and Canter (1974), and Burns and Canter (1977) shows that the nature of the articulation parameters in anterior versus posterior patients is quite distinguishable. There is an apraxic, nonfluent character in the frontal lobe subjects, whereas the temporoparietal lesion patients show a fluent and well-articulated phonemic disorder where, for instance, all allophones of substituted phonemes have their predicted phonetic shapes. This second current proposal brings to bear not only neuroanatomical questions but also LINGUISTIC questions. Much argumentation now involves determining just what is and what is not phonemic. As we shall see, the interpretations are often quite inconsistent, the reason being, I believe, that the abstract nature of the phoneme has not been fully appreciated.

A. R. Luria (1973) is surprisingly reminiscent of Liepmann in his views of apraxia. He equates Broca's aphasia (efferent motor aphasia) with a kinetic apraxia, and afferent motor aphasia with kinesthetic apraxia of speech. The phonological paraphasias of sensory aphasics are correlated with an ideational apraxia. It turns out, however, that Luria only admits of center-lesion explanations for apraxic behavior. An excellent example is taken from Luria's (1973) description of the speech problems secondary to lesions in the inferior postrolandic zones of the parietal lobe—that is, the cortical sensory area for the speech musculature. He writes,

> If a lesion of the secondary (kinaesthetic) zones of the post-central region affects the LOWER ZONES OF THIS REGION OF THE LEFT (DOMINANT) HEMISPHERE, i.e., the region of secondary organization of kinaesthetic sensation in the face, lips and tongue, the kinaesthetic apraxia may manifest itself in a special manner in the organization of movements of the speech apparatus, leading to the distinctive disorder of speech which has been called AFFERENT MOTOR APHASIA [p. 174].

Luria, in the same manner as Liepmann, views any voluntary movement as mediated by a "complex functional system" involving ideation, kinesthetic afferentiation, and kinetic organization. Each of these organizational levels has its anatomical substrate, and one or another type of apraxia will arise secondary to lesions in the respective areas. Movement parameters for speech will be disturbed in various ways depending upon the localization of damage along the posterior to frontal axis. The articulatory aspect, therefore, of the different types of aphasia will be characterized as one or another type of "apraxia of speech," from ideational to kinetic.[5] Luria (1972) provides criticism of the notion of conduction aphasia and in general is critical of disconnectionism. It is clear, therefore, that Luria would emphasize center-lesion theories of apraxia rather than disconnection theories. Consequently, it is not at all difficult for Luria to conceive of apraxia of speech, in fact, he considers several possible forms for it.

5. One could certainly argue that "ideation-to-kinetic" feedforward microgenesis schemes come dangerously close to Jackson's (1931/1878a) edict against the direct mind–brain leap taken in models that allow psychic states to fine away into physical states. This parallels the problem alluded to in footnote 2 of going from phoneme to articulation. See also Kelso & Tuller (1981, p. 227).

Jason Brown (1972) agrees with Luria to the extent that there is "inter-ference at comparable stages in microgenesis of speech and movement [p. 198]." Brown writes that "disorders of movement, like those of speech, are disturbed in a posterior–anterior fashion [p. 195]." Or, put differently, "the movement complex passes from a conceptual to a motoric form [see Footnotes 1 and 5], undergoing a progressive dif-ferentiation comparable to that which occurs in the speech system [p. 195]." More recently, Brown (1975a, 1975b, 1977) has refined his notion of microgenesis of action. For Brown (1975a) "the term microgenesis has been proposed for the continuous formative activity which underlies cognition [p. 26]." For instance, he writes (1977), "Both facial and limb apraxia can occur with frontal and temporoparietal lesions. In this re-spect, they are comparable to phonemic paraphasia, which also occurs with anterior and posterior pathology [p. 72]." Blumstein (1973) sup-ported this; in fact, in that publication she found MORE phonemic paraphasia with anterior-lesioned patients. At the phonemic level, the anterior versus posterior differences appeared to be quantitative, not qualitative—just as Poeck and Kerschensteiner (1975) found for oral ap-raxia. Similarly, De Renzi *et al.* (1966) write, "Oral apraxia characterizes patients whose speech productions may be very different from one another [p. 68]." For aphasic speech errors in anterior versus posterior populations, the qualitative distinctions do not reside in the phonemics of the errors but rather in the allophonics. There seems to be more incorrect allophonic production by frontal patients, who nevertheless at other times will also produce correct allophones of incorrectly selected phonemes as do the posterior patients. I will return to this question later. In any event, for Brown, the more anterior the lesion is, the more "maladroit" the action.

Brown now (1975a) believes, "There is little evidence for the view that language is formed posteriorly and somehow conveyed, by way of thalamus, insula or an association bundle, to Broca's area for motor speech. Rather, there appears to be simultaneous realization out of a common deep structure into the final perceptual and motoric forms of the language act [p. 26]." This means that damage along the posterior–anterior plane of the cortex at one or another location will NOT give rise to qualitatively different types of disturbed action. This is quite a dif-ferent position from the one taken in Brown (1972, chap. 17, p. 195), where the microgenesis of action took the route of the posterior–anterior axis over the cortical mantle along which distinct apraxic syndromes could be placed (i.e., more or less Liepmann's conception). In any event, Brown admits of center lesion apraxias rather than disconnecting lesion apraxias. One other important distinction is made by Brown (1975a) when he writes, "The 'centers' of traditional neuropsychology are rather to be considered as LEVELS by means of which cognition is carried one stage further [p. 29]." Pathways, for Brown, "do not serve to associate ideas, perceptions of movements, written words to spoken words, etc., but rather link up temporally transformations occuring at different points in the microgenetic sequence [p. 29]." In addition, his model incorporates distinct levels of speech apraxias. I mentioned earlier that in many cases of nonconnectionistic explanations of apraxia the concepts of "volition" and "will" play an important role. This is the case with Brown as well. For instance, "object facilitation" for transitive movements is said to bring "about a more concrete (i.e., less volitional) setting for the desired movement. In this sense, movements with objects are comparable to performance in conversational speech [Brown, 1972, p. 197]." The clear implication is that spontaneous conversational speech is less volitional than being requested to do something such as provide linguistic labels for objects, repeat a linguistic form, describe some scene, or imitate a transitive movement (without the object). Brown proposes his dynamic microgenesis model as an alternative to disconnection theory. We witness this in his discussion of conduction aphasia (Brown, 1975b). The speech paraphasia and the movement apraxia represent disturbances at comparable levels in the actualization of speech and movement. Since speech is a form of movement, the two collapse into one and thus we have (for conduction aphasia) an "ideomotor apraxia of speech." Brown avoids reference to an interruption of pathways and instead claims that the patient shows apraxic behavior because the language input stimulus (the request) presses the volitional system—not because the language area is cut off from the motor zones. Brown (personal communication 1978) would actually state this somewhat differently. Instead of a language input stimulus pressing a volitional system, he would prefer to say that it is the level of representation of an act that determines whether it has a volitional or automatic character. Therefore, in Brown's model the linguistic command does not play the essential role that it does in the disconnection model. A spontaneous act for Brown would represent a developing crystalization of that act at a more "preliminary" level and is therefore more automatic. The act executed secondary to a command to do it exists at a "higher" representational level and consequently determines the increased volitional nature of the performance. The various forms of apraxia, according to Brown, reflect or point to stages in the ontogeny of a motor act, and he parallels this with the view that the distinct forms of aphasia characterize stages in the development of a linguistic production. In Brown (1977) facial apraxia is described as a "disorder of VOLITIONAL facial action appearing in performances initiated in the test situation with no alteration of spontaneous facial motility. The more automatically elicited performances are better preserved, whereas actions elicited by written or spoken commands are impaired [p. 72, emphasis added]."

Much has been said about apraxia from supramarginal gyrus lesions (Brown, 1972; Denny-Brown, 1958; Geschwind, 1965; Mateer & Kimura, 1977). Predictably, those who admit of center-lesion explanations have considered supramarginal gyrus apraxia OF SPEECH. The supramarginal gyrus is a crucial zone for the discussion of apraxia in general AND of apraxia of speech. Although it is a CORTICAL area of the parietal lobe strategically located for the language zones, it is also anatomically quite near the arcuate fasciculus fibers traveling through opercular regions. There have been those who have preferred to call the repetition disturbance of conduction aphasia an "ideokinetic apraxia for the formation of sounds" (Kleist, 1916). Center-lesion theories of apraxia, of course, are premised on statements such as "memory for movement is stored in this area," etc. If the area is damaged, the patient will be apraxic whether or not he is TOLD TO DO anything. D. Denny-Brown (1958) seems to be representative of those investigators who emphasize posterior center-lesion theories of apraxia of speech. He writes,

> Although the complex movements of lips, tongue and larynx show disturbances that are apractic in nature, these occur in isolation from other types of body apraxia, as if the praxis of speech had developed independently in the dominant insula and parietal operculum, more removed from the parietal-occipital region concerned in other types of ideation apraxia. Thus apraxia of the tongue is a special and particular variant of motor apraxia, associated most commonly with executive aphasia, and usually dissociated from apraxia of facial expression [pp. 12–13].

There is no mention here of a relevant stimulus (the linguistic command)—a characteristic of center-lesion theories of apraxia. It should be pointed out, however, that by 1965 Denny-Brown had shifted his focus to frontal lesions (Broca's aphasia) and consequent speech disturbances. He described (Denny-Brown, 1965) a Broca's aphasic with lesions in the left third and part of the second frontal convolution. The patient (a) had difficulty initiating words; (b) had occasional substitution and anticipation of segments and syllables; (c) had a "slowing of rhythm"; and (c) showed great variability. Denny-Brown (1965) concluded, "This particular difficulty is associated with varying degrees of apraxia of the tongue, lips, face, and respiratory control [p. 462]." Denny-Brown still admits of center-lesion apraxias, but now the region involved for apraxia of speech is in the dominant frontal lobe instead of the insular and parietal opercular zones described in the 1958 paper.

In a series of articles (Kimura, 1976; Kimura, 1977a; Kimura & Archibald, 1974; Mateer & Kimura, 1977), Doreen Kimura has suggested that, "lesions of the left hemisphere impair the performance of complex motor sequences, regardless of whether the sequences are meaningful or not [Kimura & Archibald, 1974, p. 346]." Her belief is that speech disturbances and apraxia are simply distinct manifestations of a breakdown in the control of the action of motoric sequencing. The actual sequential control system is in the parietal lobe according to Kimura, although she rarely gives any details on this localization (Kimura, 1976, p. 153). Kimura's theory is that the movements need only be complexly coordinated, not necessarily meaningful (i.e., symbolic). The reasoning is extended to her hypothesis that "the left hemisphere is particularly well adapted, not for symbolic function per se, but for the execution of some categories of motor activity which happen to lend themselves readily to communication [Kimura, 1976, p. 154]."[6] The problem here, of course, is to determine just what is complex and what is not. In a sense, although it is rather uninteresting, the issue may reduce simply to the fact that multiple or sequential movements are more difficult to produce than single isolated ones. It should be pointed out that Kimura has begun to think that the problem is "a failure to achieve target motor responses when more than one is required rather than just an improper ordering of those targets [Mateer & Kimura, 1977, p. 274]." Similarly, Kimura (1977b) has stated that her analysis of apraxic errors (due to left posterior lesions) reveals that the principal difficulty rests, not with ordering the movements, but rather with selecting and/or executing new postures, whether of brachial or oral musculature.

More germane to this chapter, however, are Kimura's assumptions and explanations for apraxia. She clearly admits of center-lesion explanations of apraxia and does not support disconnection theories. Kimura's views of apraxia seem to cloud her understanding of the disconnection view, which always stipulates the linguistic command stimulus. By failing to isolate the "relevant stimulus" in Geschwind's model, she misses the point when examining his work. The following quotation from Kimura and Archibald (1974) is indicative of misunderstanding at the explanatory level. They start off by writing, "Section of the corpus callosum drastically diminishes the control of the left hemisphere over the left hand, . . . which would seem to support Geschwind's suggestion

---

6. Kimura's position might be strengthened to the extent aphasics can be shown to be capable of manipulating nonarticulatory symbolic systems such as manual signing. On the other hand, her theory would not account for the movement complexity of manual signing.

that cortico-cortical pathways are involved in the left hemisphere's bilateral control of movement [p. 347]." Left-handed "sympathetic" apraxias arise from left frontal or anterior callosal lesions that disconnect left Wernicke's area from right hemisphere motor zones. The disconnection theory is NOT that "memory for movements," etc. is located, say, in the supramarginal gyrus. In fact, Geschwind (1965, pp. 612–613) argues against this view. Kimura and Archibald (1974) continue, "However, the inadequacy of the left hemisphere control over the left hand in callosally sectioned patients has been demonstrated largely via verbal instruction [p. 347]." This quotation more than anything else demonstrates the misunderstanding of the connectionistic theory of apraxia, because it implies that nonverbal instructions should have been used. Again, for Geschwind, in order to demonstrate an apraxia in the split-brain cases, the input command should be via verbal instruction. So, it is rather pointless for Kimura and Archibald to proceed. They write, "It is quite possible that non-verbal instruction, of the kind involved in imitating movement sequences, could proceed via extra-callosal pathways [p. 347]." Geschwind would certainly agree that the movement could be produced with a nonverbal input command, but largely because the right hemisphere could get the command information from, for instance, the right visual cortex.

Geschwind's connection model certainly holds for those patients who can nevertheless perform to imitation. There are problems, however, in explaining those cases where that patient is apraxic to imitation also, since as Geschwind (1975) admits, "We are led to expect that the patient will respond correctly to non-verbal stimuli, which can reach motor regions without going through the speech areas [pp. 190–191]." Geschwind (1975) writes, "Clearly some factor other than disconnection between language and motor areas seems to be necessary to account for these findings [p. 191]." The other factor invoked by Geschwind (1975) is that of cerebral dominance for limb (arm, hand) movement that (contrary to Kimura's theory) may or may not be in the same hemisphere for speech (Heilman, Coyle, Gonyea, & Geschwind, 1973; also see Heilman, 1979a, 1979b, for excellent summaries of the apraxias in general). This addition to Geschwind's disconnectionism does not necessarily denigrate his model, since the dominant hemisphere can be said to "lead" or "drive" the nondominant hemisphere in many instances. Heilman *et al.* (1973) and Rubens, Geschwind, Mahowald, and Mastri (1977) support the model that incorporates dominance theory AND disconnectionism. Of course, in the instances of lack of improvement on imitation, the issue of a verbal language input does not play a role. Nevertheless, disconnection theory still offers the most plausible explanation for the sympathetic apraxias.

Kimura and Archibald (1974) discuss purported counterevidence for the pathway involved in sympathetic apraxia. From the outset, Liepmann (1900) and Bonhoeffer (1914) predicted the possibility of a left-handed apraxia from right frontal lobe damage, where the hemiplegia was not serious enough to render apraxia testing worthless. Geschwind has repeatedly made similar predictions. Kimura and Archibald (1974) write, "The difficulty with this view is that one would occasionally expect apraxia to appear only in the left hand, from a right hemisphere lesion . . . because the control from the left cortex to left hand had been disrupted in its passage through the right hemisphere [p. 347]." It is somewhat strange to see this wording; this is precisely what the prediction has been from the beginning! It would appear that Kimura and Archibald were unaware of the prediction. They further state that in their "own series of patients, the hypothesis was testable only in three patients who had right hemisphere damage without hemiplegia, and in these patients both hands performed equally well on movement copying [p. 347]." There are two serious problems with this statement. In the first place, all we are told is that Kimura and Archibald's patients have right hemisphere damage with no hemiplegia. In these cases it is crucial to state WHERE in the right hemisphere. For all we know, these three patients could have had postrolandic involvement, in which case the purported counterevidence collapses. Geschwind (1975) has commented on right hemisphere sympathetic apraxia. He writes,

> Such cases are rare; in most instances the area of destruction is large enough to affect the actual precentral motor regions on the right, and the resulting left-sided paralysis makes it impossible to assess the presence of apraxia. I have, however, seen one patient with a left-sided apraxia in whom radioisotope-brain-scanning showed a lesion deep in the right frontal lobe [p. 190].

In these rare cases, it is essential that the site of the right hemisphere lesion be specified. It must be frontal, be small enough so as not to occasion paralysis, and be strategically located so as to disrupt the anterior callosal fibers coming from the left. The second error, which is more to the point of the present chapter, is that Kimura and Archibald's three patients were tested on MOVEMENT COPYING. There is much tactile and visual information in the movement-copying task that can get to the right hemisphere for left-hand movement. This is not counterevidence for the connectionistic theory, since the stimulus input command is not spoken language. In fact, Geschwind (1965) has stressed that " 'apraxia' is not a unitary disturbance, since under appropriate conditions these patients could carry out complex motor tasks [p. 612]." Again, it appears that the essential aspects of a connectionistic explanation of apraxia have not been appreciated by Kimura and Archibald. I should also reiterate that Kimura's center-lesion theories of apraxia quite predictably lead her to admit of apraxias of speech. In fact, as I showed, the speech apraxias for her are simply one manifestation of complex nonsymbolic movement disorders that arise secondary to posterior left hemisphere damage.

It should be clear to the reader at this juncture that all the center lesion theories of apraxia usually admit of one or more distinct "apraxias of speech": Kleist—ideomotor apraxia of speech; Denny-Brown—ideomotor (insular–parietal operculum) and frontal lobe apraxia of speech; Luria and J. Brown—kinetic, ideomotor, and ideational apraxias of speech;[7] Kimura—posterior (supramarginal gyrus) apraxia of speech; Canter and Darley (Mayo School)—frontal lobe (around central sulcus) apraxia of speech. I would emphasize that this enumeration of different types of apraxia of speech has more serious consequences for the concept "apraxia of speech" as a whole than does the enumeration of different terminological classifications of one form of apraxia of speech (the limb-kinetic). Again, to my knowledge, one of the best reviews of this view of apraxia of speech is found in Johns and LaPointe (1976). These authors' theoretical assumption is that there is an apraxia of speech, and it is a type of limb-kinetic apraxia for the speech musculature; it is essentially Liepmann's view of that type of apraxia. Their literature survey and in-depth discussion of terminological confusion, etc. almost entirely deals with limb-kinetic center- lesion apraxia of speech and the plethora of nomenclature it has had throughout the history of aphasia. Table 1 in their article comes from the work initiated by Johns in his doctoral dissertation research on this form of apraxia of speech. Again, it is based on center-lesion theory, obviously not connection theory. Throughout history (they begin with Auburtin, 1861), this frontal lobe apraxia of speech

7. In Brown (1972, chap. 10) a strong correlation is drawn between ideational apraxia and posterior fluent paraphasic speech. He writes, "We may almost speak of ideational apraxia as a 'fluent' apraxia, contrasting it with 'non-fluent' apraxias of anterior origin. In ideational apraxia there is an abundance of partial movements, each normal in itself, and the overall movement sequence, though disorganized, has an ease and an effortless quality as is seen in the speech of posterior aphasia [p. 170]." Again, this is essentially Luria's view as well; consequently, I have grouped them together here, although as Brown has pointed out to me (personal communication, 1978) he never actually made the correlation complete by specifically referring to an ideational apraxia OF SPEECH. From the above quotation, however, it would have not been very far fetched had he done so.

has been referred to as "aphemia, Broca's aphasia, motor aphasia, anarthria, verbal aphasia, phonetic disintegration of speech, apraxia, apraxic dysarthria, cortical dysarthria, and oral verbal apraxia [Johns & LaPointe, 1976, p. 163]. The context of the actual descriptions, however, reveals that "generally good clinical agreement has existed [p. 163]." There is never much argument with the actual descriptions; I would imagine that the connectionist would give similar descriptive details of the typical Broca patient.[8]

There are, however, a few places in the Johns and LaPointe (1976, pp. 186, 191) review where they mention disconnection phenomena and where they refer to another center-lesion type of apraxia of speech. When discussing the De Renzi *et al.* (1966) findings concerning the possible (but not often obtaining) separation of limb–kinetic apraxia of speech and oral–facial apraxia, they compare the two possible anatomical explanations suggested in that paper. One is that oral non verbal movements and oral verbal (speech) movements could be mediated by two distinct frontal cortical association areas. Note that this view would NOT be in accord with Kimura's model discussed earlier, although it is clearly a center-lesion hypothesis. The second consideration of De Renzi *et al.* (1966), however, as Johns and LaPointe (1976) write, is "that apraxia from commands can result from lesions to pathways connecting frontal and temporal lobes; and apraxia from imitation can result from lesions disrupting occipital and frontal fasciculi [p. 186]." Further on in their review, they outline speech disturbances that may stem from lack of cortical sensory feedback information, and they note that perhaps there could be another type of apraxia of speech. In fact, they point out that Jay Rosenbek, one of the most influential clinicians and researchers of the Mayo tradition, has "revised the concept of apraxia of speech to include sensory-perceptual influences rather than the traditional view of it as strictly a motor, or output, speech disorder [pp. 191–192]." The various peripheral oral sensation studies in limb–kinetic apraxias of speech have shown sensory deficits. These deficits could presumably occur from lesions that extend to the lower postrolandic region, and therefore what Rosenbek discovered was that Luria's "afferent apraxia" could be an added component to limb-kinetic apraxia.

It is unfortunate that Johns and LaPointe (1976) did not include discussion of Kimura's work on posterior apraxia of speech or of the whole question of disconnection explanation in apraxia. Kimura has denied

8. I am aware that a large percentage of Broca's aphasics have more extensive lesions of "the operculum from anterior frontal through Broca's area to anterior parietal regions, the insula, both banks of the central (Rolandic) fissure . . . usually extending deep into the hemisphere [Mohr, 1976, p. 228]."

that frontal lesions result in anything more than weakness, slowness, and incoordination of movement. In addition, Geschwind (1965) writes that " 'limb-kinetic' apraxia has not been defined clearly enough to separate it from mild pyramidal disturbance [p. 617]." Certainly, there is no frontal apraxia of speech for Geschwind (or any apraxia of speech, for that matter) because of his connectionistic paradigm. Geschwind has explained Broca's aphasia as due to a disconnection between Broca's area and the motor face area on the motor strip anterior to the rolandic fissure, but he denies that anything is gained by using the term APRAXIA OF SPEECH since patients are seen with Broca's aphasia who do not have an oral-facial apraxia and others are seen with Wernicke's aphasia who do have an oral-facial apraxia. Furthermore, as mentioned above, patients with distinct aphasic outputs may have qualitatively similar oral-facial apraxias and patients with no speech problems at all may have an oral-facial apraxia. There is no frontal apraxia of speech for Kimura either, since for her complex praxis for movement is a dominant POSTERIOR function of the brain. It is these theories that have challenged the theoretical position of the Mayo tradition as to apraxia of speech. Nevertheless, what I am arguing for in this chapter is that it is hopelessly ambiguous to simply say that this or that is an apraxia of speech without further specifying the neuroanatomical explanation being used, the location of the lesion, and the stimulus conditions that evoked the behavior said to be apraxic.

General Characteristics of Limb-Kinetic Apraxia of Speech

There are at least five typically observable behaviors in patients with a limb-kinetic apraxia of speech. In attempting to articulate, patients will often show a groping behavior, which indicates that they have the underlying phonological form in mind. Although there are difficulties with initiating the articulated sequence, articulatory preposturing will quite often reveal the vocal tract configuration for the initial segments of the word to be uttered. This initial preposturing may also include some noncontiguous coarticulatory information, so that, for example, the lips may be rounded for the preposturing of /k/ when a patient is groping for the word /klu/ ('clue'). In light of the fact that these patients often manifest sequencing impairments, the coarticulated /k/, rounded by the influence of the noncontiguous high-back vowel /u/, is easier to produce than the sequential transition to the /l/, which is contiguous to the /k/. This demonstrates that coarticulation and transitionalizing are separate processes, and that coarticulated information is coded within syllable-sized units. Limb–kinetic apraxics' disturbances will often be exacerbated on elicitation, which, of course, relates to the issue of volitional level and confrontation testing.

I would now like to mention some of the difficulties I have interpreting various of the supposed linguistic and nonlinguistic diagnostic characteristics of the limb-kinetic type of apraxia of speech, that is, the frontal Broca's patient. PROGRAMMING, INCOORDINATION, and VARIABILITY are three terms that, to my way of thinking, have led to many inconsistencies and have in general not served to differentiate syndromes very well. INITIATION, SELECTION, and SEQUENCE have not been sharply enough defined, and the term PHONEME itself has caused no little confusion because of its abstract nature.

When we are told that an apraxia of speech involves disorders in the "programming" of motor speech, we need to know immediately what the units of speech are that are involved and precisely where in the encoding process we are. It is not clear that the phonemic level is motor in any sense whatsoever. Is the motor level allophonic? Are the allophones specified within broadly defined syllabic units that may straddle lexical boundaries? One should not lose sight of the fact that PROGRAM is a metaphor and may be used as a descriptor at any level of abstraction whatsoever and therefore may be used at the earliest ideational levels or at the latest output levels (see footnotes 1 and 5).

It is important to distinguish between an "incoordination" of the musculature used for speech and an "incoordination" of the set of synchronous nerve impulses that eventually impinge on different muscle groups for properly timed articulatory events. Disturbed laryngeal control is certainly a type of incoordination that is seen in frontal lobe patients; it isn't muscular, but rather neural. Nevertheless, apraxic neural incoordination may be nothing more than some mild pyramidal disturbance of which Geschwind speaks.

VARIABILITY OF BEHAVIOR is another open-ended term that not only is somewhat confusing but also can define practically any aphasic or apraxic. Presumably, this term came into use as a way to differentiate the apraxic from the dysarthric. However, using the term to distinguish an apraxic from an aphasic would be disastrous. Not only do all types of aphasics exhibit variability in their language behavior, but so do apraxics. The variability, however, is explained in two quite different ways. The connectionist, like Geschwind, as I pointed out earlier, attributes the variability to the different stimulus conditions under which the patient is requested to do something. If the request is nonverbal, the patient will often be able to carry out the movement pattern despite the fact that it could not be performed to verbal request. On the other hand, center-lesion explanation must invoke "volition," "will," etc.; limb-kinetic speech apraxias are characterized by the "islands of error-free productions" that are often thought to be more automatic, less propositional, and therefore less volitional. Recall, however, the different interpretation of center-lesion apraxic disturbances in Brown's theory to which I alluded earlier. The term VARIABILITY, therefore, does not even distinguish between theories of apraxia, rather what distinguishes them is their explanatory mechanisms.

Canter, Burns, and Trost (1975) have brought in a useful distinction for getting around the problems with the vague term SEQUENCING. They differentiate between "transitionalizing" from phoneme to phoneme (it would have been more proper to say from phone to phone) and the sequential ordering of phonemes. Therefore, we could say that the essential problem with posterior patients is with sequential ordering, whereas the problem with the Broca patient is with "sequential flow." Note that the "syntagmatic" disorder of the motor aphasic described by Luria (and linguistically characterized by Jakobson) is that of Canter's sequential flow, although until it is disambiguated in this way, SYNTAGMATIC as a descriptive term will not work, since the posterior "paradigmatic" aphasics will exhibit the sequential ordering disturbances that are clearly "syntagmatic" in nature (Buckingham, 1977).

The qualitative aspect of phonemic paraphasia in terms of substitution, deletion, addition, and linear switch is no different for ANY aphasic, including any patient with limb-kinetic apraxia of speech. The cortical system for selecting and sequencing phonemic units will show disruption at times for frontal patients as well as for posterior patients. For instance, it confuses the issue when we try to distinguish frontal from posterior syndromes by stating that only posterior cases show selection difficulties; the frontal patient does also. I have seen many posterior cases where there are addition, deletion, and linear types of phonemic paraphasia. It is not diagnostic of any group to show that substitution errors, for example, are more frequent than other error types. Buckingham and Kertesz (1976, p. 52) show that, of the analyzable phonemic paraphasias of a neologistic jargonaphasic, there were far more substitution errors. Earlier, Blumstein (1973, pp. 46–47) demonstrated that (using her classification of aphasia), when one analyzes the phonemic errors of Broca's, conduction, and Wernicke's aphasics in terms of substitution, simplification, linear switch ("environment" in Blumstein's terms), and addition, one finds that all the groups have the same relative difficulty. Each group had more substitutive errors, followed by simplifications (deletions), and next by linear switches. Least in number for all groups were addition paraphasias. Evidently, as Blumstein (1973) states, "the phonological errors characteristic of aphasic speech reflect a systematic disorganization of phonology independent of a particular lesion site [p. 47]." In addition, the fact that error sounds are usually off target by only one dimension (feature) as opposed to two or three is not diagnostic either for any one group, since, again, Blumstein's study (1973, p. 49) showed that ALL aphasics will exhibit substitutive paraphasias that in the majority of cases differ from the target phonemic unit by one distinctive feature. The distinctions that would be diagnostic for each group would be quantitative in nature, not qualitative—at least at the phonemic level.

Experimental Studies

The actual situation with substitution errors is more complex, however, and we must make some finer suBphonemic distinctions. In this way we might come up with a better diagnostic for differentiating patients with limb-kinetic apraxias of speech from the posterior patients. Let us assume that there may be two possible disturbances, one at a NONmotoric phonemic level and the other at some lower stage of speech production (see Footnotes 1 and 5). Breakdown at either level may result in a substitutive error. The problem was well stated by De Renzi *et al.* (1966): "It is hard to decide if the substitution of voiced consonantal sounds (e.g., b, v, g), by the corresponding voiceless consonants (p, f, k, respectively) is due to wrong choice of phonemes... or to lack of synergy of the vocal cords with the muscles of articulation [p. 55]."

The phonetic counterpart for the linguistic distinctive feature [voice] for syllable initial stop consonants involves the time interval between the release of the consonantal closure and the onset of vocal fold vibration of the larynx for the following vowel: VOICE-ONSET TIME (VOT). Generally speaking, the closer the voice onset occurs to the time of release, the more likely the consonant will be filtered through the linguistic system as [+voice]. The parameters are language dependent, and there will always be a range of values of onset times where variation within the range causes no perceptual differences for hearers. For instance, the VOT value of syllable initial /d/ in English may range from −180 msec to +25 msec, but most adult values range from 0 to +20 msec. Time of stop release is always zero with respect to VOT, so that a VOT of −180 msec means that the folds start vibrating 180 msec BEFORE stop release. For /t/, the VOT values range from +40 msec to +120 msec. The consonants /b/–/p/ and /g/–/k/ have different ranges, the bilabials ranging to the left of the alveolars and the velars ranging to the right. Therefore, for example,

the /k/ will have the longest VOT lag of the stops. The phonetic counterpart of the linguistic nondistinctive feature [aspiration] is the VOT lag
subsequent to closure release; the longer the voicing lag, the more aspiration. Aspiration is a characteristic of English syllable initial /p/, /t/, and
/k/, except when these segments follow /s/, in which case their VOT lags
shorten considerably. The shortened lag places them perceptually closer
to their [+voice] counterparts.

A study by Blumstein, Cooper, Zurif, and Caramazza (1977) comparing anterior subjects with posterior subjects on voice-onset timing[9] parameters has shown a "lack of synergy" for the former group. Although
at times they will produce phonemic substitutions (certainly to be expected, given Blumstein, 1973), this group produces asynergic phonetic
substitutions that in several instances turn out to be unexpected, incorrect ALLOPHONIC productions. In the case of /t/, for instance, the anterior
patient is likely to substitute the allophone of /t/ that normally occurs after
/s/, as in [stap], in syllable initial position (see Blumstein, Cooper,
Goodglass, Statlender, & Gottlieb, 1980, for the addition of conduction
aphasics and of a dysarthric speaker with brain stem damage in comparative VOT studies). To a native speaker of English with a "good
phonetic ear" or with, for example, a knowledge of a language like
Spanish (Abramson & Lisker, 1973), this will be recognized (perceived)
as a voiceless initial unaspirated stop. By many (probably most), however, it will be perceived as belonging to /d/ and not as an incorrect
allophone belonging to /t/. Accordingly, the patient will be credited with
a phonemic error, when in fact a phonetic error had been produced!

Sands, Freeman, and Harris (1978) followed the improvement over a
10-year period of a patient with a limb–kinetic apraxia of speech. They
found that, at the end of this period, errors of place and manner of
articulation as well as deletion errors were greatly reduced. What persisted were essentially errors in voicing, and thus it was concluded that
the remaining apraxic disturbance was one of temporal coordination of
the abductory (spreading) and adductory (bringing together) laryngeal
processes with upper articulatory events.

Freeman, Sands, and Harris (1978) followed up with a more detailed
study of VOT in apraxia and found that it differed markedly from productions in non-brain-damaged normals. They noted that apraxic articu-

---

9. Experimental analysis with such parameters as VOT will provide a far superior account
of phonemic versus phonetic error and will no doubt help clarify the nature of "phonetic disintegration." This is an extremely important issue, since many have claimed that
apraxia of speech (or verbal apraxia) is phonetic disintegration (Alajouanine, Ombredane, & Durand, 1939; Shankweiler & Harris, 1966; Shankweiler, Harris, & Taylor,
1968).

lations did not include voicing lead for voiced stops and that lag times for voiced stops were longer than normal. On the other hand, the lag times for voiceless stops were shorter than normal. All of these apraxic changes resulted in more closely compact VOT ranges around the point of stop release. Consequently, there was a clear overlapping of [+voice] or [−voice] perceptual categories. Apraxics produced little or no prevoicing leads or long lags. Since VOT is the acoustic cue for perceiving the [±voice] distinction for syllable initial consonants, apraxic incoordinations will trigger perceptual categorial switches in hearers. Finally, the authors note that the apraxics' VOT range constriction to the short lag area (+20 msec to +30 msec) mirrors VOT ranges in young children, but they offer no explanation for this.

Kewley-Port and Preston (1974), as discussed in Cooper (1977), offered an account of VOT acquisition in children in terms of complexity of neural control. In the first place, vocal fold vibration is brought about by three factors: (*a*) folds must be adducted; (*b*) they must be relatively relaxed; and (*c*) a sufficient drop in pressure across the larynx must be maintained in order to permit an accelerated air flow. The neural control for these three factors is different for the three VOT types—prevoicing, short lag, and long lag. It turns out that the short-lag VOT is neuromuscularly less complex, because, unlike with prevoicing and long lag, factor (*c*) is mechanically produced. For short-lag VOTs, the speaker need only adduct the folds prior to release of stop closure and keep them relatively lax. Upon release of closure, a sufficient drop in transglottal pressure takes place automatically due to the equalization of mouth pressure. This enables initiation of glottal vibration shortly after the release. For prevoicing or long-delay VOT, the maintenance or delay of cross-glottal pressure drop requires more complexly timed and controlled neural commands. Eventually, the child comes to master the more complex neuromuscular coordination. It appears that the apraxic has lost it. As we will see later, however, dysarthric speech is characterized by abnormally long voice lags for voiceless consonants, and consequently, one must be cautious when interpreting neuromuscular complexity explanations for voice-onset lag times.

Incorrect allophonic production may, in some cases, even sound like a foreign accent to some. In fact, one characterization of a foreign accent is precisely that the nonnative speaker will often produce some inappropriate phonetic variant of the target phoneme for the language he is speaking. Whitaker (1975) has described a patient with left frontal damage whose speech output gave the partial impression of being Spanish in origin. Whitaker wrote that the patient had characteristics of Broca's aphasia with apraxia of speech. This patient was from central Michigan, had not been outside the area, and had never studied a foreign language. Whitaker writes, "There were striking problems with aspiration; initial voiceless stops were often unaspirated [p. 27]." One suspects that the patient was having difficulties with temporal coordination from the description given, although no acoustic measurements were taken. There were other phonetic characteristics of this syndrome that were clearly not phonemic in nature and that gave the impression of being ataxic. This type of subphonemic foreign accent output secondary to frontal rolandic area lesions has been described by several others as a cortical dysarthria (Whitaker, 1975, pp. 23–25). This does not mean that the cortical frontal lobe patient is impossible to distinguish from the patient with upper or lower motor neuron damage, who also produces phonetic errors.

The phonetic distortions are less variable in the motor neuron group than in the cortical group, and, unlike the motor neuron dysarthrias, the limb-kinetic patients will quite often produce phonemic errors with proper allophonic realization. Blumstein *et al.* (1980) and Itoh, Sasanuma, Hirose, Yoshioka, and Ushijima (1980) have been able to distinguish dysarthric speech from limb-kinetic apraxic speech. Blumstein *et al.* showed that, unlike Broca's aphasics, whose VOT range was quite restricted, the dysarthric productions for consonants were distributed over a wider VOT range. Broca's VOT values for voiceless consonants rarely surpassed the +150 msec point, whereas the predominant voiceless productions for the dysarthrics were abnormally long. This is why dysarthric speech at times seems overly aspirated. Furthermore, unlike the Broca productions, the dysarthric productions showed no phonetic overlap between voiced and voiceless categories. This would explain why hearers rarely attribute phonemic errors to dysarthrics, but often do so to apraxics. Itoh *et al.* (1980) clearly demonstrated that the pattern and velocity of dysarthric (one patient with ataxia and the other with amyotrophic lateral sclerosis) articulations are distinct from those of limb-kinetic apraxia of speech. For the most part, VOT studies have concentrated on syllable-initial stops.

Still another type of substitutive phonetic error can be seen. It represents a phonetic problem, but unlike the [pʰ] → [p] in English, where the incorrectly substituted phone may be assigned to the same phonemic unit to which the target phone belongs, the error MUST be assigned to a different phonemic unit from that of the target, even though the phonetic error may not imply a phonemic selection error. Itoh, Sasanuma, and Ushijima (1979) studied velar movements in the speech of a limb-kinetic type of patient by fiber optic techniques. The patient's lesion involved "the cortical surface near the anterior tip of the Sylvian fissure of the left hemisphere and immediately subjacent subcortical white matter [p. 229]." Due to asynchronous velar movement, a phonetic change of [n] → [d] (i.e., improper lowering of the velum) was demonstrated. The phonetic error, however, is assigned to a phonemic unit distinct from that of the target phone. The phoneme /n/ does not have [d] as a possible allophonic alternation in Japanese, and consequently, the phonetic error [d] must be assigned to /d/. However, as the authors point out, the fiber optic measurements showed that, despite variation in the slope of velar lowering, the pattern of anticipatory lowering was constantly preserved. This was interpreted by the authors as indicating that "the observed variation of the pattern of velar movements and the resultant phonetic change do not stem from a selection or retrieval error of a target phoneme in the process of speech production, namely, an error of phonological processing [p. 235]." Obviously, then, the error is primarily [n] → [d], not /n/ → /d/, although the target phone and the error phone must be assigned to /n/ and /d/, respectively.

Itoh *et al.* (1980) again measured temporal asynchronies among articulators in apraxia; this time, however, they used a different technique. By placing radioactive pellets upon the lower lip, the lower incisor (for tracking jaw movement), the dorsum of the tongue, and the nasal surface of the velum, a computer-controlled X-ray microbeam system could track the simultaneous movements of these structures during articulation. This procedure further demonstrated the variability and temporal disorganization in the speech of limb–kinetic apraxics.

It is certainly true that the patient with limb–kinetic apraxia of speech may or may not have a concomitant oral–facial apraxia AND may or may not have a concomitant aphasia. That is, some sort of "pure" apraxia of speech may be seen. Therefore, it would be best not to claim that Broca's aphasia equals apraxia of speech. The typical Broca's aphasic clearly has more than the articulatory asynchronies we have been discussing; the apraxia is usually but one component and is most often accompanied by agrammatic production and comprehension[10] (see Chapter 6 in this volume).

Lecours and Lhermitte (1976) demonstrated that an apraxic (for them, "anarthric") phonetic disintegration can exist in isolation from aphasia and from dysarthria. Their patient had cortico-subcortical softening of the inferior half of the left precentral gyrus, with Broca's area, nevertheless, intact. Although Lecours and Lhermitte call this "pure" form of phonetic disintegration "a relatively infrequent form of aphasia [p. 109]," the patient has no other aphasic symptomatology. Although

---

10. Recall the arguments of A. Damien Martin (1974).

some of the errors in this case were at the phonemic level, the vast majority of them were subphonemic.

It should be clear to the reader that these experimental studies of apraxia are directed, not at studying what patients do on linguistic command, but rather at measuring articulatory parameters. Thus, they tacitly accept the nonconnectionistic, center-lesion view of apraxia. Disconnection explanations play no role whatsoever in the accounts of the apraxic productions in these studies. Rather, they focus upon subphonemic errors, variability and nonfluency.

VARIABILITY is often used to distinguish the dysarthric from the cortically damaged patient, but it is a nonlinguistic descriptor and need not be specifically linked to speech behavior. Furthermore, variability can only be used to distinguish apraxic distortions from dysarthric distortions. It will not serve to differentiate apraxia from aphasia, since aphasic behavior itself is quite variable. FLUENCY, in terms of struggle, may certainly be used to distinguish (within reason) between frontal and posterior cases, as long as we can be sure it is a motoric struggle and not a word-finding block, which can also cause struggling and groping behavior in the patient.

More crucially, I would argue that the actual descriptions of apraxic speech errors are only valid if they are made at the allophonic, post-phoneme selection level. Consequently, any theory that states that apraxia of speech is a motoric disturbance composed of "substitutions, additions, and repetitions of phonemes [Mayo Clinic and Mayo Foundation, 1976, p. 232]" will have to demonstrate how the substitutions, additions, and repetitions of phonemes are different from posterior aphasic errors that can be characterized in the same way. More importantly, these theories that are worded in terms of phonemes will have to show what it means for the switch (at the selection level) of /m/ to /p/, for instance, to be motoric. As mentioned earlier, it is impossible to conceive of a motor disorder at the phonemic level; no invariant articulatory (as measured by cineradiography or by electromyography) or acoustic (as measured spectrographically) pattern has ever been found that uniquely specifies some phonemic unit. Yet, the psychological reality of those units is unquestionable. Therefore, phonemes cannot be submitted to physical scrutiny, and by the same token, it is anomalous to describe motor disorders of speech in terms of them.

Concluding Remarks

In conclusion, it is safe to say that there is ample historical precedent for two different neuroanatomical explanations for apraxia—center lesion and disconnection. Whether or not one of these explanations will generally come to be accepted over the other, only time will tell. It does appear, however, that experimental studies of phonetic parameters in apraxia will not focus much on anatomical disconnection. This will be especially obvious in those cases where the speech output that is measured is not elicited by linguistic command (i.e., by repetition). The studies on the center-lesion limb–kinetic apraxias of speech predictably claim that the cortical regions damaged are those that (somehow) contain the information for proper articulatory timing; they do not necessarily stipulate the stimuli presented for the elicitation of speech. Disconnection theories label a behavior apraxic if the stimulus input is linguistic, such as *Show me how you would. . .* , *Stick out your tongue. . . .* , etc. The apraxic behavior is said to result from some disconnection between Wernicke's area in the superior temporal lobe of the dominant hemisphere and a cortical motor center. If imitation does not facilitate performance, disconnectionism must then resort to the concept of cerebral dominance, as I have mentioned. Center-lesion theories, on the other hand, do not eliminate the possibility of performing a motor act during some behavior not necessarily induced by a verbal command. Therefore, the center-lesion theories are much more likely to include apraxia of speech. VOLITION is used by the center-lesion theory as a way to explain why certain acts cannot be induced upon linguistic command but can be produced reflexively. The explanatory use of WILL is Jacksonian and stipulates that we press the human's volitional response capabilities to the highest degree when we REQUEST that he act in some fashion or other. However, recall Brown's different view of the role of volition in his center-lesion model. The center-lesion hypothesis need not make recourse to a disconnection between the language and motor areas of the brain. In addition, the language stimulus is not nearly so crucially involved in center-lesion explanations. I am not convinced that more data are necessarily needed to decide which of these theories is best. Perhaps what is needed is more reinterpretation of data and descriptions that have existed for a long time. Obviously, lines of investigation will center on newly proposed models, such as Brown's, Kimura's, and Geschwind's. At least, however, each proponent should be fully aware of the different explanatory mechanisms involved for all the theories.

The additional claim I would make is that it would be desirable indeed for those who accept center-lesion theories and, in particular, frontal lobe limb-kinetic apraxia of speech (to the exclusion of other forms of apraxia of speech) to characterize very closely the actual speech errors of that patient population in order to distinguish the errors themselves (both phonemic and phonetic) from the articulatory–behavioral context within which they are uttered. This behavioral context is NONlinguistic and includes all those struggling attempts to initiate speech and keep it going that the cortical frontal motor patient displays. It also includes the fact that the speech behavior is variable (necessary to distinguish this patient from the motor neuron patient); but, again, variability is NONlinguistic. It is part of the total behavioral context, which should not be confused with the linguistic nature of the aphasic error itself. Once this is realized, I think it will become clear that phonemic paraphasic errors alone (in terms of quality) are not a good diagnostic for the frontal cortical patient and that we must look at such phonetic parameters as VOT and velar function. Once we fully understand the phonetics of the errors, we will be in a better position to truly distinguish the frontal cortical speech errors from dysarthric speech and from posterior phonemic selection errors.

Acknowledgments

I would like to express my appreciation to Norman Geschwind, Jason W. Brown, and Leonard LaPointe for their helpful remarks on earlier drafts of this chapter. Naturally, they are not to be held responsible for any of my interpretations. This chapter is essentially reprinted from the author's paper, which appeared in *Brain and Language*, 1978, *8*, 202–226.

References

Abramson, S., & Lisker, L. 1973. Voice-timing perception in Spanish word-initial stops. *Journal of Phonetics, 1*, 1–8.
Alajouanine, T. 1960. Baillarger and Jackson: The principle of Baillarger–Jackson in aphasia. *Journal of Neurology, Neurosurgery, and Psychiatry, 23*, 191–193.
Alajouanine, T., Ombredane, A., & Durand, M. 1939. Le syndrome de la désintegration phonétique dans l' aphasie. Paris: Masson.
Auburtin, E. 1861. Sur la forme et le volume du cerveau: Sur le siége de la faculté du language. *Bulletin de la Société d' Anthropologie, Paris, 2*, 214–233.
Benton, A. L., & Joynt, R. J. 1960. Early descriptions of aphasia. *Archives of Neurology, 3*, 205–222.
Blumstein, S. 1973. *A phonological investigation of aphasic speech*. The Hague: Mouton.
Blumstein, S., Cooper, W. E., Goodglass, H., Statlender, S., & Gottlieb, J. 1980. Production deficits in aphasia: A voice-onset time analysis. *Brain and Language, 9*, 153–170.
Blumstein, S., Cooper W. E., Zurif, E. B., & Caramazza, A. 1977. The perception and production of voice-onset time in aphasia. *Neuropsychologia, 15*, 371–383.
Bonhoeffer, K. 1914. Klinischer und anatomischer befund zur lehre von der apraxie und der "motorischen sprachbehn." *Monatsschrift für Psychiatrie und Neurologie, 35*, 113–28.
Bouillaud, J. B. 1825. Recherches cliniques propres à démonstrer que la perte de la parole correspond à la lésion des lobules anterieurs du cerveau. Et a confirmer l'opinion de M. Gall sur le siege de l'organe du language articulé. *Archives of General Medicine* (Paris), *8*, 25–45.

Broca, P. 1960. Remarks on the seat of the faculty of articulate language, followed by an observation of aphemia. In G. von Bonin (Ed.), *Some papers on the cerebral cortex.* Springfield, Ill.: Thomas. (Originally published, 1861.)

Brown, J. W. 1972. *Aphasia, apraxia and agnosia.* Springfield, Ill.: Thomas.

Brown, J. W. 1975. On the neural organization of language: Thalamic and cortical relationships. *Brain and Language, 2,* 18–30. (a)

Brown, J. W. 1975. The problem of repetition: A study of "conduction" aphasia and the "isolation" syndrome. *Cortex, 11,* 37–52. (b)

Brown, J. W. 1977. *Mind, brain and consciousness: The neuropsychology of cognition.* New York: Academic Press.

Buckingham, H. W. 1977. A critique of A. R. Luria's neurodynamic explanation of paraphasia. *Brain and Language, 4,* 580–587.

Buckingham, H. W., & Kertesz, A. 1976. *Neologistic jargon aphasia.* Amsterdam: Swets & Zeitlinger.

Burns, M. S., & Canter, G. 1977. Phonemic behavior of aphasic patients with posterior cerebral lesions. *Brain and Language, 4,* 492–507.

Canter, G. 1973. Dysarthria, apraxia of speech, and literal paraphasia: Three distinct varieties of articulatory behavior in the adult with brain damage. Paper presented at the meeting of the American Speech and Hearing Association, Detroit, MI., October 1973.

Canter, G., Burns, M., & Trost, J. 1975. Differential phonemic behavior in anterior and posterior aphasic syndromes. Paper presented at the 13th Annual Meeting of the Academy of Aphasia, Victoria, British Columbia.

Cooper, W. E. 1977. The development of speech timing. In S. J. Segalowitz & F. A. Gruber (Eds.), *Language development and neurological theory.* New York: Academic Press.

Denny-Brown, D. 1958. The nature of apraxia. *Journal of Nervous and Mental Disease, 126,* 9–32.

Denny-Brown, D. 1965. Physiological aspects of disturbances of speech. *Australian Journal of Experimental Biology and Medical Science, 43,* 455–474.

De Renzi, E., Pieczuro, A., & Vignolo, L. A. 1966. Oral apraxia and aphasia. *Cortex, 2,* 50–73.

Freeman, F. J., Sands, E. S., & Harris, K. S. 1978. Temporal coordination of phonation and articulation in a case of verbal apraxia: A voice onset time study. *Brain and Language, 6,* 106–111.

Fromkin, V., & Rodman, R. 1978. *An introduction to language* (2nd ed.). New York: Holt, Rinehart and Winston.

Geschwind, N. 1965. Disconnexion syndromes in animals and man. *Brain, 88,* 237–294, 585–644.

Geschwind, N. 1969. Anatomy of the higher functions of the brain. In R. S. Cohen & M. Wartofsky (Eds.), *Boston studies in the philosophy of science* (Vol. 4). Dordrecht: D. Reidel.

Geschwind, N. 1975. The apraxias: Neural mechanisms of disorders of learned movement. *American Scientist, 63,* 188–195.

Head, H. 1926. *Aphasia and kindred disorders of speech* (Vols 1 and 2). London: Cambridge Univ. Press.

Heilman, K. M. 1979. Apraxia. In K. M. Heilman & E. Valenstein (Eds.), *Clinical neuropsychology.* New York: Oxford Univ. Press. (a)

Heilman, K. M. 1979. The neuropsychological basis of skilled movement in man. In M. S. Gazzaniga (Ed.), *Handbook of behavioral neurology* (Vol. 2, Neuropsychology). New York: Plenum. (b)

Heilman, K. M., Coyle, J. M., Gonyea, E. F., & Geschwind, N. 1973. Apraxia and agraphia in the left-hander. *Brain, 96,* 21–28.

Itoh, M., Sasanuma, S., Hirose, H., Yoshioka, H., & Ushijima, T. 1980. Abnormal articulatory dynamics in a patient with apraxia of speech: X-ray microbeam observation.
Brain and Language, 11, 66–75.
Itoh, M., Sasanuma, S., & Ushijima, T. 1979. Velar movements during speech in a patient
with apraxia of speech. *Brain and Language, 7,* 227–239.
Jackson, J. 1931. Notes on the physiology and pathology of language. In J. Taylor (Ed.),
Selected writings of John Hughlings Jackson (Vol. 2). London: Hodder & Stoughton. (Originally published, 1866.)
Jackson, J. 1931. On affections of speech from disease of the brain. In J. Taylor (Ed.),
Selected writings of John Hughlings Jackson (Vol. 2). London: Hodder & Stoughton. (Originally published, 1878.) (a)
Jackson, J. 1931. On the nature of the duality of the brain. In J. Taylor (Ed.), *Selected
Writings of John Hughlings Jackson* (Vol. 2). London: Hodder & Stoughton. (Originally
published, 1874.)
Jackson, J. 1931. Remarks on the non-protrusion of the tongue in some cases of aphasia. In
J. Taylor (Ed.), *Selected Writings of John Hughlings Jackson* (Vol. 2). London: Hodder &
Stoughton. (Originally published, 1878.) (b)
Johns, D. F., & Darley, F. L. 1970. Phonemic variability in apraxia of speech. *Journal of
Speech and Hearing Research, 13,* 556–583.
Johns, D. F., & LaPointe, L. L. 1976. Neurogenic disorders of output processing: Apraxia
of speech. In H. Whitaker & H. A. Whitaker (Eds.), *Studies in neurolinguistics* (Vol. 1).
New York: Academic Press.
Kelso, J. A. S., & Tuller, B. 1981. Toward a theory of apractic syndromes. *Brain and Language,
12,* 224–245.
Kewley-Port, D., & Preston, M. S. 1974. Early apical stop production: A voice onset time
analysis. *Journal of Phonetics, 2,* 195–210.
Kimura, D. 1976. The neural basis of language qua gesture. In H. Whitaker & H. A.
Whitaker (Eds.), *Studies in neurolinguistics* (Vol. 2). New York: Academic Press.
Kimura, D. 1977. Acquisition of a motor skill after left-hemisphere damage. *Brain, 100,*
527–542. (a)
Kimura, D. 1977. Studies in apraxia. Paper presented at the 15th Annual Meeting of the
Academy of Aphasia, Montreal. (b)
Kimura, D., & Archibald, Y. 1974. Motor functions of the left hemisphere. *Brain, 97,*
337–350.
Kinsbourne, M. 1972. Behavioral analysis of the repetition deficit in conduction aphasia.
Neurology, 22, 1126–1132.
Kleist, K. 1916. Ueber Leitungsaphasie und grammatische Störungen. *Monatsschrift für
Psychiatrie und Neurologie, 40,* 118–199.
Lecours, A. R., & Lhermitte, F. 1976. The "pure form" of the phonetic disintegration
syndrome (pure anarthria); Anatomo-clinical report of a historical case. *Brain and Language, 3,* 88–113.
Liepmann, H. 1900. Das krankheitsbild der Apraxie (motorischen asymbolie) auf grund
eines falles von einseitiger apraxie. *Monatsschrfit für Psychiatrie und Neurologie, 8,* 15–40,
102–32, 182–97. (English translation in D. A. Rottenberg & F. H. Hochberg [Eds.]. 1977.
Neurological classics in modern translation. New York: Hafner.)
Luria, A. R. 1972. Aphasia reconsidered. *Cortex, 8,* 34–40.
Luria, A. R. 1973. *The working brain: An introduction to neuropsychology.* New York: Basic
Books.
Martin, A. 1974. Some objections to the term apraxia of speech. *Journal of Speech and
Hearing Disorders, 39,* 53–64.

Mateer, C., & Kimura, D. 1977. Impairment of non-verbal oral movements in aphasia. *Brain and Language, 4,* 262–276.

Mayo Clinic and Mayo Foundation. 1976. *Clinical examinations in neurology* (4th ed.). Philadelphia: Saunders.

Mohr, J. P. 1976. Broca's area and Broca's aphasia. In H. Whitaker & H. A. Whitaker (Eds.), *Studies in neurolinguistics* (Vol. 1). New York: Academic Press.

Poeck, K., & Kerschensteiner, M. 1975. Analysis of the sequential motor events in oral apraxia. In K. J. Zülch, O. Creutzfeldt, & G. C. Galbraith (Eds.), *Cerebral localization.* New York: Springer-Verlag.

Rubens, A. B., Geschwind, N., Mahowald, M. W., & Mastri, A. 1977. Posttraumatic cerebral hemispheric disconnection syndrome. *Archives of Neurology, 34,* 750–755.

Sands, E. S., Freeman, F. J., & Harris, K. S. 1978. Progressive changes in articulatory patterns in verbal apraxia: A longitudinal case study. *Brain and Language, 6,* 97–105.

Shankweiler, D., & Harris, K. S. 1966. An experimental approach to the problem of articulation in aphasia. *Cortex, 2,* 277–292.

Shankweiler, D., Harris, K. S., & Taylor, M. L. 1968. Electromyographic studies of articulation in aphasia. *Archives of Physical Medicine and Rehabilitation, 48,* 1–8.

Stookey, B. 1963. Jean-Baptiste Bouillaud and Ernest Auburtin: Early studies on cerebral localization and the speech center. *Journal of the American Medical Association, 184,* 1024–1029.

Taylor, J. (Ed.). 1931. *Selected writings of John Hughlings Jackson* (Vols. 1 and 2). London: Hodder & Stoughton.

Trost, J., & Canter, G. 1974. Apraxia of speech in patients with Broca's aphasia: A study of phoneme production accuracy and error patterns. *Brain and Language, 1,* 63–80.

von Bonin, G. (Ed.) 1960. *Some papers on the cerebral cortex.* Springfield, Ill.: Thomas.

Wernicke, C. 1977. [The aphasia symptom-complex: A psychological study on an anatomical basis.] In G. Eggert (Ed. and trans.), *Wernicke's works on aphasia: A source-book and review.* The Hague: Mouton. (Originally published, 1874.)

Whitaker, H. A. 1975. *Levels of impairment in disorders of speech.* Paper presented at the VIIIth International Congress of Phonetic Sciences. Leeds, England.

Young, R. M. 1970. *Mind, brain and adaptation in the nineteenth century.* Oxford: Oxford Univ. Press.

10

Aphasia-Related Disorders

EDITH KAPLAN and HAROLD GOODGLASS

Aphasic disturbances of production and comprehension of spoken language are usually associated with a disruption in the encoding and decoding of written language (agraphia and alexia). In addition, disorders of gestural representation (apraxia), calculation (acalculia), right–left orientation, finger localization, and visuospatial construction ability are commonly associated with aphasia. These functions may be impaired in isolation or in selective clusters as a function of the locus, extent, and etiology of lesion of the dominant hemisphere. The severity of the dysfunction may depend on such variables as the patient's handedness, history of familial sinistrality, and premorbid capacity. Obviously a careful delineation of the nature and extent of these deficits will contribute to diagnosis and to inferences concerning localization. Equally important, such an evaluation will have impact on the choice of appropriate interventions (e.g., language and cognitive therapies) and considerations for vocational rehabilitation.

The following sections of this chapter review each of the disorders listed in the preceding paragraph, their neuroanatomic substrates and their characteristic presentation in the adult with damage to the left hemisphere.

Reading Disturbances

Reading rarely escapes unscathed in any form of aphasia, except in the relatively rare cases of PURE WORD DEAFNESS and APHEMIA. While the severity and character of reading disorders show some systematic rela-

303

tionship to lesion site and to the form of the oral language disorder, this relationship is considerably less predictable than is the case for the speech pattern. For example, while Broca's aphasics characteristically comprehend written language much better than they produce it, some of them are severely impaired in reading. Thus, it appears most profitable to describe reading disturbances in relation to the components of the reading process and refer incidentally to the predominant association of particular features with a standard syndrome. An exception will be made in the case of parietal alexia and agraphia and pure word blindness—disorders in which written language is selectively disturbed.

The reading process is obviously founded on the ability to perceive and discriminate the elementary components of the written code and to recognize their class membership as letters, words, or numerals. Loss of such recognition capacity may be regarded as a prelinguistic disorder, belonging in the category of visual agnosia. Disorders at this level are usually associated with impaired recognition of visual stimuli of other types, including objects and faces, and need not be associated with aphasia.

Assuming the integrity of this basic recognition capacity, there are a number of elementary processes that are probably operating concurrently in the process of word recognition. These are (*a*) the appreciation of the individual identity of the letters of the alphabet and the appreciation of their equivalent across styles of print and handwriting; (*b*) the ability to apply graphophonemic conversion rules so that sequences of letters are mapped by their phonological value onto an integrated sound sequence; (*c*) the association of written letter sequence, as a whole, to the total phonological representation of a word; (*d*) the direct association of a concept to a written word, without phonological mediation.

While there has been considerable controversy among reading theorists as to the relative role of each of these components in normal reading, it is easy to demonstrate that both graphophonemic conversion and direct phonological access must operate exclusively at certain points. The former process is the only means by which nonsense syllables or novel names can be sounded. The latter is the only means by which such forms as *lbs.* and *Mrs.* can be read aloud, and it probably applies as well to irregularly spelled words like *Worcester* and *reign*.

Beyond the one-word level, there is now evidence both from normal readers (Bradley, Garrett, & Zurif, 1980) and aphasics (Saffran, Bogyo, Schwartz, & Marin, 1980) that the reading of lexical words (i.e., those that refer to a semantic concept) uses a different mechanism from the reading of grammatical morphemes, and, as we will see, aphasia may produce a total dissociation between these two mechanisms. The preservation of these two different and parallel reading capacities is probably related to the ability to understand, not only isolated lexical terms, but the syntactic relationships among words in a sentence. Here, again, we will see that aphasia may produce dissociations.

Finally, before examining the clinical features of the dyslexias, it is important to distinguish between oral and silent reading and possibly between both of these and reading comprehension. Certainly, oral reading may be quite dissociated from silent reading either because of impaired articulatory capacity or because of paraphasic intrusions.

Clinical Features

Reading Comprehension

Even global aphasics retain some ability to match letters and short familiar words across various forms of script—for example, upper- and lowercase print and longhand. Global aphasics and severe mixed aphasics who are unable to select individual words on oral request or on matching to pictures are often still able to find the one word in a group of four or five that does not belong to the same category as the remaining words (e.g., a flower name among a list of foods). The ability to match objects and actions to their pictures is usually preserved in Broca's and Wernicke's aphasia, and the completeness of the patients' recognition vocabulary parallels the severity of the aphasia; that is, words of low frequency are missed more often than are common words. Given the opportunity for semantically based errors, Wernicke's aphasics are more vulnerable than Broca's aphasics. Conduction aphasics and most anomic aphasics perform well on the one-word level. Some anomic aphasics, however, having lesions in the angular gyrus, show a profound reading disorder. Transcortical sensory aphasics, who repeat well without comprehending speech, commonly have an equally severe inability to understand writing—even single words.

Differences between aphasic subgroups become more marked for sentence comprehension, particularly where the understanding of the syntax is vital for disambiguating the sentence. Broca's aphasics have been shown (Caramazza & Zurif, 1976; Samuels & Benson, 1979; Stockert & Bader, 1976) to have difficulty in using the syntactic features effectively, although they understand the content words well. In contrast, Wernicke's aphasics are usually more severely impaired across the board in sentence comprehension. There are, however, exceptional patients with Wernicke's aphasia who perform well in reading at the sentence level. Conduction aphasics and most anomics (with the noted exception) also read sentences with fairly good comprehension.

Reading at the paragraph level and beyond is almost invariably slow and laborious for aphasics of all types, until and unless they attain a high degree of recovery in oral language, probably because of the verbal memory demands of longer sentences and paragraphs.

Reading of Grammatical Words

It is a frequent finding among Broca's and mixed aphasics that they have difficulty in both reading aloud and selecting from multiple choice the small grammatical words of the language (i.e., articles, prepositions, pronouns, forms of the copula, and auxiliary and modal verbs). Their difficulty with this group of high-frequency words contrasts with their success in reading content words of much lower frequency. Gardner and Zurif (1975) have documented the interesting fact that patients may correctly select or read aloud noun or verb homonyms of these grammatical words. For example, they may read *bee* but not *be, hymn* but not *him, buy* but not *by.* This difficulty may or may not be associated with agrammatism in oral language. It is dramatically prominent in the disorder called DEEP DYSLEXIA, described later.

Oral Reading

Oral reading, much more than silent reading, parallels the pattern of spoken language. Thus, Broca's aphasics who are agrammatic in speech are most likely to read nouns and principal verbs correctly but omit or misread the small words of grammar. Their errors on content words usually involve partial application of graphophonemic rules; that is, word substitutions are usually based on similarity of the first portion of the word, while semantic substitutions are uncommon.

In contrast, many Wernicke's aphasics may read aloud as paraphasically as they speak, making semantic substitutions for both content and grammatical words.

Similarly, conduction aphasics' oral reading is usually marked by literal paraphasic errors parallel to those of their speech. Anomic aphasics (with the exception of those with parietal alexia) read well orally. Paradoxically, good oral reading is often observed in transcortical sensory aphasics, who may read aloud without comprehension much as they repeat without comprehension.

Literal Alexia

LITERAL ALEXIA, which would more accurately be termed LETTER ANOMIA, refers to the inability to name letters of the alphabet on sight in the presence of successful word reading. It is most frequently seen in Broca's aphasics (Albert, 1979).

Deep Dyslexia

Marshall and Newcombe (1966) first described a configuration of symptoms in which their patient's oral reading of lexical words was frequently paralexic—for example, *child* read as *girl*, *wed* as *marry*, *air* as *fly*, *listen* as *quiet*. In addition to semantic substitutions, like the foregoing, there were many derivational errors (*direction* for *directing*) and visual errors (*terror* for *error*). Grammatical morphemes were either totally omitted or misread with a different and irrelevant function word (e.g., *you* for *an*). The patients are totally unable to appreciate the phonic values of written letters, so that they cannot detect homonyms (e.g., *pail* and *pale*) or rhymes using different spelling (e.g., *fight* and *kite*), nor can they select nonsense words. The term DEEP DYSLEXIA referred to the fact the patients went directly to the semantic value of the word from its printed form, without any appreciation of its sound. The same disorder has been described by Shallice and Warrington (1975) with the term PHONEMIC DYSLEXIA and by Andrewsky and Seron (1975), M. F. Schwartz, Saffran, & Marin (1977), and Patterson and Marcel (1977). The two central problems are that these patients can neither use graphophonemic recoding nor access the phonology of a word directly. Their oral reading is not really reading in the normal sense. That is, they derive a semantic impression from the written form and apply a spoken word to this meaning that may or may not correspond exactly to the written word. Since grammatical morphemes have no semantic referent, they cannot be dealt with at all by this information processing route.

While the full syndrome of deep dyslexia is relatively uncommon, many of its components are encountered in aphasics of all types but most frequently in patients with the speech pattern of Broca's aphasia with agrammatism.

Pure Word Blindness (Alexia without Agraphia)

Dejerine (1892) described the syndrome in which the ability to recognize words was lost, while writing and oral language were unaffected. The lesion most commonly responsible for this syndrome has been confirmed repeatedly (Brissaud, 1900; Geschwind & Fusillo, 1966; Poetzl, 1928; Redlich, 1895; Vincent, David, & Puech, 1930). It involves the splenium of the corpus callosum, the left visual cortex, and lingual gyrus. This lesion, usually produced by occlusion of the posterior cerebral artery, deprives the language zone of the left hemisphere of all visual input, from both the left and right hemispheres. The ability to recognize words is severely impaired; recognition of numbers and letters is sometimes preserved. In these instances, patients can read laboriously through letter-by-letter spelling. A distinctive feature of alexia without agraphia is that patients understand orally spelled words perfectly, as well as letters and words traced on their palms. In many instances, this disorder is accompanied by difficulty in naming and understanding color names and by a short-term memory disorder.

Alexia with Agraphia

ALEXIA WITH AGRAPHIA has also been called PARIETAL ALEXIA (Hermann & Poetzl, 1926; Hoff, Gloning, & Gloning, 1954) and VISUAL ASYMBOLIA (Brain, 1961). Impairment in reading and writing commonly co-occurs with the fluent aphasias (PARIETAL-TEMPORAL APHASIA, Benson, 1979), particularly in Wernicke's aphasia, which has been described earlier. However, alexia with agraphia may occur in relative isolation from aphasia. Dejerine (1891) described a patient with a profound alexia and agraphia that persisted to his death despite the clearing of a mild aphasia. At postmortem the responsible deep vascular lesion involved most of the left angular gyrus. Subsequent reports confirm this localization (Benson & Geschwind, 1969).

Since the inferior portion of the angular gyrus is located in the posterior temporal region and the inferior portion of the parietal region, it is not surprising to find an associated anomia with inferior angular gyrus involvement and some or all of the components of the Gerstmann syndrome (agraphia, acalculia, right–left disorientation, and finger agnosia) as well as some visuospatial constructional difficulty.

Most patients with alexia and agraphia are incapable of either spelling aloud or comprehending spelled words. A number of cases of alexia with agraphia and preserved ability to spell and comprehend spelling have been reported (Albert, Yamadori, Gardner, & Howes, 1973; Dejerine & Andre-Thomas, 1904; Kinsbourne & Rosenfield, 1974; Mohr, 1976; Rothi & Heilman, 1981). Rothi and Heilman propose that underlying the alexia and agraphia, at least in their case, was an inability to transcode between the auditory–verbal and visual–graphic codes. The alternative strategy employed by their patient was to name the letters. They argue that there may be at least three reading strategies: (*a*) a visual code analysis (letter naming); (*b*) a whole word pattern analysis; and (*c*) grapheme–phoneme conversion. Identifying the strategy available to the patient could then more effectively direct the therapeutic approach.

Disorders of Writing (Agraphia)

Writing, like reading, is almost always impaired in aphasia, although the specific form of the writing disorder tends to show some parallels with oral language, particularly with respect to the presence of word-finding disorders, paraphasia, and agrammatism. These parallels are most easily seen in Broca's and Wernicke's aphasias.

Writing in Broca's Aphasia

Writing is usually severely impaired in Broca's aphasia. The poor motor control of the nonpreferred hand (in the presence of right hemiplegia) is not sufficient to account for the degree of awkwardness (Heilman, 1975). Block printing is more common than cursive writing. Letters are oversized, there are letter reversals, and words are misspelled through omission and substitution of letters (literal paragraphia). Recovery of writing may parallel that of speech and in these cases shows the same features of agrammatism, preponderance of substantives, and reduced output (Goodglass & Hunter, 1970). Impaired writing usually persists as the most severe residual (Kertesz, 1979).

Writing in Wernicke's Aphasia

Wernicke's aphasics usually execute the mechanics of writing easily with their dominant hand—in cursive style, with well-formed letters—showing an analogy to their facile articulation of speech. Moreover, their writing shows the same propensity for semantic paraphasia, neologistic jargon, and paragrammatic sentence forms as does their speech. It is, however, reduced in speed and quantity from normal levels. The narrative writing of Wernicke's aphasics has shorter runs of grammatically coherent words than does their speech. At the same time, the repetitious use of low-information verbs and vague nouns is reduced in their writing as compared to their speech (Goodglass & Hunter, 1970).

Parietal Agraphia

The agraphic component of alexia with agraphia may be so severe as to appear to be an apraxic disorder in forming letters (Marcie & Hécaen, 1979). However, it is not simply an impairment of motor execution, as these patients are severely impaired in spelling. In milder instances of this disorder, however, it is apparent that these patients can form grammatically correct sentences.

Pure Agraphia

Reports of isolated agraphia are sparse, and there is little consensus as to a lesion site. Exner (1881) postulated a writing center at the foot of the second frontal gyrus, separate from Broca's area. Other reports of pure agraphia (Assal, Chapuis, & Zander, 1970; Henschen, 1922; Mahoudeau, 1950; Mahoudeau, David, & Lecoeur, 1951; Morselli, 1930; Sinico, 1926; Wernicke, 1903) support a frontal localization. Penfield and Roberts (1959) observed transient agraphia following surgical excision of F2 and F3. Other investigators support a parietal locus (Kinsbourne & Rosenfeld, 1974), while a number accept a frontal and posterior localization and maintain that there are two forms of the defect, one a grapheme selection disorder and the other a spatiotemporal disorganization specific to writing (Dubois, Hécaen, & Marcie, 1969).

The demonstrated existence of cases of pure agraphia, as well as dissociations between severity of written and spoken language, argues for a functional autonomy between written and oral codes (Marcie & Hécaen, 1979). This is further supported by the less frequent association of writing disorders with deficits in oral language in left handers.

Rosati and De Bastiani (1979) consider the pure agraphia in their patient with a vascular lesion in the language zone (perisylvian region of the left hemisphere) to represent a discrete form of aphasia. However, Chedru and Geschwind (1972) do not accept pure writing disturbances as a specific language encoding disorder, but rather propose that writing is susceptible to influences from a wide variety of pathophysiological processes. In the absence of other language disorders, they noted writing to deteriorate to senseless scrawls in confusional states.

Acalculia

In 1919, Henschen introduced the term ACALCULIA to designate an acquired calculation disorder distinct from an aphasic inability to read and write numbers. Prior to Henschen, there had been a number of case reports of acquired impairment of calculation overshadowing other co-occurring impairments. Lewandowsky and Stadelman (1908) described a patient who could read and write numbers but was severely impaired in the simplest of oral arithmetic problems. In this patient all other language functions were spared except for increased latency in word finding and an inability to write words spelled aloud. The responsible lesion was a hematoma in the left occipital lobe (surgically removed), which led Lewandowsky and Stadelman to attribute this relatively isolated deficit to a specific disorder in the optic representation of numbers. Peritz (1918) proposed the left angular gyrus as the center for calculation, a localization supported by Henschen.

Hans Berger (1926) described three cases of acalculia with dominant hemisphere lesions that did NOT involve the angular gyrus (two occipital and one temporal). These "pure" cases (PRIMARY ACALCULIA) were distinct from SECONDARY ACALCULIA, that is, calculation disturbances resulting from problems in attention, memory, language (aphasia, alexia, agraphia), or general cognitive functioning. Obviously, secondary acalculia would therefore occur more frequently than pure or primary acalculia.

The co-occurrence of severe constructional difficulties noted in some cases (e.g., Singer & Low, 1933) led some investigators to consider the role of a spatial component (Critchley, 1953).

In 1961, Hécaen, Angelergues, and Houillier proposed the following classification based on a study of 183 acalculic patients with retrorolandic lesions:

1. Digit alexia and agraphia that may or may not be accompanied by an aphasia, alexia, and/or agraphia. In this type, the paralexic substitutions for presented numbers (stimuli) and the paragraphic errors during computation (response) preclude a correct answer. Benson and Denckla (1969) demonstrated intact computational ability in two patients with digit alexia and agraphia by presenting multiple-choice solutions for arithmetic problems that had been originally "solved" incorrectly.

2. Spatial acalculia—that is, incorrect solutions that result from misalignment of numbers, misordered numbers, number reversals, directional confusion, visual neglect, or oculomotor disturbances. Here, too, basic computational skills may or may not be demonstrated to be intact.

3. Anarithmetia is a fundamental, primary impairment of calculation. This does not imply an isolated impairment but rather one that does not have as its source an alexia or agraphia for numbers or a spatial organizational problem.

Of these three types of acalculia, digit alexia and agraphia and anarithmetia were found to occur predominantly with left hemisphere lesions, whereas spatial acalculia rarely occurred with left hemisphere lesions (10%) but occurred in 73.3% of right-hemisphere-lesioned patients (Hécaen & Angelergues, 1961).

Within each hemisphere, varieties of acalculic problems have been identified in virtually all regions of the brain (Grewel, 1969). Some of this variability in lesion loci has been attributed to premorbid individual differences in processing mathematical problems (Leonhard, 1979) involving different neural substrates. Conversely, the nature and severity of the calculation disorder is obviously, in good measure, determined by the specific dysfunctions referable to different lesion loci, which in turn have differential impact on various aspects of the complex function of calculation (Benson & Weir, 1972; Cohn, 1961; Gerstmann, 1940; Hécaen *et al.*, 1961). Further, the complexity of calculation may be impaired differentially as a function of the modality of presentation, modality of response (Benton, 1963), and the nature and number of operations involved. As Boller and Grafman (1980) and Levin (1979) concluded in their reviews of the acalculias, the mechanisms of anarithmetia and its regional localization require further study.

Taking the lead from Benton (1963) and Boller and Hécaen (1979), a calculation test battery could be developed that (*a*) establishes the integrity of number recognition, number reading, writing, memory span, and spatial organization; (*b*) evaluates appreciation of number values (e.g., which of two numbers is greater), number concepts, etc.; (*c*) permits a detailed analysis of stimulus parameters and modality of presentation and response; (*d*) involves a qualitative analysis of errors. Finally, a profile of spared and impaired aspects of calculation functions on a background of spared and impaired language and general neuropsychological functioning could provide insights for the development of intervention strategies.

Finger Agnosia

The inability to recognize or otherwise identify fingers on both of one's own hands, on those of the examiner, or on model hands was considered by Gerstmann (1924) to be a consequence of a more general disturbance of the body schema and attributable to a lesion in the parieto-occipital junction around the angular gyrus of the dominant hemisphere. It should be noted that the severity of the impairment in finger naming or comprehension overshadows an impairment in body-part identification in general.

As is the case in each of the specific disorders (e.g., alexia, agraphia, and acalculia described earlier), finger agnosia is manifested in a variety of ways. Schilder (1931) distinguished a finger aphasia, an optic finger agnosia, and a constructive finger apraxia. Performance may be impaired as a function of modality of presentation or response, that is, whether the modality of stimulation is auditory, visual, or tactile and the response verbal or nonverbal (Benton, 1959; Critchley, 1966; Ettlinger, 1963). Correlational studies (Matthews, Folk, & Zerfas, 1966; Poeck & Orgass, 1969; Sauguet, Benton, & Hécaen, 1971) indicate that tasks involving verbal aspects of finger identification correlate with verbal IQ and are highly associated with receptive aphasic disorders; tasks involving nonverbal aspects of finger recognition correlate more highly with performance IQ than verbal IQ and were also associated with a receptive aphasia. Though nonverbal finger recognition was found to be impaired in left (18%) and right (16%) hemisphere lesions, most of the left-hemisphere-damaged patients showed evidence of either an aphasia or general mental impairment (Gainotti, Cianchetti, & Tiacci, 1972).

Finger agnosia rarely occurs as an isolated finding. Gerstmann (1924) suggested that finger agnosia is the primary deficit in a cluster of symptoms (agraphia, acalculia, and right–left disorientation). This tetrad of symptoms, known as the Gerstmann syndrome, will be discussed later.

In a study of nine patients with nonverbal impairment in finger identification, Kinsbourne and Warrington (1962) found a high degree of association with visuoconstructive disorders. Schilder (1935) similarly had reported the frequency of co-occurrence of such constructional defects as drawings (especially of face and hands in the human drawings). Gerstmann (1940) as well recognized the frequency of co-occurrence of a CONSTRUCTIONAL APRAXIA. Goodglass and Kaplan (1972) found finger agnosia to correlate best with arithmetic (.58), three-dimensional block constructions (.52), and stick construction (.52) and a general loading of .74 with a parietal lobe factor.

Right–Left Disorientation

The inability to identify the right and left sides of one's own body, as well as those of another person, vis-à-vis has been long recognized to occur with lesions lateralized to the left hemisphere and in the presence of an aphasia (Bonhoeffer, 1923; Head, 1926). Like finger agnosia, right–

left disorientation may be selectively impaired as a function of the modality of stimulus and the required response. Verbal tasks (e.g., naming, responding to verbal command) and nonverbal tasks (e.g., imitation) should be studied separately, as should tasks of varying levels of complexity, such as identifying single lateralized parts on one's own body, executing double uncrossed and crossed commands on one's own body (e.g., uncrossed—touching RIGHT eye with RIGHT hand; crossed— touching right eye with left hand), and pointing to parts of the examiner's body (Dennis, 1976; Sauguet, Benton, & Hécaen, 1971).

Head (1926) and McFie and Zangwill (1960) attribute verbal and non-verbal (imitation) impairment in right–left orientation to a left hemisphere lesion and an associated aphasia. Sauguet, Benton, and Hécaen (1971) support this lateralization for orientation only to one's own body. They found imitation of lateral movements to occur in 38% of patients with right-hemisphere-disease as contrasted with 48% of aphasic patients. Luria (1966) considered the inability of patients with frontal pathology to make reversals on the examiner—that is, identifying the RIGHT side of the examiner as the LEFT side (especially on tasks of imitation)—as echopraxic. Benton (1979) views such errors as conceptual, that is, an inability to understand the relativistic nature of the right–left concept.

Tests of right–left discrimination in extrapersonal space, such as the Road Map Test (Money, 1965), make greater demands on visuospatial functions and are as demanding for right as for left-hemisphere-lesioned patients. Again, right–left disorientation is immediately related to the demands of the test. As is the case in acalculia and finger localization (described earlier), the complexity of the task requires sensitive sorting out of the components that may be selectively impaired as a function of the lesion site.

The Gerstmann Syndrome

The tetrad of symptoms described in the preceding sections— agraphia, acalculia, finger agnosia, and right–left disorientation—were as a complex assumed to represent a distinct neuropsychological syndrome (Gerstmann, 1930). Gerstmann assumed that finger identification is central to the development of calculation. Strauss and Werner (1938) demonstrated a definite relationship between the ability to articulate the fingers and the early development of the number concept. Finger localization and calculation are presumed to be precursors of right–left orientation and the ability to write. In addition to the prominence of this cluster of symptoms, Gerstmann noted cases with constructional problems, word-finding difficulty, mild reading difficulty, color naming problems, and/or absence of optokinetic nystagmus. The presence of any or all of these associated problems constitute a secondary syndrome implicating more extensive involvement of the parieto-occipital junction of the left hemisphere. The sudden appearance of either the primary or secondary syndrome has been associated with space occupying lesions. Kertesz (1979) identified 9 out of 556 aphasics and controls who were observed to have the four components of the syndrome distinct from other deficits. Seven of the 9 cases had a left parieto-occipital lesion, 1 had bilateral lesions, and 1 was a trauma and had a negative scan.

The infrequent occurrence of the specific tetrad of Gerstmann, and the greater frequency of the symptoms occurring separately (Heimburger, Demeyer, & Reitan, 1964), has raised the question of the existence of this syndrome. In 1961, Benton addressed this question in his paper entitled "The Fiction of the 'Gerstmann Syndrome'." He concluded, as did Poeck and Orgass (1975), that the intercorrelations between the four elements of the Gerstmann syndrome were not any greater than correlations between any one element of the syndrome and defects not included in the syndrome. Strub and Geschwind (1974), on the other hand, argue that the infrequency of occurrence of a specific combination of symptoms is what clinically defines a syndrome. For those who accept the entity of the Gerstmann syndrome, it serves to localize the lesion to the parieto-occipital region of the left hemisphere.

There have been a number of reports of a developmental Gerstmann syndrome. Benson and Geschwind (1970) reported two cases of good readers with the tetrad of symptoms along with contructional difficulties. Rourke and Strang (1978) found children referred to a clinic for deficient calculating ability demonstrated a pattern of deficits analogous to the Gerstmann syndrome—that is, problems in arithmetic, right–left orientation, writing, and finger gnosis—while reading was found to be at or above expected grade level. J. Schwartz, Kaplan, and A. Schwartz (1981) examined school records of 1438 fifth and sixth grade children and identified 22 dyscalculic students (1% of the population). The following seven tests were administered: finger gnosis, right–left orientation, Money Road Map Test, block design subtest of the Wechsler Intelligence Scale for Children–Revised, Rey–Osterrieth Complex Figure, visual reproduction subtest of the Wechsler Memory Scale, and the Wide Range Achievement spelling subtest. Ten of the 22 children (45% of the dyscalculic population) were found to have all the components of the Gerstmann syndrome and in addition (as in Rourke's population) had constructional difficulties. Qualitative analysis of their strategies and errors suggested greater compromise of RIGHT hemispheric functions than was the case in either the 12 dyscalculic children who had no evidence of finger agnosia or the nondyscalculic normal matched peer group. It is of interest that the spelling errors of the Gerstmann group in this study as well as in the Rourke study were predominantly phonemic. It would appear then that there is a developmental Gerstmann syndrome, but that, unlike in the adults, it does not indicate left hemisphere dysfunction.

Constructional Disorders

Impaired performance in producing drawings or geometric configurations is frequently referred to as constructional apraxia. However, the original conception (Kleist, 1912) was reserved for those faulty productions that were NOT the result of either impaired visual or motor executive function but rather a defect in the TRANSMISSION of the visual information to the motor system. The early descriptions (Kleist, 1912; Poppelreuter, 1914–1917) implied this disconnection mechanism. Current use of the term CONSTRUCTIONAL APRAXIA no longer reflects the original presumed underlying mechanism. For some investigators (e.g., Arrigoni & De Renzi, 1964; Piercy & Smith, 1962), constructional disorders following left and right hemisphere lesions reflect the same basic disturbance except that it is more frequent and more severe in right hemisphere than left hemisphere lesions. They may reflect larger right hemisphere lesions, since left hemisphere lesions probably come to the attention of a physician earlier because of the associated aphasic symptoms.

Benton (1969) demonstrated differences as a function of the nature of the constructional task (e.g., drawing, assembling) and concluded that constructional difficulty does not represent a unitary disorder.

During the last two decades, a number of investigators have observed distinctive lateralized differences in the quality of performance. Warrington, James, and Kinsbourne (1966) and Hécaen and Assal (1970) demonstrated that left-hemisphere-lesioned patients improve with practice, whereas right-hemisphere-lesioned patients worsen with practice. Left-hemisphere-lesioned patients produce more right angles than are given in drawing a cube; right-hemisphere-lesioned patients underestimate angles in a star; left-lesioned patients overestimate angles. In drawings right-hemisphere-damaged patients show a tendency to oversketch, produce more lines and more details, whereas left-hemisphere-lesioned patients tend to simplify drawings and delete details. Inattention to the left side of space is far more characteristic of right-hemisphere-lesioned patients.

Block design constructions (subtest of the Wechsler Adult Intelligence Scale) are performed poorly but qualitatively differently by patients with lesions lateralized to opposite hemispheres. A study by Kaplan (1980) found that patients with focal lesions tend to begin working on a block design in the hemiattentional field contralateral to the noncompromised hemisphere; that is, left-lesioned patients work significantly more often from left to right, whereas right-hemisphere-lesioned patients work significantly more often from right to left. Errors enroute to a final solution as well as in the final product are more prevalent in the hemiattentional field contralateral to the lesioned hemisphere; that is, left-hemisphere-lesioned patients make significantly more errors on the right side of the designs, and patients with right hemisphere lesions make significantly more errors on the left side.

The tendency for right-hemisphere-lesioned patients to use a piecemeal approach (Paterson & Zangwill, 1944) without integrating component parts results in a remarkable inability to maintain the 2 × 2 or 3 × 3 matrix (broken configuration). Broken configurations evident in productions of right-hemisphere-damaged patients were virtually absent in the productions of left-hemisphere-lesioned patients. Hemispheric differences were also noted in drawings (e.g., Wechsler memory visual reproductions, Rey–Osterrieth Complex Figure). Patients with left hemisphere lesions were noted to deal more effectively with contour information than with internal features or details, whereas the reverse obtained for patients with right hemisphere lesions.

Once again, qualitative analyses of the strategies that patients spontaneously use to compensate for their deficits, along with stimulus parameters that induce or preclude such behaviors, have the potential for contributing to the development of both materials and approaches for therapeutic interventions.

Apraxia: Disorders of Gestural Behavior

Liepmann (1908) defined apraxia as a disorder of the execution of learned movement that is not due to motor or sensory defects, poor comprehension, or intellectual deterioration. The responsible lesion always involves the corpus callosum either where the fibers arise from cells in the left hemisphere or by direct destruction of the corpus callosum itself. (Lesions in the right frontal lobe destroying the callosal fibers toward the premotor region have a similar effect as a midcallosal lesion.) Geschwind (1965, 1975) describes the consequences of a premotor and a callosal lesion as follows: An auditory command to perform a movement, such as *Show me how you would brush your teeth with a toothbrush*, is comprehended in Wernicke's area; however, destruction of the premotor area necessary to program and initiate the movement precludes performance with either the right hand or left hand since the information has no way of getting to the right premotor area either. Patients with a midcallosal lesion, as in the case of Geschwind and Kaplan (1962) and Gazzaniga, Bogen, and Sperry (1967), are capable of performing the movement with the right hand (left premotor region is intact) but are incapable of performing it with the left hand since the fiber tract from the left premotor to the right premotor region is destroyed. Another disconnecting lesion occurs in the left arcuate fasciculus. Here the lesion in the fiber tract deep to the parietal lobe connecting Wernicke's area to the premotor area precludes the decoded command from reaching the premotor area (as well as resulting in a conduction aphasia). Liepmann's attribution of motor programming to the dominant hemisphere for handedness as well as the earlier localization of language to the left hemisphere (in right-handed individuals) by Broca (1861) and Wernicke (1908) explain the frequent co-occurrence of apraxia with an aphasia. Despite this earlier work, Goldstein (1948) argued for a central communication disorder. Patients who could not communicate orally or in writing also could not use the gestural channel. Goodglass and Kaplan (1963) tested the notion of a central communicative disorder. The finding that the severity of aphasia did not correlate with the severity of the gestural disturbance argued against a central communication disorder.[1] Further, the finding that the inability to imitate the gestures demonstrated by the examiner supported Liepmann's position that the aphasic's gestural deficit represented an apraxic disorder. Body part as object (e.g., the use of a body part to represent an absent implement, such as using the index finger as if it were a toothbrush and then vigorously rubbing teeth with the index finger) was commonly noted in the apraxic aphasic and was later found by Kaplan (1968) to be a characteristic response of 4-year-old normal children. In her developmental study, a distinct developmental progression was noted in the acquisition of gestural representation of absent implements. Using the example of representing brushing teeth with a toothbrush,

---

1. Pickett (1974), using the Porch Index of Communicative Ability (PICA) and 10 commonly used objects in addition to the 10 items used in the PICA, concluded that gestural ability is related to severity of aphasia rather than to a limb apraxia.

young children between 2½ and 4 years rely on deictic behavior (pointing to the locus of the action, e.g., pointing to the mouth) and manipulation of the object of the action (rubbing the teeth). At age 4, body part as object is the most characteristic mode of representation. By age 8, the children are pretending to hold the absent implement, but the movement is too close to the object of the action (e.g., the teeth) and may degrade into a body part as object. By age 12, children are performing like adults, pretending to hold the implement and utilizing empty space to represent the extent of the implement. It may be inferred that the use of body part as object is employed by apraxic patients to circumvent their difficulty in positioning the hand and reproducing the movement veridically. Gestural representation in dementing patients, in intellectually inferior adults, or in the elderly tends toward more concrete representation and the use of body part as object as in the immature child.

Thus far we have discussed impairment of limb movements to command. Patients with arcuate fasciculus lesions as well as left premotor lesions will have similar difficulty carrying out buccofacial movements.

In all apraxic patients, there is a relatively spared class of movements, axial or whole body movements (e.g., stand up, turn around twice, and sit down). Geschwind (1975) suggests that axial movements are controlled by nonpyramidal systems arising from multiple regions in the cortex, whereas the pyramidal systems controlling unilateral movements arise primarily from the precentral gyrus.

Finally in support of Liepmann's proposition that praxis is localized to the hemisphere dominant for handedness, we may cite a case report by Heilman, Coyle, Gonyea, and Geschwind (1973). Their patient was left handed and sustained damage to his motor and premotor region of the right hemisphere. He sustained left-sided hemiparesis WITHOUT an aphasia and a severe apraxia involving the right limb; though this patient's intact left hemisphere was obviously dominant for language, he was apraxic secondary to the lesion of the right hemisphere (dominant for handedness). This case dramatically supports the separate functions of language and praxis and argues for their co-occurrence in aphasia as a result of the proximity of structures affected by one lesion.

Thus far we have focused on the issue of production of gesture and pantomime to verbal command. The role of a general symbolic disturbance underlying COMPREHENSION of symbolic gestures and pantomime has been separately addressed. Duffy, Duffy, and Pearson (1975) found pantomime recognition to be significantly correlated with auditory comprehension, naming ability, and overall linguistic competence and argued for the concept of a central communicative disorder. Opposing this view are the findings of Zangwill (1964) and Alajouanine and Lhermitte

(1964), who support the prevalence of defective pantomime recognition in aphasics but not a correlation with the severity of the aphasia. Gainotti and Lemmo (1976) found a high degree of relationship between the comprehension of symbolic gestures and semantic errors on a verbal comprehension test. Though it was again clear that understanding symbolic gestures was more impaired in aphasics than in other brain-damaged patients, there was a minimal relationship between comprehension and production of symbolic gestures (a finding contrary to Duffy, Duffy, & Pearson, 1975). Finally, Varney (1978) found deficits in pantomime recognition always co-occurred with reading deficit (but not vice versa). Pantomime recognition was found to be only weakly associated with auditory comprehension and naming ability. Varney concludes along with Vignolo (1969) that the possibility of modality-specific factors may underlie the relationships that have been obtained (in this study, the visual modality).

Despite severe inability to engage in gestural representation to verbal command, apraxic patients perform relatively well in the context of real action with implements. (Heilman, 1975, reports some clumsiness in the use of the nonpreferred limb.) Further, global aphasic, apraxic patients have been demonstrated to have the capacity to use nonorthographic visual stimuli for comprehension as well as for communication (Gardner, Zurif, Berry, & Baker, 1976; Glass, Gazzaniga, & Premack, 1973). Helm-Estabrooks, Fitzpatrick, and Barresi (unpublished manuscript), guided by this body of evidence, developed a therapeutic program (visual action therapy). Beginning with actual utilization of the implement, global aphasics were trained to produce symbolic gestures to represent absent stimuli. On pre–post testing, these patients showed significant improvement on PICA pantomime and auditory comprehension subtests. The results of this study hold promise for therapeutic intervention in apraxic aphasic patients.

Acknowledgment

This work was supported in part by the Medical Research Service of the Veterans Administration and in part by USPH Grants NS 07615 and 06209. The authors also wish to thank Anne Foundas and Cheryl Weinstein for their assistance in the preparation of the manuscript.

References

Alajouanine, T., & Lhermitte, F. 1964. Non-verbal communication in aphasia. In A. De Reuck & M. O'Connor (Eds.), *Disorders of language.* Boston: Little, Brown.

Albert, M. L. 1979. Alexia. In K. M. Heilman & E. Valenstein (Eds.), *Clinical neuropsychology*. New York: Oxford Univ. Press.

Albert, M. L., Yamadori, A., Gardner, H., & Howes, D. 1973. Comprehension in alexia. *Brain, 96,* 317–328.

Andrewsky, E., & Seron, S. 1975. Implicit processing of grammatical rules in a case of agrammatism. *Cortex, 11,* 379–390.

Arrigoni, G., & De Renzi, E. 1964. Constructional apraxia and hemispheric locus of lesion. *Cortex, 1,* 170–197.

Assal, G., Chapuis, G., & Zander, E. 1970. Isolated writing disorders in a patient with stenosis of the left internal carotid artery. *Cortex, 6,* 241–248.

Benson, D. F. 1979. *Aphasia, alexia, and agraphia*. New York: Churchill Livingstone.

Benson, D. F., & Denkla, M. B. 1969. Verbal paraphasia as a cause of calculation disturbances. *Archives of Neurology, 21,* 96–102.

Benson, D. F., & Geschwind, N. 1969. The alexias. In P. J. Vinken & G. W. Bruyn (Eds.), *Handbook of clinical neurology: Disorders of speech, perception, and symbolic behavior*. New York: Amer. Elsevier.

Benson, D. F., & Geschwind, N. 1970. Developmental Gerstmann syndrome. *Neurology, 20,* 293–298.

Benson, D. F., & Weir, W. F. 1972. Acalculia: Acquired anarithmetia. *Cortex, 8,* 465–472.

Benton, A. L. 1959. *Right–left discrimination and finger localization: development and pathology*. New York: Harper (Hoeber).

Benton, A. L. 1961. The fiction of the "Gerstmann syndrome." *Journal of Neurology, Neurosurgery, and Psychiatry, 24,* 176–181.

Benton, A. L. 1963. *Assessment of number operations*. Iowa City: University of Iowa Hospital, Department of Neurology.

Benton, A. L. 1969. Constructional apraxia: Some unanswered questions. In A. L. Benton (Ed.), *Contributions to clinical neuropsychology*. Chicago: Aldine.

Berger, H. 1926. Ueber Rechenstorungen bei Herderkran Kungen des Grosshirns. *Archiv für Psychiatrie und Nervenkrankheiten, 78,* 238–263.

Boller, F., & Grafman, J. 1980. Acalculia: Historical development and current significance. Paper presented at Broca Centennial Conference, Mohonk, New York.

Boller, F., & Hécaen, H. 1979. L'évaluation des fonctions neuropsychologiques: Examen standard de l'unité de recherches neuropsychologiques et neurolinguistiques (Vol. 3) I.N.S.E.R.M. *Revue de Psychologie Appliquée, 29,* 247–266.

Bonhoeffer, K. 1923. Zur Klinik und Lokalization des Agrammatismus und der Rechts-links-desorientierung. *Monatsschrift für Psychiatrie und Neurologie, 54,* 11–42.

Bradley, D., Garrett, M., & Zurif, E. B. 1980. Syntactic deficits in Broca's Aphasia. In D. Caplan (Ed.), *Biological studies of mental processes*. Cambridge: MIT Press.

Brain, R. 1961. *Speech disorders*. London: Butterworth.

Brissaud, E. 1900. Cécité verbale sans aphasie ni agraphie. *Revue Neurologique, 8,* 757.

Broca, P. 1861. Perte de la parole. Ramollissement chronique et destruction partielle du lobe antérieur gauche du cerveau. *Bulletin de la Société de l'Anthropologie, 2,* 219.

Caramazza, A., & Zurif, E. B. 1976. Dissociation of algorithmic and heuristic processes in language comprehension: Evidence from aphasia. *Brain and Language, 3,* 572–582.

Chedru, F., & Geschwind, N. 1972. Writing disturbances in acute confusional states. *Neuropsychologia, 10,* 343–354.

Cohn, R. 1961. Dyscalculia. *Archives of Neurology, 4,* 301–307.

Critchley, M. 1953. *The parietal lobes*. New York: Hafner.

Critchley, M. 1966. The enigma of Gerstmann's syndrome. *Brain, 89,* 183–198.

Dejerine, J. 1891. Sur un cas de cécité verbal avec agraphie suivi d'autopsie. *Memoires de la Societé de Biologie, 3,* 197–201.

Dejerine, J. 1892. Contribution à l'étude anatomo-pathologique et clinique des différentes variété de cecité verbale. *Memoires de la Société de Biologie, 4,* 61–90.

Dejerine, J., & Andre-Thomas, J. 1904. Un cas de cécité verbale avec agraphie suivi d'autopsie. *Revue Neurologique, 12,* 655–664.

Dennis, M. 1976. Dissociated naming and locating of body parts after left temporal lobe resection. *Brain and Language, 3,* 147–163.

Dubois, J., Hécaen, H., & Marcie, P. 1969. L'agraphie "pure." *Neuropsychologia, 7,* 271–286.

Duffy, R., Duffy, J., & Pearson, K. 1975. Pantomime recognition in aphasic patients. *Journal of Speech and Hearing Disorders, 18,* 115–132.

Ettlinger, G. 1963. Defective identification of fingers. *Neuropsychologia, 1,* 39–45.

Exner, S. 1881. *Untersuchungen über die Lokalisation der Funktionen in der Grosshirnrinde des Menschen.* Vienna: Wilhelm Braumuller.

Gainotti, G., Cianchetti, C., & Tiacci, C. 1972. The influence of hemispheric side of lesion on nonverbal tests of finger localization. *Cortex, 8,* 364–381.

Gainotti, G., & Lemmo, M. A. 1976. Comprehension of symbolic gestures in aphasia. *Brain and Language, 3,* 451–460.

Gardner, H., & Zurif, E. B. 1975. Bee but not be: oral reading of single words in aphasia and alexia. *Neuropsychologia, 13,* 181–190.

Gardner, H., Zurif, E., Berry, T., & Baker, E. 1976. Visual communication in aphasia. *Neuropsychologia, 14,* 275–292.

Gazzaniga, M. S., Bogen, J. E., & Sperry, R. W. 1967. Dyspraxia following division of the cerebral commissures. *Archives of Neurology, 12,* 606–612.

Gerstmann, J. 1924. Fingeragnosie: Eine umschriebene Störung der Orientierung am eigenen Korper. *Wiener Klinische Wochenschrift, 37,* 1010–1012.

Gerstmann, J. 1930. Zur Symptomatologie der Hirnläsionen im Ubergangsgebiet der unteren Parietal und mittleren Occipitalwindung. *Nervenartz, 3,* 691–695.

Gerstmann, J. 1940. Syndrome of finger agnosia, disorientation for right and left, agraphia, and acalculia. *Archives of Neurology and Psychiatry, 44,* 398–408.

Geschwind, N. 1965. Disconnexion syndromes in animals and man. *Brain, 88,* 237–294, 585–644.

Geschwind, N. 1975. The apraxias: Neurological mechanisms of disorders of learned movement. *American Scientist, 63,* 188–195.

Geschwind, N., & Fusillo, M. 1966. Color naming defects in association with alexia. *Archives of Neurology, 15,* 137–146.

Geschwind, N., & Kaplan, E. 1962. A human deconnection syndrome. *Neurology, 10,* 675–685.

Glass, A. V., Gazzaniga, M. S., & Premack, D. 1973. Artificial language training in aphasia. *Neuropsychologia, 11,* 95–103.

Goldstein, K. 1948. *Language and language disturbances.* New York: Grune & Stratton.

Goodglass, H., & Hunter, M. A. 1970. Linguistic comparison of speech and writing in two types of aphasia. *Journal of Communication Disorders, 3,* 28–35.

Goodglass, H., & Kaplan, E. 1963. Disturbance of gesture and pantomime in aphasia. *Brain, 86,* 703–720.

Goodglass, H., & Kaplan, E. 1972. *Assessment of aphasia and related disorders.* Philadelphia: Lea & Febiger.

Grewel, F. 1969. The acalculias. In P. J. Vinken & G. W. Bruyn (Eds.), *Handbook of clinical neurology* (Vol. 4). New York: Elsevier.

Head, H. 1926. *Aphasia and kindred disorders of speech.* Cambridge, England: Cambridge Univ. Press.

Hécaen, H., & Angelergues, R. 1961. Etude anatomo-clinique de 280 cas de lésions rétro-rolandiques unilaterales des hémisphères cérébraux. *Encéphale, 6,* 533–562.
Hécaen, H., Angelergues, R., & Houillier, S. 1961. Les varietes cliniques des acalculies au cours des lesions retrorolandiques: Approche statistique du probleme. *Revue Neurologique, 105,* 85–103.
Hécaen, H., & Assal, G. 1970. A comparison of construction deficits following right and left hemispheric lesions. *Neuropsychologia, 8,* 289–304.
Heilman, K. M. 1975. A tapping test in apraxia. *Cortex, 11,* 259–263.
Heilman, K. M., Coyle, J. M., Gonyea, E. F., & Geschwind, N. 1973. Apraxia and agraphia in a left-hander. *Brain, 96,* 21–28.
Heimburger, R. F., Demeyer, W., & Reitan, R. M. 1964. Implications of Gerstmann's syndrome. *Journal of Neurology, Neurosurgery, and Psychiatry, 27,* 52–57.
Helm-Estabrooks, N., Fitzpatrick, P. M., & Barresi, B. Visual action therapy for global aphasia. Unpublished manuscript.
Henschen, E. S. 1919. Ueber Sprach, Musik, und Rechenmechanismen und ihre Lokalisationen im Grosshirn. *Zeitschrift für die gesamte Neurologie und Psychiatrie, 52,* 273–298.
Henschen, E. S. 1922. *Klinische und anatomische Beitrage zur Pathologie des Gehirnes. VII. Uber motorische Aphasie und Agraphie.* Stockholm: E. S. Henschen.
Hermann, G., & Poetzl, O. 1926. *Ueber die Agraphie und ihre Lokaldiagnostischen Beziehungen.* Berlin: Karger.
Hoff, H., Gloning, I., & Gloning, K. 1954. Ueber Alexie. *Wiener Zeitschrift für Nervenheil-kunde, 10,* 149–162.
Kaplan, E. 1968. Gestural representation of implement usage: An organismic-developmental study. Unpublished doctoral dissertation. Clark University, Worcester, Mass.
Kaplan, E. 1980. A qualitative approach to clinical neuropsychological assessment. Paper presented at American Psychological Association, Montreal.
Kertesz, A. 1979. *Aphasia and associated disorders.* New York: Grune & Stratton.
Kinsbourne, M., & Rosenfield, D. 1974. Agraphia selective for written spelling. *Brain and Language, 1,* 215–225.
Kinsbourne, M., & Warrington, E. K. 1962. A study of finger agnosia. *Brain, 85,* 47–66.
Kleist, K. 1912. Der gang und der gegenwurtige stand der apraxieforschung. *Zeitschrift für Neurologie und Psychiatrie, 1,* 342–452.
Leonhard, K. 1979. Ideokinetic apraxia and related disorders. In Y. Lebrun & R. Hoops (Eds.), *Problems of Aphasia.* Lisse: Swets & Zeitlinger.
Levin, H. A. 1979. The acalculias. In K. M. Heilman & E. Valenstein (Eds.) *Clinical neuro-psychology.* New York: Oxford Univ. Press.
Lewandowsky, M., & Stadelmann, E. 1908. Ueber einen bemerkenswerten Fall von Hirnblutung und über Rechenströrungen bei Herderkrankung des Gehirns. *Journal für Psychologie und Neurologie, 11,* 249–265.
Liepmann, H. 1908. *Drei Aufsatze aus dem Apraxiegebiet.* Berlin: Karner.
Luria, A. R. 1966. *The higher cortical functions in man.* New York: Basic Books.
McFie, J., & Zangwill, O. L. 1960. Visuo-constructive disabilities associated with lesions of the right cerebral hemisphere. *Brain, 82,* 243–259.
Mahoudeau, D. 1950. Considerations sur l'agraphie, a propos d'un cas observe chez un traumatise du crane porteur d'une lesion des deuxieme et troisieme convolutions fron-tales gauches. *Semaine des Hopitaux, 26,* 1598–1601.
Mahoudeau, D., David, M., & Lecoeur, J. 1951. Un Nouveau, cas d'agraphie sans aphasie revelatrice d'une tumeur metastatique du pied de la deuxieme circonvolution frontale gauche. *Revue Neurologique, 1,* 159–161.

Marcie, P., & Hécaen, H. 1979. Agraphia: Writing disorders associated with unilateral cortical lesions. In K. M. Heilman & E. Valenstein (Eds.), *Clinical neuropsychology*. New York: Oxford Univ. Press.

Marshall, J. C., & Newcombe, F. 1966. Syntactic and semantic errors in apralexia. *Neuropsychologia, 4*, 169–176.

Matthews, C. G., Folk, E. G., & Zerfas, P. G. 1966. Lateralized finger localization deficits and differential Wechsler–Bellevue results in retardates. *American Journal of Mental Deficiency, 70*, 695–702.

Mohr, J. P. 1976. An unusual case of dyslexia with dysgraphia. *Brain and Language, 3*, 324–334.

Money, J. 1965. *A standardized road-map test of directional sense*. Baltimore: Johns Hopkins Press.

Morselli, G. E. 1930. A proposito di agratia pura. *Rivista Sperimentale di Freniatria, 54*, 500–511.

Paterson, A., & Zangwill, O. L. 1944. Disorders of visual space perception associated with lesions of the right cerebral hemisphere. *Brain, 67*, 331–358.

Patterson, K. E., & Marcel, A. J. 1977. Aphasia, dyslexia and phonological coding of written words. *Quarterly Journal of Experimental Psychology, 29*, 307–318.

Penfield, W., & Roberts, L. 1959. *Speech and brain mechanisms*. Princeton: Princeton Univ. Press.

Peritz, G. 1918. Zur Pathopsychologie des Rechnens. *Deutsche Zeitschrift fur Nervenheilkunde, 61*, 234–340.

Pickett, L. W. 1974. An assessment of gestural and pantomimie deficit in aphasic patients. *Acta Symbolica, 5*, 69–88.

Piercy, M., & Smith, V. O. 1962. Right hemisphere dominance for certain nonverbal intellectual skills. *Brain, 85*, 775–790.

Poeck, K., & Orgass, B. 1969. An experimental investigation of finger agnosia. *Neurology, 19*, 801–807.

Poeck, K., & Orgass, B. 1975. Gerstmann syndrome without aphasia: Comments on the paper by Strub and Geschwind. *Cortex, 11*, 291–295.

Poetzl, O. 1928. *Die Optisch-Agnostischen Storungen*. Vienna: Deuticke.

Poppelreuter, W. 1914–1917. *Die psychischen Schadigungen durch Kopfschuss in Kriege*. Leipzig: Vass.

Redlich, E. 1895. Ueber die sogenannte subcorticale Alexie. *Jahrbucher fur Psychiatrie Neurologie, 13*, 1–60.

Rosati, G., & De Bastiani, P. 1979. Pure agraphia: A discrete form of aphasia. *Journal of Neurology, Neurosurgery, and Psychiatry, 42*, 266–269.

Rothi, L. J., & Heilman, K. M. 1981. Alexia and agraphia with letter recognition abilities. *Brain and Language, 12*, 1–13.

Rourke, B. P., & Strang, J. D. 1978. Neuropsychological significance of variations in patterns of academic performance. *Journal of Pediatric Psychology, 3*, 62–68.

Saffran, E. M., Bogyo, L. C., Schwartz, M. F., & Marin, O. S. M. 1980. Does deep dyslexia reflect right hemisphere reading? In M. Coltheart, K. Patterson, & J. C. Marshall (Eds.), *Deep Dyslexia*. London: Routledge and Kegan Paul.

Samuels, J. A., & Benson, D. F. 1979. Some aspects of language comprehension in anterior aphasia. *Brain and Language, 8*, 275–286.

Sauguet, J., Benton, A. L., & Hécaen, H. 1971. Disturbances of the body schema in relation to language impairment and hemispheric locus of lesion. *Journal of Neurology, Neurosurgery, and Psychiatry, 34*, 496–501.

Schilder, P. 1931. Fingeragnosie, Fingerapraxie, Finger Aphasie. *Nervenarzt, 4*, 625–629.

Schilder, P. 1935. *The image and appearance of the human body.* London: Routledge and Kegan Paul.

Schwartz, J., Kaplan, E., & Schwartz, A. 1981. Childhood dyscolculia and Gerstmann syndrome. Paper presented at the American Academy of Neurology, Toronto.

Schwartz, M. F., Saffran, E. M., & Marin, O. S. M. 1977. An analysis of agrammatic reading in aphasia. Paper presented at the International Neuropsychological Society, Santa Fe, New Mexico.

Shallice, T., & Warrington, E. K. 1975. Word recognition in a phonemic dyslexic patient. *Quarterly Journal of Experimental Psychology, 27,* 187–199.

Singer, H. D., & Low, A. A. 1933. Acalculia (Henschen): A clinical study. *Archives of Neurology and Psychiatry, 29,* 476–498.

Sinico, S. 1926. Neoplasia della seconda circonvoluzione frontale sinistra: Agratia pura. *Gazzetta degli Ospedali e delle Cliniche, 47,* 627–631.

Stockert, T. R. von, & Bader, L. 1976. Some relations of grammar and lexicon in aphasia. *Cortex, 12,* 49–60.

Strauss, A., & Werner, H. 1938. Deficiency in the finger schema in relation to arithmetic disability. *American Journal of Orthopsychiatry, 8,* 719–725.

Strub, R. L., & Geschwind, N. 1974. Gerstmann syndrome without aphasia. *Cortex, 10,* 378–387.

Varney, N. R. 1978. Linguistic-correlates of pantomime recognition in aphasic patients. *Journal of Neurology, Neurosurgery, and Psychiatry, 41,* 564–568.

Vignolo, L. 1969. Auditory agnosia: A review and report of recent evidence. In A. L. Benton (Ed.), *Contributions to modern clinical neuropsychology.* Chicago: Aldine.

Vincent, C., David, M., & Puech, P. 1930. Sur l'alexie. Production du phenomene a la suite de l'extirpation de la sorne occiputale due ventricule lateral gauche. *Revue Neurologique, 1,* 262–272.

Warrington, E. K., James, M., & Kinsbourne, M. 1966. Drawing disability in relation to laterality of lesion. *Brain, 89,* 53–92.

Wernicke, C. 1903. Ein Fall von isolierter Agraphie. *Monatsschrift fur Psychiatrie und Neurologie, 13,* 241–265.

Wernicke, C. 1908. The symptom-complex of aphasia in disease of the nervous system. In E. D. Church (Ed.), *Modern clinical medicine: Diseases of the nervous system.* New York: Appleton.

Zangwill, O. 1964. Intelligence in aphasia. In A. DeReuch & M. O'Conner (Eds.), *Disorders of language.* Boston: Little, Brown.

11

Intelligence and Aphasia

KERRY HAMSHER

Early Controversies

The Discursive Arguments

The purpose of this chapter is to identify issues and to review the present state of knowledge concerning the relation between aphasia and intelligence. The debate surrounding this topic is far from being concluded and remains a major topic for future research in the field of aphasia. This issue has at its heart two underlying themes: First, what is the relationship between language and thought; second, to what extent does a brain event causing an aphasia syndrome transcend a mere disorder of speech. The first theme has manifold ramifications ranging from hotly contested philosophic debates to questions about vocational rehabilitation for stroke victims. The second theme is a restatement of the first using the terms and concepts of clinical neurology and neuropsychology. As we shall see, these concepts of "thought" and "language" are much like Siamese twins: At their points of interface, it may not be possible to say where one stops and the other begins; nevertheless, on the whole, each operates independently and possesses a unique character.

In Chapter 1, Benton described the history of concern with the effects of aphasia on intelligent thought, a concern that was deeply rooted in the earliest theories of aphasia. From those early clinical observations of patients with acquired aphasia were born two revelations: (*a*) that aphasia was more than a paralysis of the muscles involved in speech and therefore must involve some mental or cognitive capacity; (*b*) the prob-

327

lems in the activities of daily living and limitations in communication with others in the environment manifested by aphasics seemed greater than what could be accounted for by the speech defects alone. In response to the first revelation, hypotheses were offered to link a cognitive defect with the consequent disturbances in speech. Bouillaud and Lordat, for example, supposed there was damage to the "organ of memory for words," leading to a concept of aphasia as a specific amnestic defect. Broca, Wernicke, and Lichtheim spoke of defects in association processes that link words with their referent objects or actions. Logically, this concept would allow that both memory for words and a meaningful appreciation of the environment could be preserved though dissociated in aphasia.

In response to the second revelation come ponderings about the effect of aphasia on thought processes. Trousseau first emphasized the apparent impairment in thought processes in aphasia, followed by J. Hughlings Jackson and Baillarger. Pierre Marie spoke of the necessary impairment of limited but important aspects of intelligence in aphasia. Arnold Pick (1931/1973) declared that "speech symbols represent an important aid to thought [p. 136]." In describing thought processes as cascading events in which the early stages of formulation serve to guide the later stages, Pick suggested that a deficiency in language would degrade the formulation of thought at its earliest stages and thus could give the appearance of intellectual retardation. By this comment one may suppose that Pick felt the real substance of intelligence may remain intact in aphasia but be kept in waiting for the return of linguistic skills. Finkelnburg, Kurt Goldstein, and Head believed aphasia could be conceived as a defect in symbolic thinking. Whether printed or sounded out, words are, after all, a convenient way to refer to elements of one's environment and thus are very much symbols.

In some senses, these are all appealing concepts of aphasia. However, it is not clear that any of them can adequately account for either the variety of cognitive deficits that are associated with aphasia or the variability among aphasics in their patterns of cognitive symptomatology. For example, while language represents a special use of symbolic thinking—namely, "the use of symbols for purposes of communication [Benton, 1965, p. 298]."—this does not appear to be the only aspect of language that is vulnerable to brain disease. The four major syndromes of aphasia share the symptom of an impairment in naming: in Broca's aphasia, effortful and labored attempts to name result in phonemic paraphasias; in so-called conduction and Wernicke's aphasias, naming is noneffortful and fluent, but there are prominent phonemic and semantic paraphasic errors; in nominal aphasia, paraphasic errors are rare and the defect in naming appears to represent a failure in word retrieval (Goodglass, 1980). It is difficult to imagine how all these characteristics could be explained by one mechanism.

Empirical Formulations

An understanding of the contribution of the right hemisphere to the performance of certain intellectual tasks or functions was largely missing during the early stages of the development of a concept of aphasia. This lack of appreciation for the role of the so-called minor hemisphere persisted despite the contributions of J. Hughlings Jackson, who at the time of Broca's discoveries was suggesting that symptoms of visuospatial impairment, which he called "imperception," could result from right hemisphere lesions, particularly in the posterior zone (Benton, 1977a). Yet, even Jackson lacked a formal theory of intelligence, and certainly none of the early theorists proposed a view of intelligence as an objective and measurable behavioral capacity. The work of Weisenburg and McBride (1935), discussed in Chapter 1, ushered in both a new approach to the question of the relation between aphasia and intelligence and a new speculation. Their objective assessment of both verbal and nonverbal cognitive performances in aphasic, nonaphasic brain-damaged, and control subjects led them to believe that individual cognitive styles or strategies must play a role. Persons accustomed to solving problems by verbal means might, by this formulation, be the ones most likely to exhibit nonverbal defects in the context of aphasia. Weisenburg and McBride's contribution marked the onset of a new era in which formal conceptualizations of intelligence—and the method of assessment—were brought to bear on the question of the effect of aphasia on intelligence.

Intelligence

The Concept of Intelligence

A definition of the concept of intelligence is at once both controversial and complex. To emphasize here the points of disagreement would be self-defeating, for we cannot realistically evaluate the issues at hand if a consensus definition of intelligence is circumvented. At the same time, some of the complexity must be preserved if we are going to do justice to the term and meaningfully test the limits of the concept of intelligence in the context of aphasia.

Sir Cyril Burt (1955) ascribes the origin of the concept of intelligence to Plato and Aristotle and credits Cicero with the coinage of the term. The use of tests to assess intelligence and the application of statistics to these data was introduced by an English scientist, Sir Francis Galton. Galton was interested in supporting the theories of his first cousin, Charles Darwin, by demonstrating that the principles of hereditary descent applied to intellectual as well as physical attributes. To this end he published his study *Hereditary Genius* in 1869 (Galton, 1887). But as Zangwill (1964) has pointed out, the real work on the exploration and development of this concept began with the development of intelligence tests for the purpose of addressing socioeducational problems. This work was begun by Alfred Binet, a French lawyer and natural scientist by education, who became a psychologist largely through self-tutoring.

A misconception of the term INTELLIGENCE is sometimes encountered among the general public where it is taken to mean a state of above normal thinking capacity. Perhaps this comes from expressions describing some individuals as "intelligent" and others as "unintelligent." In scientific psychology, intelligence is conceived as a largely but not exclusively biologic characteristic that is expressed in behavior, which varies from one person to the next, and accounts for some individual differences in behavior. Therefore, it is a quantitative concept, as are the concepts of height and weight. As with height and weight, when applied to people, it is difficult to conceive of zero or very small values of intelligence in a meaningful fashion. At the same time, there appears to be some naturally occurring upper limit to human intelligence, but this limit is not explicitly defined. Unlike height and weight, intelligence cannot be directly observed, touched, or measured in physical terms. It is more well defined and less arbitrary than such concepts as beauty, ugliness, and creativity. Also, the characteristics one looks at to assess intelligence in a subjective fashion are more consistent than, say, the characteristics that might be employed to assess "athleticism" in ping-pong players, football players, gymnasts, and runners.

A distinction is made by most authorities between the application of the concept of intelligence to represent one's ability versus one's actual performance. A highly intelligent individual could on some occasions perform very poorly on an intelligence test for a variety of reasons, such as anxiety or preoccupation. Clearly one could fake a bad performance on an intelligence test, and obviously such an event would not in any real sense lower that person's intellectual competence. Thus, this distinction between capacity and performance is crucial and something to be addressed later in this chapter.

Wechsler (1958) describes general intellectual ability as the "global capacity of the individual to act purposefully, to think rationally, and to deal effectively with his environment [p. 7]." Intellectual behavior or functional intelligence, he says, depends on general intellectual ability plus the way in which specific cognitive abilities are combined and such nonintellectual factors as the person's drive and the incentive offered by the situation in which intelligence is being assessed.

So intelligence is a construct that implies an underlying reality, but this reality must be inferred from behavioral observations (Wechsler, 1971). The parallel to this is a working definition of intelligence that says intelligence is a complex trait that is measured by intelligence tests (Wechsler, 1971). Since psychology has developed methods to determine if a particular test is a measure of what we intend to call intelligence, the circularity of the working definition is no longer problematic. These methods derive from our current understanding of the structure of intelligence.

The Structure of Intelligence

Two differing views of the structure of intelligence developed during the first half of the twentieth century. One view, which was articulated by the British psychologist Spearman (1927), holds that intelligence is a unitary trait that is expressed to greater or lesser extents on most any cognitive task. The opposing view is that general intelligence is merely the sum (or average) of a collection of different primary abilities. This point of view was championed by the American psychologist Thurstone (1938). Since Thurstone's primary abilities are not independent of each other and, in fact, are intercorrelated, this position is not fundamentally different from Spearman's position that besides the general factor there are also specific intellectual factors (Piercy, 1969). Modern psychology therefore views intelligence as having both unitary and multiple or factorial aspects. The history that led to this conclusion is described by Matarazzo (1972, pp. 24–62).

Intelligence is generally conceived as being organized in a hierarchical fashion. This notion is borrowed from the facts of evolution, especially with regard to the development of the central nervous system. According to this model, in the normal brain, general ability exerts a downward influence on the next level of organization, which consists of several major or group factors (primary abilities). The group factors are, in turn, composed of several specific factors, factors that may be specific to the type of task or method of assessing performance. Whether there are two, three, or more levels of organization within the various spheres of cognitive activity has not been fixed in fact or theory. The question of the number of levels of organization is an arbitrary one, since the answer will vary depending upon the number and types of cognitive behaviors sampled, the methods of assessment, and the type of statistical analysis applied.

A concrete example may assist in appreciating the theoretical view of the structure of intelligence. To begin, an extensive battery of cognitive tests would be administered to a cross-section of the general population. The finding that all the test scores correlate positively with each other provides the basis for inferring the presence of a general factor of intelligence, often called g after the manner of Spearman. When the influence of each test's correlation with g is statistically removed, one can determine to what degree two tests are related to each other in a way not accounted for by their shared correlation with g. This leads to the observation that there are clusters of tests that tend to correlate with each other to a high degree and show a low or no correlation with the remaining tests. This is how major or group factors are identified. To determine an individual test's correlation with our statistical definition of g, each subject's score on that test would be correlated with the subject's score on the entire battery. The test battery could be purified by removing the individual tests with the lowest correlation with g and then recomputing each remaining test's correlation with summary scores derived from the new abbreviated battery. Examining these new correlations, one will find that some tests correlate with (predict) g better than others. Those tests with the strongest correlation with g are considered the best representatives of measures of general intelligence within that test's group factor. Among verbal tests, vocabulary and general information show this strong relationship with g. Among nonverbal intellectual tasks, Raven's Progressive Matrices and the block design subtest from the Wechsler Adult Intelligence Scale (WAIS) are among the best predictors of g.

The Validity of Intelligence

This psychometric framework allows behavioral scientists to develop and validate measures of intelligence within various cultures. Thus, when we speak of measures of general intelligence, we are denoting measures that predict how well a person will likely perform on a wide variety of cognitive tasks. Though eloquently conceived, this view of intelligence would be rather trivial if it were not also true that intelligence, defined and measured by objective means, predicted or coincided with other real-world events and biologic patterns.

When the concept of general intelligence is expressed as a summary score derived from an intelligence test battery, then the technical term INTELLIGENCE QUOTIENT (IQ) may be used. A quotient score is a way of expressing performance level in a standard fashion. By convention, quotient scores have a mean of 100 and a standard deviation of 15 points. The IQ score states a person's standing relative to some reference group. Since performance on intelligence tests progressively increase with age during the developmental years and may progressively decline with age during late life, separate reference groups are needed for various age categories.

Childhood IQs starting from age 7–8 correlate with adult IQ in the range of $r = .70$–.85, suggesting a fair degree of stability. Childhood IQs also are correlated with adult occupational level ($r = .50$–.60) and with adult educational attainment ($r = .40$–.60). Similarly, adult IQ scores correlate with adult educational and occupational levels in the same range (approximately $r = .50$) (McCall, 1977). We may infer from these findings that, while performance on an intelligence test battery seems to have an important relationship to adult educational and occupational achievements, other factors must also be involved that are not accounted for in the IQ score. Since our concept of intelligence does not require that it account for everything, these summary findings reported by McCall can be considered supportive of the validity of measured intelligence.

There is now substantial evidence that objective measures of intelligence are in part under hereditary control. For example, the highest correlations in IQs are found among identical twins (about $r = .90$). As expected, there are highly significant but smaller correlations between the IQs of siblings and between parents and children, all of whom share fewer genes than identical twins. There is also evidence that, while these correlations are attenuated when the pairs in these correlations live apart from each other, the pattern of correlations (e.g., identical twins versus fraternal twins) remains much the same. Moreover, the magnitude of these correlations are similar to those of other complex, multiply determined traits, such as height and weight. Since the IQ is not a perfectly reliable score and will vary within the same individual on different occasions and is subject to the influence of such personality and environmental factors as drive and incentive, the obtained correlations may be considered minimal correlations. The magnitude of the contributions of heredity and environment is a question that is still at issue; for our purposes, knowing that the IQ is in part under hereditary control is sufficient with regard to the question of the validity of the concept of intelligence expressed as an IQ score (Matarazzo, 1972, pp. 298–317; Vandenberg, 1971).

So far, we have seen that in civilized cultures the concept of intelligence has appeared self-evident, and broadly speaking this concept has remained relatively constant through the centuries. Through trials and errors, attempts were made to objectively measure intelligence, and in the end an empirical formulation was achieved. Intelligence has progressed from an abstract concept to a concrete IQ score, and this score appears valid in the sense that IQ scores tend to covary with the trappings of the abstact concept of intelligence, such as educational and occupational attainment and performance, heredity, and its susceptibility to decline with brain damage.

Intelligence and Brain Disease

When speaking of disease of the brain, one may be tempted to think of something akin to an inflammation, but DISEASE is a broad term that carries with it no particular implication for the etiology of the diseased or abnormal state. Disease of the brain may be acquired through such mechanisms as heredity, tumors of the brain, prenatal trauma or metabolic disorders, postnatal vascular events such as stroke, a shearing of the brain from sudden rotation, missile wounds such as a gunshot wound, and a secondary consequence of a disease of another organ system, such as renal failure or liver disease. Likewise, the term LESION is not a specific term. A lesion is a site of abnormality. It may be visible radiographically because it alters brain structure or causes a breakdown in the blood–brain barrier, but this is not required. A lesion may also be said to be present as a result of microscopic changes in brain tissue or even changes in intracellular metabolism. However, for the most part, the kinds of lesions referred to in studies of the effects of focal brain lesions on intelligence are ones that have been demonstrated radiographically (on X ray) or through electrophysiology (i.e., on the EEG) or have been visualized by a neurosurgeon and occasionally the neuropathologist.

General Intelligence and Brain Disease

Karl S. Lashley, a physiological and behavioral psychologist, brought together psychological and statistical concepts of intelligence, neurological concepts of dementia and mental retardation, and some sparse neuroanatomic observations. From this mixture of data and conjecture, he enunciated two major principles: EQUIPOTENTIALITY and MASS ACTION. Equipotentiality means that the cerebral cortex is considered undifferentiated in its contribution to the performance of intelligent behavior—that is, the contribution of one section of cortex is presumed to be as good as, and equal to, the contribution of some other section. Mass action means that all regions of the equipotential cortex work together, en masse as it were, to produce intelligent behaviors so that a loss in efficiency consequent to brain damage will be proportional to the loss in cortical mass (tissue) regardless of its locus. According to Lashley, these principles applied only to nonlocalized behavioral functions, such as learning and intelligence. Lashley (1929) supported these concepts with data on the maze-learning performances of rats in relation to the locus and amount of cortical tissue that was surgically removed. By today's standards, several of his correlations would not be considered statistically significant (reliably greater than zero), so in retrospect his arguments were not as sound as they were thought to be at the time. But these principles had value in that they generated research in attempts to defend or refute Lashley's laws.

In a study that was the human analogue of Lashley's classic study, Chapman and Wolf (1959) correlated IQ scores with the neurosurgeon's estimated amount of cerebral tissue removed during operations for the treatment of brain tumors and arteriovenous malformations. Evidence for mass action was found with the stricture that the relationship between intellectual and cerebral tissue loss was much more firm in those patients where the cortical excisions were postrolandic (involving the parietal, occipital, and temporal lobes). In an equally monumental study carried out by Blessed, Tomlinson, and Roth (1968), the investigators examined the brains of decreased demented patients, most of whom suffered from Alzheimer's disease. A counting was made of the number of senile plaques found in several brain regions. Senile plaques are present in excessive amounts in the brains of demented patients relative to age-matched nondemented controls. Prior to these patients' deaths, they were administered a battery of cognitive tests, and behavioral ratings were obtained from relatives. These investigators found a significant but modest correlation between mean plague count and scores on the mental test battery, while the plaque count correlated more highly with the ratings of a decline in the patients' personal and social habits. The difference in the magnitude of these correlations may be due to an artifact of assessment, since the behavioral ratings were a direct rating of decline in behavioral status, whereas the mental test scores may have been partially confounded with premorbid ability level. Nevertheless,

these and similar findings lend credence to the notion that some summary index of acquired intellectual impairment derived from a battery of
cognitive performances provides at least a rough index of the status of
the cerebrum as a whole (Benton, 1980).

Focal Brain Lesions and Intellectual Performance

So far we have seen how the concept of intelligence as having both
multifactorial and unitary aspects developed from studies of neurologically normal individuals. When a broad array of cognitive abilities are
sampled in the investigation of general intelligence, one frequently ob-
serves individual patterns of cognitive performance, that is, areas of
relative strengths and weaknesses as opposed to equivalent scores
across all samples of cognitive performance. Because of what was earlier
described as a downward influence of general ability on more specific
abilities, we find that if two individuals have broadly separated IQ
scores, even in the case where one person's weakness is the other's
strength, the person with the lower IQ will seldom surpass the higher
IQ individual on any of these more specific intellectual factors. Another
way to view this is to say that to some extent particular abilities, such as
spatial, verbal, or numerical abilities, are dissociable within the general
population. There is some evidence to suggest that an individual's pattern of specific abilities in the context of their general ability level plays a
role in occupational selection. For example, architects may outperform
mechanics on measures of general ability, while each share a relative
superiority in mechanical and visuoperceptive skills compared with
such other abilities as numerical or verbal (cf. Matarazzo, 1972, pp.
168–174).

Understanding g as a summary statement of intellectual standing in
the normal population, the concept of dementia may be viewed as a
pathological counterpart to g. In behavioral terms, dementia denotes a
generalized decline in all aspects of cognitive functioning, which neurologically is represented by widespread cerebral disease or dysfunction
(Benton, 1980). In short, dementia implies a significant decline in g from
some previous (premorbid) level due to brain disease. Between these
two extremes of an intact and devastated cerebrum are the effects of
focal brain lesions.

The Wechsler Adult Intelligence Scale (WAIS), like its predecessor
the Wechsler–Bellevue Intelligence Scale, consists of a collection of 11
tests covering a variety of different cognitive abilities. Scores from 6 of
the subtests are grouped together to yield a verbal IQ score (VIQ), and

the remaining 5 subtests are grouped to yield a performance IQ score (PIQ). The full-scale IQ (FSIQ) represents the sum of performances across all the subtests. Several statistical studies using factor analysis (see Matarazzo, 1972, pp. 261–276) suggest the VIQ is composed of two factors, one of which could be called verbal–conceptual abilities (information, comprehension, similarities, vocabulary) and the other could be called attention–concentration (arithmetic reasoning, digit span). The PIQ is composed of tests assessing perceptual–constructional abilities (block design, picture arrangement, object assembly, picture completion) and psychomotor speed (digit symbol substitution).

The selection and grouping of the WAIS subtests into the verbal and performance scales was largely done on a rational rather than on an empirical basis. While it was not specifically designed to detect or localize brain disease, this test battery has some usefulness along these lines (Benton, 1977b; Fogel, 1964; McFie, 1975; Wilson, Rosenbaum, & Brown, 1979). For the sake of argument, we will consider the VIQ and PIQ to represent two major intellectual factors. Studies of the WAIS performances of patients with focal or at least largely unilateral brain lesions suggest that lesions of the left hemisphere often result in a VIQ deficit, whereas lesions of the right hemisphere result in greater impairment of the PIQ. Not all studies are in agreement with this summary statement, but the trend has appeared often enough in many separate clinical settings that it has become accepted with qualifications (G. Goldstein, 1974; Klove, 1974; Lezak, 1976, pp. 181–224; Smith, 1975; Walsh, 1978, pp. 282–331). Furthermore, McFie (1960, 1969; McFie & Thompson, 1972) has reported specific patterns of deficits on the Wechsler subtests that are associated with the intrahemispheric locus of focal brain disease (e.g., frontal versus temporal versus parietal lobes). While these latter findings with the Wechsler tests have not been fully substantiated, the fact that patterns of specific cognitive deficits may be associated with lesions in specific brain areas (foci) is well established (McFie, 1969; Newcombe, 1974; Piercy, 1964; Walsh, 1978).

These illustrative points help to build a conceptual framework for understanding how focal brain lesions may affect intellectual performance. First, depending upon its locus, the lesion may severely compromise a given test performance. Because that test shares some properties with the other tests with which it is factorially grouped—which is the nature of factorial grouping—the effect of that lesion may be seen as partially affecting related test performances. Both the specific test defect and shared deficits on related tests would act to lower the major factor or test group score (e.g., the PIQ). This, in turn, would result in a lowering of the summary or general intellectual score. According to this model, in pathological conditions, specific cognitive defects may exert an upward influence through the structure of intelligence, and its influence would tend to be diminished at higher stages in the hierarchy. To take the analogy one step further, suppose there were a single test that incorporated several of the more specific cognitive abilities, all of which were required for the successful performance of the task. First, in the general population we may expect such a task to have a high correlation with g because of its multifactorial composition. Second, we might expect that focal lesions in different regions of the brain may impair test performance because of impairment of one or another or several of the more specific abilities incorporated in the test. Studies of the effects of focal brain lesions on cognitive performance may also provide an alternative method to factor analysis to identify the structure and hierarchial organization of intellectual abilities.

It has been asserted that, when g is conceived as the composite sum of various performances that individually may be sensitive to aphasic, apraxic, and agnosic disorders, it may not be possible to assess general intelligence meaningfully in the presence of cerebral disease (Messerli & Tissot, 1974). Given a patient who has suffered a stroke resulting in aphasia who had a premorbid IQ of 110 but who after the stroke obtained a VIQ of 78 and a PIQ of 108 with a resulting FSIQ of 93, can we say the full-scale IQ represents a fair and adequate assessment of the patient's general intelligence? It certainly would not reflect the patient's spatial strengths nor the severity of the verbal deficits. At this point we reach a theoretical and empirical impass, for to date we are without an adequate conceptualization of intelligence that can accommodate the findings obtained from normals, demented patients, and patients with focal lesions. As an attempt to arrive at a pragmatic solution, the custom that is sometimes adopted for patients with cerebral disease is to use an IQ score derived from nonverbal tests for patients with aphasic disorders and to use a measure of verbal IQ for patients with visuoperceptive or spatial disorders. The supporting reasoning is that specific cognitive defects, such as aphasia or constructional apraxia, are considered to be acquired disabilities much like acquired blindness, deafness, or hemiplegia, which interfere with the usual method of assessing general intelligence. Automatically this would appear to deny that aphasia or constructional apraxia are in any sense intellectual defects, but at the same time there is no reason to suppose that either the VIQ or the PIQ loses its relationship with g when one or the other is specifically impaired because of brain disease.

Language and Intellectual Development

Deafness and Illiteracy

Because of the intimate relationship between language and thought in our everyday experiences, it may take a moment of reflection to disengage the two concepts. True, much of our thought processes are expressed verbally, as in the classroom or when writing an exam or in talking to ourselves to work through solutions to various problems (so-called inner speech). But we can also recall situations and social relations in the form of visual memories, like silent movies, and in this mode we may use visual imagery to replay and rearrange events in our mind. We may find the best route on a map by visual inspection with the aid of spatial judgments, and we may conceive of repairing an automobile engine or an electric appliance without aid of words but not without thought. To refrain from attempting to put a large square peg through a small round hole surely represents not only perceptual discrimination but also some form of conceptual thought (Piaget, 1936).

Through the use of pantomime, we can communicate such nonverbal thoughts to others, although, granted, this may be a tedious and inefficient process when compared to oral speech. Infrahuman animals, such as dogs, can be trained to perform many tasks, for example, to fetch a stick and return it to the master in exchange for a pat or some treat. When the same dog spontaneously brings an object in an effort to initiate the game or to receive a reward, we must assume this, too, represents thought as well as learning in the absence of language. Yet these examples do not reveal what level of complexity can be achieved by humans without the aid of words.

Pitner and Lev (1939) examined the intellectual performances of partially deaf children in comparison with hearing children in grades 5–8. The mean performance of the hearing-impaired children was 8 IQ points below that of normal children on verbal intellectual measures but only 3 IQ points below on nonverbal tests. Upon a review of the literature, Furth (1964; Furth & Youniss, 1975) noted that on a variety of tests of reasoning and problem solving, deaf children are often able to perform very closely to the level of hearing children of the same age. While the retardation in oral and written language acquisition that results from deafness is a formidable obstacle, the many points of intellectual similarity between the deaf and their hearing peers would seem to negate the necessity of language for the development of normal—or near normal—intelligence and conceptual thinking. It has also been noted that environmental circumstances may be pivotal in the degree to which deafness and other forms of sensory deprivation may retard or place limits on learning processes (Kodman, 1963). One must ask to what extent others in the deaf person's environment have tried to communicate using preserved sensory channels, such as the visual, tactile, and proprioceptive modalities. The developmental history of Helen Keller provides strong testimony to the importance of this environmental issue.

The assumption that deaf children, who are without oral or written language, actually lack ANY form of language, however, may not be valid. Since deafness is a peripheral sensory impairment, there is no reason to suppose the deaf lack or have an impairment of the neural structures that subserve language in the hearing and speaking population. Pilot observations of deaf children between 1.5 and 4 years of age who have not been exposed to a manual sign language suggest they may spontaneously develop their own structured sign system that contains the basic properties of spoken language (Goldin-Meadow & Feldman, 1977). The lack of aural exposure to language with the consequent failure to develop oral speech or its graphic representation may not preclude the development of the fundamental properties of language, nor does it preclude the capacity for intelligent thought.

Illiteracy (due to social rather than intellectual restrictions) represents a similar but more limited form of environmental deprivation for an aspect of language in the context of presumably normal neurological mechanisms to acquire it. Despite the incompleteness of the illiterate's language repertoire, thinking, linguistic processing, hemispheric specialization for language, and vulnerability to neurological impairments of language, for the most part, do not appear to differ from those of literate individuals (A. R. Damasio, Castro-Caldas, Grosso, & Ferro, 1976; A. R. Damasio, Hamsher, Castro-Caldas, Ferro, & Grosso, 1976; H. Damasio, A. R. Damasio, Castro-Caldas, & Hamsher, 1979).

Developmental Aphasia and Intelligence

DEVELOPMENTAL APHASIA (or CONGENITAL APHASIA) is a term that is used to describe the condition in which a child shows a relatively specific failure in the acquisition of language functions and manifests abnormalities in either expressive speech alone or in both comprehension and oral speech (Benton, 1964). With rare exceptions—for instance, congenital auditory imperception (Worster-Drought & Allen, 1929)—language functions are similarly affected in the auditory, visual, and tactile modalities. By definition, language abilities must be more severely impaired than other cognitive functions so as to distinguish this specific syndrome from general mental impairment (mental retardation, or amentia). Likewise, other causes for a failure to exhibit normal language for age must be excluded (Benton, 1964; Zangwill, 1978), such as deafness or more pervasive neuropsychiatric disease in which disturbances in verbal communication represent but a subset of core symptoms as in childhood autism (A. R. Damasio & Mower, 1978).

It is reasonable to query whether the criteria for this behavioral diagnosis begs the question of intellectual deficit in the context of developmental aphasia. To a limited extent it does, since investigators are not likely to argue points of concern to developmental aphasia using data from subjects who are also severely impaired in nonverbal intellectual performance. Also, at very low levels of cognition, numerous technical problems adhere to mental measurements. Inasmuch as the diagnosis requires only a relative disparity between verbal and nonverbal abilities, rather than some absolute level of nonverbal intelligence, the case material reported in the literature can still be informative on this point.

The issue of the status of cognitive functioning in the presence of developmental aphasia is as complex as in the case of adult acquired aphasia. The rarity of the childhood disorder makes it particularly difficult to arrive at statistically reliable empirical formulations. The failure of investigators to describe adequately the symptomatology of the subjects under study makes comparisons across different studies tenuous at best, as does the failure to report or account for demographic variables that influence expected intellectual values, as discussed earlier in the section on the validity of intelligence. The indiscriminate lumping together of children with quite variable patterns of speech and language impairments certainly clouds and may confound experimental findings as well. Two broad classifications are minimally indicated: children with primarily expressive speech defects and children with expressive and receptive language deficits (Benton, 1978).

From the available findings, it may be concluded that children with developmental aphasia (or developmental dysphasia), in addition to speech defects, are impaired in verbal intelligence relative to their performance on nonverbal intellectual measures and are more variable than normals in their nonverbal IQs, which tend to be lower than expected given the child's family background (Benton, 1978). Some of these children do obtain high average to superior nonverbal IQs, but a larger proportion are in the low average to dull normal categories. Although the evidence is insufficient to make a definitive statement, generally children in the primarily expressive speech defect category show little impairment in nonverbal intelligence, whereas those in the receptive–expressive group are at much greater risk for these additional deficits.

Benton (1978) has reviewed three hypotheses to account for nonverbal intellectual deficits in developmental aphasia. The first view holds that the two types of deficits are fundamentally independent. The extent to which developmental aphasics are impaired in nonverbal intelligence depends upon the extension of the underlying neurological disease to areas beyond the language zone. This places developmental aphasia on a neurological continuum with mental retardation, the latter manifesting cognitive symptoms of bilateral and more symmetric hemispheric dysfunction.

The second hypothesis is similar to that discussed earlier in the section on the concept of intelligence—namely, that developmental aphasia is a handicap that limits and may distort the child's appreciation of his environment and his communication with others and, in turn, this may have a retarding influence on intellectual development. This implies that through special environmental intervention the handicapping factor may be minimized. On the whole, the evidence does not strongly support this concept. Yet there is a case report by Landau, Goldstein, and Kleffner (1960) of a child with receptive–expressive language impairments who showed a 19-point increment in nonverbal intellectual performance following intensive and protracted language training.

The third hypothesis holds that developmental aphasia represents the expression of a more general or higher-order cognitive function that is not strictly verbal and may encompass certain nonverbal abilities. Accordingly, the language deficits are not seen as the core disturbance but rather as a reflection of a disability in a more major cognitive function. This position finds support of the concept in the case of the receptive–expressive form of developmental aphasia in which a higher-level auditory–perceptual deficit has been held to be primarily responsible for the failure in language development (Benton, 1964; Tallal & Piercy, 1978; Worster-Drought & Allen, 1929). However, agreement on the specificity of the defect to the auditory modality is controversial (Zangwill, 1978), and others insist that developmental aphasia is specifically a defect in the structure of language (Cromer, 1978).

It is well known that language is acquired on the basis of audition and that the infant must first learn that the mother's spoken language has symbolic significance before the instrumental use of expressive language develops. It is fundamental that we must first be able to perceive something before we can come to know it, let alone make use of it for our own purposes. It must be very frustrating and perhaps confusing to children with expressive developmental aphasia to be able to hear and come to understand language without being able to imitate it faithfully and effortlessly. Considerably more sympathy and understanding must be held out for the child with receptive–expressive developmental aphasia who is deprived of these early experiences demonstrating the symbolic and communicative uses of language. Furthermore, because "communicating with oneself is an important aspect of thinking and that to this extent language is also a tool of thinking [Benton, 1965, p. 299]," it is not surprising that a receptive–expressive disorder will hamper the development of nonverbal problem-solving skills. What is remarkable is how little impairment some of these children show. These observations suggest the tentative conclusion that the neural mechanisms that subserve nonverbal intelligence must be independent of those that subserve language. However, inasmuch as the two cerebral hemispheres and their various lobes work together in concert (Zangwill, 1974)—usually a harmonious one—brain lesions affecting language operations, particularly receptive ones, that have the consequence of disrupting internal communications may also have a disharmonious impact on nonverbal operations. To overcome this, one may have to learn to disattend to faulty "verbal" insights and selectively rely on nonverbal perceptions, reasoning, and innate intuitions. This is likely a far easier task for the deaf child, who has the neurological mechanisms for language, than for the aphasic child, whose apparatus for language is partly nonfunctional or functioning abnormally.

Acquired Aphasia and Cognition

Performance on Tests of Intelligence

Weisenburg and McBride (1935) provided sound evidence that some aphasics show defects in visuoperceptive and spatial abilities and thus seem to have acquired cognitive deficits that exceed the concept of aphasia as strictly a disorder of language. On the other hand, Weinstein and Teuber (1957) reported that the patients who showed the greatest deficit on the Army General Classification Test in their studies of soldiers with missile wounds were those with left temperoparietal lesions, some of whom were aphasic and some of whom were not. Perhaps, then, these extralinguistic symptoms are not so much an expression of aphasia as they are a coincidence of anatomy. If there were areas in the left hemisphere that mediated nonverbal cognitive abilities and if these were situated near the language zone (e.g., Newcombe, 1969, pp. 98–102) or overlapping with it (Basso, De Renzi, Faglioni, Scotti, & Spinnler, 1973; Goodglass, 1974), then it would seem that some aphasics are at risk for extralinguistic cognitive deficits by virtue of the size and locus of their lesions. This formulation would deny that these extralinguistic defects are psychologically (i.e., functionally) related to the aphasic symptoms. Such cognitive symptoms could be as incidental to aphasia as are visual field defects, hemiplegia, or sensory-discriminative impairments. If aphasia, or some forms of it, were psychologically related to nonverbal mental impairment, then language may be viewed as having some supraordinate role in intelligent thought—perhaps. If not, as suggested by the anatomical explanation, then we could conceive of the cerebrum as composed of several compartments, each of which subserves some different and relatively independent primary mental ability. To try to link aphasic symptoms to nonverbal cognitive deficit would be pure folly if the anatomical hypothesis were correct.

Many investigators have reported that aphasics are more impaired than nonaphasic left-brain-damaged patients on the nonverbal portions of the Wechsler intelligence scales (Orgass, Hartje, Kerschensteiner, & Poeck, 1972). Particularly, it appears to be those aphasics who manifest signs of constructional apraxia who are at greatest risk for nonverbal intellectual impairment (Alajouanine & Lhermitte, 1964). However, this association between constructional apraxia and nonverbal intellectual impairment seems to hold for patients with both left- and right-sided lesions (Arrigoni & De Renzi, 1964; Klove & Reitan, 1958) and therefore is not peculiar to aphasia. Given that the block design subtest from the WAIS is often employed to assess constructional praxis (Warrington, 1969), it is not clear how one can separate constructional praxis from nonverbal intelligence. It is also not clear that constructional praxis is as unitary a concept as some clinical investigators would have us believe. The various ways an examiner may test for constructional apraxia, such as by having the patient copy drawings or geometric designs or build forms out of sticks or models out of blocks, are not highly correlated in brain-damaged patients (Benton, 1969). Each one of these tests for apraxia may be tapping one or more specific abilities that belong to a more general spatial factor that may not be fundamentally different from the spatial factor composing the nonverbal intellectual measure. Therefore, there is no compelling reason to attach special significance to the observation that the symptom of constructional apraxia is predictive of impairment in nonverbal intelligence.

Raven's Progressive Matrices (RPM) test has been demonstrated to be a measure of general intelligence obtained through nonverbal means. The test requires subjects to examine a visual array from which a subsection appears to have been cut out. Via either an oral or a pointing response, the subject then indicates which of several multiple-choice alternatives is the correct one. Some items involve the simple completion of a pattern, such as diagonal stripes, while other items incorporate a progression or sequence of figures, such as the systematic rotation or elaboration of figures, which must be discerned and understood in order to make the correct choice. This task calls upon various cognitive abilities, including visuoperception, abstract reasoning, spatial relation, counting, and mental flexibility.

Significant impairment in the performance of the RPM test is seen in patients with both right and left hemisphere lesions, particularly in association with constructional apraxia (Arrigoni & De Renzi, 1964; Zangwill, 1975). In right hemisphere disease, impairment on this task is associated with defects in block building and visual pattern matching, but not in left hemisphere disease. Among patients with left brain damage, impairment on the RPM test is associated with the presence of aphasia (Basso *et al.*, 1973), and among aphasics, such defects are primarily restricted to patients with language comprehension impairment (Archibald, Wepman, & Jones, 1967; Costa, Vaughan, Horwitz, & Ritter, 1969; Zangwill, 1969). However, there are patients with severe receptive language deficits who may perform rather well on this task (Kinsbourne & Warrington, 1963; Zangwill, 1964).

Constructional Apraxia

Constructional apraxia was originally viewed as a symptom of cerebral disease in the left posterior quadrant, but numerous studies have since shown that patients with lesions in the right posterior quadrant have the highest incidence and produce the most severe forms of this cognitive symptom (see Benton, 1967; Warrington, 1969). When present, it is often associated with general mental impairment (Benton, 1962; Benton & Fogel, 1962). While general mental impairment may result in the appearance of constructional apraxia, this is not a consistent consequence, and constructional apraxia may occur as a relatively isolated cognitive defect, that is, outside the context of general mental impairment. Obviously, there is no relationship between language impairment and constructional apraxia among patients with right hemisphere lesions as there is in patients with left hemisphere lesions. Specifically, in left hemisphere disease, constructional apraxia is associated with the presence of receptive language impairment, and the more severe the receptive disorder, the more likely constructional apraxia will occur (Benton, 1973). The relationship between constructional apraxia and receptive language disorders with left hemisphere disease may be described as a one-way relationship. There is a high probability of receptive impairment when constructional apraxia is present, but only about one-half of patients with moderate to severe comprehension defects manifest constructional apraxia (Benton, 1973). This probabilistic relation between the severity of the linguistic defect and the likelihood of constructional apraxia, while consistent with the notion of a functional relation between the two, does not contradict the anatomical hypothesis described earlier.

Visuoperceptive and Visuospatial Performances

Nonverbal intellectual measures, such as the performance scale from the WAIS or the RPM test, as well as measures of constructional apraxia are all in part dependent upon visuoperception. Whether on the left or on the right, brain lesions producing constructional disabilities typically result in associated visuoperceptive deficits (Dee, 1970). One standardized visuoperceptive task is a facial recognition test that calls for the matching of photographs of unfamiliar persons taken from different angles and under different lighting conditions (Benton & Van Allen, 1968; Benton, Van Allen, Hamsher, & Levin, 1975). In patients with focal brain lesions who show no evidence of general mental impairment, defective performance on this test is associated with right hemisphere lesions and with lesions of the left hemisphere but only in the context of an aphasia syndrome in which language comprehension is significantly impaired (Hamsher, Levin, & Benton, 1979). Aphasic patients without significant comprehension deficits as assessed by objective tests (Benton & Hamsher, 1976) and nonaphasic left brain damaged patients perform on a par with hospital control subjects who are without history or evidence of neurological disease. Similarly, a disturbance in perceptual association involving colors is associated with aphasic impairments in language comprehension and not with "pure" measures of color perception (such as color matching or color discrimination); the opposite pattern is obtained with right hemisphere lesions (De Renzi, Faglioni, Scotti, & Spinnler, 1972; De Renzi & Spinnler, 1967). The ability to associate colors with objects may be assessed by having patients select colored pencils to shade in a drawing of, say, an apple. Interestingly, impairment on this performance in the setting of aphasia is correlated with deficits in conceptual performances rather than on tests of facial matching or identifying figures hidden in complex drawings (De Renzi *et al.*, 1972).

One example of a visuoperceptive performance that is not apparently disrupted in the context of receptive aphasia is global stereopsis. Stereopsis is the ability to appreciate that two objects lie at different distances from the observer based on the fact that each eye receives slightly different retinal images of these objects. If one looks through a stereoscope, which presents separate images to the two eyes, and sees two forms with one eye and the same with the other except with a different horizontal separation, then when both eyes are used one form will appear closer than the other. This is steropsis. Global stereopsis is similar, except that the two images must be extremely complex, being composed of such things as randomly placed dots. It is impossible to see any forms at all with either eye alone, but when viewed binocularly, part of the background stands out from the rest and the viewer then perceives a form in space. To achieve this visual feat, one must call upon certain higher-level visuoperceptive abilities (Hamsher, 1978a). Lesions of the right hemisphere can impair one's capacity to achieve global stereopsis, whereas patients with left hemisphere lesions perform at the level of hospital control patients (Carmon & Bechtoldt, 1967) even in the context of objectively demonstrated receptive language impairment (Hamsher, 1978b).

Aphasics have been reported to perform more poorly that other brain-damaged groups on a task involving the use of maps, both in the visual and tactile modalities (Semmes, Weinstein, Ghent, & Teuber, 1963). In aphasia this type of apparent spatial deficit is not associated with generalized spatial disorientation as it is in right hemisphere disease (McFie & Zangwill, 1960). Yet, on what must be considered a rather pure measure of "spatial thinking," which merely calls for matching of lines having the same spatial orientation, aphasics perform very nearly at the level of non-brain-damaged control patients, whereas a sizable proportion of patients with right hemisphere lesions show severe impairment (Benton, Hannay, & Varney, 1975; Benton, Varney, & Hamsher, 1978). These findings are in accord with previously described observations suggesting aphasics show little or no impairment on simple and direct measures of visuoperceptive and spatial capacities, whereas on more complex tasks that often involve an amalgam of spatial, perceptual, and conceptual abilities, very severe cognitive disability may emerge in some forms of aphasia, especially in the context of language comprehension deficits. Regrettably, as yet, we cannot say why this is so. Perhaps in receptive forms of aphasia, the victim loses the ability to integrate several specific mental processes though individually these processes are retained. The difficulty levels of the more specific tests do not seem to provide a useful explanation since, for example, normal persons describe the spatial orientation task as more difficult than the constructional praxis task, the opposite of the order of difficulty in aphasia.

Conceptual Performances

Conceptual thinking is something of an amorphous concept that has been applied in such various ways that it is difficult to separate it from either general intelligence or some specific verbal ability. In fact, some theorists, for example Bay (1962), would subsume the nonverbal cognitive deficits in aphasia under the rubric of a defect in conceptual or categorical thinking. It is only when we restrict our usage of the term to its basic elements that we can employ it in a definable and tractable fashion. So we shall use CONCEPTUAL ABILITY to mean the fundamental ability to generate a concept of a class of things and to discriminate those things that belong to the class from those that do not. Tasks calling for the sorting of objects, colors, forms, etc. were thought by Kurt Goldstein to be good representatives of conceptual thinking (Goldstein, 1948; Goldstein & Scheerer, 1941). One often-used task is the Weigl Color-Form Sorting test. The test uses tokens of several colors in the shape of circles, squares, and triangles. The subject's task is to form a principle and sort the tokens accordingly and then form a second principle and re-sort the tokens to fit it. So the task also involves a conceptual shift.

In an early study using the Weigl sorting task, McFie and Piercy (1952) reported that defective performance was associated with left hemisphere lesions, based on the observation that failure on this task occurred in 52% of 42 patients with unilateral left-sided lesions and in only 6% of 32 patients with right-sided lesions. Within the left hemisphere cases, these investigators reported there was no relationship between conceptual failure and aphasia. A reanalysis of their data, however, suggests this conclusion may be inaccurate if one considers frontal lobe patients separately. In the left frontal lobe group, there were 7 defective performances out of 12, and 6 of the patients with defective performances were nonaphasic. Statistically, there was only a trend for aphasia and defective sorting to be dissociated in left frontal lobe disease (the Fisher exact probability of chance association was $p = .14$). On the other hand, in patients with lesions outside the frontal lobe, aphasia was positively associated with impaired sorting (Fisher exact probability $= .047$), that is, only 2 of the 15 defective performances were produced by nonaphasic patients (one of whom had a frontoparietal meningioma). Excluding aphasics, there were 8 cases with left-sided lesions and defective sorting out of 17, and 6 of these patients had frontal or frontoparietal lesions. Thus, in the absence of aphasia, it is likely there exists a positive association between defective performance and frontal lobe involvement (Fisher exact probability = .041).

These new analyses highlight an interesting point: Within a single hemisphere, lesions in different loci may result in the same defective cognitive performance but for different reasons. It is now well known that lesions in certain regions of the frontal lobes outside the language zone produce disturbances in sorting behaviors and the ability to perform conceptual shifts (Milner, 1963). These reanalyses also bring McFie and Piercy's classic study in line with the results of other investigators who find, on the whole, defects on sorting tasks are related to the presence of aphasia and, more specifically, aphasia involving receptive language impairment (De Renzi, Faglioni, Savoiardo, & Vignolo, 1966).

Language Comprehension Impairment

Nonverbal Communicative Performances

Up to now we have followed the usual custom of thinking of, or at least referring to, language comprehension impairment and its synonyms as if it were a single entity. However, this may no longer be justified, as suggested by recent findings. It is fitting to conclude this chapter on intelligence and aphasia with a discussion of language comprehension impairments since it is primarily in association with such defects that nonverbal intellectual performance is most variable and most vulnerable to impairment. The emphasis here shall be on processes leading to, or occurring with, receptive impairment, with special attention being given to the types of errors made by aphasics. We shall be looking for clues that might help resolve the enigma of nonverbal intellectual impairments in aphasia. If the anatomical hypothesis is correct, then this is largely for naught. At the present, there are no technically adequate studies to resolve the validity of the anatomical hypothesis that may be resolved through detailed clinicopathological correlation studies. With the advent of CT scanning and the aid of an atlas approach for localizing lesions (H. Damasio & A. Damasio, 1979; Mazzocchi & Vignolo, 1978) and with advances in aphasia assessment, such studies have become quite feasible.

In attempting to explain the basis for the occurrence of nonverbal intellectual deficits in receptive aphasia, both the anatomical hypothesis and the psychological hypothesis suffer from certain inconsistencies. It is often stated that if a symptom of cognitive impairment occurs with equal frequency with lesions of either hemisphere then it bears no essential relationship with language, which in most individuals resides in the domain of the left hemisphere. That the symptom may have a close association with aphasia in the context of left-sided lesions could be attributed to a coincidence of anatomy. However, this dictum may not be warranted unless the investigator can demonstrate that the cognitive symptom has the same correlates regardless of whether the lesion is on the right or left. Of course, because of anatomical coincidence, there may be different additional correlates depending on the side of the lesions, but, at the same time, there should remain a core set of related cognitive disabilities that is invariable. This requirement is derived from the concepts of the structure of intelligence as described earlier, and it is on this point that the anatomical hypothesis is in conflict with the data. The psychological hypothesis stresses the position that behaviors, especially complex cognitive behaviors, have multiple determinants and therefore are subject to distortions for various reasons and from several sources. Exactly what psychological (cognitive, mental) process is the cause of the nonverbal symptoms is the subject of much debate. It may lie in the ability to manipulate symbols or, more basically, in the ability to formulate symbols or categories. However, if this were the root cause of both the linguistic and the nonverbal symptoms, then it is difficult to explain the substantial proportion of patients with apparently severe receptive deficits and no evidence of a compromise of nonverbal abilities. To postulate the existence of some conceptual center that lies near, or partially overlaps with, the language zone would provide a compromise to the two countervailing hypotheses, but it would also require the assumption of the existence of a set of cognitive abilities that have not previously been shown to have unique properties. For these reasons the issue of the status of intelligence in aphasia remains unresolved.

Language, as a more or less codified system of symbols used to express or communicate ideas and information, has several forms for expression (e.g., oral speech, written language, gesture). For each mode of expression, there must exist a corresponding mode of reception for communication to take place. LANGUAGE is usually used to refer to the use of verbal symbols (words), but we may also think of a nonverbal form of language that allows an individual to communicate with his environment.

That defects in the recognition of nonverbal meaningful sounds, such as thunder, the ringing of a door bell, and animal sounds, are associated with aphasia and specifically with impairment in aural comprehension of spoken language was experimentally demonstrated by Spinnler and Vignolo (1966). By using a multiple-choice assessment technique, they were also able to show that the types of errors made by aphasics were not random; instead they were predominantly errors involving semantic slippage. For example, if an error were to be made by an aphasic patient in response to a stimulus such as a canary singing, the most likely response choice would be one from the same semantic class, such as a cock crowing, rather than an acoustically similar response, such as a man whistling, or an irrelevant response, such as a train in motion. This impairment is not due to an acquired hearing loss nor does it represent a defect in sound discrimination, since receptive aphasics who are impaired on this measure show no defect in the discrimination of meaningless sounds, while patients with right hemisphere lesions may show the opposite pattern (Faglioni, Spinnler, & Vignolo, 1969). Not all aphasics with receptive deficits show a defect in the recognition of meaningful environmental sounds. Those who do, however, have a high frequency of impairment on the Weigl sorting task and the RPM test. These findings have been interpreted as demonstrating the presence of a "cognitive-associative" deficit in comprehension impaired aphasics (Vignolo, 1969).

Subsequently, Varney (1980) replicated these findings and added three new observations. First, sound recognition impairment is specifically associated with aural comprehension as opposed to the comprehension of written language in the visual modality (reading). Second, sound recognition deficits, when present, appear to represent a primary determinant of aural comprehension impairment rather than an expression of it, because defects in aural comprehension of at least equal severity always accompany sound recognition deficits, while there are patients with severe impairments in the understanding of oral speech who are not impaired in recognizing the meaning of environmental sounds. Third, Varney and Benton (1979) demonstrated that a defect in the ability to discriminate phonemes represents another, relatively independent, source of aural comprehension deficits. Thus, the aural comprehension of speech may be impaired for either semantic-associative or for perceptual-linguistic reasons.

Deficits in the ability to comprehend the meaning of pantomimes represents another form of nonverbal comprehension impairment in aphasia. Goodglass and Kaplan (1963) observed such impairments in the context of aphasia. Because there was not a close association between the severity of aphasia and the severity of the disturbances in gestures and pantomime, they were led to the conclusion that such deficits must in some sense be independent of aphasia. Subsequently, Varney (1978) demonstrated that, while there was no special correlation between pantomime recognition defects and the severity of the disorder in aural comprehension or verbal expression (naming), failure in pantomime recognition was closely allied with disturbances in reading comprehension (that is, reading for meaning rather than reading aloud). Impairment in the comprehension of pantomimes always occurred in association with defects in reading comprehension of at least equal severity. However, one could be alexic, even severely so, without showing any impairment in the recognition of pantomimes. Thus, in the visual modality, there is likely to be more than one determinant for an acquired impairment in the comprehension of written language. Varney (1978) also demonstrated that the major error type committed by aphasics was to select from among four response alternatives a response that was semantically associated with the pantomimed stimulus rather than selecting an irrelevant item or one that was visually similar but semantically unrelated to the stimulus. These findings suggest a parallel organization of verbal and nonverbal language processing in the visual and auditory modalities.

Nonverbal Intelligence and the Receptive Aphasias

Do these defects in sound and pantomime recognition in association with aphasia tell us anything about the fundamental structure of language, or are they merely instances of a host of findings of nonverbal deficits in comprehension impaired aphasics? It has been argued that the ability to comprehend gestural communication and to appreciate the significance of environmental sounds represent the selective advantages that fostered the evolutionary development and refinement of the neural structures in humans that serve these functions. They are considered selective advantages because they may be directly related to one's ability to survive in a primitive and hostile environment. Thus, the human brain may have become preadapted for language through the evolutionary development of these pristine nonverbal communicative abilities (Varney & Vilensky, 1980). Arguments of this sort are necessarily discursive, for when empirical proof cannot be obtained, one must rely on analytic reasoning. Since oral speech arises from audition, it would be natural to expect that mechanisms for understanding sounds as meaningful stimuli must precede the development of speech. Also, it would be difficult to maintain, in view of the very recent and rapid development of reading abilities in human evolution, that the capability for understanding written language in the visual modality was acquired on the basis of a selective advantage that augmented one's probability of surviving.

The final task before us is to relate these recent developments in identifying modality-related subtypes of comprehension impairments to the problem of explaining nonverbal intellectual deficits in aphasia. In our present and limited state of knowledge, it is more reasonable to look for clues rather than solutions to the puzzle. We owe to J. Hughlings Jackson the concept of two classes of behavioral symptoms of brain disease: the negative and the positive. Negative symptoms represent the loss of an ability to produce behaviors that were previously in one's behavioral repertoire. An example would be an inability to recall the name of an object. Positive symptoms represent the emergence of new behaviors that were not previously in the behavioral repertoire. An example of a positive symptom would be misnamings, such as the utterance of semantic or phonemic paraphasias in the attempt to name an object (e.g., calling a knife a fork). Whether the errors described here as semantic (conceptual, associative, symbolic) slippages are negative or positive symptoms may be more an academic argument than a real distinction. If characterized as a loss in the ability to discriminate among members of the same semantic class, they could be considered negative symptoms; if characterized as an active error tendency, perhaps as the result of a derailment in thinking, they could be considered positive symptoms. Since aphasic patients who show these errors of semantic slippage may make their response choices with great conviction and an air of success, it may be convenient to think of these errors as positive symptoms resulting from an active process that causes one to err in a particular direction.

If we were to accept the proposition that some comprehension impaired aphasics suffer from some form of semantic slippage, we may then begin to provide explanations for the occurrence of nonverbal intellectual deficits in aphasia. Applying this model to the problem at hand, we could conceptualize nonverbal intellectual deficits as the consequence of a newly acquired active error tendency that disrupts performance on complex tasks rather than as the result of a loss in the cognitive abilities the tasks were intended to measure. To restate this, the nonverbal deficits associated with aphasia may represent faulty response selection rather than a degraded form of stimulus processing. One convenience of this model is that it does not require the postulation of the bilateral representation of visuoperceptive, spatial, and constructional abilities or other components of nonverbal intelligence.

The demonstration that there are at least two types of acquired deficits that may result in language comprehension impairment may help to explain the exceptional cases of patients who do not understand oral speech but show none of the deficiencies in nonverbal intellectual performance that are associated with receptive language impairment. Finally, these hypotheses may help to explain the high degree of variability in the pattern of nonverbal deficits exhibited by groups of aphasic patients who previously were thought to share the same, unitary symptom of comprehension impairment. Should these hypotheses find significant empirical support in the future, then we may be forced to redefine the syndromes of aphasia to include nonverbal symptomatology that heretofore has been omitted in the assessment and classification of aphasic disorders.

Summary

Intelligence, conceived abstractly, represents one's innate ability to generate ideas and solve problems of varying complexity and to communicate effectively with others and with one's environment. In an effort to approximate this abstract concept, psychologists have developed batteries of cognitive tests from which an IQ score can be obtained. Evidence gathered from various sources shows that intelligence, expressed concretely as an IQ score, meets psychometric criteria and predicts demographic characteristics of individuals that are incorporated in the abstract notion of intelligence.

Neurological disease affecting the cerebrum often results in corresponding impairments in intellectual functioning. In the usual case, disease of the right hemisphere may be reflected in acquired impairments of nonverbal intelligence, whereas disease of the left hemisphere may result in verbal intellectual deficits. However, in a significant proportion of aphasic patients having receptive language defects, nonverbal intellectual performance appears to be compromised. Such findings are in conflict with our current understanding of the functional and neurological structure of intelligence.

The hypotheses offered to account for these incongruous findings fall into two general classes. One general hypothesis is that some portion of the cerebral cortex in the left hemisphere, which lies near or overlaps with the language zone, subserves the same general mental functions as mediated by the right hemisphere. If lesions resulting in aphasia happen to invade this region as well, then nonverbal intellectual deficits will result. This hypothesis denies the existence of a functional relation between nonverbal intelligence and aphasia. The other general hypothesis suggests the opposite and links disturbances in language with disturbances in thought processes. So far, the evidence brought to bear on this issue is mixed and so if sampled selectively allows one to support or refute either hypothesis.

It is argued that linguistic aspects of language were derived from pristine nonverbal communicative abilities. Recent investigations of the capacity of aphasics to comprehend environmental sounds and pantomimes has disclosed the presence of error tendencies, described here as semantic slippage, in both the auditory and visual modalities. In aphasia, these error tendencies may disrupt response selections in the performance of nonverbal intellectual tasks, whereas in right hemisphere disease, acquired deficits in stimulus processing may be the root causes of nonverbal intellectual impairment. This conciliatory hypothesis may help explain how nonverbal intelligence can be affected by acquired disturbances of language. Empirical support for this hypothesis has not yet been provided nor have neuroanatomic correlates of these nonverbal communicative deficits been investigated.

References

Alajouanine, T., & Lhermitte, F. 1964. Non-verbal communication in aphasia. In A. de Reuck & M. O'Connor (Eds.), *Disorders of language*. Boston: Little, Brown.

Archibald, Y. M., Wepman, J. M., & Jones, L. V. 1967. Nonverbal cognitive performance in aphasic and nonphasic brain-damaged patients. *Cortex, 3,* 275–294.

Arrigoni, G., & De Renzi, E. 1964. Constructional apraxia and hemispheric locus of lesion. *Cortex, 1,* 170–197.

Basso, A., De Renzi, E., Faglioni, P., Scotti, G., & Spinnler, H. 1973. Neuropsychological evidence for the existence of cerebral areas critical to the performance of intelligence tests. *Brain, 96,* 715–728.

Bay, E. 1962. Aphasia and non-verbal disorders of language. *Brain, 85,* 411–426.

Benton, A. L. 1962. The visual retention test as a constructional praxis task. *Confinia Neurologica, 22,* 141–155.

Benton, A. L. 1964. Developmental aphasia and brain damage. *Cortex, 1,* 40–52.

Benton, A. L. 1965. Language disorders in children. *Canadian Psychologist, 7a,* 298–312.

Benton, A. L. 1967. Constructional apraxia and the minor hemisphere. *Confinia Neurologica, 29,* 1–16.

Benton, A. L. 1969. Constructional apraxia: Some unanswered questions. In A. L. Benton (Ed.), *Contributions to clinical neuropsychology*. Chicago: Aldine.

Benton, A. L. 1973. Visuoconstructive disability in patients with cerebral disease: Its relationship to side of lesion and aphasic disorder. *Documenta Ophthalmologica, 34,* 67–76.

Benton, A. L. 1977. Historical notes on hemispheric dominance. *Archives of Neurology, 34,* 127–129. (a)

Benton, A. L. 1977. Psychologic testing. In A. B. Baker & L. H. Baker (Eds.), *Clinical neurology* (Vol. 1). Hagerstown: Harper. (b)

Benton, A. L. 1978. The cognitive functioning of children with developmental dysphasia. In M. A. Wyke (Ed.), *Developmental dysphasia*. London: Academic Press.

Benton, A. L. 1980. Psychological testing for brain damage. In H. I. Kaplan, A. M. Freed-
    man, & B. J. Sadock (Eds.), *Comprehensive textbook of psychiatry* (Vol. 1, 3rd ed.). Balti-
    more: Williams & Wilkins.
Benton, A. L., & Fogel, M. L. 1962. Three-dimensional constructional praxis. *Archives of
    Neurology, 7*, 347–354.
Benton, A. L., & Hamsher, K. 1976. *Multilingual Aphasia Examination.* Iowa City: Depart-
    ment of Neurology, University of Iowa.
Benton, A. L., Hannay, H. J., & Varney, N. R. 1975. Visual perception of line direction in
    patients with unilateral brain disease. *Neurology, 25*, 907–910.
Benton, A. L., & Van Allen, M. W. 1968. Impairment in facial recognition in patients with
    cerebral disease. *Cortex, 4*, 344–358.
Benton, A. L., Van Allen, M. W., Hamsher, K., & Levin, H. S. 1975. *Test of Facial Recogni-
    tion, Form SL.* Iowa City: Department of Neurology, University of Iowa.
Benton, A. L., Varney, N. R., & Hamsher, K. de S. 1978. Visuospatial judgment: A clinical
    test. *Archives of Neurology, 35*, 364–367.
Blessed, G., Tomlinson, B. E., & Roth, M. 1968. The association between quantitative
    measures of dementia and of senile change in the cerebral grey matter of elderly
    subjects. *British Journal of Psychiatry, 114*, 797–811.
Burt, C. 1955. The evidence for the concept of intelligence. *British Journal of Educational
    Psychology, 25*, 158–177.
Carmon, A., & Bechtoldt, H. 1967. Dominance of the right cerebral hemisphere for
    stereopsis. *Neuropsychologia, 7*, 29–39.
Chapman, L. F., & Wolf, H. G. 1959. The cerebral hemispheres and the highest integrative
    functions of man. *Archives of Neurology, 1*, 357–424.
Costa, L. D., Vaughan, H. G., Jr., Horwitz, M., & Ritter, W. 1969. Patterns of behavioral
    deficit associated with visual spatial neglect. *Cortex, 5*, 242–263.
Cromer, R. F. 1978. The basis of childhood dysphasia: A linguistic approach. In M. A.
    Wyke (Ed.), *Developmental dysphasia.* London: Academic Press.
Damasio, A. R., Castro-Caldas, A., Grosso, J. T., & Ferro, J. M. 1976. Brain specialization
    for language does not depend on literacy. *Archives of Neurology, 33*, 300–301.
Damasio, A. R., Hamsher, K. de S., Castro-Caldas, A., Ferro, J., & Grosso, J. T. 1976.
    Brain specialization for language: Not dependent on literacy. *Archives of Neurology, 33*,
    662.
Damasio, A. R., & Maurer, R. G. 1978. A neurological model for childhood autism. *Ar-
    chives of Neurology, 35*, 777–786.
Damasio, H., & Damasio, A. 1979. "Paradoxic" ear extinction in dichotic listening: Possible
    anatomic significance. *Neurology, 29*, 644–653.
Damasio, H., Damasio, A. R., Castro-Caldas, A., & Hamsher, K. de S. 1979. Reversal of
    ear advantage for phonetically similar words in illiterates. *Journal of Clinical Neuro-
    psychology, 1*, 331–338.
Dee, H. L. 1970. Visuoconstructive and visuoperceptive deficits in patients with unilateral
    cerebral lesions. *Neuropsychologia, 8*, 305–314.
De Renzi, E., Faglioni, P., Savoiardo, M., & Vignolo, L. A. 1966. The influence of aphasia
    and of hemispheric side of the cerebral lesion on abstract thinking. *Cortex, 2*, 399–420.
De Renzi, E., Faglioni, P., Scotti, G., & Spinnler, H. 1972. Impairment in associating
    colour to form, concomitant with aphasia. *Brain, 95*, 293–304.
De Renzi, E., & Spinnler, H. 1967. Impaired performance on color tasks in patients with
    hemispheric damage. *Cortex, 3*, 194–217.
Faglioni, P., Spinnler, H., & Vignolo, L. A. 1969. Contrasting behavior of right and left
    hemisphere-damaged patients on a discriminative and a semantic task of auditory
    recognition. *Cortex, 5*, 366–389.

Fogel, M. L. 1964. The intelligence quotient as an index of brain damage. *American Journal of Orthopsychiatry, 34,* 555–562.

Furth, H. G. 1964. Research with the deaf: Implications for language and cognition. *Psychological Bulletin, 62,* 145–164.

Furth, H., & Youniss, J. 1975. Congenital deafness and the development of thinking. In E. H. Lenneberg & E. Lenneberg (Eds.), *Foundations of language development: A multidisciplinary approach* (Vol. 2). New York: Academic Press.

Galton, F. 1887. *Hereditary genius: An inquiry into its laws and consequences* (New and rev. ed., with an American preface). New York: D. Appleton & Co.

Goldin-Meadow, S., & Feldman, H. 1977. The development of language-like communication without a language model. *Science, 197,* 401–403.

Goldstein, G. 1974. The use of clinical neuropsychological methods in lateralisation of brain lesions. In S. J. Dimond & J. G. Beaumont (Eds.), *Hemisphere function in the human brain.* New York: Halsted Press.

Goldstein, K. 1948. *Language and language disturbances.* New York: Grune & Stratton.

Goldstein, K., & Scheerer, M. 1941. Abstract and concrete behavior: An experimental study with special tests. *Psychological Monographs, 53,* 1–151 (Whole No. 239).

Goodglass, H. 1974. Nonverbal performance. In Y. Lebrun & R. Hoops (Eds.), *Neurolinguistics,* Vol. 2. *Intelligence and aphasia.* Amsterdam: Swets & Zeitlinger B. V.

Goodglass, H. 1980. Disoders of naming following brain injury. *American Scientist, 68,* 647–655.

Goodglass, H., & Kaplan, E. 1963. Disturbance of gesture and pantomime in aphasia. *Brain, 86,* 703–720.

Hamsher, K. de S. 1978. Stereopsis and the perception of anomalous contours. *Neuropsychologia, 16,* 453–459. (a)

Hamsher, K. de S. 1978. Stereopsis and unilateral brain disease. *Investigative Ophthalmology and Visual Science, 17,* 336–343. (b)

Hamsher, K. de S., Levin, H. S., & Benton, A. L. 1979. Facial recognition in patients with focal brain lesions. *Archives of Neurology, 36,* 837–839.

Kinsbourne, M., & Warrington, E. K. 1963. Jargon aphasia. *Neuropsychologia, 1,* 27–37.

Klove, H. 1974. Validation studies in adult clinical neuropsychology. In R. M. Reitan & L. A. Davison (Eds.), *Clinical neuropsychology: Current status and applications.* Washington, D.C.: V. H. Winston & Sons.

Klove, H., & Reitan, R. M. 1958. Effect of dysphasia and spatial distortion on Wechsler-Bellevue results. *Archives of Neurology and Psychiatry, 80,* 708–713.

Kodman, F. Jr. 1963. Sensory processes and mental deficiency. In N. R. Ellis (Ed.), *Handbook of mental deficiency.* New York: McGraw-Hill.

Landau, W. M., Goldstein, R., & Kleffner, F. R. 1960. Congenital aphasia: A clinicopathologic study. *Neurology, 10,* 915–921.

Lashley, K. S. 1929. *Brain mechanisms and intelligence. A quantitative study of injuries to the brain.* Chicago: Univ. of Chicago Press.

Lezak, M. D. 1976. *Neuropsychological assessment.* New York: Oxford Univ. Press.

McCall, R. B. 1977. Childhood IQ's as predictors of adult educational and occupational status. *Science, 197,* 482–843.

McFie, J. 1960. Psychological testing in clinical neurology. *Journal of Nervous and Mental Disease, 131,* 383–393.

McFie, J. 1969. The diagnostic significance of disorders of higher nervous activity: Syndromes related to frontal, temporal, parietal and occipital lesions. In P. J. Vinken & G. W. Bruyn (Eds.), *Handbook of clinical neurology.* Vol. 4. *Disorders of speech, perception, and symbolic behaviour.* Amsterdam: North-Holland Publ.

McFie, J. 1975. *Assessment of organic intellectual impairment.* New York: Academic Press.

McFie, J., & Piercy, M. F. 1952. The relation of laterality of lesion to performance on Weigl's sorting test. *Journal of Mental Science, 98,* 299–305.

McFie, J., & Thompson, J. A. 1972. Picture arrangement: A measure of frontal lobe function? *British Journal of Psychiatry, 121,* 547–552.

McFie, J., & Zangwill, O. L. 1960. Visual-constructive disabilities associated with lesions of the left hemisphere. *Brain, 83,* 243–260.

Matarazzo, J. D. 1972. *Wechsler's measurement and appraisal of adult intelligence* (5th ed.). Baltimore: Williams & Wilkins.

Mazzocchi, F., & Vignolo, L. A. 1978. Computer assisted tomography in neuropsychological research: A simple procedure for lesion mapping. *Cortex, 14,* 136–144.

Messerli, P., & Tissot, R. 1974. Operational capacity and aphasia. In Y. Lebrun & R. Hoops (Eds.), *Neurolinguistics.* Vol. 2. *Intelligence and aphasia.* Amsterdam. Swets & Zeitlinger B. V.

Milner, B. 1963. Effects of different brain lesions on card sorting. *Archives of Neurology, 9,* 90–100.

Newcombe, F. 1969. *Missile wounds of the brain: A study of psychological deficits.* London: Oxford Univ. Press.

Newcombe, F. 1974. Selective deficits after focal cerebral injury. In S. J. Dimond & J. G. Beaumont (Eds.), *Hemisphere function in the human brain.* New York: Halsted Press.

Orgass, B., Hartje, W., Kerschensteiner, M., & Poeck, K. 1972. Aphasie und nichtsprachliche intelligenz. *Nervenarzt, 43,* 623–627.

Piaget, J. 1936. *La naissance de l'intelligence chez l'enfant.* Neuchâtel: Delachaux & Niestlé. (English translation by M. Cook. 1952. New York: International Univ. Press.)

Pick, A. 1931. Aphasie. In A. Bethe, G. von Bergman, G. Emblem, & A. Ellinger (Eds.), *Handbuch der normalen und pathologiochen physiologie* (Vol. 15, Pt. 2). Berlin: Springer-Verlag. (English translation by J. Brown. 1973. Springfield, Ill: Thomas.)

Piercy, M. 1964. The effects of cerebral lesions on intellectual function: A review of current research trends. *British Journal of Psychiatry, 110,* 310–352.

Piercy, M. 1969. Neurological aspects of intelligence. In P. J. Vinken & G. W. Bruyn (Eds.), *Handbook of clinical neurology.* Vol. 3. *Disorders of higher nervous activity.* Amsterdam: North-Holland Publ.

Pitner, R., & Lev, J. 1939. The intelligence of the hard of hearing school child. *Journal of Genetic Psychology, 55,* 31–48.

Semmes, J., Weinstein, S., Ghent, L., & Teuber, H.-L. 1963. Correlates of impaired orientation in personal and extra-personal space. *Brain, 86,* 747–772.

Smith, A. 1975. Neuropsychological testing in neurological disorders. In W. J. Friedlander (Ed.), *Advances in neurology.* Vol. 7. *Current reviews of higher nervous system dysfunction.* New York: Raven.

Spearman, C. 1927. *The abilities of man.* New York: Macmillan.

Spinnler, H., & Vignolo, L. A. 1966. Impaired recognition of meaningful sounds in aphasia. *Cortex, 2,* 337–348.

Tallal, P., & Piercy, M. 1978. Defects of auditory perception in children with developmental dysphasia. In M. A. Wyke (Ed.), *Developmental dysphasia.* London: Academic Press.

Thurstone, L. L. 1938. Primary mental abilities. *Psychometric Monographs,* No. 1.

Vandenberg, S. G. 1971. What do we know today about the inheritance of intelligence and how do we know it? In R. Cancro (Ed.), *Intelligence: Genetic and environmental influences.* New York: Grune & Stratton.

Varney, N. R. 1978. Linguistic correlates of pantomime recognition in aphasic patients. *Journal of Neurology, Neurosurgery, and Psychiatry, 41,* 564–568.

Varney, N. R. 1980. Sound recognition in relation to aural comprehension and reading comprehension in aphasic patients. *Journal of Neurology, Neurosurgery, and Psychiatry, 43,* 71–75.

Varney, N. R., & Benton, A. L. 1979. Phonemic discrimination and auditory comprehension in aphasic patients. *Journal of Clinical Neuropsychology, 1,* 65–74.

Varney, N. R., & Vilensky, J. A. 1980. Neuropsychological implications for preadaptation and language evolution. *Journal of Human Evolution, 9,* 223–226.

Vignolo, L. A. 1969. Auditory agnosia: A review and report of recent evidence. In A. L. Benton (Ed.), *Contributions to clinical neuropsychology.* Chicago: Aldine.

Walsh, K. W. 1978. *Neuropsychology: A clinical approach.* New York: Churchill Livingstone.

Warrington, E. K. 1969. Constructional apraxia. In P. J. Vinken & G. W. Bruyn (Eds.), *Handbook of clinical neurology,* Vol. 4. *Disorders of speech, perception, and symbolic behaviour.* Amsterdam: North-Holland Publ.

Wechsler, D. 1958. *The measurement and appraisal of adult intelligence* (4th ed.). Baltimore: Williams & Wilkins.

Wechsler, D. 1971. Intelligence: Definition, theory, and the IQ. In R. Cancro (Ed.), *Intelligence: Genetic and environmental influences.* New York: Grune & Stratton.

Weinstein, S., & Teuber, H.-L. 1957. Effects of penetrating brain injury on intelligence test scores. *Science, 125,* 1036–1037.

Weisenburg, T. H., & McBride, K. E. 1935. *Aphasia: A clinical and psychological study.* New York: Commonwealth Fund.

Wilson, R. S., Rosenbaum, G., & Brown, G. 1979. The problem of premorbid intelligence in neuropsychological assessment. *Journal of Clinical Neuropsychology, 1,* 49–53.

Worster-Drought, C., & Allen, I. M. 1929. Congenital auditory imperception (congenital word-deafness): With report of a case. *Journal of Neurology and Psychopathology, 9,* 193–208.

Zangwill, O. L. 1964. Intelligence in aphasia. In A. V. S. de Reuck & M. O'Connor (Eds.), *Disorders of language.* Boston: Little, Brown.

Zangwill, O. L. 1969. Intellectual status in aphasia. In P. J. Vinken & G. W. Bruyn (Eds.), *Handbook of clinical neurology.* Vol. 4. *Disorders of speech, perception, and symbolic behavior.* Amsterdam: North-Holland Publ.

Zangwill, O. L. 1974. Consciousness and the cerebral hemispheres. In S. J. Dimond & J. G. Beaumont (Eds.), *Hemisphere function in the human brain.* New York: Halsted Press.

Zangwill, O. L. 1975. The relation of nonverbal cognitive functions to aphasia. In E. H. Lennenberg & E. Lennenberg (Eds.), *Foundations of language development: A multidisciplinary approach* (Vol. 2). New York: Academic Press.

Zangwill, O. L. 1978. The concept of developmental dysphasia. In M. A. Wyke (Ed.), *Developmental dysphasia.* London: Academic Press.

12

Artistry and Aphasia

HOWARD GARDNER and ELLEN WINNER

Language is our central mode of communication. Accordingly, psychologists interested in the problem of human communication have concentrated on the study of language to the virtual exclusion of other forms of communication. Thus, although the symbol systems of the arts are almost as universal and as well developed among humans as is language, much less is known about the representation of artistic skills in the brain. Moreover, little is known about the relationship of language and artistic modes of communication. For instance, while it is well known that damage to the left hemisphere entails a loss of linguistic capacities, less information is available on whether a breakdown in language entails—or occurs independently of—a breakdown in one or more of the symbol systems of the arts. An understanding of the fate of artistic skills after damage to the brain that has either spared or impaired language should clarify the relationship that obtains between the symbol systems of language and those of the arts.

Any investigation of artistry and aphasia must be built upon a way of thinking about the arts. Work in our laboratory at the Boston University Aphasia Research Center has been guided by a point of view first put forward by the philosopher Nelson Goodman (1968, 1972, 1979) and developed over the past decade at Harvard Project Zero (Gardner, 1976, 1979; Gardner, Howard, & Perkins, 1974; Perkins & Leondar, 1977). According to this point of view, involvement in the arts entails the ability to "encode" and to "read" symbols, whether these be verbal, pictorial, musical, gestural, or some combination thereof. Rather than simply an arena of entertainment or of emotional gratification, the arts are thus seen as fundamentally cognitive: Mental processes are needed

361

to make sense of artistic symbols just as they are required to interpret symbols functioning in a scientific, journalistic, or conversational vein. In brief, works of art must be "read," and literacy in the arts is no less demanding than literacy in the scientific domain.

Such a cognitive approach to the arts serves here as a point of departure for a psychology (and a neuropsychology) of art, as well as an investigation into the relationship between linguistic and artistic symbols and symbol systems. In what follows, we review certain lines of evidence about the nature of artistry. We consider the visual and literary arts but have chosen to focus on music simply because more is known about the psychology of music than about other forms of art.

Three general questions are posed with respect to each art form. What is the relationship between language and the artistic skill in question? What is the predominant mode of information processing in the art form under consideration? And what difference exists between those artistic skills that are highly developed and displayed by only a few individuals and those artistic abilities possessed by most normal human beings in our culture?

Music

Preliminary Considerations

Music is a logical candidate for initial consideration in any neuropsychology of the arts. Some form of music is evident in all human cultures, and musical performances and rites date back thousands of years. Music is not only universal, it is also unique among the arts because, unlike literature and nonabstract visual art, it lacks representational content. Representational forms of art have an immediately obvious relation to the "real" world and thereby possess a less "free-standing existence" than music. Indeed, the survival of music in the face of the "triumph" of language poses a riddle for evolutionary theorists: Why has such an apparently "nonadaptive" symbol system continued to figure so importantly in human culture?

Other reasons motivating a neuropsychology of music merit brief mention. Music offers a particularly rich set of roles. In addition to audience member and critic, individuals can participate through singing, playing works produced by others, or creating works of their own, for voice, for instrument, or even for electronic realization by a computer. There are numerous types of music, ranging from folk music to high art, a myriad of styles, and a complex notation that is understood, at least in part, by many literate individuals. This variegated symbolic domain raises a multitude of questions about how competence can be organized in the human brain.

Even to mention the many approaches to music developed over the centuries by musicians, scholars, and, most recently, behavioral scientists would take many pages (for reviews, see Cooper & Meyer, 1960; Langer, 1953; Lerdahl & Jackendoff, forthcoming; Meyer, 1956). Rather than offering a necessarily superficial review of what has been said before, it seems preferable to introduce those organizing principles that have most often emerged in current efforts to study music.

To begin with, one may (following current usage in the cognitive sciences) distinguish two primary approaches in conceptualizing the domain of music. Taking a "bottom–up" approach, one may focus on the elementary components of music—pitch, rhythm, timbre—and gradually build up from these individual components to that complex interplay that constitutes a musical composition. Adopting the contrasting "top–down" approach, one takes as a point of departure the organized piece of music. According to this approach, it is assumed that musical analysis, like the perception of a musical work, should begin by approaching the organized musical form, or gestalt, with subsequent analysis into components an optional (and possibly advisable) ploy on the part of the analyst or the observer.

Neither approach is wholly adequate. Those researchers who adopt a "top–down" approach often have difficulty specifying the components of music that contribute to understanding. Those who embrace a bottom–up approach are often unable to effect the bridge from artificial musical stimuli to more naturalistic "whole pieces" of music.

To be sure, a few researchers have exhibited ingenuity in bridging the gap between the building blocks of music and more holistic patterns of perception and production. The most effective methods have utilized a strategy whereby a specific musical fragment is viewed as an instance within a more general musical vocabulary. Thus, Krumhansl (1979) has provided musical contexts to subjects and then asked them to judge the similarity of stimuli presented within these contexts; and Dowling (1978, 1979) has studied the abilities of individuals to discern similarities and differences among musical passages that differ systematically in the kinds of tonal relationships that are featured. While such efforts still lean heavily on judgments of brief, somewhat contrived stimuli, their incorporation of musical contexts and their focus on musical (as opposed to acoustic) modes of analysis suggest a fruitful way of integrating the two approaches sketched here.

While the aforementioned strategies characterize the range of investigations, certain issues have proved particularly germane for those researchers working in the neuropsychological tradition. As mentioned,
we will focus on three organizing issues:

1. *The relationship between linguistic and musical processing.* At least in
certain superficial aspects (e.g., the processing of sequential materials
over time, the existence of a basic "syntactic component," division into
perceptual and productive capacities), music can be analogized to
natural language (cf. Kleist, 1962). But the utility of this comparison
remains to be demonstrated.

2. *The predominant mode of musical processing.* Echoing the distinctions
raised in the preceding discussion, it is possible to view the apprehension of music primarily in terms of gestalt or holistic processes, primarily
in terms of elementary or atomistic factors, or through some amalgam of
these two approaches. This issue assumes particular aptness in view of
current discussions about processing strategies favored by the two cerebral hemispheres.

3. *Contrasting pattern of skills across levels of talent or accomplishment.*
Because of the wide range of competence in the music domain, due to
differences in genetic endowment and/or training, it becomes crucial to
establish whether superior performances by some individuals are due
simply to a greater facility in processing musical elements or whether
they reflect qualitatively different strategies.

Components of Music

Most studies in the neuropsychology of music have focused on the
extent to which specific musical capacities and skills can be dissociated
by brain damage (cf. Benton, 1977). A pioneering study of this kind was
published in 1962 by Milner. Subtests of the Seashore test battery were
administered both pre- and post-operatively to epileptic patients who
underwent removal of one of their temporal lobes. Following removal of
the right temporal lobe, there was a significant drop in scores on subtests measuring sensitivity to timbre, sensitivity to intensity, and tonal
memory. Other subtest scores revealed no significant drop. Of greater
importance, the performances of patients with left temporal lobe removal were generally comparable to their preoperative levels. Here,
then, was early documentation of the relatively greater importance of
the right hemisphere in the processing of musical stimuli, as well as a
provisional demonstration that musical abilities could be dissociated on
a neurological basis.

Subsequent studies utilizing different patient populations and testing techniques have validated the greater importance of the right hemisphere in the processing of musical stimuli and have documented an important division in the organization of musical skills. As summarized in a major review article by Gates and Bradshaw (1977), rhythmic processing, a temporal sequencing task, draws particularly on intact left hemisphere structures. In contrast, the processing of pitch presupposes major participation on the part of the right hemisphere (H. Gordon, 1970; Kimura, 1973; Shankweiler, 1966; Zattore, 1979). More recent evidence suggests further a decisive role played by the anterior portions of the right frontal lobes in the processing of tonal material (Shapiro, Grossman, & Gardner, 1981).

While most experimental research has focused on the perception of musical components, there is some documentation of lateralization in the production of musical entities. Injecting sodium amytal into the carotid arteries of presurgical patients, Bogen and Gordon (1971) were able to mimic (in a reversible manner) the effects of hemispherectomies. After paralysis of the right hemisphere, singing was reduced to a monotone. Following injection of the left hemisphere, words were omitted and the melody was distorted but still recognizable. Contrary to what might have been expected, rhythm remained relatively intact under both procedures.

These findings are consistent with scattered clinical impressions. Many aphasiologists have reported a relative sparing of singing capacities following severe aphasia (Goodglass & Kaplan, 1972), and one promising form of aphasia therapy, in fact, exploits this preserved singing ability as a basis for reconstructing propositional speech (Sparks, Helm, & Albert, 1974). Our own observations indicate that, in left-hemisphere-damaged patients, singing a melody aids in the utterance of articulated words; in contrast, among right-hemisphere-damaged patients, it is the production of the verbal components of music that actually aids in the accurate rendition of melodies (see also Ross & Mesulam, 1979).

Some researchers have asked whether musical capacities may be organized differently in talented or trained individuals. While the data are still far from conclusive, some intriguing possiblities have been suggested. Thus, Bever and Chiarello (1974) devised a task that required the analysis of the internal structure of musical fragments. Individuals with musical training not only performed better on this task but also displayed a stronger right ear (left hemisphere) advantage than musically naive subjects. In a supporting study, Shanon (1980) documented a greater amount of left hemisphere involvement in tasks requiring complex musical decisions. However, another study, in which patients were

required to recognize dichotically presented chords, yielded a contrasting pattern of results (H. Gordon, 1970): Here musicians demonstrated a
right hemisphere advantage, while nonmusicians exhibited no ear preference (see also H.W. Gordon, 1980). These latter studies dictate caution
in inferring a universal pattern in the performances of musically trained
(as against musically naive) subjects: Effects may prove specific to certain stimuli, tasks, or subject groups.

Occasional efforts have been undertaken to examine the "meaning"
of musical fragments. In one study, Gardner, Silverman, Denes,
Semenza, and Rosenstiel (1977) asked patients to match a simple musical fragment with one or two contrasting geometric patterns. The sets of
pictures were varied systematically on a number of graphic dimensions
hypothesized to reflect different connotative aspects of musical patterns.
Thus, for example, an ascending passage should be paired with an up-
pointing line, while a descending passage should be paired with a descending line; a continuous tone "matches" an intact circle, while a broken
tone "matches" a fragmented circle.

Though levels of performance varied considerably across groups of
organic patients, a revealing dichotomy emerged: Right hemisphere patients proved better able to link a musical passage to a pattern that
portrayed the temporal course of the piece (such as regularity–
irregularity) than to a pattern that captured gestalt aspects (such as
continuity–discontinuity). In contrast, left anterior patients proved better able to match sounds to pictures that captured holistic properties of
the piece, while performing less adequately on those stimuli that depicted temporal aspects. Here, then, understanding of the connotative
(or expressive) aspects of a piece of music proves consistent with certain
hypotheses about preferred modes of information processing in the two
hemispheres (Galin, 1974; Kaplan, 1980; Nebes, 1974).

Studies of Larger Musical Fragments

A few investigators have asked subjects to make judgments about
actual musical works. For instance, in an effort to document comprehension of the denotative meanings of familiar pieces, Gardner and Denes
(1973) asked patients to pick out which picture from a set of four "went
with" a familiar piece of music. In half of the instances, the correct
answer was based upon the lyrics (not given) of a song; for example, in
order to match the melody of "Row, Row, Row Your Boat" with the
correct illustration (a boat), knowledge of the lyrics or title would be
called for. For the other half of the items, knowledge of lyrics was un-

necessary: Thus, to match the tune of "Hail to the Chief" with the correct illustration (the president), a patient merely had to know that the piece was usually played at official ceremonies, but did not have to know its unfamiliar title.

Results documented the extent to which musical performance by right-hemisphere-injured patients depends upon verbal information. On those items where correct performance necessitated knowledge of lyrics, right hemisphere patients outperformed those with left hemisphere damage. On the other hand, on those items where knowledge of lyrics was irrelevant, and identification could proceed simply on the basis of knowledge of the situation in which such a piece was ordinarily heard, left hemisphere patients surpassed those with injury to the right hemisphere. Here, then, is further documentation that purely musical components cohere and can be dissociated from verbal aspects of musical stimuli.

Following another line of investigation, Shapiro, Grossman, and Gardner (1981) asked whether the effects found with atomistic musical stimuli are also in evidence with familiar compositions. Experimenters played familiar pieces and asked subjects merely to judge whether they sounded "right" or "wrong." Groups of subjects proved differentially skilled at this task. Thus, left anterior patients evinced skill at detecting the major kinds of errors, having slight difficulty only with those pieces that were played unusually rapidly or unusually slowly. Left posterior and left central patients performed somewhat more poorly, particularly on items probing sensitivity to tempo. Patients with right anterior damage performed at the lowest level, responding at chance level on every kind of item except the control pieces (pieces that were correctly performed). Counter to the prevalent notion that the left hemisphere is dominant for rhythmic processing, it was the right hemisphere patients who proved poor at detecting rhythmic errors.

This pattern of results may be interpreted as evidence that right hemisphere patients have a fragile or impaired internal representation of all aspects of the melody. In the absence of such an internal representation, which indicates what the piece is supposed to sound like, it would of necessity prove difficult to determine whether or not it had been performed correctly. Further evidence for a possible deficit in the overall internal representation (or auditory imagery) of musical material comes from a recent case study at the Boston University Aphasia Research Center. An amateur musician suffering from auditory agnosia secondary to major right hemisphere involvement proved able to answer challenging theoretical questions about music. Yet the same patient could not indicate whether the first note of a familiar piece of music was higher or lower than the second. Such evidence suggests that his internal auditory imagery for known melodies had been severely degraded.

Case Studies

By far the richest and most important information about the organization of musical skills has come from the study of talented individuals who have sustained brain damage. The existence of such a population has made it possible to examine the organization of the highest level of musical skill. Moreover, in cases where examples of premorbid artistry can be examined, it proves possible to make crucial comparisons that may illuminate the effect of the brain damage on the organization of music.

In this review, we will retain the organizing themes that have guided our presentation of more traditional empirical investigations. We will examine the relationship between aphasia and musical achievement, the kinds of strategies used by individuals who have suffered brain disease, and the fate of various discrete and holistic capacities in the light of brain damage. In addition, we will comment on the fate of originality, creativeness, and overall sense of form in musical achievements following injury to the brain.

A well-known pair of case studies has highlighted the relationship between the components of linguistic and musical competence. Botez and Wertheim (1959) studied an accordion player who, following removal of a tumor in the second right frontal convolution, suffered several severe amusic disturbances. While able to sing individual pitches, he could not combine them into a song. His repetition of rhythmic and melodic material was poor, and, most importantly, he was unable to play his accordion. Despite these difficulties, the subject had perfectly preserved perceptual and receptive capacities for music. He recognized pieces, spotted deliberate errors introduced in them, and was highly critical of his own performance. Suggesting an analogy to expressive aphasia, Botez and Wertheim spoke of their patient as exhibiting expressive amusia secondary to damage in the right frontal lobe.

Wertheim and Botez (1961) also reported a case of receptive amusia in a concert violinist who became severely aphasic, apparently as a result of left hemisphere injury. In contrast to their other patient, this violinist lost his absolute pitch, had difficulty in appreciating tempo changes, was unable to analyze chord structure, and could not name familiar pieces. His performance was far from perfect, but he was able to pick out pieces on the violin with his nonparetic hand. Moreover, when accompanied on the piano, his performance improved. Thus, pursuing the analogy to the aphasias, here was a patient whose receptive problems were more striking than his expressive ones. Yet, while this dichotomy may aid in an effort to organize complex findings, the distinction between receptive and expressive remains problematic, particularly with reference to the violin player.

A second topic that can be probed only with case studies of musically talented individuals is the fate of music reading following damage to the brain. Intuitively, it might seem that linguistic and musical alexia should be closely allied. In fact, however, these two forms of reading have been dissociated from one another in a number of instances. Thus, Soukes and Baruk's (1930) patient, a severe Wernicke's aphasic, was wholly unable to read text while still able to read music at the piano. In contrast, Dorgueille (cited in Benton, 1977) reported a patient who, after a left hemisphere stroke, was no longer able to read music but could still read text.

A few other generalizations can be offered on the basis of the dozens of case studies carried out since the turn of the century. It is very rare to encounter individuals who have sustained significant aphasia without some loss in musical competence (Feuchtwanger, 1930; Ustvedt, 1937), even though the overlap between aphasia and amusia is very far from complete. There may be a rough association between receptive factors on the one hand and expressive on the other, but in general no set of factors is completely impaired without there being correlative difficulty with other factors. In nearly all cases, individuals prove better able to handle old, overlearned materials than new, unfamiliar materials. In fact, in some cases, patients perform almost perfectly with well-known materials, while showing little or no capacity to master new materials (Judd, Gardner, & Geschwind, 1980). This result may simply reflect the well-documented phenomenon that brain-damaged individuals have an inordinate amount of difficulty learning to master any new kinds of materials.

Of numerous case studies that have been conducted with competent musicians, several stand out in terms of the detail of reporting and the significance of the results. In the five reviewed here, relatively complete information existed about the premorbid level of skill; moreover, the examiners probed relevant issues about the organization of artistic capacities.

In three cases, a major composer suffered a stroke in the posterior region of the left hemisphere, thereby developing significant aphasic disturbance. The first, the renowned Russian composer Shebalin, became severely aphasic following a stroke; nonetheless, he continued his composing and teaching activities as before and was considered by critics to be as brilliant a composer as ever (Luria, Tsvetkova, & Futer, 1965).

A second individual was a major American composer of choral works. He initially suffered a fluent aphasia, which later cleared to the level of a moderate anomia. Like Shebalin, this musician's capacities to compose and to criticize performances of music returned rather quickly to a level approaching that of his premorbid skills (Judd *et al.*, 1980). The condition of this composer is instructive in that he remained completely alexic for written language. As a result he had to institute various innovations to permit him to set text to music; for example, memorizing the text or having it read aloud as needed. His ability to read and write musical notation was much less severely impaired. Often, when unable to identify exact notes, he was still able to make shrewd guesses about what was wanted in a particular circumstance, and he could readily recognize scores, even when he could name neither the pitches nor the compositions. Here, then, is an instructive instance where the mechanics of musical performance and composition were impaired because of particular difficulty in the processing of visual symbols, while underlying musical intelligence was spared.

The well-known French composer Maurice Ravel had a tumor in the left hemisphere that left him with a permanent Wernicke's aphasia (Alajouanine, 1948). Ravel presented an interesting pattern of musical breakdown. He was able to recognize pieces he had known before his illness and could detect even minor faults in a performance. He still enjoyed listening to music after his illness and remained able to evaluate new pieces critically. However, he was never able to write or compose another piece, and he had great difficulty in playing the piano. Whether Ravel's inability to compose was due to mechanical difficulties of the sort that obtain in the Judd *et al.* case or to a more fundamental impairment of musical intelligence could not be determined with certainty, although it seems likely that his musical intelligence was at least to some extent compromised.

Another case provides further information on the relationship between left hemisphere disease and amusia. A 64-year-old Swiss pianist suffered a form of Wernicke's aphasia in which word deafness was particularly pronounced. Despite this difficulty with language, his musical capacities remained essentially intact. He could instantly recognize pieces of music and make all necessary corrections in a performance. Moreover, he was able to play even new pieces with no noticeable mistakes. Only when tasks involved a linguistic capacity, such as identification of notes by names, did the patient exhibit difficulties (Assal, 1973).

A final and highly instructive contrasting case is presented by a composer who suffered a stroke involving the right frontoparietal and temporal regions (Judd, Arslenian, Davidson, & Locke, unpublished research). Following his stroke, this composer's musical understanding remained intact. In fact, he wrote a musical textbook and also mastered two foreign languages after his stroke. Although musical testing uncovered some subtle perceptual defects, he was able to continue teaching at a school of music. In sharp contrast to the other musicians reviewed, however, he lost his interest in the creative process. He no longer felt motivated to compose; as he put it, he could no longer conjure up the appropriate atmosphere. He even reported that he could no longer "conceive of a whole piece." He indicated that he no longer listened to music for enjoyment as much as he had in the past and that he no longer experienced the rich set of associations while listening to music. His own postmorbid compositions he correctly judged as uninspired and uninspiring.

This case helps to clarify results obtained from individuals who have suffered an aphasia. With the possible exception of Ravel, musicians with language impairment caused by left hemisphere disease have retained the capacity and the desire to engage in creative musical activity. In contrast, an individual with significant right hemisphere disease, whose language remained on an extraordinarily high level and whose musical technique and technical skill had been largely spared, seemed to have undergone an alteration in his relationship to musical material and proved able to compose only in a very limited and uninspiring way.

On the basis of studies conducted with musicians who have suffered unilateral brain damage, and in light of studies conducted with both brain-damaged and healthy nonmusicians, complicated and sometimes conflicting patterns of findings have been reported. Nonetheless, a number of generalizations can be made. The most general statement that should be made is that both hemispheres are involved in music but that each hemisphere makes a different kind of contribution. Although the right hemisphere plays the most important role, it is rare to encounter an individual with severe aphasia who has not also suffered some loss in musical capacity.

The right hemisphere seems to be particularly important in four areas: the processing of the components of music (e.g., recognizing pitch, timbre); the internal representation of a melody that allows error detection; the production of music (e.g., combining notes into a recognizable melody, playing an instrument); and the individual's emotional relationship to music (e.g., motivation, inspiration, gratification sustained). The left hemisphere seems to be particularly important in those aspects of music most closely allied to language: reading musical notes and naming notes and entire pieces. It should be mentioned that the ability to read musical notation is dissociable from the ability to read linguistic text: Either one alone may be impaired as a result of left hemisphere damage. It should also be stressed that, while the ability to read music and name pieces may be severely impaired, the individual's underlying musical intelligence may be spared. On the basis of this review, then, it seems possible to distinguish between a capacity to carry out tasks involving musical notation, and a capacity to engage in musical creation and to sustain certain kinds of emotional gratification from a relationship with works of music.

Drawing

The bulk of research on graphic competence conducted with both normal and gifted individuals documents a high degree of dissociation between graphic and linguistic capacity. Indeed, with the exception of Bay (1962, 1964), nearly all authorities agree that graphic competence can exist at a high level despite a significant aphasia and, correlatively, that graphic competence can be compromised even when language is spared.

A more promising way of conceptualizing graphic competence highlights the different contributions made to the graphic process by each cerebral hemisphere. As formulated by Kaplan (1980), the left hemisphere proves particularly important for providing the details in a copied or original graphic production; in contrast, the right hemisphere assumes a significant role in providing the overall form, or external configuration, of a target object. Thus, individuals with left hemisphere disease are prone to make drawings whose overall configuration is correct or at least recognizable but whose details and internal structure are impoverished. In contrast, individuals with unilateral right hemisphere disease tend to fashion drawings with rich internal detail but with an impaired external configuration and, not infrequently, a relative neglect of the left side of space.

Other lateralized dissociations have also been reported. For instance, according to Jones-Gotman and Milner (1977), the right hemisphere seems to play a role of particular importance in the fluency with which drawings are produced. And, when asked to draw an instance of a category (e.g., to draw a vegetable), injury to the right hemisphere leads to bizarre drawings that incorporate incorrect or extraneous information (e.g., a picture of a potato with a stem when asked to draw a vegetable).

In contrast, individuals with left anterior injury are able to draw prototypical members of a category, although various defects may also attend the performance of these language-impaired patients. Fluent
aphasics, despite profound word-finding deficits, encounter little difficulty producing large numbers of pictures, although they often cannot
name perfectly recognizable pictures that they have drawn (Grossman,
1980).

It is important to indicate that, while these differences in drawing
performance can be documented in certain clearcut instances, in many
other cases, overall level of drawing deteriorates to such an extent that
the site of damage and the kind of drawing deficit become difficult to
specify.

On the receptive side, there is ample evidence to suggest that the
right hemisphere plays a principal role in the "reading of pictorial information," including paintings and drawings. Little information has
been gathered on the abilities of brain-damaged patients to attend to
those aspects of graphic symbols that contribute to their aesthetic significance, such as composition, balance, or expressiveness. However,
one study (Gardner, 1975a) does document the role of the right hemisphere in "reading" the style of a work of art. Asked to put together
those paintings that were made by the same artist, right-hemisphere-
injured patients classify not by style but by subject matter. Patients
with left hemisphere damage, in contrast, show a normal or even a
superior capacity to sort paintings by style, quite possibly because their
orientation to the subject matter has been diminished by their pathology.

Examination of skilled artists who have suffered brain disease uncov-
ers a number of suggestive phenomena. Studies of painters with left
hemisphere damage have revealed that the left hemisphere of the skilled
individual may play a less crucial graphic role than it does in the unskilled. For instance, a major French painter studied by Alajouanine
(1948) was rendered severely aphasic by a left hemisphere stroke. After
the stroke, his artistic activity did not decline nor did it seem to change
in its technique or tone. The painter poignantly described this split between his artistic self and his other selves:

> There are in me two men, the one who paints, who is normal while he is
> painting, and the other one who is lost in the mist, who does not stick to
> life. . . . I am saying very poorly what I mean. . . . There are inside me the
> one who grasps reality, life; there is the other one who is lost as regards
> abstract thinking. . . . These are two men, the one who is grasped by real-
> ity to paint, the other one, the fool who cannot manage words any more
> [Alajouanine, 1948, p.238.].

And the case of a Bulgarian painter, Z. B., described by Zaimov, Kitov, and Kolev (1969), confirms the finding that the ability to paint is not affected by the loss of linguistic skills. Z. B. suffered a severe aphasia as well as paralysis of the right side of the body. Because of the paralysis, the painter began to teach himself to draw with his left hand. He gradually regained his fluency but, unlike the French painter described here, Z. B. had developed an entirely new style. In his prestroke work, he depicted events occurring over time—in the past, present, and future. His poststroke work was no longer in such a narrative style but instead was characterized by strange and fantastic dreamlike images, clear colors, and symmetrical patterns. While his style was clearly new, it was in no way worse than his prestroke style.

These two case studies reveal that in skilled painters, graphic skills can function independently of language and other left hemisphere skills. As we saw earlier, this is not the case with unskilled individuals, in whom left hemisphere damage results in an impoverishment of detail in their drawings. Whether the visual analysis of detail is preserved in the left hemisphere damaged artist because it is overlearned, or whether it is preserved because it is represented more widely in the brain, is not known. But of course, since the two groups of patients were not matched in terms of lesion site, no strong conclusions can be drawn as to the difference between the role of the left hemisphere in normal and gifted draughtsmen.

Another case demonstrates that graphic ability may be impaired despite intact linguistic capacities and also that the ability to draw may be composed of two separable components. An investigation of a visually agnostic artist documented a striking dissociation of drawing skills (Wapner, Judd, & Gardner, 1978). This individual was unable to recognize objects that were presented to him, although he remained able to draw quite accurately from memory those objects as he had once known them. When asked to copy an object or picture placed in front of him, he was able to make exceedingly slavish copies of that object, ones of almost photographic accuracy; at the same time, he was unable to identify or name the object in question. In those rare cases where identification was possible or where the name was provided, he drew the objects in a very different, more schematic, and less slavish way.

This patient documents two separate forms of graphic competence in an artist: (*a*) a photographic copying mechanism in which every detail of an object is rendered just the way that it is perceived retinally, even at the cost of distortion (cf. Gombrich, 1960, who demonstrates that photographically accurate pictures may appear distorted); and (*b*) a more schematic way of rendering, in which the patient exploits some established pattern for representing an object. In the latter instance, the painter is prepared to sacrifice particular identifying features of the object in question in order to produce a more generally recognizable version of that object. Further confirmation of this dissociation can be found in the remarkable drawings by the autistic child Nadia (Selfe, 1977). This young girl could produce slavishly realistic representations, but she had no apparent knowledge of the objects involved and no generalized schemata that could be used to denote an entire class of objects.

The small amount of research carried out with major visual artists who have suffered strokes permits certain tentative generalizations. If a gifted artist suffers a left hemisphere stroke, and is not completely paralyzed, he should be able to continue to draw in the same style and also exhibit the same skills as in his premorbid state. In the case of regression, the style of depiction is likely to become more primitive but still recognizable. Indeed, the clinical literature contains several descriptions of individuals who were allegedly able to draw better than before; however, a certain romanticism may stimulate such claims (Gardner, 1975b).

It has proved possible to study the paintings of a few individuals who suffered significant right hemisphere disease and yet still continued to paint (Jung, 1974). Two German expressionists, Lovis Corinth and Anton Räderscheidt, both resumed painting after partial recovery from significant right hemisphere strokes. Initially, their paintings included neglect of the left side of space, irregular contours, misplaced detail, and general fuzziness in depiction. With recovery, the neglect of space was reduced; however, the drawings continued to exhibit fundamental differences in style. Specifically, the drawings became much more emotional, primitive, and bizarre, featuring rough lines and grotesque effects (Gardner, 1975b).

At the time that these drawings were first produced, art historians and critics spoke of a general change in style, one perhaps reflecting the patient's reaction to his severe illness. However, it is possible to put forward an alternative explanation. Suppose, as several studies have suggested, that the right hemisphere is essential for emotional appropriateness; it may be that, as a result of their significant pathology, these patients were now affected by a different set of emotional concerns. Reflecting these concerns, they went on to produce paintings that were much more sensual and "raw" in appearance.

It is important to ascertain which account of the changed style of these painters is correct. If it is the case that painters, irrespective of their variety of brain damage, begin to paint in anomalous styles, then the "general reactive" interpretation gains in persuasiveness. If, however, as we believe, such painting changes will only occur in individuals with significant right hemisphere pathology, then the style alteration can be traced directly to a certain form of brain damage.

In sum, studies of both normal individuals who have suffered unilateral brain damage and gifted artists with brain damage reveal that, while both hemispheres play a role in the visual arts, the right hemisphere is dominant. In the case of average individuals, the left hemisphere is important for rendering the details of a represented object; the right hemisphere is important in enabling the artist to draw fluently, in capturing the overall form of an object, and in knowing what is and is not appropriate to include in a drawing.

In the case of gifted visual artists, the left hemisphere seems to play little or no role. Painters with severe aphasia consequent to left hemisphere damage have been able to continue painting with no decrement in the quality of their output. Here is strong evidence that graphic skills can function independently of linguistic and other left hemisphere skills. When a painter suffers right hemisphere damage, on the other hand, the paintings become altered in at least two ways: At first there is a noticeable neglect of the left side of the pictorial space; and, more importantly, the style of painting may become more emotional and direct.

Language and Literary Creativity

Research into the basic components of language—phonology, semantics, and syntax—has demonstrated that language is one of the most strongly lateralized functions. The central role of the left hemisphere in language is beyond dispute, and it is well known that damage to the left brain causes aphasias in the case of right-handed individuals. For a long time, it was commonly believed that ONLY the left hemisphere was involved in language processing. But there is by now a great deal of evidence that the right hemisphere also plays some role in language: The right brain is capable of uttering overlearned phrases (such as *How are you?*) (Taylor, 1932); it can process vowels, intonation contours, and affectively tinged language (Blumstein & Cooper, 1974; Cicone, Wapner, & Gardner, 1980; Heilman, 1976; Kimura, 1973); and it may even possess some vocabulary and syntax (Gazzaniga, 1970; Sperry, 1974; Zaidel, 1973, 1977, 1978a, 1978b).

However, despite all that is known about the organization of basic language skills, we cannot predict with confidence what will happen to literary skills after left brain damage. Dealing with literature requires far more than syntax, semantics, or phonology. Indeed, the abilities most central to literary competence appear to lie in another area. For instance, to write or to appreciate a piece of literature, one must go beyond the literal and appreciate figurative forms of language involving metaphor, irony, or humor. And to perceive or produce a fictional work requires a sensitivity to the rules of narrative structure and an awareness of the boundary between fact and fiction. Thus, in evaluating the effects of left hemisphere damage on literary skill, the important questions do not concern performance on standard linguistic tasks. Rather, one wants to know whether individuals understand metaphor, whether they know what a story is, and whether they grasp that a story is fundamentally different from a journalistic account of an actual event. Put simply, do the abilities of the right hemisphere allow these individuals to grasp figurative language or to apprehend a story?

Two predictions are plausible. On the one hand, one might expect poor performance on literary tasks because such tasks tap higher-order levels of language. However, clinical observations suggest that the right hemisphere may be particularly important in attending to the context and nuance. Given this, one might expect that just such artistic verbal abilities are spared after left brain damage.

Presented with a description of a person having a "heavy heart," aphasics have difficulty explaining the meaning of this metaphor (Winner & Gardner, 1977). But this difficulty stems simply from an inability to put their understanding into words. Provided with a nonlinguistic response mode in which they may simply point to a picture that goes with such a metaphoric statement, patients with left-sided damage perform nearly as well as normal individuals (Winner & Gardner, 1977). The pictures that they were shown for "heavy heart" included a "literal" picture of a person staggering under the weight of a heavy, heartshaped object; the correct choice was a picture of a person crying.

Left-hemisphere-damaged patients, thus, retain some literary sensitivity, suggesting that the right hemisphere contributes to the understanding of figurative language. Nevertheless, damage to the left hemisphere cripples the writer. The French poet Baudelaire, after suffering a left hemisphere stroke, was never able to write again, and the only words that he could utter were an oath, *cré-nom*. In situations where the aphasia recedes and some recovery is evidenced, the individual may go on to write again. The poet William Carlos Williams was able to write some poetry after his partial recovery from aphasia (Plimpton, 1977). And a number of physicians who have become aphasic and then recovered went on to write about their experience (Gardner, 1975b). But, not surprisingly, in no case has an aphasic writer demonstrated the ability to write in the face of a loss of ordinary language ability.

What happens to literary skill after right hemisphere damage? On the surface, right hemisphere patients appear to possess intact language. Yet closer inspection reveals subtle language difficulties. For instance, such individuals are often unable to relate a statement to its context and thus tend to misinterpret the speaker's meaning. Upon hearing someone reject an offer of help in hanging a picture by saying that "too many cooks spoil the broth," a right-hemisphere-damaged patient may fail to recognize that the import of this statement has to do with hanging pictures and not with cooking. Failure to relate this statement to its appropriate context leads to a literal interpretation.

The role of the right hemisphere in attending to context and intention suggests that this hemisphere may make an important contribution in the domain of the literary arts. For when language is functioning aesthetically, it is often its nonliteral aspects that are the most crucial to apprehend. An inability to relate sentence to context ought to result in a tendency to interpret figurative language literally (taking "heavy hearted" to mean physically heavy) and to confuse the boundary between a fictive narrative and a straightforward description of actually occurring events (believing, for instance, that a story can only contain descriptions of events that may occur in reality). And, indeed, investigation of the role of the right hemisphere in both metaphoric and narrative uses of language reveals just such difficulties.

Unlike left damaged patients, those with right damage often speak in a manner that sounds metaphoric (e.g., a patient might joke about a paralyzed arm, calling it his *old fin*). Yet, asked to paraphrase the metaphoric sentence *He had a very heavy heart,* they are initially resistant, often insisting that such language is not proper English. However, after a bit of prodding, they reveal no difficulty in paraphrasing the sentence, explaining that it means that someone is sad. But, asked to point to the picture that goes with the description, right hemisphere patients are as likely to choose the literal depiction as to choose the metaphoric one. Moreover, unlike left hemisphere patients and non-brain-damaged individuals, they fail to find the literal pictures amusing. Nor do they notice the conflict between their verbal paraphrase and their literal picture choice (Winner & Gardner, 1977).

How can such results be explained? One way to understand these findings is to think of the left hemisphere as a "language machine," able to supply verbal paraphrases and definitions of any sentences or words it is given. Thus, the patient with a damaged right hemisphere and an intact left hemisphere has no problem paraphasing metaphors. Where the right hemisphere appears to be particularly crucial is in alerting the listener to context—recognizing situations in which uttering a particular statement would or would not be appropriate. Thus, those with right hemisphere damage are unable to select the picture depicting the situation in which one would ordinarily say *He had a very heavy heart.*

Sensitivity to context is not only important in understanding the kind of language used in the verbal arts; it is also important in understanding fictional narrative. Understanding a narrative requires, among other things, that one suspend disbelief, willingly enter into the story, and yet all the time retain a clear awareness of the boundary between the fantasy of the story, on the one hand, and reality, on the other. And it appears that these abilities are impaired after right hemisphere damage.

A study of various aspects of story sensitivity in right hemisphere patients has been carried out by Wapner, Hamby, and Gardner (in press). In this study, patients heard a series of brief stories. After hearing each tale, they were asked to retell it and were then posed a set of questions about the main points of the story. Overall, the responses of these patients underscored the importance of the right hemisphere in narrative comprehension. First of all, although in retelling the story these patients had no difficulty using appropriate phonology and syntax, they revealed considerable difficulty both in integrating the elements of the story and in grasping the narrative structure. For instance, when asked to assemble given story components in their logical order, these patients were markedly impaired. Thus, while unhindered in "straight" linguistic processing, right hemisphere patients could not organize linguistic information at the discourse level.

Further evidence of a lack of sensitivity to narrative form was the abundance of extraneous additions to the story on the retelling task. A number of these embellishments indicated an unwillingness to accept the story on its own terms and to respect the boundary between fiction and "real life." Upon hearing a story about a fireman, one patient insisted that the story was "incorrect." The reason that he gave for this odd statement was that the story mentioned an alleyway, and alleyways could not be located near a firehouse. Similarly, commenting on a part of the story describing a little girl who sneaks a ride on the engine, he insisted that this was an impossible occurrence. Other patients retold the story and changed it so that there was no fire; or they retold the story adding the experimenter as one of the characters.

Such instrusions suggest that the patients failed to respect the story as a separate and integral entity. Constantly violating the boundary between fiction and actuality, they seemed uncertain about the difference between the events related in the story and the events that typically occur in actuality.

Another dramatic finding concerned the right hemisphere patients' reaction to certain bizarre elements that were inserted into several of the stories. For instance, in a story about a lazy hired hand, it was stated that his boss had decided to give him a raise. While normal individuals as well as left hemisphere patients found such a statement odd (and even, perhaps, amusing) and recognized that is was at variance with the description of the employee as lazy, the right hemisphere patients did not react in this way. Moreover, in retelling the story, they related such elements just as if they were canonical elements of the story.

The right hemisphere patients thus refused to accept some aspects of stories that normal people have no difficulty accepting (such as the description of a girl sneaking a ride on a fire engine), but they also went out of their way to make sense of truly bizarre aspects of stories that healthy people would find jarring. Overall, the right hemisphere patients exhibited striking difficulties in handling complex linguistic materials, in grasping the basic structure of a story, and in recognizing the story as a fictional entity.

The right hemisphere patients' performance on these narrative tasks is mirrored by their performance on humor tasks. These patients often fail to grasp the point of a verbal joke: They do not laugh at jokes that normal and left brain-damaged patients find amusing and, when asked to select an appropriate punch line, they tend to choose a non sequitur (Gardner, Ling, Flamm, & Silverman, 1975; Michel, 1981). Thus, in the realm of humor as well as narrative, damage to the right hemisphere alters the ability to integrate verbal material and grasp the main point—a skill crucial in the apprehension of verbal art.

With respect to the literary arts, we can conclude that literary creativity requires both an intact right and an intact left hemisphere. Severe aphasia, of course, cripples the literary artist. Nonetheless, despite the left hemisphere's undisputed dominance for language, the right hemisphere also plays a very important role in the literary arts. In particular, the right hemisphere is important in determining the intention behind an utterance and in relating an utterance to its linguistic and situational context. Because patients with right hemisphere damage are often unable to recognize the context and the intention behind an utterance, they tend to interpret figurative statements, such as metaphors and proverbs, quite literally. Moreover, because of the right hemisphere's attention to context, this hemisphere plays a critical role in story understanding: Without a sensitivity to context, the right-hemisphere-damaged patient is unable to accept a story as a fictional entity that must be taken on its own terms yet must also be clearly distinguished from "reality."

Concluding Remarks

The symbol system of language has been shown to bear a different kind of relationship to each of the three art forms considered here. The relationship is never a simple one, and the pattern found often differs, depending on whether gifted or average individuals are under discussion. Still, despite the complexity of the findings, a few generalizations can be tentatively put forth.

Disorders of language appear in many cases to leave musical skill relatively unaffected. It is the right hemisphere that has a particularly important role to play, contributing not only to technical skill but also to the individual's affective relationship to music. Yet, it may well be that, in the case of the highly trained individual, left hemisphere damage impairs the ability to perceive a piece of music in an analytic mode. Further, the representation in the brain of musical abilities may differ greatly from one talented individual to another.

In the case of the visual arts, aphasias in the average individual appear to entail some loss of graphic ability. However, in the artist, in whom painting and drawing are overlearned skills, graphic ability continues to function largely independently of language and other left hemisphere abilities. Once again, it is right hemisphere damage that yields the most potent effects: While it does not necessarily curtail artistic activity, it sometimes alters the style in which the artist paints.

It is, of course, in the case of the literary arts that one would expect the strongest relationship between aphasia and artistry. And, indeed, left hemisphere damage affects the language of the writer no less than that of the average individual. Overlearning appears to be no protection against the ravages of aphasia, and the language abilities of the writer are indisoluably tied to linguistic competence *per se.*

The critical role of the left hemisphere in the case of the literary arts does not, however, mean that the right hemisphere is not involved. Indeed, the right hemisphere has been shown to be essential in governing attention to linguistic and extralinguistic context. Lacking such sensitivity to context, the right hemisphere injured individual is likely to find figurative language perplexing and to fail to respect the implicit boundary between a fictional realm and the "real" world.

The picture of symbolic functioning obtained from the study of organic patients yields certain implications for language therapy. Individuals with unilateral right hemisphere lesions may well benefit from efforts to sensitize them to figurative or fictive uses of language, even as communication with these patients may initially proceed most effectively if their proclivity to take messages literally is borne in mind. Correlatively, even aphasic patients with severe compromise of ordinary language functions may retain basic understandings of verbal humor and narrative constructions (Gardner, Ling, Flamm, & Silverman, 1975; cf. Stachowiak, Huber, Poeck, & Kerschensteiner, 1977). Upon these spared capacities, it may be possible to build, or to resurrect, enhanced understanding of the messages of daily life as well as provide an entry to simple works of literature.

Acknowledgments

Preparation of this chapter was supported by the Veterans Administration; the National Institutes of Neurological Diseases, Communication Disorders, and Stroke (MS 11408); and Harvard Project Zero. We thank Hiram Brownell, Andrew Ellis, and Dee Michel for their thoughtful comments on an earlier version.

References

Alajouanine, T. 1948. Aphasia and artistic realization. *Brain, 71,* 229–241.

Assal, G. 1973. Aphasie de Wernicke chez un pianiste. *Revue Neurologique, 29,* 251–255.

Bay, E. 1962. Aphasia and non-verbal disorders of language. *Brain, 85,* 411–426.

Bay, E. 1964. Present concepts of aphasia. *Geriatrics, 19,* 319–31.

Benton, A. L. 1977. The amusias. In M. Critchley & R. A. Henson (Eds.), *Music and the brain.* London: Heinemann.

Bever, T., & Chiarello, R. 1974. Cerebral dominance in musicians and non-musicians. *Science, 185,* 357–359.

Blumstein, S., & Cooper, W. E. 1974. Hemispheric processing of intonation contours. *Cortex, 10,* 146–158.

Bogen, J., & Gordon, H. 1971. Musical tests for functional lateralization with intra-carotid amabarbital. *Nature, 230,* 524–525.

Botez, M. I., & Wertheim, N. 1959. Expressive aphasia and amusia following right frontal lesion in a right handed man. *Brain, 82,* 186–201.

Cicone, M., Wapner, W., & Gardner, H. Sensitivity to emotional expressions and situations in organic patients. *Cortex, 1980, 16,* 145–158.

Cooper, G., & Meyer, L. 1960. *The rhythmic structure of music.* Chicago: Univ. of Chicago Press.

Dowling, W. J. 1978. Scale and contour. Two components of a theory of memory for melodies. *Psychological Review, 85,* 341–354.

Dowling, W. J. 1979. Mental structures through which music is perceived. Paper presented at the National Symposium on the Applications of Psychology to the Teaching and Learning of Music, Ann Arbor, Michigan.

Feuchtwanger, E. 1930. *Amusie.* Berlin: Springer-Verlag.

Galin, D. 1974. Implications for psychiatry of left and right cerebral specialization. *Archives of General Psychiatry, 35,* 572–583.

Gardner, H. 1975. Artistry following aphasia. Paper presented at the Academy of Aphasia, Victoria, British Columbia, October. (a)

Gardner, H. 1975. *The shattered mind.* New York: Alfred Knopf. (b)

Gardner, H. 1976. Promising paths to knowledge. *Journal of Aesthetic Education, 10,* 201–207.

Gardner, H. 1979. Developmental psychology after Piaget: An approach in terms of symbolization. *Human development, 22,* 73–88.

Gardner, H., & Denes, G. 1973. Connotative judgments by aphasic patients on a pictorial adaptation of the semantic differential. *Cortex, 9,* 183–196.

Gardner, H., Howard, V., & Perkins, D. 1974. Symbol systems: A philosophical, psychological, and educational investigation. In D. Olson (Ed.), *Media and symbols.* Chicago: Univ. of Chicago Press.

Gardner, H., Ling, K., Flamm, L., & Silverman, J. 1975. Comprehension and appreciation of humor in brain-damaged patients. *Brain, 98,* 339–412.

Gardner, H., Silverman, J., Denes, G., Semenza, C., & Rosenstiel, A. 1977. Sensitivity to musical denotation and connotation in organic patients. *Cortex, 13,* 243–256.

Gates, A., & Bradshaw, J. 1977. The role of the cerebral hemispheres in music. *Brain and Language, 4,* 403–431.

Gazzaniga, M. 1970. *The bisected brain.* New York: Appleton.

Gombrich, E. H. 1960. *Art and illusion.* Princeton: Bolligen.

Goodglass, H., & Kaplan, E. 1972. *The assessment of aphasia and related disorders.* Philadelphia: Lea and Febiger.

Goodman, N. 1968. *Languages of art.* Indianapolis: Bobbs-Merrill.

Goodman, N. 1972. *Problems and projects.* Indianapolis: Bobbs-Merrill.

Goodman, N. 1979. *Ways of worldmaking.* Indianapolis: Hackett Publishing.

Gordon, H. 1970. Hemispheric asymmetries in the perception of musical chords. *Cortex, 6,* 387–398.

Gordon, H. W. 1980. Degree of ear asymmetries for perception of dichotic chords and for illusory levels of competence. *Journal of Experimental Psychology: Human Perception and Performance, 6,* 516–527.

Grossman, M. 1980. Figurative referential skills after brain damage. Paper presented at the International Neuropsychological Society, San Diego, February.

Heilman, K. 1976. Affective disorders associated with right hemisphere disease. Invited address to Aphasia Academy, Miami, Florida, October.

Jones-Gotman, M., & Milner, B. 1977. Design fluency: The invention of nonsense drawings after local cortical lesions. *Neuropsychologia, 15,* 653–674.

Judd, T., Arslenian, A., Davidson, L., & Locke, S. Unpublished research.

Judd, T., Gardner, H., & Geschwind, N. 1980. *Alexia without agraphia in a composer.* Project Zero Technical Report #15. Harvard University.

Jung, R. 1974. Neuropsychologie und Neurophysiologie des Kontur—Formensehens in Zeichung und Malerei. In H. M. Wieck (Ed.), *Psychopathologie Musischer Gestaltungen.* Stuttgart: Schattauer-Verlag.

Kaplan, E. 1980. Process and achievement revisited. Presidential address, International Neuropsychological Society, San Diego, February.

Kimura, D. 1973. The asymmetry of the human brain. *Scientific American, 228,* 70–78.

Kleist, K. 1962. *Sensory aphasia and amusia.* Oxford: Pergamon.

Krumhansl, C. 1979. The psychological representation of musical pitch in a tonal context. *Cognitive Psychology, 11,* 346–374.

Langer, S. 1953. *Feeling and form.* New York: Scribners.

Lerdahl, F., & Jackendoff, R. *A generative theory of total music.* Cambridge, Mass.: MIT Press, forthcoming.

Luria, A. R., Tsvetkova, L. S., & Futer, D. S. 1965. Aphasia in a composer. *Journal of Neurological Science, 2,* 288–292.

Meyer, L. 1956. *Emotion and meaning in music.* Chicago: Univ. of Chicago Press.

Michel, D. 1981. *Sensitivity to humor in brain damaged patients.* Unpublished research.

Milner, B. 1962. Laterality effects in audition. In V. B. Mountcastle (Ed.), *Interhemispheric relations and cerebral dominance.* Baltimore, Md.: Johns Hopkins Press.

Nebes, R. 1974. Hemispheric specialization in commissurotomized man. *Psychological Bulletin, 81,* 1–14.

Perkins, D., & Leondar, B. (Eds.) 1977. *The arts and cognition*. Baltimore, Md.: Johns Hopkins Press.

Plimpton, G. (Ed.) 1977. *Writers at work* (Vol. 3). New York: Penguin Books.

Ross, E., & Mesulam, M. 1979. Dominant language functions of the right hemisphere: Prosody and emotional gesturing. *Archives of Neurology, 36*, 144–148.

Selfe, L. 1977. *Nadia*. New York: Academic Press.

Shankweiler, D. 1966. Effects of temporal lobe damage on perception of dichotically presented melodies. *Journal of Comparative and Physiological Psychology, 62*, 115.

Shanon, B. 1980. Lateralization effects in musical decision tasks. *Neuropsychologia, 18*, 21–31.

Shapiro, B., Grossman, M., & Gardner, H. 1981. Selective musical processing deficits in brain damaged populations. *Neuropsychologia, 19*, 161–169.

Soukes, A., & Baruk, H. 1930. Autopsie d'un case d'amusie (avec aphasie) chez un professeur de piano. *Revue Neurologique, 1*, 545–556.

Sparks, R., Helm, N., & Albert, M. 1974. Aphasia rehabilitation resulting from melodic intonation therapy. *Cortex, 10*, 303–316.

Sperry, R. 1974. Lateral specialization in the surgically separated hemispheres. In F. O. Schmitt & F. Worden (Eds.), *The neurosciences third study program*. Cambridge, Mass.: MIT Press.

Stachowiak, F.J., Huber, W., Poeck, K., & Kerchensteiner, M. 1977. Text comprehension in aphasia. *Brain and Language, 4*, 177–195.

Taylor, J. (Ed.). 1932. *Selected writings of John Hughlings Jackson* (Vols. 1 and 2). London: Hodder & Stoughton.

Ustvedt, H. 1937. Über die untersuchung der musikalischen funktionen bei patienten mit gerhirnleiden, besonders bei patienten mit aphasie. *Acta Medica Scandinavia Supplement, 86*.

Wapner, W., Hamby, S., & Gardner, H. The role of the right hemisphere in the organization of complex linguistic materials. *Brain and Language*, in press.

Wapner, W., Judd, T., & Gardner, H. Visual agnosia in an artist. *Cortex, 14*, 343–364.

Wertheim, N., & Botez, M. 1961. Receptive amusia. *Brain, 84*, 19–30.

Winner, E., & Gardner, H. 1977. The comprehension of metaphor in brain damaged patients. *Brain, 100*, 719–727.

Zaidel, E. 1973. Linguistic competence and related functions in the right hemisphere of man following cerebral commissurotomy and hemispherectomy. Unpublished doctoral dissertation, California Institute of Technology.

Zaidel, E. 1977. Unilateral auditory language comprehension on the Token Test following cerebral commissurotomy and hemispherectomy. *Neuropsychologia, 15*, 1–8.

Zaidel, E. 1978. Auditory language comprehension in the right hemisphere following cerebral commissurotomy and hemispherectomy: A comparison with child language and aphasia. In A. Caramazza & E. B. Zurif (Eds.), *Language acquisition and language breakdown: Parallels and divergences*. Baltimore, Md.: Johns Hopkins Press. (a)

Zaidel, E. 1978. The elusive right hemisphere of the brain. *Engineering and Science, 42* California Institute of Technology, September–October. (b)

Zaimov, K., Kitov, D., & Kolev, N. 1969. Aphasie chez un peintre. *Encephale, 68*, 377–417.

Zattore, R. J. 1979. Recognition of dichotic melodies by musicians and nonmusicians. *Neuropsychologia, 17*, 607–617.

13

Language in the Elderly Aphasic and in the Dementing Patient

LORAINE K. OBLER and MARTIN L. ALBERT

To write about language in the elderly aphasic and in the dementing patient is to write about two different but related topics. When we speak about language in the elderly aphasic, we are in fact, for the most part, considering an aphasic population with which we are already familiar: the Wernicke's aphasics, since Wernicke's aphasia is most common in the elderly. When we turn to language in dementia, however, we are covering new and relatively unexplored territories. Thus, our approach in this chapter will be to treat the two populations somewhat differently.

With respect to language in the elderly aphasic, we may reframe the questions that have traditionally been asked about the relation between age and aphasia. Thus, the relation between age and severity of aphasia becomes a less conspicuous issue, while the issue of age and benefit from speech therapy may be considered in a new light. That is to say, the extent to which symptoms of dementia may interact with aphasia becomes pertinent. Symptomatology of aphasia in the elderly and the capacity to respond to traditional language rehabilitation, we will argue, are both influenced by the normal cognitive changes of aging.

With respect to language disturbances in the dementias, on the other hand, we feel it important to spend some time documenting the patterns of deficit, precisely because so much less is generally known about language profiles in the various dementias. One dimension of particular relevance here is the distinction between those dementias that affect predominantly cortical regions and those that affect predominantly subcortical regions. In patients with cortical dementias, for example, the differential diagnosis that must often be made is between Wernicke's aphasia and Alzheimer's Dementia–Senile Dementia Complex. Patients

385

with subcortical dementias, by contrast, would never be confused with
Wernicke's aphasics; rather one's interests lie in (*a*) distinguishing them
from patients with subcortical aphasias; and (*b*) considering how the
nonlanguage cognitive deficits of attention and memory and pacing that
are disturbed in these patients may contribute to their speech and language disorders.

Aphasia in the Elderly

Traditionally, the questions about how age interacts with aphasia
have concerned whether or not aphasia is more severe as one gets older
and whether recovery is worse with advanced age. In fact, there is
controversy around these questions in the literature. Some researchers,
such as Smith (1971), claim that severity of aphasia increases with age,
whereas other researchers, such as Culton (1971), argue that severity is
no worse with age (at least if one compares older and younger adults,
excluding childhood aphasics). As to recovery, one school of researchers
demonstrates that advancing age correlates with poorer recovery
(Sands, Sarno, & Shankweiler, 1969, Vignolo, 1964) while another
school reports that age per se is not a strong predictor of recovery
(Basso, Capitani, & Vignolo, 1979; Kertesz & McCabe, 1977; Sarno &
Levita, 1971; see Sarno, 1980, for a review of these studies).

Clearly, these debates have pragmatic consequences, because in the
event that elderly aphasics are more severely impaired or less likely to
recover than younger patients, one might be tempted to choose to direct
rehabilitative efforts away from the elderly. Of course, the counterar-
gument could be made, that if elderly aphasics are more severely impaired or less likely to recover SPONTANEOUSLY than younger aphasics,
then we must direct the greater weight of our rehabilitative efforts toward working with the older aphasic. Thus, it becomes important to
dissociate spontaneous recovery from recovery in response to therapy.

We have developed two other approaches to asking questions about
aphasia in the elderly. In one approach, we ask how the different
aphasia syndromes distribute across the life span and what the implications of age differences for aphasia types are. In the second, we ask how
aphasia interacts with the cognitive changes of normal aging and of the
dementias. In the following sections, we consider these questions in
greater detail.

Aphasia in the Aging Brain

Sarno (1980) reported on response to therapy in aphasic patients over
age 50 and observed that the differences across age, whereby the

younger patients did slightly better than the older patients, are nonsignificant. What is important to note is that patients with cognitive, attentional, or other symptoms associated with senile dementia were excluded from her study. Previous findings of more severe aphasia with age, or worse recovery from aphasia with age, may well be attributable to higher incidence of symptoms of dementia in the elderly populations studied. In fact, we would maintain that such syndromes as multiinfarct dementia, which may not lead to observable cognitive deficits in an individual before his or her aphasia-producing lesion, may interact with the aphasia when it occurs. Since incidence of most dementias increases with age, the poorer spontaneous recovery reported in certain studies may reflect greater numbers of mildly dementing patients in those studies.

As to the reports of poorer recovery among the elderly aphasics who are given speech therapy, this finding (when it occurs) may also relate to increased incidence of dementias in the elderly population. Holland (1980) has reported a decline in all aspects of communicative abilities in daily living among noninstitutionalized aphasic patients, most strikingly after age 46. Institutionalized aphasics perform worse than noninstitutionalized patients on her test, and, unlike for the noninstitutionalized patients, evidence is seen of decrement between those aged 56–65 and those over age 65. These findings further support our position that an increase in the cognitive decline associated with aging interacts with and influences aphasia in all its dimensions. This is not to suggest, of course, that elderly aphasic patients should not be given language therapy, rather that their aphasias may call for nontraditional forms of language and cognitive therapy.

Aphasia Types and Aging

Cognitive decline associated with normal aging or with early dementia, then, must be taken into account when asking how age interacts with severity of aphasia and recovery from aphasia. The second major factor that must be considered is how aphasia types interact with age. Until 1978 it was generally believed that the various classical aphasic syndromes occurred in all but children and adolescents. Our 1978 study (Obler, Albert, Goodglass, & Benson, 1978) demonstrated that the different aphasia types distribute differently across older adulthood. Most markedly, Broca's or nonfluent aphasias are most prevalent among patients in their early 50s, whereas Wernicke's or fluent aphasias are most prevalent in patients in their early 60s. In that population of 167 right-handed males who had suffered strokes and had unequivocal diagnosis in one of the standard aphasia categories, the patients with global aphasias with a mean age of 56 were intermediate to the Brocas ($\bar{X} = 51$) and the Wernickes ($\bar{X} = 63$) aphasics. That study has since been replicated with at least 11 populations (Castro-Caldas, Ferro, & Grosso, 1979; Harasymiw, Halper, & Sutherland, in press; Holland, 1980; Kertesz, 1979; Miceli, Caltagirone, Gainotti, Silveri, & Villa, 1981; Obler, Albert, Caplan, Mohr, & Geer, 1980; Sarno, 1980), and no evidence has surfaced to contradict the basic finding that, among males at least, Wernicke's aphasics are significantly older than the average aphasic, whereas Broca's aphasics are significantly younger. For women aphasics the findings are less clear, although the tendencies are in the same direction, with fluent aphasics somehwat older than nonfluent aphasics (Harasymiw *et al.*, 1981; Obler *et al.*, 1980).

In the follow-up study that we conducted to test explanations for these findings (Obler *et al.*, 1980), it became clear that both the age differences for aphasia type and the sex differences were related to the location and type of stroke that produced the aphasia. Thus, the reason one sees more male Wernicke's aphasics among 60 year olds than among younger aphasics is that 60 year olds are more prone to evidence strokes affecting posterior language zones. For the women aphasics in our population, on the other hand, there is less discrepancy between the ages for anterior ($\bar{X} = 62$) and posterior ($\bar{X} = 61$) strokes; hence, one sees less difference between the ages of women with Wernicke's aphasia and women with Broca's aphasia.

These facts, then, can explain the contradictions discussed here around whether elderly aphasics do or do not suffer more severe aphasias and whether or not they benefit as younger aphasic patients do from language rehabilitation. In particular, we argue that populations with great numbers of patients having global aphasias and few patients with Wernicke's aphasics WILL BY DEFINITION show greater severity of aphasia with age, whereas populations with predominantly milder aphasics will not show greater severity with age. Of course, clinicians will be more concerned with the type of aphasia the patient has and its severity than they will be with the age of the patient, but because there is a literature on age and aphasia, we believe it important to expose the problems with studies that might bias clinicians to ignore the older patient.

One further point must be made in this regard. All the studies discussed here have been GROUP studies, but the clinician is regularly faced with an individual aphasic to diagnose and treat. More important than the group studies, for clinical purposes, are the studies that demonstrate that SOME very elderly individuals profit from language therapy (e.g., Vignolo, 1964). From this fact we must conclude that there are individual differences in recovery from aphasia AT ANY AGE and that each patient who desires therapy (Holland, 1980) must be given at least the chance to benefit from it.

Moreover, to the extent that dementias, or the cognitive decline of normal aging, may interact with recovery from aphasia, thus frustrating the clinician who cannot succeed with traditional therapies, new forms of rehabilitation must be developed.

Language Disturbance in the Dementias

Any study that simply groups all patients with different sorts of de- menting illness is bound to report vague and even contradictory lan- guage deficits. Thus, Gustafson, Hagberg, and Ingvar, (1978) report both MUTENESS and LOGORRHEA to be characteristic of dementing pa- tients. And few researchers go into great depth on the NAMING DISTUR- BANCE reported for dementia. (The case study reported by Schwartz *et al.*, 1979, is an important exception.) A certain EMPTINESS OF SPEECH may be evidenced by different dementing groups, again, for different reasons in the different groups. Finally, two neuropsychological behaviors characteristic of the dementias impinge on language tasks: impaired attention and perseveration. These behaviors can often be seen most clearly in AGRAPHIAS in the early stages of dementia, reflected in omis- sions or repetitions of letters, morphemes, and words. Only when we begin to discriminate among the various types of dementing diseases can we draw more detailed pictures of the language disturbances that characterize them. For our purposes, we will describe two representa- tive classes of dementing patients. First we will discuss language in Alzheimer's disease, which typifies those dementing diseases with pre- dominantly cortical dysfunction; then we will discuss language in pro- gressive supranuclear palsy, which typifies those dementing diseases with predominantly subcortical dysfunction.

Language Disturbance in Cortical Dementias

Criterial to the definition of Alzheimer's disease are emotional or personality changes, memory impairment, visuospatial deficit, and in- adequacies in information processing. Some believe language distur- bance may or may not accompany these features. We maintain language disturbance is ALWAYS present in a more or less severe form. In fairly advanced stages, patients with Alzheimer's disease resemble true aphasics of the Wernicke sort. But even in the early stages, language- related deficits may be manifest with careful testing. Thus, the early dementing patient may circumlocute like the healthy elderly person in order to arrive eventually at a correct response on a naming task, but he or she will take more time on the average than the healthy control to arrive at the word and will benefit less from phonemic cuing. In spontaneous speech, the Alzheimer's patient is likely to insert verbal paraphasias, but in the early stages will self-correct them.

In discourse, too, the patient in the early stages of Alzheimer's dementia will digress more than a healthy control and will be less likely than the healthy person to pull him- or herself back to the earlier train of thought. Speech will be personalized and somewhat repetitious and vague at the same time. In response to questions in conversation, the early Alzheimer's patient will sometimes do what a later-stage patient does more frequently—namely, respond NOT to the specific question asked, but rather to a related question. This behavior suggests that the patient has understood from the intonation and facial gestures of the interlocutor that a question was asked and has decided to respond to a likely question that contains certain of the key words he or she has picked up. Also in the early stages, patients will express verbally their unsureness, adding *perhaps* or commenting *I'm not sure, but . . .* or asking *Did I already say that?*

With more specific tests of language comprehension in the early stages, the patient with Alzheimer's dementia responds somewhat better than in conversation. Thus, the patient in the early stages of Alzheimer's disease will respond well on such standard aphasia-battery tasks as pointing to named items among a set or answering yes–no questions. If required to listen to a brief paragraph and repeat it or respond to questions, the early Alzheimer's patient experiences more difficulty and is likely to resort to a strategy of describing a picture if one is included in the task, or answering questions based on general logic rather than on the story at hand, or apologizing for being unable to perform the task. In proverb interpretation, these patients will give vague responses that are neither altogether concrete by standard measures nor intelligently abstract. For example, when asked what we mean when we say *Rome wasn't built in a day*, one patient responded *It takes a long time to build something.*

On repetition tasks, the patient will be able to repeat long sentences that contain elements with a high probability of co-occurrence (e.g., *They heard him speak on the radio last night*) but will break down on shorter sentences containing words with lower frequency and probability of co-occurrences (e.g., *He pried the tin lid off*, or, *The spy fled to Greece*). With these low-probability sentences, patients will look confused and repeat related sounds or words of the same, or slightly shorter syllable length as the stimulus item (e.g., *He bride the tid lid*, or, *The fly fed to geese*).

In the intermediate stages of the disease, more verbal paraphasias are evident in discourse, and literal paraphasias also occur and go uncorrected. Jargon terms will eventually become frequent. On directed naming tasks, subjects will be much more verbose than is necessary, will again produce paraphasias (in addition to an increase in misnamings due to misperception—e.g., calling a picture of an escalator a *cucumber* or a picture of a scissors *spoons*), and will rarely respond well to phonemic or semantic cuing. Production of nouns on picture naming tasks will be revealed as more deficited than production of verbs, although these too will suffer. A wide range of functors, on the other hand, will be expressed on discourse, even if they do not bear their full semantic content.

On repetition tasks, the middle-stage patients with Alzheimer's disease will break down on longer high-probability items as well as low-probability items. They will omit words and produce paraphasias for the high-probability stimuli and be frustrated at their inability to remember these sentences, asking for numerous repetitions.

Comprehension diminishes in this stage, and subjects are likely to respond incorrectly to yes–no questions or to questions about the agent in a passive construction (e.g., *The lion was killed by the tiger; who died?*). If asked to point to words in one of several categories, mid-stage patients with Alzheimer's disease will start to select items out of category.

In discourse these patients digress severely, from both their own points and those of the examiner. They fail on many metalinguistic tasks (e.g., *Give the opposite of* **comfortable, equal,** etc., or, *Tell me the past tense of* **He sings today**), perhaps because it is so hard to get them to understand what is expected. With automatic sequences, they may continue for a second run through or may omit items (e.g., *Monday, Tuesday, Wednesday, Thursday, Friday, Sunday, Monday, Tuesday*).

In the later stages of Alzheimer's dementia, it is primarily pragmatics that breaks down. Thus, patients may be mute or restricted to palilalia or echolalia (Haiganoosh Whitaker, 1976, describes in careful detail the echolalia of a dementing 63-year-old). What discourse is emitted is relatively fluent; it is certainly not agrammatic. Discourse emptiness at this stage results from the fact that propositional speech is barely attempted, and jargon predominates the little speech emitted. Repetition to command is poor, perhaps because it is a metalinguistic task. On a naming task, the patient may give the correct label in the course of talking but not even indicate awareness that the name has been produced.

From these caricatures, abstracted from our clinical series, it becomes clear that the patient with early Alzheimer's disease resembles the mild Wernicke's aphasic, whereas the patient with mid-stage Alzheimer's disease looks like the more florid Wernicke's aphasic. Certainly, the differential diagnosis between these two syndromes is difficult at present, as both are becoming more prevalent with the increased age of our population. Several nonlinguistic observations may be used to distinguish the dementing patient from the aphasic patient, and the pragmatics of communication will be more appropriate in the aphasic than in the dementing patient. For example, eye contact is diminished in later stages of Alzheimer's disease. Also, the dementing patient will touch the test objects more than is appropriate. Our best linguistic indicator to date seems to be the use of conjunctions; the Wernicke's aphasic will use a fairly limited set, mostly *ands* and a few *buts* (Gleason, Goodglass, Green, Obler, Hyde, & Weintraub, 1980), whereas the patient with Alzheimer's dementia will freely use the logical functors (*so, because, although*) albeit without necessarily respecting their logical entailments.

By way of example, consider the oral responses of two patients (Examples 1, 2, and 3) with moderately advanced Alzheimer's disease when asked to describe the story of what is happening in the Cookie Theft Picture (see Figure 13.1) of the Boston Diagnostic Aphasia Examination (Goodglass & Kaplan, 1972), and in conversation.

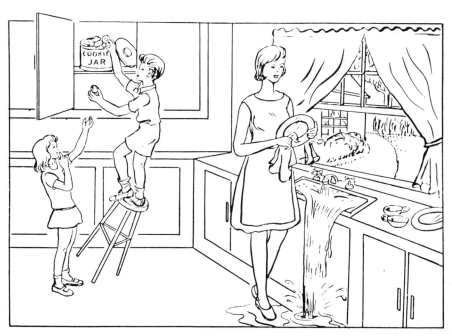

FIGURE 13.1. *Cookie Theft Picture of the Boston Diagnostic Aphasia Examination.* [*From H. Goodglass and E. Kaplan. 1972.* The Assessment of Aphasia and Related Disorders. *Philadelphia: Lea and Febiger. Reproduced by permission.*]

EXAMPLE 1

**Early mid-stage dementia in
a 70-year-old woman with Alzheimer's disease**

Let's see now, this is a little boy, in the pantry, uh, with his hands in the cookie jar, his hands in the cookie jar, whether or not he takes them I don't know, and he's up on a stool here he had to, but up here in the dangerous position for a youngster and this is his mother here in the kitchen area, I believe, and, uh, I don't know what else you want to know.

EXAMPLE 2

**Late mid-stage dementia in a 73-year-old man
with Alzheimer's disease**

There is nothing /ægbi/ that's bothering with those kids except she's in a turmoil of /smɪn/ if she didn't know what it was, but she doesn't believe it because she's believing to see something that doesn't know I'm to do it. So, over here, she see's this torrential picture although not torrential here, she sees that, she might not but she's going to see over this picture, and he'll get a . . . punch in the kisser and there th-that one's out of it and there that one's out of it.

EXAMPLE 3

Conversation with the same 73-year-old man

E: *What kind of work do you do?*
P: *Oh, when I first laughed along, I lived, uh, worked in Boston.
When I second I worked the whole crew, I worked together.*
E: *Are you married? Do you have a family?*
P: *No, I don't have any married thing at all.*
E: *What kind of building is this that we are in?* [Answer: hospital]
P: *Well they each have a sep, sep separate part of the thing here, and whatever they do, they sublimate it or do something to it, to hold up for it. And they, each one does its own part; that's what I would think.*

Language Disturbance in Subcortical Dementias

Progressive supranuclear palsy is a typical example of a dementing illness with neuropathological changes limited to subcortical nuclear structures. Neurobehaviorally this disease is characterized by (*a*) emotional or personality changes (typically inertia or apathy); (*b*) memory disorders; (*c*) defective ability to manipulate acquired knowledge; and (*d*) striking slowness in rate of information processing. Speech disturbances consist of dysarthria, monotony, and equal stress for each syllable. The patient may begin a long word or phrase intelligibly, and with good volume, but will trail off to a murmur by the end. Difficulties in controlling exhalation limit the amount of speech the patient is able to express on any given breath. Thus, when we first saw one 64-year-old retired ophthalmologist with this disease, his phrasing in describing the Cookie Theft Picture was markedly distorted, with breaks at unnatural syntactic junctures (see Example 4).

EXAMPLE 4

Dr. T., Tested before medication

The children have	*[Excuse me?]*
found the cookies	*stuffing her*
and/in the cookie jar	*face with the*
is open	*?stuffing her face with the cookies*
and the lid is off.	*And*
The boy is	*Mama*
standing on	*is drying*
a stool	*dishes*
which is	*at/and the sink*
almost	*is overflowing*
tipped over.	*its bank*
[mumble]	*on the floor.*
doesn't seem	*It's hard to determine*
paying	*whether this*
attention to	*valence*
[mumble]	*is according to*
stuffing her face	*scale or not.*

After a course of levodopa, his phrasing improved, which permitted his language disturbance to reveal itself (see Example 5):

EXAMPLE 5

Dr. T., Tested after medication

That is a boy with cookies
and he is stealing them two handedly
and the stool he is
stepped on
is a 3 legged
stool which is tipping over
strangely enough on one leg.
The young lady he is hang up
in his mischief seems to be more inclined to feed her
face than to yell "Thief, Stop!"
Meanwhile her mother is washing dishes
at the sink which is overflowing in [mumble]
   apparently water onto her stockings.
She has an open window.

Subtle naming disturbances occur in the patient with progressive supranuclear palsy, which are more evident in speech than on naming-to-confrontation or picture naming tasks. The verbal paraphasias that obtain in the speech of these patients may be termed close semantic coordinates; they are invariably related to the intended word, but slightly "off." Thus, we know what the patient meant who reported that the boy was *hang(ing)* the girl *up* in his mischief; he meant *involving* her. Unable to locate the precise word he intended, a closely related phrase was produced. For these patients, we find, nouns are not preferentially affected, as they appear to be in the cortical aphasias. As in the example, verbs and verb phrases as well as idioms may be "off." Moreover, it would appear that the lexical substitutions employed result in paragrammatisms not unlike those of the fluent aphasics. Thus one patient reported that the wolf *took a liking towards* Little Red Riding Hood's basket, in telling us her story. Two points are evidenced in this paraphasia:

1. Lexical co-occurrence constraints are broken: *Take a liking to* demands an animate object in English, but *basket* is inanimate.
2. The idiom *take a liking to* is broken with the substitution of *towards* for *to*.

This idiombreaking, not uncommon in dementing patients, deserves further analysis, since it is generally believed (e.g., Ajuriaguerra & Tis-

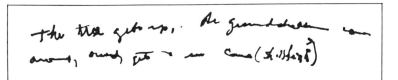

*The tree gets up, ·The grandchildren comes
around, and gets a new cane (shillelegh)*

FIGURE 13.2. *Writing sample of patient with progressive supranuclear palsy. Instructions were to write what happened in his house at Christmas.*

sot, 1975) that automatic forms are generally spared in the language of dementia.

While reading is relatively unimpaired, in the writing samples of patients with progressive supranuclear palsy, agraphic errors can be seen not unlike those of patients in confusional states (Cummings, Hebben, Obler, & Leonard, 1980). Errors are most prominently additions or omissions of inflectional endings, as demonstrated in Figure 13.2.

Unlike the patients with early cortical dementias, explanation of proverbs is concrete in patients with progressive supranuclear palsy. Our patient, tested both before and after treatment with levodopa, was able to give more abstract responses after treatment. This improvement was not attributable merely to the fact that he could produce longer phrases more comfortably and remains to be explained.

Conclusion

The life-span approach we embrace in viewing the language disturbances of aphasia and of dementia, we believe, has numerous advantages over earlier perspectives. Most importantly, it permits us to look for interactions between the natural processes of aging and the disturbed behaviors resulting from specific brain lesions. With aphasics, it aids us in diagnosis and treatment to realize that more fluent aphasias are linked to the later end of the lifespan. Moreover, as we have stressed, increasing knowledge of how dementing diseases and the cognitive decline of normal aging interact with aphasia should permit us to explore new modes of therapy for the elderly aphasic patient.

As for the dementing patient with language disturbance, we should recognize that there are numerous dementing illnesses that will each have a range of characteristic language behaviors associated with it. As neurologists and neuropsychologists detail the diverse forms of dementia, neurolinguists will document the associated language disorders, and speech pathologists will explore new modes of treatment in the hope that, even with irreversible disease, communicative function may be maintained at the highest possible level.

References

Ajuriaguerra, J. de, & Tissot, R. 1975. Some aspects of language in various forms of senile dementia. In E. Lenneberg & E. Lenneberg (Eds.), *Foundations of language development* (Vol. 1). New York: Academic Press.

Basso, A., Capitani, E., & Vignolo, L. 1979. Influence of rehabilitation on language skills in aphasic patients. *Archives of Neurology, 36*, 190–96.

Castro-Caldas, M., Ferro, J., & Grosso, J. 1979. Age, sex and type of aphasia in stroke patients. Paper presented at International Neurolopsychological Society.

Culton, G. 1971. Reaction to age as a factor in chronic aphasia in stroke patients. *Journal of Speech and Hearing Disorders, 36*, 563–64.

Cummings, J., Hebben, N., Obler, L., & Leonard, P. 1980, "Non-aphasic misnaming" and other neurobehavioral features of an unusual toxic encephalopathy: Case study. *Cortex, 16*, 315–324.

Gleason, J., Goodglass, H., Green, E., Obler, L., Hyde, M., & Weintraub, S. 1980. Narrative strategies in aphasic and normal subjects. *Journal of Speech and Hearing Disorders, 23*, 370–382.

Goodglass, H., & Kaplan, E. 1972. *The assessment of aphasia and related disorders*. Philadelphia: Lea and Febiger.

Gustafson, L., Hagberg, B., & Ingvar, D. 1978. Speech disturbances in presenile dementia related to local cerebral blood flow abnormalities in the dominant hemisphere. *Brain and Language, 5*, 103–118.

Harasymiw, S., Halper, A., & Sutherland, B. 1981. Sex, age and aphasia type. *Brain and Language, 12*, 190–198.

Holland, A. 1980. Working with the aging aphasic patient. In L. Obler & M. Albert (Eds.), *Language and communication in the elderly*. Lexington, Mass.: D. C. Heath.

Kertesz, A. 1979. *Aphasia and associated disorders*. New York: Grune & Stratton.

Kertesz, A., & McCabe, P. 1977. Recovery patterns and prognosis in aphasia. *Brain, 100*, 1–18.

Miceli, G., Caltagirone, C., Gainotti, G., Masullo, C., Silveri, M., & Villa, G. 1981. Influence of sex, age, literacy, and pathologic lesion on incidence, severity, and type of aphasia. Manuscript submitted for publication.

Obler, L., Albert, M., Caplan, L., Mohr, J. P., & Geer, D. 1980. Stroke type, aphasia type, sex differences, and aging. Paper presented at the Academy of Aphasia.

Obler, L., Albert, M., Goodglass, H., & Benson, D. F. 1978. Aphasia type and aging. *Brain and Language, 6*, 318–322.

Sands, E., Sarno, M. T., & Shankweiler, D. 1969. Long term assessment of language function in aphasia due to stroke. *Archives of Physical Medicine and Rehabilitation, 50*, 203–207.

Sarno, M. 1980. Language rehabilitation outcome in the elderly aphasic patient. In L. Obler & M. Albert (Eds.), *Language and communication in the elderly*. Lexington, Mass.: D. C. Heath.

Sarno, M. T., & Levita, E. 1971. Natural course of recovery in severe aphasia. *Archives of Physical Medicine and Rehabilitation, 52,* 175–79.

Schwartz, M., Marin, O., & Saffran, E. 1979. Dissociations of language function in dementia: A case study. *Brain and Language, 7,* 277–306.

Smith, A. 1971. Objective indices of severity of chronic aphasia in stroke patients. *Journal of Speech and Hearing Disorders, 36,* 167–207.

Vignolo, L. 1964. Evolution of aphasia and language rehabilitation: A retrospective study. *Cortex, 1,* 344–367.

Whitaker, H. 1976. A case of the isolation of the language function. In H. Whitaker & H. A. Whitaker (Eds.), *Studies in neurolinguistics.* (Vol. 2). New York: Academic Press.

14

Acquired Aphasia in Children

PAUL SATZ and CAROL BULLARD-BATES

The present chapter reviews the incidence, clinical picture, and prognosis of childhood aphasia. The term CHILDHOOD APHASIA, as used in this chapter, should be differentiated from the term DEVELOPMENTAL APHASIA. McCarthy (1963) has provided a useful working definition:

> By DEVELOPMENTAL APHASIA (sometimes called congenital aphasia) one refers to a condition in which either poor endowment or brain injury occurring before, during, or after birth prevents the child from acquiring language. By CHILDHOOD APHASIA one refers to language impairment occurring after language has been acquired in the normal manner [p.21].

The following review of the literature on childhood aphasia will draw on comparisons to the adult aphasias only in cases where differences seem to exist and only as they shed light on mechanisms that might underlie these putative differences.

The subject of acquired aphasia in children has received considerably less attention than has acquired aphasia in adults. The difference has persisted since the first reports on childhood aphasia, which emerged soon after the classic reports of Paul Broca (1861) and Carl Wernicke (1874). These early reports (Bernhardt, 1885; Clarus, 1874; Cotard, 1868; Freud, 1897/1968), although equally meritorious, have been overshadowed by Broca's and Wernicke's reports because of the disproportionate interest directed to the adult aphasias, especially in the twentieth century. This state of affairs is also evident in the publications, symposia, and conferences on the acquired aphasias. The subject of childhood aphasia is either infrequently addressed or is relegated to a brief subscript in a journal article or book chapter. The last major conference on

399

childhood aphasia, to our knowledge, was held in 1960 at Stanford University under the sponsorship of the California Society for Crippled Children and Adults and the Easter Seal Research Foundation. In his introductory remarks, Robert West (1960) ventured the hopeful remarks that "this meeting will go down in history as a very important one [p. 1]." Unfortunately, this has not been the case. The proceedings are seldom referenced, and the impact on 2 decades of subsequent research has been negligible. In a review, Martha Denckla (1979) states that "within the past decade, little has been added to the literature on acquired aphasia in preadolescence [p. 537]." Answers as to why the literature on childhood aphasia has been so unproductive are not readily apparent. A frequent explanation is the RARITY of the disorder. This explanation dates back to Cotard (1868), a pupil of Charcot, who first reported the preservation of speech in infantile hemiplegia with complete atrophy of the left cerebral hemisphere. This report represents the first evidence in support of the equipotentiality hypothesis later championed by Basser (1962) and Lenneberg (1967). Cotard (1868) said: "Il est extremement remarquable que, quel qui soit le côté de la lésion cerebrale, les individus hemiplégiques depuis leur entrance ne présentent jamais d'aphasie et cela même quand tout hémisphère gauche est atrophis." Cotard's interpretation was shared by Bayley (1939) and more recently by Martha Denckla (1979), who said; "As the sole 'cortical function' consultant in a large neurological institute, between 1969 and 1976 I saw only seven cases of acquired aphasia in children under 10 years of age [p. 537]."

These observations pertaining to the rarity of the disorder, however need further clarification. Does one mean that the unilateral lesion is rare, or the aphasia, given a unilateral lesion? Also, one might ask whether the presence (or absence) of aphasia represents an appropriate model for children whose brains modulate a volatile and partially acquired linguistic system (Dennis & Whitaker, 1977). A more appropriate model than adult aphasia syndromes might relate to delayed acquisition of word relationships. More on this point later.

Unilateral lesions of the cerebral cortex do occur in children, and the infantile hemiplegias are one typical example (Annett, 1973; Dennis & Whitaker, 1977). However, the prevalence of these lesions is far less common than in adults; this is especially true of the neoplastic and vascular lesions associated with the adult aphasias (Heilman & Valenstein, 1979). Hence, there is good reason to believe that the lesions etiologically responsible for the adult aphasias are RARE in children. One might then ask whether the risk of aphasia (or delayed language acquisition) is also rare in children with unilateral brain insult. This question addresses a different and more substantive issue—namely, whether the neural substrate for speech is organized differently in children and adults. If so, it would affect the risk probabilities of aphasia (or language delay) in children with unilateral brain injury. The reason is that, if the speech mechanisms are more diffusely and incompletely represented in the brain, then one might predict a lower risk of aphasia given a unilateral insult. Or, alternatively, if there is equipotentiality between the hemispheres in terms of speech representation, then one might predict a higher risk of aphasia but a more dramatic recovery.

The literature on child aphasia has typically noted a difference, not only in the INCIDENCE of aphasia but also in the TYPE and PROGNOSIS. The first report was made by Bernhardt (1897), who challenged the earlier report by Cotard (1868). His observations have remained essentially unchallenged throughout the twentieth century. Bernhardt stated, "True aphasia is not rare in childhood: it is a frequent symptom of infantile cerebral hemiplegia, mostly transient, rarely permanent. It is mostly motor in type [cited in Guttmann, 1942, p. 205]."

This position, in summary, states that when a unilateral lesion occurs during childhood (which is rare), the risk of aphasia (incidence) is not rare. In fact, the pattern of childhood aphasia departs significantly from the adult form in terms of incidence, type, and prognosis.

The following sections present a review of the empirical findings and theoretical rationale underlying each of these phenomena.

Incidence

A raised incidence of aphasia has typically been reported in children with unilateral brain disease (Hécaen, 1976). This raised incidence has largely been explained by the higher risk of aphasia in children than in adults with right hemisphere disease.[1] Such cases are referred to as examples of crossed aphasia, assuming that the child is right handed. Among right-handed adults, the incidence of crossed aphasia is extremely infrequent, ranging between 1% and 4% of the population (Rasmussen & Milner, 1977). Reports of the incidence among right-handed children in contrast, have ranged from a low of 7% (Woods & Teuber, 1978) to a high of 47% (Basser, 1962).

---

1. Lesions to the left cerebral hemisphere have been shown to produce aphasia equally in children and adults. Hence, the raised incidence is due to the occurrence of the crossed aphasias.

What is the basis for this presumed risk of crossed aphasia in children? The most popular explanation is that during childhood the cerebral specialization of speech is more diffusely represented in both hemispheres (i.e., the equipotentiality hypothesis). With age and maturation of the cerebral cortex, there is a progressive shift from bilateral representation to unilateral specialization on the left (Basser, 1962; Lenneberg, 1967). This position thus posits an ontogenetic development in cerebral speech dominance—namely, that speech and language functions are progressively lateralized with age. As a construct, it purports to account for differences in the incidence, type, and prognosis of aphasia in children and adults.

Naturally, support for this equipotentiality position must rest on evidence of an increased risk of aphasia and/or disordered language in right-handed children with lesions of the right hemisphere. As Dennis and Whitaker (1977) have shown, the equipotentiality hypothesis postulates an equivalence of language skills in the two infant hemispheres. Hence, the risk of aphasia and/or disordered language should be significantly higher in children than in adults with right hemisphere injury; in fact, the incidence among children should be approximately the same as for lesions to the left cerebral hemisphere. We can turn to two sources of clinical data for evaluation of this hypothesis: (*a*) the incidence of disordered language in hemiplegic children; and (*b*) the incidence of crossed aphasia in unilaterally brain-injured children.

Disordered Language

A review of this literature has been compiled by Dennis and Whitaker (1977). The review comprises all of the known studies on hemiplegia and language since the original report by Cotard (1868). Table 14.1 presents a summary of the 14 studies that report the proportion of language impairment as a function of hemiplegic side. Inspection of this table shows a significantly higher risk of impaired language following left hemisphere damage (right hemiplegia). The probability values are as follows: left hemisphere damage, $p = .40$; right hemisphere damage, $p = .18$. Thus, these data are discrepant with the equipotentiality hypothesis. As with adults, the left hemisphere seems to be at greater risk for language impairment when injured.

What about age effects and language status in childhood hemiplegia? Answers to this question can be found in the most recent study in the preceding survey (Annett, 1973). Table 14.2 presents the proportion of cases with language impairment from infancy through childhood for left and right hemiplegics. Inspection of this table shows a dramatic difference in the incidence of speech defects between left and right hemi-plegics at each age, with right hemiplegics being at greater risk. This hemispheric difference, however, was more marked in cases where the onset of hemiplegia occurred after 13 months of age. Prior to age 1 year, there was approximately a 2:1 risk for language impairment in right hemiplegics compared to left hemiplegics (30% versus 15%, respectively). However, after age 1, the risk of language impairment disappeared in left hemiplegics and dramatically increased in right hemi-

TABLE 14.1
Language Disorder as a Function of Laterality of Childhood Hemiplegia

Study	N language disordered/ N cases (%)	N language disordered right hemiplegics/ N right hemiplegics (%)	N language disordered left hemiplegics/ N left hemiplegics (%)
Cotard (1868)	9/23 (38.1)	8/13 (61.5)	1/10 (10.0)
Gaudard (1884/1968)	33/80 (41.3)	25/55 (45.4)	8/25 (32.0)
Bernhardt (1885)	11/18 (61.1)	11/14 (78.6)	0/4 (0.0)
Lovett (1888)	7/26 (26.9)	3/13 (23.1)	4/13 (30.8)
Wallenberg (1886)	62/160 (38.8)	45/94 (47.9)	17/66 (25.8)
Osler (1888)	13/120 (10.8)	12/68 (17.6)	1/52 (1.9)
Sachs and Peterson (1890)	17/105 (16.2)	10/52 (19.2)	7/53 (13.2)
Wulff (1890)	8/24 (33.3)	6/9 (66.7)	2/15 (13.3)
Freud and Rie (1891/1968)	10/35 (28.6)	7/23 (30.4)	3/12 (25.0)
Dunsdon (1952)	39/64 (61.0)	31/34 (91.2)	8/30 (37.5)
Basser (1962)	34/102 (33.3)	16/48 (33.3)	18/54 (33.3)
Ingram (1964)	12/75 (16.0)	11/44 (25.0)	1/31 (0.03)
Bishop (1967)	9/17 (53.0)	5/7 (71.4)	1/8 (12.5)
Annett (1973)	31/108 (28.7)	24/59 (40.7)	7/47 (14.9)

NOTE: Probability of language disorder after right hemiplegia = .401; probability of language disorder after left hemiplegia = .183.

TABLE 14.2
Percentage of Speech Defects by Side of Hemiplegia and Age of Onset

| | Side of hemiplegia | | | |
| | Right | | Left | |
Age at onset (presumed)	N	Percentage with speech problem	N	Percentage with speech problem
Unknown (prenatal?)	17	29.4	18	16.7
Perinatal	24	33.3	22	13.6
0–13 months	9	33.3	1	0.0
14–44 months	7	85.7	5	0.0
5½–11½ years	2	100.0	1	Speech problem in a left-handed child before onset?

plegics. Annett (1973) concluded that "after the age of 13 months, right and left hemiplegic children show a difference in the incidence of speech problems which is as marked as that found in adults; almost invariable presence following left sided lesions and absence after right sided ones [p. 11]." These results, in summary, lend further disconfirmation to the equipotentiality hypothesis, at least after the first year of age.

Aphasia

Until recently, there has been no critical review of the childhood aphasia literature. Much of this literature has been marred by anecdotal reports, biased samples, vague definitions of aphasia, and frequent failure to define hand preference, age of lesion, time of assessment following lesion onset, or even lesion side. Ambiguity regarding lesion side or the failure to separate out left handers could easily produce misleading information with respect to crossed aphasia. Evidence now points to a different form of cerebral speech specialization in left handers, at least in adults (Hécaen, 1976; Satz, 1979). The childhood aphasia studies, in addition, have often reported only the presence of aphasia for one lesion side without comparable reports for the other side. The classic study by Alajouanine and Lhermitte (1965) is subject to this criticism; only left hemisphere cases were selected, all of whom were aphasic. Other studies, while reporting the presence of aphasia, fail to report the proportion of nonaphasics either within or between lesion sides. Many of these studies have also comprised cases of mixed etiology, some of which could produce bilateral hemispheric damage (e.g., trauma and neoplasm). This is certainly true of most of the classic twentieth-century studies (e.g., Alajouanine & Lhermitte, 1965; Basser, 1962; Brown & Hécaen, 1976; Ford, 1937; Guttmann, 1942; Hécaen, 1976). Finally, many of the early twentieth century studies, especially those conducted prior to the use of antibiotics (1940), may have been flawed by the presence of systemic infectious diseases that could have produced bilateral cerebral dysfunction. Bilateral disease, of course, could spuriously inflate the overall incidence of aphasia, especially crossed aphasia. Woods and Teuber (1978) pointed out that cases selected prior to the era of antibiotics and mass immunization may have been subject to systemic bacterial infections that could have produced encephalopathic changes in both hemispheres. In fact, when they compared studies done before 1942 with later studies, they found that the proportion of crossed aphasias dropped from a high of 35% to a low of 7%.

The following section presents a review of the childhood aphasia literature that was undertaken in light of the preceding problems (Bullard, Satz, & Speedie, in press). The survey was based on reports since 1940 only. This date was chosen on the basis of Woods and Teuber's (1978) recommendations. Single case studies were rejected as not being representative, since they report the unusual or atypical case and might skew the results. One such case study was considered, however, because it reviewed 16 similar studies (Fisher & Friedmann, 1959).

Twenty-one studies comprising 929 cases were reviewed. Most cases did not meet the criteria required for use in clearly determining the incidence of aphasia after unilateral lesions for right- and left-handed children. The following criteria for case selection were employed:

1. Some speech reported before the lesion onset, regardless of how minimal. (In some cases this involved the expression of several words only.)
2. Hand preference reported before lesion onset.
3. Patient under 16 years of age BEFORE lesion onset.
4. Evidence that lesion was unilateral only. (In some cases the only evidence cited was unilateral hemiplegia.)
5. Comparison of presence versus absence of aphasia following unilateral injury. Aphasic symptoms included any one or more of the following: mutism, paraphasia, and problems in comprehension, expression, reading, writing, and naming. Cases that were reported with ONLY dysarthria or articulation difficulties were classified as nonaphasic.

Scrutiny of the 21 studies revealed problems in the examination of subjects and the description of methods employed. Only 13 studies (comprising 494 cases) reported any handedness data; the 8 that did not were immediately eliminated (Aicardi, Ansili & Cherrie, 1969; Dunsdon, 1952; Fisher & Friedmann, 1959; Guttmann, 1942; Kinsbourne, 1977; Lenneberg, 1967; McCarthy, 1963; Shillito, 1964). In 2 of these 8 studies, the lack of handedness data was not the only reason for rejection. McCarthy (1963) studied athetoids and children with spastic cerebral palsy, most of whom had in all probability suffered brain damage before they had acquired speech. In addition, they ALL showed some language difficulties. The data were therefore not felt to be applicable. Similarly, in Dunsdon's (1952) study of children with cerebral palsy, most of the patients probably had brain abnormalities at birth. Also, the author defined SPEECH DEFECTS in left and right hemiplegics as "lack of necessary control of speech mechanism muscles [p. 48]"—that is, difficulty in articulation.

Of the 13 remaining studies, those of Branco-Lefèvre (1950, 5 cases), Alajouanine and Lhermitte (1965, 32 cases), Annett (1973, 108 cases), and Byers and McLean (1962, 12 cases) were rejected because they reported results on only those patients who became aphasic, thereby precluding an assessment of the incidence of aphasia. Isler's study (1971, 82 cases) was rejected because in only 3 of 82 cases was handedness reported, although the case study reports were extensively detailed. Ingram (1964, 75 cases) also reported insufficient handedness data and described only 16 patients who were over 1 year of age when hemiplegia developed. McFie's study (1961, 40 cases) was also rejected for insufficient handedness data and because the primary focus concerned the effects of unilateral injury on intellectual performance rather than aphasia. The study by Lansdell (1969, 18 cases) was rejected because the age at onset of the lesions in his cases was unclear. In addition, it was difficult to determine whether all of his subjects had suffered aphasic symptoms at the time of the cerebral damage.

Only the authors of five studies attempted to report handedness for all their cases, which probably reflects the inadequacy of medical records. These studies (Basser, 1962, Collignon, Hécaen, & Angelerques, 1968; Hécaen, 1976, 1977; Woods & Teuber, 1978) yielded a total of 120 cases. Of these, only 68 were appropriate for classification. In 17 of 30 cases of acquired aphasia reported by Basser (1962), handedness was not specified, leaving only 13 cases that could be reliably classified. Only 34 of 65 cases had handedness and lesion side data in the Woods and Teuber study (1978). Hécaen (1976, 1977) reported that he had taken 10 of his cases from Collignon _et al._ (1968), and several of the Collignon cases showed clear bilateral abnormalities although they had been classified as unilateral in the three studies (Collignon *et al.*, 1968; Hécaen, 1976, 1977). One case (L. J. P.) was omitted because in one study the patient was classified as left handed (Collignon *et al.*, 1968) and in the other studies as right handed (Hécaen, 1976, 1977). When these factors were considered, 21 cases remained from the three studies (Collignon *et al.*, 1968; Hécaen, 1976, 1977).

It must be stated that the 68 cases found suitable for this review (Bullard *et al.*, in press) may still be faulted on several counts. Often evidence of lateralization is poor. The time at which the patients were examined was not specified; assessment during the postacute phase could have lowered the observed frequencies. Although preference for a certain hand was specified in very young children who were included in the survey, this classification may be of questionable accuracy in children who had not established a strong preferential usage of one hand for such activities as writing. The authors nevertheless attempted to be as stringent in their criteria for classification and selection of subjects as was reasonable considering the methods of reporting and the limitations already discussed.

CHILDHOOD APHASIA

The results of this survey can be seen in Table 14.3 which reports the proportion of aphasia [$P(A)$] across studies by lesion side and handedness. The data have been recalculated to show the probability of aphasia separately for lesion side [$P(A/L)$, $P(A/R)$]. The overall mean incidence of aphasia, $P(A)$, is based on the proportion of aphasia cases across lesion side (L, R) and studies ($N=3$) within each handedness group. Collignon *et al.* (1968) and Hécaen (1976, 1977) were collapsed into one study group. In interpreting the table, it is also important to note whether a bias exists in the frequency of left- versus right-sided lesions [$P(L)$, $P(R)$, respectively].

An inspection of Table 14.3 shows that the overall mean incidence of aphasia [$P(A)$] was .56 (32/57) for right handers and .64 (7/11) for left handers. A chi-square test of independence (proportions) was not significant ($p > .30$), suggesting that the incidence of aphasia was similarly high for both right and left handers. A closer inspection of the data, however, suggests that this null finding may be due to two artifacts in the reports of right-handed children. This can be seen more clearly at the bottom of the table.

In the reports for right handers, there was an extreme bias in favor of left-sided lesions [$P(L) = .61$ versus $P(R) = .39$] as well as a high probability of aphasia given a left-sided injury [$P(A/L) = .80$]. These two fac-

TABLE 14.3
Observed Incidence of Aphasia in Right- and Left-Handed Children from a Unilateral Lesion to the Left or Right Hemisphere

| Handedness and study | N of cases | Left-sided lesions | | | | Right-sided lesions | | | | Total aphasia frequency |
| | | Aphasia | | No aphasia | | Aphasia | | No aphasia | | |
		N	%	N	%	N	%	N	%	
Left handers										
1	4	2	100	0	0	1	50	1	50	3
2	6	1	33	2	67	2	67	1	33	3
3	1	1	100	0	0	0	0	0	0	1
Totals	11	4		2		3		2		7
Right handers										
1	17	11	79	3	21	0	0	3	100	11
2	28	14	88	2	12	1	8	11	92	15
3	12	3	60	2	40	3	43	4	57	6
Totals	57	28		7		4		18		32

Left handers: $P(A) = .64(7/11)$; $P(A/L) = .67(4/6)$; $P(A/R) = .60(3/5)$; $P(L) = .55(6/11)$; $P(R) = .45(5/11)$.

Right handers: $P(A) = .56(32/57)$; $P(A/L) = .80(28/35)$; $P(A/R) = .18(4/22)$; $P(L) = .61(35/57)$; $P(R) = .39(22/57)$.

tors would tend to spuriously inflate the overall incidence of aphasia [$P(A)$] in these reports.[2] One should also note that the risk of aphasia in the right handers was disproportionately higher for left- versus right-sided lesions [$P(A/L) = .80$ versus $P(A/R) = .18$]. These hemispheric differences in aphasia correspond closely to those obtained for language impairment (*LI*) in hemiplegic children [$P(LI/L) = .40$ versus $P(LI/R) = .18$] (Dennis & Whitaker, 1977). Both data sets are discrepant with the equipotentiality hypothesis (Lenneberg, 1967). In right-handed children, the left hemisphere is at much greater risk for aphasia than is the right when damaged. But this was not so for the left-handed children; although the sample size was small ($N=11$), the hemispheric risk of aphasia was more symmetrical [$P(A/L) = .67$ versus $P(A/R) = .60$].

2. The same artifact exists in the paper by Hécaen (1976). He found an even higher overall probability of childhood aphasia [$P(A) = .74$]. Unfortunately, his study contained an extreme bias in favor of left-sided lesions [$P(L) = .74$ versus $P(R) = .26$] as well as a high probability of aphasia given a left-sided injury [$P(A/L) = .88$]. Although he reported a 33% incidence of crossed aphasia, this percentage was based on only 2 of 6 cases, one of whom was left handed.

ADULT APHASIA

The preceding results on left- and right-handed children might be elucidated by a more direct comparison to the aphasia literature for left- and right-handed adults. A review of this literature was reported by Satz (1979), with revisions by Carter, Hohenegger, and Satz (1980). The review comprised all the known studies ($N = 12$) between 1935 and 1973. These results can be seen in Table 14.4 which reports the proportion of aphasia by lesion side and handedness across studies.

The overall incidence of aphasia for right-handed adults was .33 (736/2206) and for left handers was .58 (180/313). This difference was

TABLE 14.4

Observed Incidence of Aphasia in Left- and Right-Handed Adults from a Unilateral Lesion to the Left or Right Hemisphere

Handedness and study	N of cases	Left-sided lesions				Right-sided lesions				Total aphasia frequency
		Aphasia		No aphasia		Aphasia		No aphasia		
		N	%	N	%	N	%	N	%	
Left handers										
1	8	4	67	2	33	2	100	0	0	6
2	12	5	83	1	17	6	100	0	0	11
3	20	5	50	5	50	5	50	5	50	10
4	10	5	100	0	0	4	80	1	20	9
5	9	6	86	1	14	2	100	0	0	8
6	14	7	59	5	41	0	0	2	100	7
7	13	5	83	1	17	5	70	2	30	10
8	33	13	72	5	28	1	7	14	93	14
9	63	11	37	19	63	8	27	25	73	19
10	58	28	85	5	15	20	80	5	20	48
11	59	22	59	15	41	11	50	11	50	33
12	14	2	50	2	50	3	30	7	70	5
Totals	313	113		61		67		72		180
Right handers										
8	353	115	73	42	27	1	0.5	195	99.5	116
9	704	218	56	170	44	19	6	297	94	237
10	650	—		—		—		—		234
11	299	81	50	82	50	0	0	136	100	81
12	200	—		—		—		—		68
Totals	2206	414		294		20		628		736

Left handers: $P(A) = .58(180/313)$; $P(A/L) = .65(113/174)$; $P(A/R) = .48(67/139)$; $P(L) = .56(174/313)$; $P(R) = .44(139/313)$.

Right handers: $P(A) = .33(736/2206)$; $P(A/L) = .58(414/708)$; $P(A/R) = .03(20/648)$; $P(L) = .52$ (708/1356); $P(R) = .48(648/1356)$.

significant based on a chi-square test of independence ($p < .001$). Although there was a slight bias favoring left-sided lesions in the left-handed reports [$P(L) = .56$, $P(R) = .44$], this trend was not associated with a high probability of aphasia following left-sided lesions [$P(A/L) = .65$], which would have spuriously inflated the $P(A)$. Also, the percentage of left handers in these reports, based on a much larger sample size (313/2519), was 12%, which is compatible with prevalence estimates in the population (Hardyck & Petrinovitch, 1977; Satz, 1972).

CHILDHOOD VERSUS ADULT APHASIA

If maturational changes in hemispheric specialization are hypothesized to occur during childhood, then one might expect to find a difference in the incidence of aphasia between children and adults, especially in right handers. An inspection of Tables 14.3 and 14.4 show that the $P(A)$ was .33 in adults and .56 in children, which when subjected to a chi-square test of independence is significant ($p < .01$). This test, however, is subject to the same artifacts noted earlier for the data on right-handed children. The extreme bias of left-sided lesions in these reports [$P(L) = .61$ versus $P(R) = .39$] coupled with the high incidence of aphasia following left-sided lesions [$P(A/L) = .80$] would spuriously inflate the $P(A)$ value. In the reports for right-handed adults, the $P(A/L)$ was much lower, based on over 2000 cases [$P(A/L) = .58$]. Failure to recognize these flaws could lead to false rejection of the null hypothesis (type 1 error) and an unwarranted claim for maturational differences in hemispheric specialization.

It should also be noted that the raised incidence of aphasia reported for right-handed children was due in part to the larger number of CROSSED aphasias. In children, the $P(A/R)$ was .18(4/22); in adults, the $P(A/R)$ was .03(20/648). The risk of aphasia with right brain injury, while higher in children than in adults, is still much lower than the risk of aphasia following left-sided injury, regardless of age. In children, the $P(A/L)$ was .80; in adults, the $P(A/L)$ was .58. Also, the number of crossed aphasia cases among children, while higher than that among adults, was only 4 out of a total of 22 with right-sided injury. One must suspect a possible bias in selective reporting. Kinsbourne and Hiscock (1978) have stated that "there is a probability that noteworthy cases (for example, aphasia after right hemisphere damage) will be reported more often than the common case (for example, aphasia after left hemisphere damage and absence of aphasia after right hemisphere damage) [p. 213]." Indeed, the crossed aphasias are noteworthy and a subject of considerable clinical interest. But one must be assured that such cases are real and not due to artifacts of sample selection, etiology, and/or handedness.[3] The presence of bilateral disease or left handedness in the study sample would spuriously raise the incidence of aphasia following right-sided injury. Each of these factors have marred previous efforts, including the insightful paper by Hécaen (1976). The survey by Bullard *et al.* (in press) is no exception. Although efforts were made to control for handedness, presence of bilateral systemic disease, aphasia frequency by lesion side, and the like, problems still remain, particularly regarding lesion specification. One cannot be sure that the lesions were truly unilateral. As such, the raised incidence of crossed aphasia in children, while still low, could more parsimoniously be attributed to several of the procedural artifacts noted here.

SUMMARY

The preceding results, including two large-scale surveys, raised serious questions concerning presumed differences in the INCIDENCE of aphasia between children and adults. The following conclusions seem warranted. First, the childhood aphasias are not rare if the lesion is unilateral and encroaches on the speech areas. There is, however, a lower prevalence of unilateral vascular disease in children. Second, the risk of aphasia or language impairment is approximately the same in right-handed children and adults if the left hemisphere is damaged. Third, this risk is substantially greater following left- versus right-sided brain injury regardless of age—at least after infancy. This finding challenges the equipotentiality hypothesis and its corollary, the progressive lateralization hypothesis. As such, it lends additional support to the developmental invariance hypothesis, which postulates a preprogrammed asymmetry favoring left hemisphere specialization from birth or early infancy (Geschwind, 1973; Kinsbourne & Hiscock, 1977; Witelson, 1977). Fourth, cases of crossed aphasia exist, but they are rare, particularly after ages 3–5 years in the right handed and perhaps earlier. Even when present at these young ages, they could still reflect artifacts of selection bias, ambiguous lesion side, and/or handedness. Fifth, the crossed aphasias are more commonly observed in the left handed, re-

---

3. Age of lesion is another factor that could also alter the frequency of crossed aphasias. Krashen (1973) showed that in Basser's (1962) study, which reported the largest number of such cases, there were no cases of crossed aphasia after age 5. One should note that this critical period is higher than the one reported by Annett (1973) for childhood hemiplegia and language impairment. Unfortunately, the age factor was not available for study in the review by Bullard *et al.* (in press).

gardless of age, and may reflect a more diffuse or bilateral mode of speech representation.

Clinical Picture (Type)

A second distinguishing feature attributed to the childhood aphasias is the language pattern. In contrast to the adult pattern, childhood aphasia has long been characterized by its nonfluency. This position dates from the early reports of Bernhardt (1885) and Freud (1897/1968), who both noted the poverty of spontaneous speech and the telegraphic expression following unilateral brain injury. They described the aphasia as primarily motor in type, with initial mutism followed by reduced initiative for speech, hesitations, dysarthria, and impoverishment of lexical stock. These early reports also noted the absence or rarity of logorrhea, paraphasia, and auditory comprehension defects in the childhood aphasias, which suggested a dissociation between output (expression) and input (comprehension) mechanisms. This position has largely prevailed throughout the twentieth century (Assal & Campiche, 1973; Basser, 1962; Benson, 1972; Branco-Lefèvre, 1950; Byers & McLean, 1962; Denckla, 1979; Geschwind, 1973; Guttmann, 1942; Poetzl, 1926).

The first major twentieth-century study was conducted by Guttmann (1942) on 30 cases (ages 2–14) of mixed etiology (trauma, neoplasm, abscess, thrombosis). He observed a distinctive pattern in 14 of the 16 cases who became aphasic. This pattern included "absence of spontaneous speech, unwillingness to speak, poverty of speech, telegram style, hesitancy and dysarthria [p. 208]." Comprehension was seemingly spared in these cases. However, Guttmann (1942) observed that this pattern changed with age. Under age 10, every lesion in the speech field reduced the output of spontaneous speech; after age 10, the pattern more closely resembled the adult picture, particularly the increased speech fluency (HYPEPRODUCTIVE APHASIA). Similar observations were noted in an earlier report by Poetzl (1926), who found a predominant nonfluent pattern before age 10 and a more mixed pattern, including hypespontaneity of speech, after age 10. In both of these studies, the status of the children's auditory comprehension was unclear, although a later report by Branco-Lefèvre (1950) found disorders of verbal comprehension to be rare.

Subsequent studies have essentially confirmed the predominant nonfluent pattern in aphasic children, particularly the absence or rarity of logorrhea and paraphasias. However, the presence of auditory comprehension defects have been observed in a portion of these children, which contradicts the strict dissociation between expression and comprehension previously noted. These later studies have also observed a severe disorder of writing in a majority of their aphasic children (Alajouanine & Lhermitte, 1965; Collignon *et al.*, 1968; Hécaen, 1976).

The study by Alajouanine and Lhermitte (1965) is particularly salient, in light of the Guttmann (1942) findings, because it provided additional information on age. The authors studied 32 children who ranged in age from 6 to 15; all were aphasic following injury to the left hemisphere that was caused by trauma, neoplasm, or stroke. Under 10 years of age, the aphasic pattern was characterized by a severe reduction in spontaneous speech, dysarthria, impoverished verbal stock, simplified syntax, and impaired comprehension (spoken language) and writing. No cases of logorrhea or paraphasia were noted in this younger age group. After 10 years of age, the pattern revealed an increased frequency of fluency disorder, including paraphasia, jargonaphasia, and impaired comprehension of written language. Disorders of articulation were less frequent in this older age group.

Disorders of auditory comprehension and writing were also noted in a study by Hécaen (1976), although he failed to replicate the relationship between age and clinical pattern observed by Guttmann (1942) and Alajouanine and Lhermitte (1965). His sample included 26 children who ranged in age from 3½ to 15 years. The sample, as with previous studies, comprised children with mixed etiologies (trauma, hematoma, neoplasm), most of whom had left hemisphere disease. Three of the cases had known bilateral involvement. Hécaen (1976) observed the characteristic pattern of nonfluency in the majority of his patients, including mutism, loss of initiation of speech, and the absence or rarity of paraphasias and logorrhea. Disorders of auditory verbal comprehension appeared in approximately a third of the cases, primarily during the acute period, while disorders of writing appeared in the majority of cases. In contrast to previous studies, Hécaen (1976) managed to relate clinical pattern to lesion site in some of the cases. Mutism was observed in three out of four cases with anterior lesions and in only one of four cases with a temporal lesion. The temporal lesion case, however, had evidence of brain stem involvement. Comprehension problems were observed with temporal lesions only and occurred in three of the four cases. No relationship was observed between lesion site and disorders of naming, writing, or reading.

What do these studies tell us with respect to the clinical picture of childhood aphasia? Answers to this question are not easily forthcoming, except for those features that are common to each of the studies. They all uniformly characterize the aphasia as primarily nonfluent in type, marked by initial mutism followed by reduced initiative for speech, hesitations, dysarthria, and impoverishment of lexical stock. In some of the studies, this pattern is characteristic of younger children, up to age 10 (Alajouanine & Lhermitte, 1965; Guttmann, 1942; Poetzl, 1926), whereas in other studies, the pattern is characteristic of both younger and older children, up to ages 13–15 (Assal & Campiche, 1973; Basser, 1962; Benson, 1972; Branco-Lefèvre, 1950; Byers & McLean, 1962; Collignon *et al.*, 1968; Hécaen, 1976). A second common feature across studies is the rarity or absence of paraphasias and logorrhea, especially in children under age 10. Virtually all studies have noted the rarity of these symptoms.

Despite these similarities, differences in the clinical picture still exist across studies. The most notable example is the issue of auditory comprehension ability. In some of the studies, disorders of auditory verbal comprehension are reported to be rare, at least up to age 10 (Assal & Campiche, 1973; Basser, 1962; Bernhardt, 1885; Branco-Lefèvre, 1950; Freud, 1897/1968; Guttmann, 1942; Poetzl, 1926), whereas in other studies, comprehension defects have been reported in a minority (Collignon *et al.*, 1968; Hécaen, 1976) or even majority of cases (Alajouanine & Lhermitte, 1965). Disorders of writing, written comprehension, and naming have also been reported with some frequency (Alajouanine & Lhermitte, 1965; Collignon *et al.*, 1968; Hécaen, 1976). The presence of these symptoms clearly challenges earlier reports on the dissociation between output (expression) and input (comprehension)—at least for some proportion of childhood aphasics. It also challenges the unitary symptom pattern that has long been attributed to the childhood aphasic. Although the clinical pattern is predominantly nonfluent and marked by the absence or rarity of paraphasias and logorrhea, disorders of auditory comprehension, naming, and writing may coexist. Three other reports have also demonstrated the presence of symptoms that depart from the traditional nonfluency pattern. Dennis (1980) described the case of a 9-year-old female child who suffered a vascular injury to the left middle and anterior cerebral arteries. Linguistic testing revealed marked deficits in communicative intent, comprehension, and output. Woods and Teuber (1978) described the case of a 5-year-old epileptic boy who showed acute onset of right-sided weakness and jargonaphasia. Comprehension was severely impaired, and his speech was fluent and unintelligible. Van Dongen and Loonen (1979) described the case of a 9-year-old boy who had "all characteristic features of a sensory aphasia. He spoke fluently without disorders of articulation. Paraphasias were sometimes noted [p. 212]."

This variability in language behavior should caution against any premature attempts to infer qualitative differences between the childhood and adult aphasias. One should first attempt to account for the differences that currently exist among the childhood aphasics. These linguistic differences, if real, could be due to a number of factors, including lesion site, etiology, age of lesion, lesion size, type of lesion (acute versus chronic), time of language assessment postonset, and the linguistic stage of the child. With respect to linguistic stage, we do not know how the postinfantile brain, where injured, modulates a volatile and partially acquired linguistic system. As such, comparisons to the adult aphasias may be inappropriate, if not misleading (Dennis, 1980). Unfortunately, few of the childhood aphasia studies have addressed these issues, either conceptually or methodologically. Hécaen (1976) managed to relate some of the aphasic patterns with lesion site. He found that mutism, which is frequent in the early phase, was more commonly associated with anterior lesions, whereas disorders of comprehension were only associated with temporal lobe lesions. However, no relationship was observed between lesion site and disorders of naming, writing, or reading. Nor have other studies confirmed his results on mutism and disorders of comprehension. Guttmann (1942) suggested that lesion size, rather than site, could be a factor in producing disordered comprehension. Unfortunately, this inference was based on only one case of sensory aphasia. It would be tempting to extrapolate on the relationship between mutism–nonfluency and anterior lesions because most of the childhood aphasia cases have been selected by the presence of hemiparesis. However, such extrapolation is speculation at best.

Whether differences exist in the clinical picture of aphasia between children and adults cannot be answered at this time. Evidence is still unclear as to whether a unitary pattern (i.e., nonfluency) characterizes the childhood picture. Certainly, other symptoms may coexist with the nonfluency, but their origins remain obscure. Answers to these questions will depend on more rigorous investigation in the future, with attention to some of the preceding methodological and conceptual issues. Finally, more objective testing, including the special linguistic procedures employed by Dennis (1980), may well reveal clusters of deficits that heretofore masked as a unitary disorder.

Prognosis

A third and perhaps most distinguishing feature attributed to the childhood aphasias is the recovery course. It has long been reported that the symptoms are transient and rarely permanent. Recovery from child-hood aphasia is much more dramatic in comparison to the adult aphasias. These observations date from the early reports by Clarus (1874), Bernhardt (1885), and Freud (1897/1968) and have been accepted generally by most twentieth-century clinicians (Alajouanine & Lhermitte, 1965; Assal & Campiche, 1973; Basser, 1962; Benson, 1972; Byers & McLean, 1962; Collignon *et al.*, 1968; Denckla, 1979; Geschwind, 1974; Guttmann, 1942; Hécaen, 1976; Lenneberg, 1967; Woods & Teuber, 1978). In light of discrepancies seen earlier between traditional claims and observable fact, it might help to examine more critically the data that purport to show a more dramatic recovery in childhood aphasia.

The first major twentieth-century paper was by Guttmann (1942). This study comprised 30 unilateral cases, aged 2–14 years, of mixed etiology (trauma, neoplasm, abscess, thrombosis). Only 10 cases were available at follow-up, which ranged from several months (4 cases) to several years (6 cases). Six of the follow-up cases were trauma, 3 were abscess, and 1 was vascular. A robust recovery in speech was observed for 5 of the 6 trauma cases, each of whom had an initial motor type of aphasia (i.e., nonfluent). Improvement, although less marked, was observed in 2 of the 3 abscess cases; the third showed complete recovery. In contrast, little improvement was observed for the vascular case, who showed a gross disturbance in both output and comprehension several months following onset (motor and sensory aphasia). Guttmann also noted that the lesion was more extensive in this case and may have been responsible for the more protracted recovery. He also predicted a more guarded prognosis when aphasic signs were still present after 4 weeks. No information was provided on the relationship between age of lesion occurrence and recovery, nor on school outcome results.

One of the most widely quoted reports on the recovery from child-hood aphasia is that of Basser (1962). His follow-up data were based largely on 30 children who sustained an acute hemiplegia (left=15, right=15) after the onset of speech. An initial nonfluent aphasia was observed in 13 of the 15 left hemisphere cases (right hemiplegia) and in 7 of the 15 right hemisphere cases (left hemiplegia). At follow-up (3 months–2 years), Basser (1962) reported the following:

> The speech loss was not permanent in any case, recovery always taking place after varying periods with subsequent improvement. Recovery either took place very quickly when once speech had begun to reappear or more usually slowly, the patient having to relearn to speak as an infant does passing through the stages of using single words, then phrases and then sentences [p. 435].

Basser (1962) noted that the recovery course was related to age at lesion occurrence. A more protracted recovery was observed in those cases in which the lesion occurred prior to age 2. Recovery was not associated with severity of the hemiplegia or with lesion side. Despite the robust recovery in speech, the intellectual levels were in the retarded range for a majority of the sample, regardless of lesion side. Unfortunately, no additional information was available with respect to school placement or achievement.

Similar recovery results were reported in a subsequent paper by Lenneberg (1967). The sample included eight cases examined at the Children's Hospital Medical Center of Boston. Age at insult ranged from 3 to 18 years. Etiology was mixed and included cases of trauma ($N=4$), stroke ($N=3$), and neoplasm ($N=1$). Seven of the cases were due to left hemisphere injury. Each of the cases were examined between 3 months of the insult and 2 years later. All of the children were aphasic at the initial examination, but only two were aphasic at follow-up. These two were in adolescence when the lesion (one trauma, one neoplasm) occurred (ages 15 and 18, respectively). Recovery was complete for all children who were under age 11 at the time of injury. Lenneberg (1967) concluded that aphasia runs a different course before the end of the first decade. During this period, recovery from aphasia is complete," with no permanent residue [p. 146]." By the time of puberty, however, a turning point is reached. Residual symptoms are the rule, as with adults. Lenneberg (1967) provided no data on intellectual level or school achievement in his sample.

Alajouanine and Lhermitte (1965) conducted a 1-year follow-up of 32 children (ages 6–15 years), all of whom were aphasic at initial contact following injury to the left hemisphere (trauma, neoplasm, stroke). At follow-up 24 of the children had regained "a normal or nearly normal language [p. 659]." No agrammatism was observed in these children. In contrast, the remaining 8 children showed a more unfavorable course. Most of these children had large cerebral lesions. The authors found no relationship between age and speed of recovery. Nor was a relationship found between severity of hemiplegia and recovery course. A majority of the children were still hemiplegic. On the basis of these results, Alajouanine and Lhermitte concluded that recovery is an indisputable fact and one very particular to children. This conclusion, however, should be tempered by an additional finding concerning intellectual level and school achievement. The authors were the first to note that, despite a dramatic remission in aphasia, none of the children could follow a normal progress in school:

In spite of a normal language—the children have great difficulty in learning lessons, understanding the general meaning of a course and in applying to a new problem a logical system which they have been taught. In short, they were able to regain what had been learned but were unable to acquire new data. Such an inability exists in the most favorable cases in the adult but then it is less conspicuous since the adults are less often bound to progress and acquire new data. Aphasia is not directly responsible for the intellectual impairment. It is only one of the consequences of cerebral lesions which disturb cerebral mechanisms subserving many other activities than language [p. 661].

Byers and McLean (1962) also observed persisting cognitive impairments, despite restitution of speech functions in their follow-up study. The authors followed 10 children (ages 3–15 years) with hemiplegia and aphasia (mostly of vascular origin). At follow-up (1–4 years later), all had regained speech spontaneously, despite the persistance of hemiplegia. However, 7 of the children showed moderate to severe impairment on tests of verbal and/or nonverbal cognitive function.

Hécaen (1976) reported some follow-up data on the language status of 17 children (ages 3½–19 years) who became aphasic following unilateral brain injury. The sample included cases of mixed etiology (trauma, hematoma, neoplasm), 15 of whom were left hemisphere damaged. Spontaneous recovery was noted in a majority of the cases. However, most of the patients continued to show long-term difficulties in writing and naming. Disorders of auditory comprehension, which were observed initially in a third of the cases, recovered spontaneously. In contrast to Lenneberg (1967), Hécaen observed 3 cases of complete recovery in subjects 14 years of age. However, as with many of the previous studies, no relationship between age and recovery course was found. Unfortunately, Hécaen (1976) provided no data on the relationship between etiology or aphasia type and recovery course. Nor was there any information on the academic status at follow-up. He did suggest that lesion size may be associated with slower recovery.

Woods and Teuber (1978) reported follow-up data on 25 aphasic patients who ranged in age from 2 to 15 years at onset. The cases were mostly of vascular origin but included trauma cases as well. At follow-up 4 years later, 21 of the cases showed spontaneous recovery of speech. The 4 cases who remained aphasic, ranged in age from 8 to 13 years at the time of the lesion. Of these cases, 3 were vascular in origin and 1 was epileptic and hemiparetic. Inspection of Woods and Teuber's tables revealed, however, that an equal number of cases of spontaneous recovery occurred in older children with vascular injury. Also, spontaneous recovery was observed in a number of younger vascular cases. Thus, this study failed to show a relationship between age of lesion or etiology and prognosis. As with previous studies, prognosis bore no relationship to severity or presence of hemiparesis. No information was provided on school achievement outcome.

A final study on prognosis was presented by van Dongen and Loonen (1979). The study comprised 14 right-handed children with acquired aphasia who ranged in age from 4 to 14 years at onset. Nine of the cases were trauma, 4 were vascular, and 1 was convulsive. The children were reexamined variably for up to 3 years. Spontaneous recovery was observed in half of the cases; the majority of these children had sustained head trauma. Little or no recovery was observed in those children with vascular malformation or convulsive disorder. The authors also found a relationship between aphasia type and recovery. Amnesic aphasics showed greater remission of symptoms at follow-up, whereas mixed aphasics (with comprehension defects) fared more poorly. This latter outcome suggests an interaction between etiology (i.e., vascular) and aphasia type (i.e., mixed). Of interest, the 1 case of sensory aphasia (Wernicke type) recovered completely within 2 years. This study provided no information on the relationship between age of lesion and recovery. Academic status at follow-up was also not reported.

What do the results of the preceding eight studies tell us about the recovery course in childhood aphasia? First, spontaneous recovery is dramatic in a majority of cases across studies. Recovery from aphasia ranged from a low of 50% (van Dongen & Loonen, 1979) to a high of 100% (Basser, 1962; Byers & McLean, 1962). Most of the studies reported spontaneous recovery in approximately 75% of the cases. Second, spontaneous recovery is unrelated to the presence or severity of hemiparesis. A majority of the cases improved despite the residual presence of hemiparesis (Alajouanine & Lhermitte, 1965; Basser, 1962; Byers & McLean, 1962; Woods & Teuber, 1978). No studies disconfirmed this finding. Third, spontaneous recovery, while the rule, is by no means invariant. Six of the studies reported persistence of the aphasia beyond 1 year of the insult for 25–50% of the cases (Alajouanine & Lhermitte, 1965; Guttmann, 1942; Hécaen, 1976; Lenneberg, 1967; van Dongen & Loonen, 1979; Woods & Teuber, 1978). In fact, those studies that reported intellectual, cognitive, or achievement data at follow-up each reported significant impairments in a majority of their cases, most of whom had recovered from their aphasias (Alajouanine & Lhermitte, 1965; Basser, 1962; Byers & McLean, 1962). No studies disconfirmed this finding, with the exception of Lenneberg (1967) who PRESUMED the absence of cognitive sequelae. Fourth, factors predictive of recovery are not discernible from this review. The results suggested that four variables may be related to recovery, including ETIOLOGY (Guttmann, 1942; van Dongen & Loonen, 1979; Woods & Teuber, 1978), APHASIA TYPE at onset (Guttmann, 1942; van Dongen & Loonen, 1979), LESION SIZE (Alajouanine & Lhermitte, 1965; Guttmann, 1942; Hécaen, 1976), and AGE at lesion occurrence (Basser, 1962; Lenneberg, 1967). Unfortunately, conflicting results were also reported for each of these factors as they relate to prognosis. Confirmatory results were also marred because of confounding between factors. This was particularly true for etiology and aphasia type in Guttmann (1942) and van Dongen and Loonen (1979), where spontaneous recovery was related to both nonfluent aphasia and trauma and poor recovery was related to mixed aphasia and stroke. A similar confound between etiology and age was also seen in Woods and Teuber (1978), where poor recovery was related to stroke and later age of lesion (8–13 years). These confounds, in the presence of conflicting re-sults between studies, obscures those factors predictive of recovery.

Conclusions

The preceding sections examined some of the traditional claims at-tributed to the childhood aphasias. These claims, which have enjoyed widespread and often uncritical acceptance in the literature, have postu-lated qualitative differences between children and adults in the inci-dence, clinical picture, and recovery course. On the basis of these claims, neuromaturational explanations have been advanced to account for these differences. These theoretical explanations, however, have continued to conflict with data derived from studies of nonaphasic sub-jects, which have uniformly indicated a preprogrammed structural asymmetry of the brain at birth (Wada, Clark, & Hamm, 1975; Witelson & Pallie, 1973). Electrophysiological and behavioral studies of infants have also demonstrated a functional hemispheric asymmetry favoring the left that is apparently invariant with age (Barnet, Vincentini, & Cam-pos, 1974; Eimas, Siqueland, Jusczyr, Vigorito, 1971; Hiscock & Kinsbourne, 1978; Molfese, Freemann, & Palermo, 1975). These studies, in sum, raise serious questions concerning the equipotentiality hypothesis and its corollary, the progressive lateralization hypothesis (Basser, 1962; Lenneberg, 1967; Luria, 1973).

Why the discrepancy between these two data sources (aphasics and nonaphasics)? The present review suggests that this discrepancy may be more apparent than real. An examination of the results disclosed the following general findings:

1. The risk of aphasia or language impairment is approximately the same in right-handed children and adults if the left hemisphere is damaged.
2. The risk of aphasia or language impairment is substantially greater following left- versus right-sided brain injury regardless of age—at least after infancy.
3. The risk of aphasia after right hemisphere injury (crossed aphasia) is rare in both right-handed adults and children, particularly after ages 3–5 years and perhaps earlier.
4. The aphasia pattern, while predominantly nonfluent in a majority of children, is by no means invariant. As with adults, other aphasic patterns can coexist or appear independently, including disorders of auditory comprehension, writing, reading, and naming. We do not know whether these patterns are related to age and maturational mechanisms or to factors independent of age (i.e., lesion site, lesion size, etiology, type of lesion, and/or time of language assessment postonset).
5. Spontaneous recovery, while dramatic in a majority of children, is by no means invariant. A majority of studies disclosed a number of unremitting cases (25–50%) after 1 year postonset. Furthermore, even in cases of recovery from aphasia, serious cognitive and academic sequelae were found. Finally, factors independent of age could also be predictive of recovery (i.e., etiology, aphasia type, and lesion size), although these factors are not easily discriminable at the present time.

On the basis of these findings, one should be cautious about invoking neurological explanations to account for presumed differences between the child and adult aphasias. The differences are not that consistent or clear, especially with respect to the incidence and clinical picture. They certainly lend little evidence to the equipotentiality hypothesis or its corollary, the progressive lateralization hypothesis (Basser, 1962; Lenneberg, 1967; Luria, 1973). These hypotheses have long been advanced to account for differences in the incidence, clinical picture, and prognosis of aphasic children. Rejection of these hypotheses does help to resolve some of the discrepancy between the aphasic and nonaphasic studies that Hécaen (1976) tried to explain.

At the same time, regardless of the cognitive and academic sequelae that ensue, one cannot help but be struck by the rapid recovery from aphasia in a majority of the children. This recovery rate is certainly more dramatic than in the adult aphasias. This difference, while not invariant, nevertheless requires an explanation at the level of mechanism. If one rejects the equipotentiality hypothesis, or its corollary, then on what neural basis could this differential recovery course be explained? Kinsbourne and Hiscock (1977) have suggested that this difference could be explained parsimoniously by the concept of neuronal plasticity in which varying degrees of ipsilateral and contralateral capacity exist following insult to the immature left hemisphere. Unfortunately this assertion, as Geschwind (1974) has argued, tells us little about mechanism. Moreover, the central nervous system is not always plastic, as the large number of severely aphasic adults prove. One likely mechanism concerns the displacement phenomenon (speech transferability) in which the ntact "minor" hemisphere possesses the capacity to subserve speech when the "leading" hemisphere is damaged early in life. The mechanism underlying this displacement may relate to a possible release-from-inhibition effect that is extremely time dependent. The critical period for this release may extend only up to 2–4 years of age. The studies of Lansdell (1969), Dennis and Kohn (1975), Dennis and Whitaker (1976), and Rasmussen and Milner (1977) provide convincing support for this displacement hypothesis. This hypothesis, however, should not be confused with the equipotentiality hypothesis. Nor should it imply that the right hemisphere relearns language originally acquired by the left hemisphere. Geschwind (1974) has already shown that the speed of recovery in many child aphasics is incompatible with a relearning process. Most likely, the right hemisphere was learning language during this early critical period but, because of inhibitory effects, was constrained in its expression.

The displacement hypothesis unfortunately fails to account for those cases of spontaneous recovery in children after the critical period. Recently, it has been suggested that the concept of committed versus uncommitted cortex for a particular function, either intrahemispherically or interhemispherically, may play a part in recovery. This position (Goldman, 1972) postulates different rates of maturation in the brain that allow for reorganization or displacement of a given function (e.g., speech) depending on its level of organization or commitment to structure. According to Hécaen (1976):

> If these intact cortical systems are functionally immature at the time of ablation of the given area, that is 'uncommitted', they are able, by reason of their own plasticity, to assume those functions of the given area. In contrast, if the remaining tissue is already 'committed', it will have lost the capacity to guarantee this reorganization and will no longer be able to assume a new responsibility [p. 131].

This explanation, while heuristic, has yet to be confirmed or disconfirmed. At least it provides an additional framework in which to search for brain mechanisms that might help explain differences between the childhood and adult aphasias. The present chapter has largely been addressed to a determination of whether these differences, individually or in combination, permit the search for underlying explanatory mechanisms. Hopefully, in this spirit, parsimony will prevail.

Acknowledgment

This work was supported in part by funds from the National Institute of Health (NS 16347–01).

References

Aicardi, J., Ansili, J., & Cherrie, J. J. 1969. Acute hemiplegia in infancy and childhood. *Developmental Medicine and Child Neurology* (London), *11*, 162–173.

Alajouanine, T. H., & Lhermitte, F. 1965. Acquired aphasia in children. *Brain, 88,* 653–662.

Annett, M., 1973. Laterality of childhood hemiplegia and the growth of speech and intelligence. *Cortex, 9,* 4–33.

Assal, G., & Campiche, R. 1973. Aphasie et troubles du language chez l'enfant après contusion cerebrale. *Neuro-Chirurgie, 19,* 399–406.

Barnet, A. B., Vincentini, M., & Campos, M. 1974. EEG sensory evoked responses (E.R.) in early infancy malnutrition. *Neuroscience Abstracts*, No. 43, p. 130. Annual meeting of the Society for Neuroscience, St. Louis, MO., October 20–24.

Basser, L. S. 1962. Hemiplegia of early onset and the faculty of speech with special reference to the effects of hemispherectomy. *Brain, 85,* 427–460.

Bayley, P. 1939. *Intercranial tumours of infancy and childhood.* Chicago: Univ. of Chicago Press.

Benson, D. F. 1972. Language disturbances of childhood. *Clinical Proceedings Children's Hospital of Washington, 28,* 93–100.

Bernhardt, M. 1885. Ueber die spastiche cerebralparalyse im Kindesalter (Hemiplegia spastica infantilis), Nebst einem Excurse uber: "Aphasie bei Kindern". *Archiv fur Pathologische Anatomie und Physiologie und fur Klinische Medecin, 102,* 26–80.

Bernhardt, M. 1897. Ueber die spastiche cerebralparalyse im Kindesalter. *Virchow's Archiv, 102,* S. 26.

Bishop, N. 1967. *Speech in the hemiplegic child.* Proceedings of the Eighth Medical Conference of the Australian Cerebral Palsy Association. Melbourne, Victoria: Tooronga Press.

Branco-Lefèvre, A. F. 1950. Contribuicão para o estudo da psicopatologia da afasia en criancas. *Archivos Neuro-Psiquiatria* (Sao Paulo), *8,* 345–393.

Broca, P. 1861. *Sur le siège de la faculté de language articule avec deux observations d'aphemie* (Porte de Parole). Paris.

Brown, J. W., & Hécaen, H. 1976. Lateralization and language representation: Observations on aphasia in children, left-handers, and "anomalous" dextrals. *Neurology, 26,* 183–189.

Bullard, P. C., Satz, P., & Speedie, L. Cerebral dominance and handedness: A review and comparison of the childhood and adult aphasia studies. *Brain and Language,* in press.

Byers, R. K., & McLean, W. T. 1962. Etiology and course of certain hemiplegias with aphasia in childhood. *Pediatrics, 29,* 376–383.

Carter, R., Hohenegger, M., & Satz, P. 1980. Handedness and aphasia: An inferential method for determining the mode of cerebral speech specialization. *Neuropsychologia, 18,* 569–575.

Clarus, A. 1874. Uber Aphasie bei Kindern. *Jahresb. Kinderheilkd. 7,* 369–400.

Collignon, R., Hécaen, H., & Angelerques, G. 1968. A propos de 12 cas d'aphasie acquise chez l'enfant. *Acta Neurologica et Psychiatrica Belgica, 68,* 245–277.

Cotard, J. 1868. Etude sur l'atrophie partielle du cerveau. Thèse de Paris.

Denckla, M. 1979. Childhood learning disabilities. In K. Heilman & E. Valenstein (Eds.), *Clinical neuropsychology.* New York: Oxford Univ. Press.

Dennis, M. 1980. Strokes in childhood I: Communicative intent, expression, and comprehension after left hemisphere arteriopathy in a right-handed nine-year-old. In R. W. Reiber (Ed.), *Language development and aphasia in children.* New York: Academic Press.

Dennis, M., & Kohn, B. 1975. Comprehension of syntax in infantile hemiplegics after cerebral hemidecortication: Left hemisphere superiority. *Brain and Language, 2,* 472–482.

Dennis, M., & Whitaker, H. A. 1976. Language acquisition following hemidecortication: Linguistic superiority of the left over the right hemisphere. *Brain and Language, 3,* 404–433.

Dennis, M., & Whitaker, H. A. 1977. Hemispheric equipotentiality and language acquisition. In S. J. Segalowitz & F. A. Gruber, (Eds.), *Language development and neurological theory.* New York: Academic Press.

Dunsdon, M. I. 1952. *The educability of cerebral palsied children.* London: Newnos.

Eimas, P. D., Siqueland, E. R., Jusczyk, P., & Vigorito, J. 1971. Speech perception in infants. *Science, 171,* 303–306.

Fisher, R. G., Friedmann, K. R. 1959. Carotid artery thrombosis in persons fifteen years of age or younger. *Journal of the American Medical Association, 170,* 1918–1919.

Ford, F. R. 1937. *Diseases of the nervous system in infancy, childhood, and adolescence.* London.

Freud, S. 1968. [*Infantile cerebral paralysis*] (L. A. Russin, trans.). Coral Gables: Univ. of Miami Press. (Originally published, 1897.)

Freud, S., & Rie, 1968. (Article title). (Originally published, 1891.) In S. Freud, [*Infantile cerebral paralysis*] (L. A. Russin, trans.). Coral Gables: Univ. of Miami Press. (Originally published, 1897.)

Gaudard, 1968. (Article title). (Originally published, 1884.) In S. Freud, [*Infantile cerebral paralysis*] (L. A. Russin, trans.). Coral Gables: Univ. of Miami Press. (Originally published, 1897.)

Geschwind, N. 1973. Late changes in the nervous system: An overview. In D. G. Stein, J. J. Rosen, & N. Butters (Eds.), *Plasticity and recovery of function in the central nervous system.* New York: Academic Press.

Geschwind, N. 1974. Disorders of higher cortical function in children. In N. Geschwind (Ed.), *Selected papers on language and the brain.* Dordrecht-Holland: D. Reidel.

Goldman, P. S. 1972. Developmental determinants of cortical plasticity. *Acta Neurobiologiae Experimentalis, 32,* 495–511.

Guttmann, E. 1942. Aphasia in children. *Brain, 65,* 205–219.

Hardyck, C., & Petrinovitch, L. 1977. Left-handedness. *Psychological Bulletin, 84,* 385–405.

Hécaen, H. 1976. Acquired aphasia in children and the autogenesis of hemispheric functional specialization. *Brain and Language, 3,* 114–134.

Hécaen, H. 1977. Language representation and brain development. In S. R. Berenberg (Ed.), *Brain, fetal and infant.* The Hague: Martinus Nijhoff, 112–123.

Heilman, K., & Valenstein, E. 1979. *Clinical neuropsychology.* New York: Oxford Univ. Press.

Hiscock, M., & Kinsbourne, M. 1978. Ontogony of cerebral dominance; evidence from time-sharing asymmetry in children. *Developmental Psychology, 14,* 321–329.

Ingram, T. T. S. 1964. *Paediatric aspects of cerebral palsy.* Edinburgh: Livingstone.

Isler, W. 1971. Acute hemiplegias and hemisyndromes in childhood. *Clinics in Developmental Medicine,* No. 41/42. Philadelphia: Lippincott.

Kinsbourne, M. 1975. The ontogony of cerebral dominance. In D. Aaronson & R. W. Rieber (Eds.), *Developmental psycholinguistics and communication disorders. Annals of the New York Academy of Sciences, 263,* 244–250.

Kinsbourne, M. 1977. Commentary. In B. T. Woods & H. L. Teuber (Eds.), Changing patterns of childhood aphasia. *Transactions of the American Neurological Association, 102,* 38.

Kinsbourne, M., & Hiscock, M. 1977. Does cerebral dominance develop? In S. J. Segalowitz & F. A. Gruber (Eds.)., *Language development and neurological theory.* New York: Academic Press.

Kinsbourne, M., & Hiscock, M. 1978. Cerebral lateralization and cognitive development. *Education and the Brain,* 77th yearbook, pt. 2, 169–122.

Krashen, S. D. 1973. Lateralization, language learning and the critical period: Some new evidence. *Language Learning, 23,* 63–74.

Lansdell, H. 1969. Verbal and nonverbal factors in right hemisphere speech. *Journal of Comparative Physiological Psychology, 69,* 734–738.

Lenneberg, E. 1967. *Biological foundations of language.* New York: Wiley.

Lovett, R. 1888. A clinical consideration of 60 cases of cerebral paralysis in children. *Boston Medical Surgical Journal, 118,* 641–646.

Luria, A. R. 1973. *The working brain.* New York: Basic Books.

McCarthy, J. J. 1963. Clinical diagnosis and treatment of aphasia: Aphasia in children. In C. E. Osgoon & M. S. Miron (Eds.), *Approaches to the study of aphasia.* Urbana: Univ. of Illinois Press.

McFie, J. 1961. Intellectual impairment in children with localized post-infantile cerebral lesions. *Journal of Neurology, Neurosurgery and Psychiatry, 24,* 361–365.

Molfese, D. L., Freeman, R. B., & Palermo, D. S. 1975. The ontology of brain lateralization for speech and non-speech stimuli. *Brain and Language, 2,* 356–368.

Osler, W. 1888. The cerebral palsies of children. *The Medical News, 53,* 29–35.

Poetzl, T. 1926. Ueber sensorische Aphasie in Kindersalter. 2. *Hals N. Ohrenklin, 14,* 109–118.

Rasmussen, T., & Milner, B. 1977. The role of early left-brain injury in determining lateralization of cerebral speech functions. In S. J. Dimond & D. A. Blizard (Eds.), *Evolution and lateralization of the brain. Annals of the New York Academy of Sciences.* New York: Academic Press.

Sachs, B., & Peterson, R. 1890. A study of cerebral palsies of early life, based upon an analysis of one hundred and forty cases. *Journal of Nervous and Mental Disease, 17,* 295–332.

Satz, P. 1972. Pathological left handedness; an explanation. *Cortex, 8,* 121–135.

Satz, P. 1979. A test of some models of hemispheric speech organization in left-and right-handers. *Science, 203,* 1131–1133.

Shillito, J., Jr. 1964. Carotid arteritis: A cause of hemiplegia in childhood. *Journal of Neurosurgery, 21,* 540–551.

van Dongen, H. R., & Loonen, M. C. 1979. Neurological factors related to prognosis of acquired aphasia in childhood, In Y. Lebrun & R. Hoops (Eds.), *Recovery in aphasics.* Amsterdam: Swets and Zeitlenger, B. V.

Wada, J. A., Clarke, R., & Hamm, A. 1975. Cerebral hemispheric asymmetry in humans. *Archives of Neurology, 32,* 239–246.

Wallenberg, A. 1886. Ein Beitrag zur Lehre von den cerebralen Kinderlahmungen. *Jahrbuch fur Kinderheilkunde, 24,* 384–439.

Wernicke, C. 1874. *Der aphasische Symptomenkomplex.* Breslau: Max Cohen and Weigert.

West, R. 1960. What we must learn about childhood aphasia. *Childhood aphasia:* Proceedings of the Institute on Childhood Aphasia. San Francisco: California Society for Crippled Children and Adults.

Witelson, S. F. 1977. Early hemisphere specialization and interhemisphere plasticity: An empirical and theoretical review. In S. J. Segalowitz & F. A. Gruber (Eds.), *Language development and neurological theory.* New York: Academic Press.

Witelson, S. F., & Pallie, W. 1973. Left hemisphere specialization for language in the newborn: Neuroanatomical evidence of asymmetry. *Brain, 96,* 641–646.

Woods, B. T., & Teuber, H. L. 1977. Changing patterns of childhood aphasia. *Transactions of the American Neurological Association, 102,* 36–38.

Woods, B. T., & Teuber, H. L. 1978. Changing patterns of childhood aphasia. *Annals of Neurology, 3,* 273–280.

Wulff, D. 1890. Cerebrale Kinderlahmung und Geistesschwache. *Neurol. Centralbl., 9,* 343–344.

15

Aphasia in Closed Head Injury

HARVEY S. LEVIN

Closed Head Injury and Missile Wounds of the Brain

Epidemiology and Mechanisms of Injury

In contrast to the frequent occurrence of penetrating missile wounds (e.g., bullets, shell fragments) in casualties of war, closed head injury (CHI) predominates in civilian head trauma. The primary cause of CHI is vehicular accident, although falls are a common cause of head injury in children. Caveness (1977) reported incidence data based on hospital records for craniocerebral trauma in the United States as part of the study by the Department of Health, Education, and Welfare. A total of 9,760,000 cases of head injury, or 4.6% of the population, were recorded in 1975. This figure included 633,000 patients (6.5% of the series) with severe injuries (e.g., cerebral laceration, contusion, or intracerebral hematoma).

The incidence of CHI is particularly high among children, adolescents, and young adults (18–30 years of age). Males predominate in hospital admissions of adults with CHI, whereas the male–female disparity in head injury is less in young children and in adults over 70 years old (Field, 1976). In a epidemiologic study of head injury in Minnesota, with criteria for case ascertainment being loss of consciousness, posttraumatic amnesia, or skull fracture, the age-adjusted incidence rate per 100,000 was 274 in males and 116 in females (Annegers, Grabow, Kurland, & Laws, 1980).

Neuropathological investigation of the traumatized human brain (cf. Adams, Mitchell, Graham, & Doyle, 1977) and studies employing experimental models of head injury in animals (cf. Ommaya & Gennarelli, 1974) have suggested that a primary mechanism of CHI is rotational acceleration of the skull that produces shear strains within the intracranial contents. Histological study of the brains of patients dying soon after CHI has disclosed diffuse injury to the cerebral white matter that apparently results from shearing and stretching of nerve fibers at the moment of impact (Adams *et al.*, 1977). Pertinent to the development of hemispheric disconnection, the corpus callosum is especially vulnerable to diffuse mechanically induced shear strains. Ommaya and Gennarelli (1974) postulated that the severity of diffuse CHI follows a centripetal gradient; that is, the injury extends to the rostral brain stem only in cases with severe diffuse hemispheric injury. The bulk of cerebral white matter may be reduced further by delayed degeneration that results in ventricular enlargement. Complications contributing to the severity of generalized CHI include brain swelling, increased intracranial pressure, hypoxia, and infection.

Focal lesions after CHI result from contusion of the brain surface by transient in-bending of the skull or by penetration of bone fragment in cases of depressed skull fracture that may also produce brain laceration (Gurdjian & Gurdjian, 1976). Focal areas of ischemia are frequently present in the neocortex and basal ganglia (Graham & Adams, 1971). Stresses of the impact may cause arterial and venous tears resulting in intracerebral (see Figure 15.1) or extracerebral hematomas. The orbital surface of the frontal and temporal lobes are particularly vulnerable to contusion by impaction against the bony sphenoid wing. Formation of hematomas is also common in this area. Large mass lesions may produce contralateral shift of midline structures and tentorial herniation of the temporal lobe; possibly involving the uncus and hippocampus.

Blunt head injury often produces a period of amnesia, if not loss of consciousness, immediately after impact. The acute severity of diffuse CHI is measured by the degree and duration of altered consciousness. Teasdale and Jennett (1974) developed the Glasgow Coma Scale (see Table 15.1) for the assessment of coma, which consists of three components: the minimal stimulus necessary to elicit eye opening, the best motor response to command or to painful stimulation, and the best verbal response. Summation of the component scores of the Glasgow Coma Scale yields a total score, which can range from 3 to 15. Jennett *et al.* (1977) define a severe acute CHI as one that results in no eye opening, inability to obey commands, and no comprehensible speech—that is, a Glasgow Coma Scale 8 or less for a period of at least 6 hr.

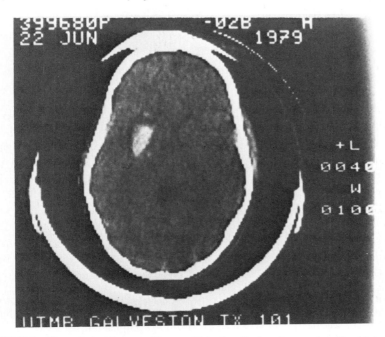

FIGURE 15.1. *Computerized tomographic scan obtained on the day of severe closed head injury in a 12-year-old girl struck by a car. The scan shows a left hemisphere intracerebral hematoma in the putamen and anterior limb of the internal capsule. This left-handed patient had a right hemiplegia and was mute for 6 weeks after regaining consciousness.*

Confusion and anterograde amnesia (i.e., inability to consolidate information about ongoing events) usually persist for varying durations after the patient emerges from coma (Russell & Smith, 1961). The duration of posttraumatic amnesia (PTA) may range from a few minutes after mild CHI that produces no coma to several months following severe CHI. The duration of PTA is directly assessed by questioning the patient concerning orientation and recent events (Levin, O'Donnell, & Grossman, 1979) and estimated retrospectively by inquiring of the

TABLE 15.1
The Glasgow Coma Scale

Best eye opening	Best motor response	Best verbal response
4 Spontaneous	6 Obeys commands	5 Oriented
3 To speech	5 Localizes to pain	4 Confused
2 To pain	4 Flexion–withdrawal to pain	3 Inappropriate words
1 None	3 Abnormal flexion to pain	2 Incomprehensible
	2 Extension to pain	1 None
	1 None	

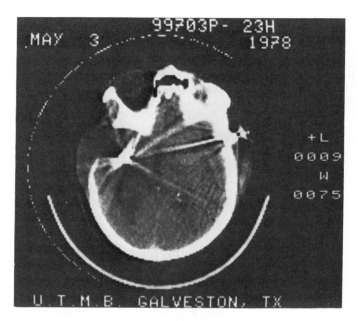

FIGURE 15.2. *Gunshot wound of the right frontotemporal region visualized by computerized tomography. Note the path of the bullet and bone fragments which traversed to the left temporal area. Wernicke's aphasia with jargon persists 18 months postinjury in this woman.*

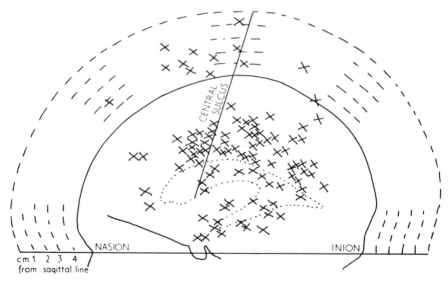

FIGURE 15.3. *Chart indicating the center of injury for missile wounds that entered the left hemisphere and caused aphasia. Cases with foreign bodies in remote regions of the brain were excluded from this map. Localization of missile wounds on the outline of a normal lateral skull was based on skull X rays and surgical findings.* [*From Russell, W. R. & Espir, M. L. E. 1961.* Traumatic Aphasia. A Study of Aphasia in War Wounds of the Brain. *London: Oxford Univ. Press. Reproduced with permission from the publisher.*]

period for which the patient has no remembrance (Russell & Smith, 1961). Focal brain lesions (e.g., hematoma) may occur in the presence of relatively mild or moderate diffuse CHI, as reflected by the period of coma and PTA.

Missile injury causes tearing of the scalp, depression or fracture of the skull, and possibly wounding of brain tissue in the track of the foreign body (see Figure 15.2). A small shower of bone fragments is often projected into the brain from the point of impact, the extent of dural penetration and loss of brain tissue being indices of injury severity (Newcombe, 1969). As a consequence of dural penetration, posttaumatic seizure disorder is more strongly associated with aphasia secondary to missile wounds than in cases of CHI (Russell & Espir, 1961).

In order to determine the locus of lesion, Russell and Espir (1961) used surgical findings and lateral and anteroposterior skull X-rays to chart the entry wound and missile track on a lateral sagittal diagram of the hemisphere (see Figure 15.3). Verification of lesion localization by postmortem data suggested that this was a fairly accurate method. Although missile wounds tend to be more circumscribed than diffuse CHI and produce little or no coma, metal fragments can spread far from the primary locus of injury. Furthermore, Mohr *et al.* (1980) found that missile injury that produced language disorder was frequently associated with a period of unconsciousness, suggesting that diffuse effects were contributory. Missile injury that results in aphasia also commonly produces motor and/or sensory deficit contralateral to the dominant hemisphere; this association is stronger than in the case of CHI (Levin, Grossman, & Kelly, 1976).

From this summary of the pathophysiology of head injury, we may infer that clinical data concerning the extent of focal brain injury and the severity of diffuse cerebral disturbance are pertinent to the assessment of posttraumatic aphasia.

Distinctive Features of Traumatic Aphasia

One of the distinctive features of acute aphasia after CHI is the predominance of anomia (Heilman, Safran, & Geschwind, 1971). Fluent speech is often associated with verbal paraphasia and circumlocution; comprehension and repetition are relatively spared, whereas naming is markedly defective, especially to confrontation. Anomic errors include semantic approximation (e.g., *snout* for the tusks of an elephant), circumlocution (e.g., *to make music* for pedals of a piano), and concrete representation (e.g., *orange* for a circle). Anomic aphasia after CHI is distinguished from nonaphasic misnaming (Weinstein & Kahn, 1955) insofar as the former is not restricted to names of objects related to the patient's illness (e.g., wheelchair) and may be apparent during spontaneous speech (Heilman *et al.*, 1971).

Apart from anomic disturbance, Wernicke's aphasia is the second most common language disorder after CHI. Although an acute picture of fluent paraphasic speech, poor comprehension for oral and written language, and impaired repetition has been described in CHI cases with left temporal lesions (Heilman *et al.*, 1971; Stone, Lopes, & Moody, 1978; Thomsen, 1976), restoration of comprehension may be rapid after a hematoma resolves or is surgically removed (cf. Stone *et al.*, 1978). A case of transient Wernicke's aphasia was observed after a relatively mild diffuse injury (as reflected by the Glasgow Coma Scale) concomitant with a suspected left hemisphere mass lesion that was not directly visualized by computerized tomography.

A 17-year-old, right-handed student sustained blunt head trauma in a motorcycle accident on 23 December 1979. When admitted to the neurosurgery service in Galveston on the day of injury, he had a Glasgow Coma Scale score of 11 and no focal motor or sensory deficit. CT showed compression of the left lateral ventricle, which resolved during the course of hospitalization. The patient's speech was fluent at a rate faster than normal and was contaminated by jargon (e.g., *ruby baby*). Comprehension was grossly impaired, and the patient's mood was one of excitement and agitation. Throughout the first two weeks of his hospitalization he was grossly disoriented and continued to exhibit Wernicke's aphasia. Stereotyped phrases and expletives were relatively spared. The patient's orientation began to improve during the third postinjury week and reached a normal level by 14 January. Although a clinical interview showed substantial improvement in his comprehension, the Multilingual Aphasia Examination on 17 January disclosed defective visual naming (e.g., a rectangle was described as a *long square*), inability to repeat sentences presented orally, and decreased word finding. Follow-up assessment six months postinjury revealed total recovery of language (see Figure 15.4).

Most published studies of aphasia after missile wounds of the brain are based on detailed observations of servicemen who were treated at the Military Hospital for Head Injuries in Oxford, England, during and after World War II (Newcombe, 1969; Russell & Espir, 1961; Schiller, 1947). Mohr *et al.* (1980) have extended this research to servicemen who sustained penetrating head injury in Vietnam. These authors have frequently described linguistic disturbance characteristic of Broca's aphasia that is typically seen after occlusion of the left middle cerebral artery.

Russell and Espir obtained information on localization of injury by separately studying aphasics who had circumscribed left hemisphere

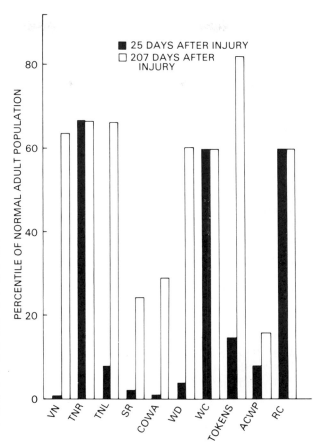

FIGURE 15.4. *Profile of language test scores obtained 1 and 6 months postinjury in a 17-year-old student who had a Wernicke's aphasia that completely resolved. VN = visual naming; TNR = tactile naming, right hand; TNL = tactile naming, left hand; SR = sentence repetition; COWA = controlled word association; WD = writing to dictation; WC = writing–copying; TOKENS = Token Test; ACWP = auditory comprehension of words and phrases; RC = reading comprehension.*

wounds without foreign bodies in remote areas of the brain (see Figure 15.3). In contrast to the rare occurrence of nonfluent agrammatic language disturbance after CHI, Russell and Espir (1961) reported that 12% of aphasics with missile wounds had Broca's aphasia that was typically associated with right-sided weakness and a focal injury to the frontal or rolandic area. In a related study, Schiller (1947) linked a disturbance of articulation, inflection, and rate of speech with a wound at the foot of the precentral convolution. He observed that agrammatism, disturbed prosody, and perseveration were present in patients with left frontotemporal missile wounds. Focal missile wounds in the dominant parietal lobe were found by Russell and Espir to result frequently in a global aphasia, though specific anomia, alexia, and agraphia were present in patients with small posterior parietal lesions. Similarly, Mohr *et al.* (1980) noted that parietal injury was more likely to produce aphasia than a focal wound of any other lobe. Global aphasia with jargon, prolonged posttraumatic amnesia, and residual memory deficit have been observed during the early stage of recovery from penetrating injury of the left temporal lobe (Russell & Espir, 1961). Focal temporal wounds damaging the optic radiations resulted in a visual field defect in addition to global aphasia. Impairment of reading was common in these patients.

Russell and Espir analyzed the occurrence of aphasia after unilateral brain wounds separately for right and left handers. The authors defined handedness in terms of preference for a majority of motor skills. As anticipated from other sources of data concerning cerebral dominance, only 1% of right handers became aphasic after a right hemisphere wound, whereas the corresponding figure in left handers was 17%. Also consistent with other lines of evidence for cerebral dominance, unilateral left hemisphere wounds more frequently produced aphasia in right handers (65%) than in sinistrals (38%). The overall figures for aphasia after unilateral injury of either hemisphere were 37% for right and 27% for left handers. Although these figures are incompatible with the concept that sinistrals are more likely to become aphasic, the comparative data presented by Russell and Espir included right-handed patients with lesions outside the speech territory. Of the right hemisphere wounds that resulted in aphasia in sinistrals, the frontal or parietal lobes were involved in all cases.

In summary, the pattern of aphasia observed after missile wounds of the brain conforms fairly well to the localization of language in patients with cerebrovascular disease (the reader is referred to Chapter 2 of this volume for background). The localizing significance of missile wounds is greatly enhanced by identifying cases in whom there is no evidence of additional brain penetration by fragments in remote areas (see Figure 15.3).

Prognosis for Recovery

Reports based on large series of servicemen with penetrating missile wounds suggest a favorable prognosis for recovery from aphasia (Mohr *et al.*, 1980; Russell & Espir, 1961). Although the results of these studies suggest more rapid restitution of language than in aphasia secondary to cerebral vascular disease, the young age of brain-injured servicemen may also be a contributing factor. Recovery of language after missile wounds has been especially rapid and complete in cases of nonfluent, expressive aphasia ("motor aphasia") produced by focal left frontal injury or lesions situated in the lower part of the rolandic area (Mohr *et al.*, 1980;

Russell & Espir, 1961). Although resolution of right-sided weakness generally parallels the recovery of language in dysfluent aphasics, motor deficit may persist after restitution of language. Russell and Espir noted that rolandic lesions also frequently resulted in residual sensory defect.

Mohr *et al.* (1980) observed that over the course of at least a year the aphasia produced by left parietal injury evolved into a residual expressive disorder characterized by reduced fluency. In patients with left posterior parietal lesions, Russell and Espir observed that anomia, alexia, and impaired spelling were the characteristic sequelae. The follow-up findings in patients with acute Wernicke's aphasia secondary to left temporal missile injury have shown, however, that impaired comprehension persists in more than three-fourths of these patients (Mohr *et al.*, 1980).

Studies reporting on the rate of recovery from aphasia after left hemisphere missile wounds have not been in close agreement. This disparity may reflect differences in the site of injury and follow-up interval across the various series. Whereas Mohr *et al.* contended that most recovery of language occurs within the first year after injury, Walker and Jablon (1961) observed recovery of language within 9 months after injury in nearly one-third of their cases. By 7–8 years postinjury, however, more than half of the servicemen who had been aphasic continued to exhibit language disturbance.

In a broader study of long-term outcome after missile injury, Newcombe (1969) found that nearly a third of the Oxford patients with left hemisphere wounds continued to evidence aphasic symptoms when examined at the time of follow-up. Word fluency, measured by retrieval of items from a given category (e.g., colors), was reduced in the total series of left hemisphere injured patients, though the deficit was more severe in patients with residual aphasic symptoms. Defects in vocabulary, reading, spelling, and writing were confined to patients considered to be aphasic. In contrast, more than half of the total series (including nonaphasic patients with left hemisphere wounds) continued to complain of "being at a loss for a word." Residual impairment of verbal memory was found in patients with left hemisphere injury, including those who were nonaphasic at the time of follow-up. In summary, most patients rendered aphasic by missile injury exhibit relatively permanent aphasic symptoms or more subtle defects in verbal skills and memory.

Investigators have only recently studied the early recovery of communicative skills after prolonged coma in patients with severe CHI. Najenson, Sazbon, Fiselzon, Becker, and Schechter (1978) plotted recovery curves for communicative skills during the first 18 months after severe CHI in 15 patients with prolonged coma (undefined) who were

TABLE 15.2
Assessment of Communication Functions after Prolonged Coma[a]

Auditory comprehension	*Oral expression*
Awareness of gross environmental sounds	Voicing
Awareness of speech	Saying vowels
Ability to indicate yes and no	Saying consonants
Understanding own name	Saying own name
Recognition of family names	Saying nouns
Understanding simple verbal orders	Saying verbs
Recognition of names of familiar objects	Saying noun–verb combinations
Recognition of colors	Saying short sentences (automatic)
Recognition of forms	Saying short sentences (nonautomatic)
Understanding use of familiar objects	Conversational speech
Visual comprehension	*Reading*
Awareness of visual stimulation	Reading own name
Understanding gesture direction	Reading family names
Association of identical objects	Reading single words
Association of identical forms	Reading simple sentences
Association of similar objects	Reading newspaper headlines
Categorization	Reading newspaper articles
Speech	*Writing*
Articulation	Writing own name
Respiration	Writing family names
Voice	Writing words
	Writing simple sentences
	Writing a letter

[a] From Najenson, T., Sazbon, L., Fiselzon, J., Becker, E., & Schecter, I. 1978. Recovery of communicative functions after prolonged traumatic coma. *Scandinavian Journal of Rehabilitation Medicine,* 10:15–21. Reproduced with permission of the authors and publisher.

referred to a rehabilitation unit. The authors developed a scale (see Table 15.2) to rate expressive and receptive functions because the patients were unable to cooperate with standardized tests usually employed during later stages of recovery. As shown in Table 15.2, this scale consists of six major functions, and each is divided into specific communicative skills. At evaluation, each specific test is assigned a score ranging from 0 to 4. The total score for each major function is summed and expressed as a percentage of the maximum possible score. Najenson *et al.* plotted the percentage scores monthly to depict the course of recovery. Six patients in this study remained in a vegetative state, whereas nine cases had partial or full restitution of language. They observed a consistent sequence of recovery; comprehension of gestures and oral language appeared first, usually between 3 weeks and 5 months after trauma. Oral expression, reading, and writing were slower to recover, and motor defects in speech (e.g., articulation, respiratory control, and phonation) were often persistently impaired. Of the nine patients who recovered communication, eight had dysarthric speech. The authors observed that the recovery of communicative ability corresponded to progressive improvement in locomotion.

In a study of outcome after severe diffuse CHI (coma > 24 hr), Thomsen (1975) administered a follow-up (mean interval of 31–33 months after injury) language examination of her own design to 12 patients who had been acutely aphasic. Four patients, including two sinistrals, had no signs of recovery of language. In the others, amnestic aphasia (slow rate of speech, slow repetition of words or phrases, verbal paraphasia, and perseveration) was frequently present. Thomsen noted a residual decline in such complex verbal skills as detailed verbal description and the use of antonyms, synonyms, and metaphors. Impaired reading was found in four cases, but no patient was totally alexic. Although these findings agree with the view that aphasia secondary to CHI has a good prognosis, Thomsen emphasized that residual linguistic defects and dysarthria were present. Moreover, she pointed out that the manifestations of "subclinical" language problems depend on the recovery of memory and general cognitive function.

In a second investigation, Thomsen (1976) reexamined the language of 15 patients with focal mass lesions (in which temporal lobe damage predominated) or extensive destruction of the left hemisphere who had been aphasic during the initial hospitalization. When tested at least 1 year after injury (mean interval = 29 months), there was an overall trend of improvement, though all patients exhibited residual language deficit. The course of recovery was characterized by improved comprehension of oral and written language and less severe agraphia. As was the case in Thomsen's study of diffuse CHI patients, amnestic aphasia and perseveration persisted in nearly all patients. Global aphasia with gross impairment of all language functions typically evolved into receptive aphasia, whereas patients who initially had a receptive aphasia frequently evidenced improvement in comprehension despite residual anomia. Although Thomsen concluded that nearly all patients with focal left hemisphere lesions made some improvement, she noted that "half the patients had severe or moderate aphasia two and a half years after the trauma and a few had not been able to pass the level of automatic language (e.g., expletives, stereotyped phrases) [p.376]."

Groher (1977) administered the Porch Index of Communicative Ability to 14 consecutively admitted, comatose CHI patients at 1-month intervals beginning shortly after termination of coma (mean duration of

17 days). He reported progressive improvement in expressive and receptive skills over a 4-month period. Naming to confrontation recovered in
all patients, whereas errors in spelling, incomplete sentence construction, and syntax persisted. The degree of recovery suggested by this
study appears to be greater than the impression conveyed by other
investigators of aphasia after severe CHI. This finding may be attributed
to Groher's inclusion of a consecutive series of comatose patients rather
than confining the study to acutely aphasic cases.

When consecutive referrals of CHI patients to a rehabilitation program are considered, a different view of outcome emerges, which may
reflect the severity of injuries requiring intensive retraining. Sarno (1980)
has described the findings for clinical examination of language and reported the results of administering the Neurosensory Center Comprehensive Examination for Aphasia (NCCEA) to 56 cases about 7
months postinjury. The series was divided nearly equally between focal
mass lesions or depressed skull fractures and patients with diffuse CHI.
Consistent with Thomsen's findings, Sarno reported that language disorder and/or dysarthria was present in all patients. Of interest was Sarno's distinctions among subclinical language disorder (e.g., defective
test scores), aphasia diagnosed on the basis of spontaneous speech and
comprehension during an interview, and dysarthria. Applying this
broad classification, she found that all patients in the series had residual
speech or language defects and that these general patterns were represented in nearly equal proportions. The quantitative test results obtained by Sarno are illustrated in Figure 15.5 and described later in the
chapter. At this point, it is useful to observe that Sarno's data confirm
Thomsen's findings in showing that subtle language disturbance is
common after CHI even in the absence of unequivocal aphasia.

In the course of a long-term study of patients with severe CHI who
had been acutely aphasic, Levin, Grossman, Sarwar, and Meyers (1981)
assessed recovery from aphasia in 21 patients. The results of initial CT
and findings from surgery disclosed evidence of primary left hemisphere injury in 8 cases, focal lesions of the right hemisphere in 4 cases,
bilateral injury in 2 patients, and diffuse CHI in the remainder of the
series. The Multilingual Aphasia Examination (MAE) (Benton, 1967) and
portions of the aphasia battery of Spreen and Benton (1969) were administered at the time of follow-up. Nine patients fully recovered from
acute aphasia, as reflected by uniformly normal scores and intact conversational speech. The 12 patients with residual language deficit (indicated by at least one grossly defective score) were equally divided
between those with a persistent impairment of both expressive and recep-

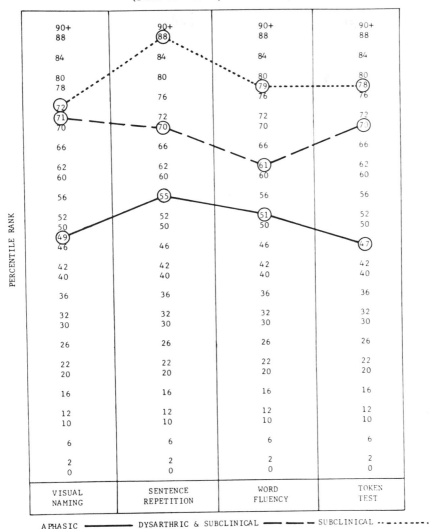

NEUROSENSORY CENTER COMPREHENSIVE EXAMINATION FOR APHASIA
(Based on Adult Aphasic Profile)

APHASIC ⎯⎯⎯⎯⎯ DYSARTHRIC & SUBCLINICAL ⎯ ⎯ ⎯ SUBCLINICAL ·········

FIGURE 15.5. *Mean percentile rank of aphasic and subclinical language disorder groups on subtests of the Neurosensory Center Comprehensive Examination for Aphasia, based on adult aphasic profile. Solid line = aphasic; broken line = dysarthric and subclinical; dotted line = subclinical.* [*From Sarno, M. T. 1980. The nature of verbal impairment after closed head injury.* Journal of Nervous and Mental Disease, *168, 685–692. Reproduced with permission of the author and publisher.*]

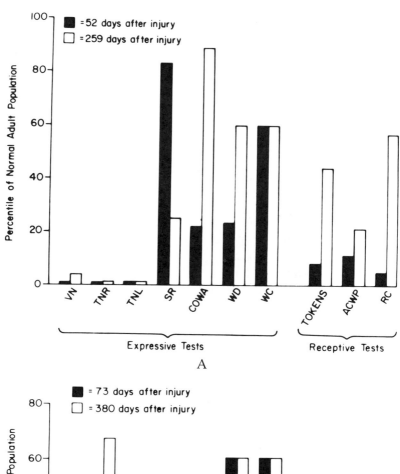

A

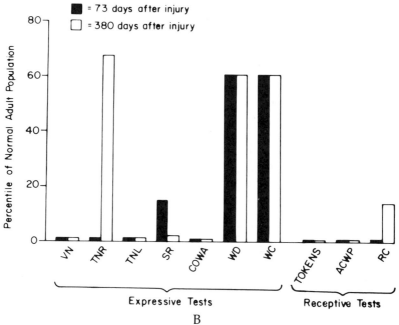

B

tive abilities and those with a specific language deficit. Anomia and decreased word finding were the most common isolated defects. Patients who fully recovered from acute aphasia or exhibited a specific language disturbance at the time of follow-up were generally functioning within the average range of intelligence, whereas patients with generalized language impairment evidenced intellectual deficit on both the verbal and performance sections of the Wechsler Adult Intelligence Scale (WAIS).

In accord with the course of recovery observed in an earlier study by Thomsen, acute global aphasia in this series of patients frequently evolved into a specific anomia. This pattern is illustrated by the serial findings in a 17-year-old student (see Figure 15.6A) who had a left temporal mass lesion and a diffuse injury of mild to moderate severity. She initially exhibited impairment of naming, word association, and alexia, whereas residual language deficit was confined to anomia. In contrast, Figure 15.6B depicts persistent, generalized language defects in an 18-year-old patient who sustained a severe CHI (coma = 21 days) complicated by bilateral frontoparietal subdural hematomas. He evidenced a concomitant decline in cognitive ability, as reflected by a disparity between follow-up results on the WAIS and his high school test scores.

To summarize, the studies of long-term recovery of language after CHI show an overall trend of improvement that may eventuate in restoration of language or specific defects ("subclinical" language disorder) in naming or word finding in about two-thirds of the patients who are acutely aphasic. Generalized language deficit, which is associated with global cognitive impairment, persists in patients who sustain severe CHI.

FIGURE 15.6. *A. Baseline and follow-up language profiles of a 17-year-old student with residual anomia that was initially accompanied by a receptive impairment after surgical evacuation of a left temporal intracerebral hematoma. B. The baseline and follow-up findings for a 19-year-old student show persistent impairment of expressive and receptive language that was associated with cognitive deficit and progressive ventricular enlargement. He sustained a severe diffuse injury (coma of 21 days) complicated by bifrontal subdural hematomas. VN = visual naming; TNR = tactile naming, right hand; TNL = tactile naming, left hand; SR = sentence repetition; COWA = controlled word association; WD = writing to dictation; WC = writing-copying; TOKENS = Token Test; ACWP = auditory comprehension of words and phrases; RC = reading comprehension. [From Levin, H. S., Grossman, R. G., Sarwar, M., & Meyers, C. A. Linguistic recovery after closed head injury. Brain and Language, 1981, 12, 360-374. Reproduced with permission of the publisher.]*

Assessment of Aphasia after Closed Head Injury

Clinical Evaluation of Conversational Speech

SPEECH DURING THE PERIOD OF POSTTRAUMATIC AMNESIA

As mentioned in the preceding review of mechanisms of injury, the early postcomatose stage of recovery from CHI is typically characterized by an amnesic condition during which the patient is confused. Reduplicative paramnesia (Benson, Gardner, & Meadows, 1976)—that is, the mistaken identification of a person, place, or event for one previously experienced, confabulation, and profound impairment of memory— may be misinterpreted as signs of language disorder. The distinction may be particularly difficult in a patient whose fluent speech is disconnected and perseverative. Confused, nonaphasic speech after CHI was evident in a patient studied in Galveston.

A 24-year-old, right-handed woman was transferred from a community hospital to the University of Texas Medical Branch 3 hr after she sustained a CHI in a motor vehicle accident on 28 January 1978. The Glasgow Coma Scale score was 8 when she was initially examined. The cerebral ventricles and cisterns were poorly visualized on CT, suggesting the presence of diffuse cerebral swelling. Although she obeyed commands after 4 days, her disorientation persisted until 5 March. Spontaneous speech during the confusional period was continuous, rambling, and disorganized in this fearful, agitated woman. When queried on 27 February regarding the reason for her hospitalization, she responded *Something that came up natural being born somewhere in here.* Later in the day, the patient elaborated that she was in the hospital *to have a baby* and that the year was 1952 (she was born in 1953). Reminiscent of the patients described by Weinstein and Kahn (1955), examination the following day elicited another theme pertinent to her hospitalization, that is, she was hospitalized because of *being stabbed.* This statement was interpreted as a reference to her intravenous tubes. Assessment of language on 19 April, however, disclosed completely normal findings on the MAE.

Analysis of this patient's utterances provided little evidence of consistent paraphasic errors, particularly when she was asked structured questions that focused on specific objects rather than expository material. Repeated questioning within the limits of her short attention span disclosed no evidence of receptive impairment similar to that found in patients with Wernicke's aphasia. Administration of tests of naming and word finding to this patient during PTA would have likely yielded defective scores. Weinstein and Kahn (1955) described patients with brain damage of diverse etiologies, including diffuse cerebral disturbance, who exhibited misnaming that was qualitatively atypical for aphasia. Anomic errors were frequently associated with objects that bore a relation to the patient's illness and frequently occurred during a period of disorientation, confabulation, and denial of illness. In contrast to cases of classical anomic aphasia, the authors observed that patients exhibiting nonaphasic misnaming frequently showed no evidence of groping for words in their spontaneous speech nor did their naming necessarily improve when correction was offered.

Conversely, the presence of paraphasic errors in conversational speech after CHI may be misinterpreted as evidence for disorientation and confusion. This condition is likely to be found in CHI patients with mass lesion or depressed skull fracture involving the left hemisphere. In such cases, a multiple-choice format of testing orientation may be useful as well as relatively nonverbal tests during the early stages of recovery.

POSTCONFUSIONAL STAGE OF RECOVERY

Few studies of aphasia during the early stages of recovery from CHI have concurrently assessed orientation. Consequently, there is a possibility that PTA had not completely resolved at the time language was evaluated.

Clinical examination of language in consecutive CHI admissions at the Boston City Hospital was found by Heilman *et al.* (1971) to yield 13 cases of aphasia, including 9 patients with anomic aphasia and 4 cases of Wernicke's aphasia. Aphasics accounted for 2% of the Boston series, a base rate very close to that obtained in a previous study of consecutive CHI admissions (Arseni, Constantinovici, Iliescu, Dobrota, & Gagea, 1970). In the Boston study, the authors defined anomic aphasia as a fluent aphasia in which the patient demonstrates verbal paraphasia for all kinds of material especially to confrontation. Wernicke's aphasia was defined as a fluent aphasia with paraphasia, impaired comprehension for spoken and written language, and poor repetition. Broca's aphasia was defined as nonfluent aphasia with relatively intact comprehension. No patient had a Broca's aphasia or exhibited total disruption of language. Heilman *et al.* excluded patients with intracranial surgery (other than evacuation of subdural hematoma); this selection may have restricted aphasic patients with mass lesions.

Heilman *et al.* distinguished the anomia in their CHI patients from nonaphasic misnaming (Weinstein & Kahn, 1955). In contrast to the narrow range of anomic errors (e.g., related to illness) in cases of nonaphasic misnaming, the anomic CHI patients described by Heilman *et al.* exhibited diverse naming defects in spontaneous speech and writing. We have also been able to distinguish anomic aphasia from nonaphasic misnaming by delaying evaluation of language until the injured patient recovers to a normal level of orientation. This strategy revealed initial findings characteristic of Wernicke's aphasia in a patient who later evidenced anomic aphasia.

On 17 October 1975 this 17-year-old student was transferred to the University of Texas Medical Branch, 3 hr after a motor vehicle accident in which she received a CHI. The Glasgow Coma Scale score on admission was 8. Although the patient obeyed commands on the day of admission, delayed neurological deterioration was reflected by the development of a right hemiparesis and progressive aphasia. Three days postinjury a partial left temporal lobectomy was performed with evacuation of an intracerebral hematoma. The patient remained confused for a month after injury but exhibited gradual improvement of receptive language. Administration of the MAE 2 months after injury disclosed findings consistent with an anomic aphasia. There were frequent errors of circumlocution (e.g., an island was described as *a place where you fish*), semantic approximation (e.g., the trunk of an elephant was described as a *nose*), and a tendency to substitute names of concrete objects for geometric designs (e.g., a triangle was described as *the thing you use when you play pool*). As shown in Figure 15.6A, the patient's long-term recovery of language was complete, with the exception of a subtle residual anomic disturbance that was evident only under testing conditions.

Anomic aphasia may also persist after resolution of PTA in patients with severe diffuse CHI who evidence no other focal neurological signs. In a study of 26 CHI patients without mass lesions who had been in coma for at least 24 hr, Thomsen (1975) found that aphasic symptoms were present during the first 2 or 3 weeks after injury in 12 cases. Verbal paraphasia (i.e., substitution of inappropriate words) and anomia were the most common defects; receptive impairment and dysgraphia were also frequently observed, whereas paragrammatism and other symptoms suggestive of Broca's aphasia were rarely seen. We have observed a patient who bears a close resemblance to the series of diffuse head injuries described by Thomsen.

A 20-year-old, right-handed man was admitted to the University of Texas Medical Branch with a severe CHI (Glasgow Coma Scale score of 5) but no focal motor deficit. The CT scan suggested generalized brain swelling without a mass lesion. Baseline assessment 4 months after injury disclosed anomic errors that deteriorated into jargon (e.g., the handle of a fork was described as a *forkline* and the posterior aspect of the leg was described as a *negline*). Circumlocution was evidenced by his response when the examiner pointed to the pedals of a piano: *If you want a different sound, push them down.* Word finding was defective on a test of letter–word association.

Clinical examination of language has disclosed a broad range of language defects in CHI patients. Thomsen (1976) characterized the findings in a series of patients with left hemisphere mass lesions as MULTISYMPTOMATIC APHASIA. She used this term to describe patients who exhibited anomia, agraphia, and impaired comprehension; a third of the patients in her series had global or receptive aphasia. Anomic aphasia was less common, whereas there were no cases of Broca's aphasia. Posttraumatic dyslexia and dysgraphia have also been reported by other authors (Morsier, 1973).

NONAPHASIC DISORDERS OF SPEECH

Posttraumatic speech disorders that may occur without aphasia include mutism, stuttering, echolalia, palilalia, dysarthria, and nonaphasic misnaming.

Mutism. Total abolition of speech may occur after termination of coma in patients capable of following commands during the transition between spontaneous eye opening and recovery of orientation. As described earlier in this chapter, transient mutism is characteristic of aphasia after head injury in children.

Prolonged if not permanent speechlessness is observed in adults who are persistently vegetative or exhibit akinetic mutism (Cairns, 1952; Plum & Posner, 1980). The akinetic type is a form of subacute or persistent mutism with little or no vocalization. Behaviorally, this condition is distinguished from the vegetative state by its immobility. The features common to both conditions include apparent wakefulness with restoration of the sleep–wake cycle and inability to demonstrate cognitive function through interaction with the environment. When akinetic mutism is a sequel to CHI, diffuse cerebral injury is to be suspected.

Geschwind (1974) distinguishes between nonaphasic and aphasic mutism. The aphasic type, which rarely occurs in adults with CHI (cf. Morsier, 1973), is accompanied by linguistic errors in writing. Nonaphasic mutism is associated with acute onset of right hemiplegia; writing is normal, and there are no signs of aphasia when speech is restored. Following Bastian 1898, Geschwind referred to this condition as aphemia rather than aphasia. In such cases, mutism may arise from focal lesions, often involving the basal ganglia. We have studied a case of subcortical mutism, which is described later.

Stuttering. Published studies suggest that stuttering is a more common sequel of penetrating missile wound than of CHI (Peacher, 1945). Morsier (1973), however, noted a fluency disorder in more than half of his series of CHI patients, including four cases with posttraumatic stuttering. Helm, Butler, and Benson (1978) implicated bilateral injury in patients with acquired stuttering after CHI.

Echolalia and Palilalia. Echolalia is the repetition of words spoken by others, whereas palilalia is the automatic repetition of one's own words. Echolalia may follow a period of mutism in cases with diffuse cerebral dysfunction (CHI) or may occur in patients with transcortical motor aphasia, that is, disturbed expressive and receptive language with preserved repetition. Apart from generalized cerebral disturbance, these disorders have been associated with large frontal lesions. According to Geschwind (1974), echolalia and palilalia are uncommon in patients with lesions primarily involving the perisylvian region of the dominant hemisphere.

Stengel (1947) distinguished between the automatic and mitigated forms of echolalia. The former is parrotlike with no elaboration of the input. Mitigated echolalia is the questioning repetition of words spoken by others, often with a change of the personal pronoun. Stengel postulated that mitigated echolalia may facilitate comprehension in patients with receptive language disturbance. Accordingly, the transition from automatic to mitigated echolalia may be a sign of clinical improvement that parallels the developmental sequence in children. Stengel also observed that the mitigated type may be confined to social conversation and less evident when the patient is directly questioned by an unfamiliar speaker.

Thomsen and Skinhøj (1976) reported three cases of echolalia in a series of 50 patients with severe CHI. Of the two echolalic patients with left hemisphere mass lesions, one initially had a global aphasia and the second had minimal spontaneous speech. The third patient, who sustained a severe diffuse CHI with residual hydrocephalus, evidenced echolalia and palilalia. In contrast to the general association of echolalia with impoverished spontaneous speech (cf. Geschwind, 1974), Thomsen commented that the patient with diffuse CHI "talked almost constantly without any inhibition [p. 220]." We have studied a patient who developed a similar echolalia after CHI.

This 18-year-old, right-handed student was brought to the emergency room of the University of Texas Medical Branch shortly after an automobile accident on 11 May 1980. Initial examination disclosed a Glasgow Coma Scale score of 6, fixed and dilated pupils, and a right hemiparesis. A CT scan on the day of injury was normal. She slowly improved and eventually followed commands on 9 June. After transfer to the Del Oro Rehabilitation Hospital in Houston on 16 June, she remained confused and disoriented until 26 June. During this period, the patient's spontaneous speech changed from an overall impoverishment to a greater than normal flow in which automatic echolalia was prominent. Observations by Mary Ellen Hayden and Ron Levy during the course of rehabilitation showed a transition to mitigated echolalia that resolved by the middle of July. Repetition was most evident in the presence of persons familiar to the patient. Aphasia examination on 16 July disclosed intact spontaneous speech and relatively normal naming. Echolalia had resolved, but repetition of sentences and verbal associative fluency were markedly impaired. Comprehension of complex commands on the Token Test was also defective, whereas the patient could read and comprehend single words and phrases. Further progress in rehabilitation was complicated by her disinhibited behavior, a finding in agreement with Stengel's (1947) interpretation of echolalia as a failure of inhibitory control.

In summary, echolalia and palilalia are infrequent sequelae of CHI that are found in cases with severe diffuse CHI or large mass lesions in the dominant hemisphere. The absence of any reference to echolalia and palilalia in several studies supports the contention that they rarely occur after CHI (Levin *et al.*, 1976; Najenson *et al.*, 1978; Sarno, 1980).

Dysarthria. Sarno (1980) defined dysarthria as a speech disorder arising from pathology in the motor speech system that is evident in defects of the acoustic aspects of the speech stream (i.e., articulation, resonance, stress, and intonation). The severity of dysarthria varies from articulatory imprecision to completely unintelligible speech. Dysarthria may be due to a lesion of either the central or peripheral nervous system. Peacher (1945) reviewed the cases of dysarthria recorded by U.S. Army hospitals during World War II. Of the injuries producing dysarthria, which were primarily missile wounds, 69% involved a lesion of the peripheral nerves. Trauma to the facial nerve was the most common site of lesion, although Peacher did not distinguish between central and peripheral facial nerve injuries.

Investigators of speech disorder after CHI have frequently reported dysarthria in patients with focal mass lesion of the left hemisphere

(Alajouanine, Castaigne, Lhermitte, Escourolle, & Ribaucourt, 1957; Morsier, 1973; Thomsen, 1975) and in cases of diffuse cerebral injury (Sarno, 1980; Thomsen, 1976). Dysarthric patients are frequently hemiparetic or may be quadriplegic. Serial assessment of language after severe CHI has suggested that dysarthria often accompanies aphasia during the early stage of recovery from CHI and may persist after restoration of language. This dissociation is illustrated in a patient admitted to the University of Texas Medical Branch, Galveston.

A 33-year-old, right-handed carpenter sustained a severe CHI in a motorcycle accident on 17 December 1977. Evaluation in the emergency room shortly after injury disclosed a Glasgow Coma Scale score of 4. A CT scan showed a large left parietotemporal epidural hematoma, which was evacuated on the day of admission. Although he progressively improved and followed commands on 20 December, a left facial palsy and right hemiparesis remained. The combined aphasia and severe dysarthria rendered his speech unintelligible. By the first week in January, the patient's language and speech disorder partially resolved, though he continued to evidence anomia and impaired comprehension. A CT scan (10 months postinjury) disclosed a large hypodense area at the site of the operated hematoma and a small hypodense area in the genu of the left internal capsule, which was interpreted as a small lacunar infarct. He was transferred to a rehabilitation center prior to neuropsychological evaluation but returned a year later for testing. Despite frequent articulatory defects, expressive and receptive language skills had uniformly recovered, as reflected by normal scores on all subtests of the MAE.

In contrast to this patient's findings, Sarno (1980) reported that subclinical language deficit (e.g., decreased word fluency) was present in all dysarthric patients in her series of CHI cases. The findings in the Galveston patient suggest that the correspondence between language skills and motor speech varies depending upon the interval between injury and assessment.

Nonaphasic Misnaming. Nonaphasic misnaming is frequently found in patients with diffuse cerebral disturbance who exhibit gross confusion, drowsiness, and memory deficit, although there may be only subtle alteration of consciousness in some cases. Geschwind (1974) distinguishes nonaphasic misnaming on the basis of well-preserved spontaneous speech as contrasted to the word-finding difficulty and circumlocution characteristic of anomic aphasia in patients with focal lesions of the left parietal lobe. Weinstein and Kahn (1965) noted that nonaphasic misnaming may selectively affect words related to the patient's medical disorder or hospitalization (e.g., a hospital is referred to as a "hotel") and be associated with denial of illness. The nonaphasic misnaming reported by these authors is similar to the "subclinical" language deficit disclosed by quantitative assessment as described in the following section.

We may conclude from these studies that assessment of communicative disorder after CHI should include evaluation of dysarthria. The tests for articulatory agility and rating speech characteristics that are included in the Boston Diagnostic Aphasia Examination (Goodglass & Kaplan, 1972) are brief and useful for this purpose.

Quantitative Findings on Aphasia Examination

The administration of standardized examinations for aphasia has yielded a characteristic profile of language disturbance after CHI. This strategy has disclosed that "subclinical" aphasic disorder—that is, evidence of language processing deficit on testing in the absence of clinical manifestations of classical aphasia (Sarno, 1980)—is a frequent sequel of CHI. Moreover, quantitative assessment has facilitated the study of long-term recovery (cf. Levin *et al.*, 1981).

Profiles of language disorder after CHI have been developed using the MAE (Benton, 1967; Benton & Hamsher, 1978) and the NCCEA developed by Spreen and Benton (1969). The MAE evaluates expressive language on tests of naming pictures of objects (visual naming), sentence repetition, digit repetition, and retrieving words beginning with a designated letter (controlled word association). Benton and Hamsher (1978) included a spelling test in their 1978 revision of the MAE. Comprehension of oral language is evaluated by the Token Test and a receptive test in which the patient points to the picture corresponding to a word or phrase presented orally (aural comprehension of words and phrases). Reading comprehension is tested using a similar format. The NCCEA (Spreen & Benton, 1969) includes similar tests, in addition to tests of naming objects presented tactually (tactile naming), construction of sentences (sentence construction), identification of objects by name, oral reading, writing names, writing to dictation and copying, and articulation. Both examinations yield a percentile score based on normative data for each subtest; the manual for the NCCEA also provides percentile scores based on performance of aphasics. Gaddes and Crockett (1973) published normative data for children on the NCCEA. The Boston Diagnostic Aphasia Examination (Goodglass & Kaplan, 1972) also provides a profile of language abilities. It incorporates tests for articulation, repetition of automatized sequences, and rating of spontaneous speech.

We administered portions of the Multilingual and Neurosensory Center aphasia examinations to a consecutive series of patients with CHI of varying severity (Levin *et al.*, 1976). In this study, injury that produced no neurological deficit or loss of consciousness longer than a few minutes was designated as grade I; grade II referred to an injury producing coma not longer than 24 hr; and grade III designated an injury that resulted in a period of coma exceeding 24 hr. A language subtest score that fell below the second percentile of the normative population was considered defective. Whereas clinical examination of spontaneous speech disclosed evidence of aphasia in only eight patients (16% of the series), nearly one-half of the patients were impaired in naming objects (see Figure 15.7). Word-finding difficulty (controlled word association) and impaired writing to dictation were also common expressive defects in this series. In contrast, Figure 15.7 shows that repetition of sentences was well preserved. Nearly a third of the patients had difficulty in comprehension of complex oral commands on the Token Test. The results provided strong support for the presence of subclinical language deficit in apparently nonaphasic CHI patients, including cases with injuries of moderate severity.

Sarno (1980) elucidated the characteristics of subclinical aphasia and speech disorder after CHI in a study of 56 patients with severe head injury who were referred to the Institute for Rehabilitation Medicine in New York. On the basis of clinical evaluation and administration of subtests of the NCCEA (median injury–test interval of 7 months), the author classified the patients into categories of grossly obvious aphasia, dysarthria, and no clinically observed language deficit. However, the two latter groups reflected subclinical aphasia on test scores. The author found that the proportion of patients with each category of language disturbance was approximately equal. The aphasic group consisted of 7 patients with fluent aphasia, 7 with nonfluent aphasia, 2 anomic cases, and 2 with global aphasia.

Most aphasics had defective scores on all four language subtests that were administered, whereas the subclinical patients typically failed only one or two tests. No CHI patients in this series, however, obtained completely normal scores.

Figure 15.5 shows the test results of the CHI patients in Sarno's study transformed into percentile scores for an aphasic population. Accordingly, any score below the ninetieth percentile is impaired in relation to normal subjects. The mean scores indicate reduced word fluency in the subclinical groups, although visual naming is also compromised. Consistent with the results of the Galveston study, Sarno's subclinical patients without dysarthria had adequate sentence repetition, whereas the dysarthric patients exhibited difficulty on this task. Impaired com-

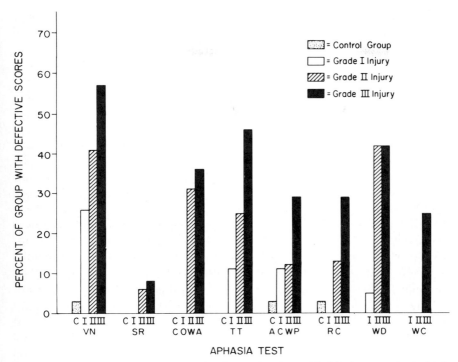

FIGURE 15.7. *Percentage of head-injured and control patients with defective scores in the Multilingual Aphasia Examination. VN = visual naming; SR = sentence repetition; COWA = controlled word association; TOKENS = Token Test; ACWP = auditory comprehension of words and phrases; RC = reading comprehension; WD = writing to dictation; WC = writing–copying. [From Levin, H. S., Grossman, R. G., & Kelly, P. J. 1976. Aphasic disorder in patients with closed head injury.* Journal of Neurology, Neurosurgery, and Psychiatry, *39, 1062–1070. Reproduced with permission of the publisher.]*

prehension of complex oral commands was also found in patients without obvious aphasia. In a discussion of the results obtained in the Galveston study and her own investigation of language disturbance after CHI, Sarno concluded that "the use of sophisticated, neurolinguistic measures with this population is needed to detect subtle deficit which can permit enlightened clinical judgment [p. 691]."

Aphasia in Children after Closed Head Injury

CEREBRAL PLASTICITY AND RECOVERY OF FUNCTION

Investigations of early insult to the human brain have suggested that it possesses considerable plasticity for language development. Lenneberg (1967) proposed that recovery from aphasia parallels the degree to which specialization for language has become lateralized, that is, the commitment of the left hemisphere. From observations of aphasia in children, he postulated that cerebral dominance is established from 2 to 10 years of age. Young children would thus be able to displace language to the right hemisphere after injury to the left hemisphere. This postulation is also consistent with the observation that a right hemisphere lesion produces aphasia more frequently in young children than in older patients. Recent evidence suggests that the development of hemispheric dominance is a gradual process beginning at age 2 (Woods & Carey, 1979). In addition to interhemispheric plasticity, Hécaen has suggested that intrahemispheric reorganization may subserve the rapid recovery from expressive aphasia in children. Studies of infantile hemiplegia have shown no evidence of residual aphasia and only transient or mild aphasia when hemispherectomy is performed on young children with hemiplegia who have acquired language prior to surgery (Basser, 1962; Teuber, 1978). The integrity of language after early brain injury may be achieved, however, at the expense of functions primarily subserved by the right hemisphere (Teuber, 1978). For a more detailed discussion of the relationship between brain maturation and recovery from aphasia in children, the reader is referred to the chapter by Satz and Bullard-Bates in this volume.

The impression of greater capacity for recovery from CHI in children has received support from a study at the Children's Hospital in Philadelphia, which showed a mortality of only 6% in cases with a severe injury defined by an initial Glasgow Coma Scale score of 8 or less (Bruce *et al.*, 1979). Whereas Bruce *et al.* reported that 90% of the children achieved a good recovery or were only moderately disabled, more detailed studies employing psychological assessment have documented permanent cognitive deficit in more than a third of children who sustain a severe head injury (Brink, Garrett, Hale, Woo-Sam, & Nickel, 1970). In summary, it may be anticipated that cognitive impairment contributes to the clinical picture in children who are referred for assessment of aphasia after severe CHI.

DESCRIPTION AND CLINICAL COURSE OF APHASIA AFTER HEAD INJURY IN CHILDREN

Guttmann (1942) published one of the earliest systematic studies of aphasia in children. In his review of previous descriptions, he commented that childhood aphasia was historically viewed as a congenital disorder, whereas acquired aphasia was less well known. The author attributed the prevailing concept of acquired aphasia as a rare disorder in children to a lack of familiarity with its distinctive features.

In a series of 30 children (2–14 years of age) that included 9 cases of head injury, Guttmann pointed out that his patients generally did not exhibit obvious paraphasic errors and were less likely than adults to complain of difficulty in speech. Consequently, Guttmann suggested that acquired aphasia in children may be overlooked or misinterpreted as an unwillingness to speak. Of the 16 children with left hemisphere lesions, 14 were aphasic; 1 of the 13 children with a right hemisphere lesion was also aphasic, as was a single case with bilateral injury. The author characterized their initial language disturbance as an absence of spontaneous speech followed by a poverty of expression, hesitancy, and dysarthria when speech returned. In view of incomplete follow-up data and technical limitations, Guttmann refrained from definitive statements regarding prognosis or localization of lesion.

Alajouanine and Lhermitte (1965) studied 32 aphasic children with left hemisphere lesions, including 13 cases with head injury who ranged in age from 6 to 15 years. Consistent with Guttmann's earlier observations, the most striking feature of the aphasic disorder was poverty of expression, including oral and written language and gestures. Dysarthria, which was present in two-thirds of the children, was associated with hemiplegia. In contrast to aphasia in adults, the authors found that fluent paraphasic speech was rare and that perseveration was absent even in cases with temporal lesions. The 7 children with paraphasic errors were older than 10 years of age. In agreement with Guttmann's findings, only one-third of the children had a receptive deficit for oral speech, although nearly two-thirds were alexic. Comparison of the aphasic children who were under 10 years of age with those from 10 to 15 years of age disclosed that the younger patients had a more profound reduction of verbal expression and a more consistent disruption of articulation. Follow-up examinations at 6 months and 12 months after the appearance of aphasia disclosed normal or nearly normal language in 22 and 24 cases, respectively. The authors observed subtle alterations of language in 14 children on tests of narration, construction of sentences, and definition of words.

Hécaen (1976) described 26 children (3½–15 years of age) with focal cortical lesions of whom 16 (7 left, 6 right, 3 bilateral), sustained a CHI. Nineteen children were aphasic, including 88% of the cases with a left hemisphere lesion and 33% of the children with a right hemisphere lesion. Consistent with previous reports of acquired aphasia in children, Hécaen considered the two essential features of language disorder in his patients to be the loss of initiation of speech (if not mutism) and the absence of paraphasia. Articulation disorder was also common. Impaired auditory verbal comprehension was found only in children with temporal lobe lesions. Alexia resolved rapidly, whereas disturbance of writing was the most common symptom during the acute period and the least likely to resolve. Acalculia was also frequently present in the aphasic children. Although Hécaen's findings lend support to the impression of more rapid resolution of aphasia in children, only one-third of his cases recovered fully.

Insofar as Hécaen investigated acquired aphasia, he confined his study to children who had developed language prior to injury (the youngest aphasic in Hécaen's series was 3½ years of age). We had the opportunity, however, to study serially the recovery of a 2½-year-old girl in whom language development was advanced (e.g., she spoke in sentences, could recite the alphabet, and write her name prior to injury) and a decided manual preference for the right hand had been established. This child sustained a CHI in a motor vehicle accident on 20 March 1975. Examination in the emergency room shortly after injury disclosed a Glasgow Coma Scale score of 6; she had a right hemiparesis and a third-nerve palsy. An angiogram showed no evidence of mass lesion. She followed commands after 10 days but remained mute. The patient gradually vocalized and uttered the *b* sound on 9 April when shown the alphabet. She verbalized single words and brief phrases and joined in singing but failed to initiate speech. Clinic visits over the subsequent 5 years disclosed progressive improvement in language to a nearly normal level within 1 year after injury. During the 6 months following injury the only residual noted in a speech evaluation was a slight hesitancy. The patient shifted her manual preference to the left hand and left foot, though strength on her right side was greatly improved.

Recent studies of pediatric head trauma have focused on quantitative assessment of language (Levin & Eisenberg, 1979). We administered the NCCEA to a consecutive series of 22 children (6–12 years) and 42 adolescents (13–18 years) after they regained orientation. No child was mute or unresponsive at the time of testing. The series was comprised of 60% mild injuries (no coma) and 40% with more severe CHI (coma duration ranged from an hour to more than 3 weeks). The results showed that residual language defect was present in about one-third of the patients. Consistent with findings in adults with CHI, anomia was the most prominent deficit and verbal repetition was least affected. Comprehension of oral language was impaired in 11% of the children studied. Our results suggest that subclinical language disorder occurs after CHI in children with a frequency comparable to that found in adults.

Effects of Severity of Injury

Severity of Diffuse Injury

The duration of coma and persistence of PTA are widely viewed as indices of diffuse injury severity. The divergence in findings on the effects of duration of coma on language may reflect differences in the definition of coma and the interval between injury and assessment. Brooks, Aughton, Bond, Jones, & Rizvi (1980) defined duration of coma in reference to the Glasgow Coma Scale showing no eye opening, failure to obey commands, and the absence of comprehensible speech. In contrast, we employed the interval during which the patient was unable to follow commands (Levin *et al.*, 1976).

Most investigators have reported no relationship between duration of coma and severity or persistence of language disturbance (Brooks *et al.*, 1980; Groher, 1977; Morsier, 1973; Sarno, 1980). The data of patients with mass lesions, however, are typically merged with those of diffuse CHI cases. We reported significant correlations between duration of coma and test scores on visual naming, word fluency, comprehension of aural language, and reading comprehension. Review of individual scores on scatterplots disclosed cases with brief coma and a patient with a left hemisphere mass lesion who evidenced language disturbance. The correlations were nonsignificant on other subtests of the MAE. In a follow-up study of long-term recovery (median interval of 1 year) of language, we confirmed that persistent impairment of both expressive and receptive abilities was related to a prolonged period of coma (Levin *et al.*, 1981). Brooks *et al.* (1980) found that residual word fluency was correlated with the duration of PTA, which was estimated by retrospectively questioning the patient.

Severe diffuse CHI is frequently presumed in patients with a long period of coma in the face of a normal CT scan. Severity of generalized injury may also be reflected by an acute CT scan showing compression of the ventricles and cisterns by cerebral swelling. The possibility of differential recovery of language in patients with this CT pattern has not been studied. In summary, we may conclude that prolonged coma is neither a necessary nor sufficient condition for residual aphasia.

Focal Brain Lesions

Localization of lesion in aphasia is reviewed by Damasio in Chapter 2 of this volume. This section provides a cursory summary of findings in patients with head injury. In acute CHI the presence of a focal mass lesion (i.e., hematoma or contusion) is visualized in most cases by a CT scan. Figure 15.1 is a CT scan obtained on the day of injury that shows an area of increased density consistent with an intracerebral hematoma. Smaller lesions, such as hemorrhagic contusions, are also appreciated by CT.

In general, the type of aphasia associated with a specific locus of lesion corresponds to the language disorder produced by nontraumatic vascular lesions in the same region (Alajouanine *et al.*, 1957). This generalization has received support from studies of adults with left temporal intracerebral hematoma who exhibit fluent, paraphasic speech and impaired comprehension (Debray-Ritzen, Hirsch, Pierre-Kahn, Bursztejn, & Labbe, 1977; Stone *et al.*, 1978). Injury to the dominant temporal lobe or extensive left hemisphere damage accounted for most of the aphasic CHI patients with focal lesions described by Thomsen (1976). The presence of a focal lesion concomitant with diffuse injury may result in an apparent "crossed aphasia." From neurological findings, CT results, and observations made during surgery, we recorded six patients with a predominant right hemisphere lesion who exhibited a linguistic defect on at least one subtest of the MAE (Levin *et al.*, 1976). In contrast to aphasics with major involvement of the left hemisphere, contralateral hemiparesis was not present in these patients. We also observed that clinical evidence of injury to the rostral brain stem was more closely associated with linguistic disturbance than were signs of hemispheric injury, a finding consistent with Ommaya and Gennarelli's (1974) model of CHI discussed earlier in this chapter.

Subcortical Lesions

Evidence for the participation of subcortical structures in language is reviewed in Chapter 2. We have been impressed by the long periods of mutism in three patients, including two adolescents and an adult, in whom CT disclosed a subcortical intracerebral hematoma. The findings in one patient are summarized (see Figure 15.1).

A 12-year-old, left-handed girl (inconsistent familial sinistrality) was evaluated 20 min after sustaining a CHI on 22 June 1979, when she was struck by a car. Examination in the emergency room disclosed a Glasgow Coma Score of 6; she began to obey commands on 30 June but had a right hemiplegia and uttered no words or sounds. The CT scan disclosed a hemorrhagic contusion of the left putamen and anterior limb of the internal capsule (see Figure 15.1). She remained mute until 15 July. Throughout the mute period she was dysgraphic; her spelling was impaired, and she wrote in block letters. A repeat CT scan showed density changes suggesting resolution of the hemorrhagic lesion in the basal ganglia. Detailed assessment of language on 13 August when she was fully oriented, disclosed an impoverished lexical stock with infrequent initiation of spontaneous speech. The MAE showed a decrement in verbal associative fluency and defective comprehension (Token Test). Spontaneous speech was grossly intact when she was examined a year later. The follow-up tests disclosed a residual impairment in word fluency and impaired comprehension of complex commands (Token Test), although there was a trend of improvement.

Concomitant Neuropsychological Deficits

Hemispheric Disconnection

In view of the shearing and stretching of axons and resultant injury to the corpus callosum, hemispheric disconnection syndrome would appear to be a likely consequence of severe CHI. The first description of a hemispheric disconnection after CHI was the case reported by Lhermitte, Massary, and Huguenin (1929) of a jockey who developed alexia without agraphia after falling off a horse. He had a right homonymous hemianopsia and a left inferior quadrantopsia. The patient could not read words but was capable of reading single letters. The second case study of hemispheric disconnection after CHI was published 40 years later (Schott, Michel, Michel, & Dumas, 1969), but there was no anatomical confirmation of injury to the callosum. The authors described tactile anomia, ideomotor apraxia, and agraphia confined to the left hand. A case of posttraumatic disconnection syndrome with neuropathological verification was found to evidence ideomotor apraxia and agraphia confined to the left hand (Rubens, Geschwind, Mahowald, & Mastri, 1977). Neuropathological findings showed marked thinning of the corpus callosum with demyelination and loss of axons.

We tested interhemispheric transfer of information by comparing naming of objects placed in the left or the right hand in a study of long-term recovery from acute aphasia following CHI (Levin *et al.*, 1981). There was disproportionate impairment of naming objects placed in the left hand, a finding consistent with callosal dysfunction. Two cases with residual expressive and receptive deficits also exhibited ideomotor apraxia, as they could not do better than approximate familiar gestures when they were requested orally to perform them. We postulated that ideomotor apraxia in these patients may have resulted from interruption of intrahemispheric connections.

The presence of hemispheric disconnection may be clinically investigated by detailed assessment of ideomotor apraxia, testing writing in both hands, and examining the patient's ability to name objects placed in either hand. It is necessary to exclude the possibility of a primary sensory defect by determining whether the patient can visually match objects that are incorrectly named.

Other Neuropsychological Deficits

Descriptive studies after CHI have emphasized the frequent finding of concomitant neuropsychological deficits. Associated verbal impairment, which may be viewed as an integral aspect of aphasia, includes alexia, agraphia, and acalculia (Heilman et al., 1971; Morsier, 1973). Heilman et al. observed that anomic patients frequently exhibit right–left confusion, finger agnosia, and difficulties in calculation, writing, and reading. The authors also found reversible amnesic disorder in four of the nine anomic patients.

Thomsen (1977) compared verbal learning and memory for words, sentences, and numbers in CHI patients with persistent aphasic symptoms to nonaphasic CHI cases who had a comparable duration of PTA. This study, which tested patients more than 2 years after injury, disclosed that both groups had impaired verbal memory for information beyond immediate span when their performance was compared to a control group. Residual impairment of immediate memory (e.g., digit span) was confined to the aphasic CHI patients, whose learning and retention of unrelated words were inferior to that of nonaphasic head-injured patients.

In a quantitative study of language defects after CHI, we considered related deficits on visuoperceptive and visuomotor tasks (Levin et al., 1976). Although we found a trend suggesting an association, it was not significant when compared to other CHI patients who were spared linguistic disturbance.

The relationship between aphasia, of any etiology, and intellectual function has been a controversial issue historically. We approached the problem by differentiating acutely aphasic CHI patients whose language fully recovered, from cases with specific residual defects or chronic impairment of both expressive and receptive abilities (Levin et al., 1981). Patients with persistent aphasic disorder also had marked cognitive deficit on both verbal and visuospatial subtests of the Wechsler Adult Intelligence Scale, whereas the other patients recovered to a low normal if not average intellectual level.

Behavioral Disturbance

The sequelae of CHI frequently include alterations in behavior (cf. Levin & Grossman, 1978). Severe head injury may result in a thinking disturbance reflected by intrusion of irrelevant material into spontaneous speech. Patients disabled by CHI often lack insight into the severity of their deficits and inappropriateness of their verbalizations. Motor retardation and withdrawal to isolated activities are also common in these patients. To a lesser degree, depression and anxiety may be present and affect the course of speech therapy, although these sequelae are not closely related to the severity of initial injury.

Special Aspects of Speech Therapy

The general topic of speech therapy for aphasia is discussed by M. T. Sarno in Chapter 17 of this volume. Although the techniques for remediation of aphasic symptoms after head injury may not differ fundamentally from the methods used for aphasics with cerebral vascular disease, the speech therapist should be particularly sensitive to related problems in young patients recovering from CHI. Providing feedback to assist the head-injured patient in monitoring linguistic errors and appropriateness of content may facilitate psychosocial functioning. This aspect of speech therapy assumes a prominent role when we consider that neuropsychological impairment and behavioral disorder far overshadow the contribution of focal motor deficit to chronic disability in head-injured patients. The intrusion of irrelevant and unrealistic statements into the conversational speech of brain-injured patients has been mentioned by various authors (cf. Levin & Grossman, 1978). Although there is no firm evidence that monitoring of speech content may respond favorably to therapeutic intervention, this potential role of the speech therapist warrants further study.

The application of techniques for memory training of head-injured patients may also broaden the role of the speech therapist. Instruction of the patient to evoke visual images to integrate and retrieve verbal material has been the most widely studied technique (Jones, 1974), although other methods have been proposed. The employment of visual imagery as a mnemonic aid would be ostensibly useful in patients with focal left hemisphere injury. This possibility, however, awaits confirmation by definitive outcome studies.

Summary

There is considerable heterogeneity in the mechanisms of brain injury produced by penetrating missile wounds and closed head injury, which is reflected by differences in the aphasic symptoms. Nonfluent expressive aphasia is common in patients with left hemisphere missile injury but rarely found in adults with closed head injury. Anomic disturbance predominates in clinically obvious aphasia after closed head injury and may be demonstrated by appropriate testing in patients with relatively intact spontaneous speech. In contrast, acquired aphasia produced by closed head injury in children is characterized by a reduction in output, with hesitancy, failure to initiate speech, and possibly mutism. Although the prognosis for recovery from aphasia is generally better in patients with closed head injury than in patients with cerebral vascular disease, residual defects in complex verbal skills are frequently present. Patients with closed head injury who become aphasic frequently exhibit concomitant neuropsychological deficits, including hemispheric disconnection syndrome, verbal memory impairment, and acalculia.

Acknowledgments

The author is indebted to Dr. A. L. Benton for providing valuable advice and reviewing the manuscript, and to Sarah A. De Los Santos for typing the manuscript. Preparation of this manuscript was supported by DHEW 5PO1 NS 07377–11, Center for the Study of Nervous System Injury grant, and NO1 NS 9-2314, Comprehensive Central Nervous System Trauma Center Contract.

References

Adams, J. H., Mitchell, D. E., Graham, D. I., & Doyle, D. 1977. Diffuse brain damage of immediate impact type. *Brain, 100,* 489–502.

Alajouanine, T., Castaigne, P., Lhermitte, F., Escourolle, R., & Ribaucourt B. De. 1957. Étude de 43 cas d'aphasie posttraumatique. *Encéphale, 46,* 1–45.

Alajouanine, T., & Lhermitte, F. 1965. Acquired aphasia in children. *Brain, 88,* 653–662.

Annegers, J. F., Grabow, J. D., Kurland, L. T., & Laws, E. R. 1980. The incidence, causes, and secular trends of head trauma in Olmsted County, Minnesota. *Neurology, 30* (9), 912–919.

Arseni, C., Constantinovici, A., Iliescu, D., Dobrota, I., & Gagea, A. 1970. Considerations on posttraumatic aphasia in peace time. *Psychiatria Neurologia Neurochirurgia, 73,* 105–115.

Basser, L. S. 1962. Hemiplegia of early onset and the faculty of speech with special reference to the effects of hemispherectomy. *Brain, 85,* 427–460.

Bastian, H. C. 1898. *A treatise on aphasia and other speech defects.* London: H. K. Lewis.

Benson, D. F., Gardner, H., & Meadows, J. C. 1976. Reduplicative paramnesia. *Neurology, 26,* 147–151.

Benton, A. L. 1967. Problems of test construction in the field of aphasia. *Cortex, 3,* 32–58.

Benton, A. L., & Hamsher, K. 1978. *Manual for the multilingual aphasia examination.* Iowa City: Univ. of Iowa.

Brink, J. D., Garrett, A. L., Hale, W. R., Woo-Sam, J., & Nickel, V. L. 1970. Recovery of motor and intellectual function in children sustaining severe head injuries. *Developmental Medicine and Child Neurology, 12,* 565–571.

Brooks, D. N., Aughton, M. E., Bond, M. R., Jones, P., & Rizvi, S. 1980. Cognitive sequelae in relationship to early indices of severity of brain damage after severe blunt head injury. *Journal of Neurology, Neurosurgery, and Psychiatry, 43*, 529–534.

Bruce, D. A., Raphaely, R. C., Goldberg, A. I., Zimmerman, R. A., Bilaniuk, L. T., Schut, L., & Kuhl, D. E. 1979. Pathophysiology, treatment and outcome following severe head injury in children. *Child's Brain, 5*, 174–191.

Cairns, H. 1952. Disturbances of consciousness with lesions of the brain-stem and diencephalon. *Brain, 75*, 8–146.

Caveness, W. F. 1977. Incidence of craniocerebral trauma in the United States, 1970–1975. *Annals of Neurology, 1*, 507.

Debray-Ritzen, P., Hirsch, J.-F., Pierre-Kahn, A., Bursztejn, C., & Labbe, J.-P. 1977. Atteinte transitoire du langage écrit en rapport avec un hématome du lobe temporal gauche chez une adolescente de quatorze ans. *Revue Neurologique, 133*, 207–210.

Field, J. H. 1976. *A study of the epidemiology of head injury in England and Wales.* London: Department of Health and Social Security.

Gaddes, W. H., & Crockett, D.J. 1973. The Spreen-Benton aphasia tests, normative data as a measure of normal language development. *Research Monograph*, No. 25, 1–76. Neuropsychology Laboratory, Univ. of Victoria.

Geschwind, N. 1974. *Selected papers on language and the brain.* Dordrecht, Holland: D. Reidel.

Goodglass, H., & Kaplan, E. 1972. *The assessment of aphasia and related disorders.* New York: Lea and Febiger.

Graham, D. I., & Adams, J. H. 1971. Ischaemic brain damage in fatal head injuries. *Lancet 1*, 265–266.

Groher, M. 1977. Language and memory disorders following closed head trauma. *Journal of Speech and Hearing Research, 20*, 212–223.

Gurdjian, E. S., & Gurdjian, E. S. 1976. Cerebral contusions: Reevaluation of the mechanism of their development. *Journal of Trauma, 16*, 35–51.

Guttmann, E. 1942. Aphasia in children. *Brain, 65*, 205–219.

Hécaen, H. 1976. Acquired aphasia in children and the ontogenesis of hemispheric functional specialization. *Brain and Language, 3*, 114–134.

Heilman, K. M., Safran, A., & Geschwind, N. 1971. Closed head trauma and aphasia. *Journal of Neurology, Neurosurgery, and Psychiatry, 34*, 265–269.

Helm, N. A., Butler, R. B., & Benson, D. F. 1978. Acquired stuttering. *Neurology, 28*, 1159–1165.

Jennett, B., Teasdale, G., Galbraith, S., Pickard, J., Grant, H., Braakman, R., Avezaat, C., Maas, A., Minderhoud, J., Vecht, C. J., Heiden, J., Small, R., Caton, W., & Kurze, T. 1977. Severe head injuries in three countries. *Journal of Neurology, Neurosurgery, and Psychiatry, 40*, 291-298.

Jones, M. K. 1974. Imagery as a mnemonic aid after left temporal lobectomy: Contrast between material-specific and generalized memory disorders. *Neuropsychologia, 12*, 21-30.

Lenneberg, E. 1967. *Biological foundations of language.* New York: Wiley.

Levin, H. S., & Eisenberg, H. M. 1979. Neuropsychological impairment after closed head injury in children and adolescents. *Journal of Pediatric Psychology, 4*, 389–402.

Levin, H. S., & Grossman, R. G. 1978. Behavioral sequelae of closed head injury: A quantitative study. *Archives of Neurology, 35*, 720-727.

Levin, H. S., Grossman, R. G., & Kelly, P. J. 1976. Aphasic disorder in patients with closed head injury. *Journal of Neurology, Neurosurgery, and Psychiatry, 39*, 1062–1070.

Levin, H. S., Grossman, R. G., Sarwar, M., & Meyers, C. A. 1981. Linguistic recovery after closed head injury. *Brain & Language, 12,* 360–374.

Levin, H. S., O'Donnell, V. M., & Grossman, R. G. 1979. The Galveston orientation and amnesia test: A practical scale to assess cognition after head injury. *Journal of Nervous and Mental Disease, 167,* 675–684.

Lhermitte, J., Massary, J. de, & Huguenin, R. 1929. Syndrome occipital avec alexie pure d'origine traumatique, par. *Revue Neurologique, 2,* 703–707.

Mohr, J. P., Weiss, G., Caveness, W. F., Dillon, J. D., Kistler, J. P., Meirowsky, A. M., & Rish, B. L. 1980. Language and motor deficits following penetrating head injury in Vietnam. *Neurology, 30,* 1273–1279.

Morsier, G. de. 1973. Sur 23 cas d'aphasie traumatique. *Psychiatria Clinica, 6,* 226–239.

Najenson, T., Sazbon, L., Fiselzon, J., Becker, E., & Schechter, I. 1978. Recovery of communicative functions after prolonged traumatic coma. *Scandinavian Journal of Rehabilitation Medicine, 10,* 15–21.

Newcombe, F. 1969. *Missile wounds of the brain.* London: Oxford Univ. Press.

Ommaya, A. K., & Gennarelli, T. A. 1974. Cerebral concussion and traumatic unconsciousness: Correlation of experimental and clinical observations on blunt head injuries. *Brain, 97,* 633–654.

Peacher, W. G. 1945. Speech disorders in World War II. II. Further studies. *Journal of Nervous and Mental Disease, 102,* 165–171.

Plum, F., & Posner, J. B. 1980. *The diagnosis of stupor and coma.* Philadelphia: Davis.

Rubens, A. B., Geschwind, N., Mahowald, M. W., & Mastri, A. 1977. Posttraumatic cerebral hemispheric disconnection syndrome. *Archives of Neurology, 34,* 750–755.

Russell, W. R., & Espir, M. L. E. 1961. *Traumatic aphasia. A study of aphasia in war wounds of the brain.* London: Oxford Univ. Press.

Russell, W. R., & Smith, A. 1961. Posttraumatic amnesia in closed head injury. *Archives of Neurology, 5,* 4–17.

Sarno. M. T. 1980. The nature of verbal impairment after closed head injury. *Journal of Nervous and Mental Disease, 168,* 685–692.

Schiller, F. 1947. Aphasia studied in patients with missile wounds. *Journal of Neurology, Neurosurgery, and Psychiatry, 10,* 183–197.

Schott, B., Michel, F., Michel, D., & Dumas, R. 1969. Apraxie idéomotrice unilatérale gauche avec main gauche anomique: Syndrome de déconnexion calleuse? *Revue Neurologique, 120,* 359-365.

Spreen, O., & Benton, A. L. 1969. *Neurosensory center comprehensive examination for aphasia: Manual of directions.* Victoria, B.C.: Neuropsychology Laboratory, Univ. of Victoria.

Stengel, E. 1947. A clinical and psychological study of echo-reactions. *Journal of Mental Science, 93,* 598–612.

Stone, J. L., Lopes, J. R., & Moody, R. A. 1978. Fluent aphasia after closed head injury. *Surgical Neurology, 9,* 27–29.

Teasdale, G., & Jennett, B. 1974. Assessment of coma and impaired consciousness: A practical scale. *Lancet, 2,* 81–84.

Teuber, H.-L. 1978. The brain and human behavior. In R. Held, H. W. Leibowitz & H.-L. Teuber (Eds.), *Perception.* Berlin: Springer-Verlag.

Thomsen, I. V. 1975. Evaluation and outcome of aphasia in patients with severe closed head trauma. *Journal of Neurology, Neurosurgery, and Psychiatry, 38,* 713–718.

Thomsen. I. V. 1976. Evaluation and outcome of traumatic aphasia in patients with severe verified focal lesions. *Folia Phoniatrica, 28,* 362–377.

Thomsen, I. V. 1977. Verbal learning in aphasic and non-aphasic patients with severe head injury. *Scandinavian Journal of Rehabilitation Medicine, 9,* 73–77.

Thomsen, I. V., & Skinhøj, E. 1976. Regressive language in severe head injury. *Acta Neurologica Scandinavica, 54,* 219–226.

Walker, A. E., & Jablon, S. 1961. A follow-up study of head wounds in World War II. *V. A. Medical Monograph.*

Weinstein, E. A., & Kahn, R. L. 1955. *Denial of illness.* Springfield, Ill.: Thomas.

Woods, B. T., & Carey, S. 1979. Language deficits after apparent clinical recovery from childhood aphasia. *Annals of Neurology, 6,* 405–409.

16

Emotional Aspects of Aphasia

JOHN SARNO

A textbook on acquired aphasia would not be complete without some attention to the emotional dimensions of the disorder, first because the emotional reactions of the individual so afflicted may represent an important determinant of the outcome of his rehabilitation and, second, because the pathological lesion resulting in aphasia may also be responsible for alterations in emotional responses on a purely anatomical–physiological basis. If these represent two major areas for study, what is the foundation for future research?

There is little in the literature on disturbances in emotionality and personality specifically associated with aphasia. Of the few reports extant, most deal with broader categories, such as the emotional concomitants of stroke and closed head injury. These will be reviewed, however, so that we may extract from them whatever is relevant to this topic. The majority of specific references to aphasia are anecdotal but will be reported nevertheless for the same reason.

If we separate the two processes in which we are interested—that is, emotionality and human communication—there is an extensive literature in both fields. Interest in aphasia dates to the latter part of the nineteenth century; knowledge of the brain mechanisms underlying human emotion is of more recent vintage but of increasing interest to brain scientists. There appears to be a conjunction, however, which will be discussed in this chapter. It is speculative but could not be otherwise, given the current state of knowledge.

Let us first consider some contributions of historical interest. Kurt Goldstein focused on what he identified as the CATASTROPHIC REACTION

ACQUIRED APHASIA

(CR), characteristic of many patients with aphasia, and argued that it resulted from a disturbance in the patient's ability to maintain "biologic homeostasis" rather than from a sense of inadequacy (Goldstein, 1942). He based this conclusion on the immediacy of the CR and the patient's lack of awareness of the reason for it. Neglecting the concept of the unconscious, which had been well formulated by that time by Freud and his followers, he postulated that brain damage produced a failure of the entire organism, a "biologic" rather than a psychic response, and that the patient's reactions represented his attempts to maintain biologic homeostasis. A student of Freudian psychology could, of course, argue for the concept that these same behaviors represented a desperate effort of the individual's psychic apparatus to maintain equilibrium (sanity, emotional stability) in the face of insults to his higher functions (language, cognition, perception) and that psychic stability was an integral aspect of biologic homeostasis rather than a thing apart. His biologicophilosophic ideas aside, the description of the CR has been of great value to clinicians (Schuell, Jenkins, & Jiménez-Pabón, 1964).

Later, Goldstein (1952, 1959) further theorized on the effect of brain damage on language and the personality, continuing to focus on the catastrophic reaction but further developing his concepts to include what he called the ABSTRACT ATTITUDE, lost in many patients with brain damage and responsible for personality changes. Since the abstract attitude refers to cognitive ability, this would appear to be an example of the impact of intellectual function on personality.

In retrospect, Goldstein's greatest contribution vis-à-vis conceptualization of the impact of brain damage on emotional function may have been his willingness to engage the problem and draw its attention to the world of neurology. He theorized and wrote prolifically on both emotional and language function and can appropriately be considered one of the "fathers" of the field of neuropsychology.

Luria (1963), although he did not systematically study the impact of brain damage on emotionality, stated that premorbid personality played an important part in the process of recovery from aphasia.

A number of well-known clinicians have called attention to the importance of the emotional concomitants of aphasia. Schuell and her colleagues (1964), Wepman (1951), and Eisenson (1973) all made frequent references to emotional phenomena in their writings and emphasized the necessity of considering them in therapeutic interaction with patients. Both Wepman and Eisenson stressed the occasional need for psychotherapy. More recently, Benson (1979, 1980) has discussed emotional disorders in a systematic way and has made suggestions for the management of the aphasic patient.

Review of the Literature

A review of the basic literature on communication and emotional behavior suggests that one is most likely to see a point of convergence by considering the function of the limbic system. Study of language has been limited almost entirely to neocortical systems, but there have been recent allusions to the phylogenetically older and primarily subcortical limbic areas that are intriguing and attractive.

The term LIMBIC SYSTEM refers to a group of structures deep within the substance of the brain that have gradually come to be associated in humans with emotional behavior and attitudes and more recently with communication drives. It incorporates both cortical and subcortical structures that in lower animals primarily serve the sense of smell and that as biologic imperatives changed with evolution became converted to other functions. A publication by Papez in 1937 is credited with having provided a theoretical base for the idea that the phylogenetically old rhinencephalon was the source of emotional and motivational behavior. Since then there has been a great deal of research activity corroborating this concept. This includes the work of Bard and Mountcastle (1947), Brodal (1947), Pribram and Kruger (1954), and Maclean (1952), who was the first to use the term limbic system.

Lamendella's Review

Motivated by the desire to draw attention to the role of the limbic system in human communication, Lamendella (1977) has done a detailed review of the subject and presented some original concepts as a result of his study. Because they bear so closely on the subject matter of this chapter, some of his observations and conclusions will be reported.

It is Lamendella's major thesis that the limbic system plays an important role in human social and communicative behavior. In fact, he suggests that this system may be responsible for most human non-propositional communication activity. He sees the limbic system as poised between and acting upon both vegetative (species preserving) functions, through its connections with the hypothalamus, and the neocortex, which is involved with those higher-level functions that define the human species—social and communicative behavior. Following a review of the anatomy, physiology, and phylogeny of the system as it is presently conceptualized, Lamendella presents evidence linking the limbic system to primate social and communication function and then identifies five levels of forebrain activity that participate in human communication, three of which are included within the limbic system. The highest level, that of propositional communication, incorporates the dominant and nondominant hemispheres, the latter of which he suggests is closely related to nonpropositional processes that originate in the limbic system and are intertwined with affective subsystems. He suggests that the dominant left hemisphere, in addition to being the locus of propositional speech, appears to play an inhibitory role vis à-vis affective function.

The emotional lability of patients with left hemisphere lesions, many of whom are aphasic, is given as evidence of the loss of this inhibitory function. On the other hand, the indifference behavior of patients with right hemisphere lesions would point to an impairment of the limbic–right hemisphere system, which underlies affective function, according to his concepts.

What is most relevant to the subject of this chapter is the section of Lamendella's paper relating limbic and linguistic communication.

He presents two ideas in this regard. First, AUTOMATIC speech is to be distinguished from PROPOSITIONAL speech, the latter being represented in the left hemisphere and, therefore, often disordered when there is damage to that area. He believes that automatic speech may be processed in multiple loci, including limbic, basal ganglia, thalamic, or midbrain structures and, therefore, may be relatively preserved in a patient with classical aphasia (Bay, 1964; Critchley, 1970; Head, 1926; Jackson, 1932; Luria, 1970;). Second, Lamendella states that one type of automatic speech has referential meaning: that which has emotional content. He believes that such speech (including obscenities and vulgarisms) actually originates in the limbic system because of its affective nature and that these utterances have the dual purpose of relieving affective pressures within the individual as well as of evoking "limbic" responses in the person being spoken to. These affective pressures, in his view, include all of the primitive vegetative functions with which the limbic system is involved, colorfully identified by Pribram (1971) as the four Fs.

One final reference should be made, which surely suggests a powerful relationship between emotional and communication functions. This is the observation of Robinson (1976) concerning a patient who was severely aphasic and right hemiparetic and who subsequently developed a manic–depressive psychosis. During the manic phase, both his motor deficit and aphasia disappeared only to return when the mania was controlled with medication. This remarkable pattern could be repeated by manipulating the medication; that is, when the medication was stopped and the patient became depressed again, aphasia and the motor deficit returned.

Robinson interpreted this phenomenon to suggest the existence of two separate speech systems, but Lamendella advances the hypothesis that strong emotional stimuli originating in the limbic system might possibly overcome or circumvent the loss of control over speech and motor systems normally exercised by the left hemisphere.

Summarizing his concept, Lamendella suggests that, though high-level neocortical systems may be largely responsible for communication now enjoyed by human beings, there is reason to believe that the complex systems for communication developed at lower brain levels down through phylogenetic strata continue to play a role in human communication. And, most germane to our topic, this role is most relevant where emotions and speech conjoin.

Gainotti's Study

A report by Gainotti (1972), though primarily designed to explore the differences in emotional behavior associated with the hemispheric side of a lesion, is the only one of which we are aware in which reported data make specific reference to the emotional reactions of the patient with aphasia. Emotional reactions are identified in four groups: a category of seven reactions under the heading CATASTROPHIC REACTIONS, five affective states characterized as DEPRESSIVE MOODS, four INDIFFERENCE REACTIONS, and a category of OTHER REACTIONS, which included confabulations, delusions, and hate for limbs. Patients with left hemisphere lesions manifested catastrophic or anxiety–depression symptoms more frequently than did patients with lesions of the nondominant hemisphere, while indifference reactions were more common among the latter group. When he subdivided the left hemisphere patients according to the presence or absence of aphasia, further differences were noted. So-called Broca's aphasics had statistically more dramatic, sudden, short-lived emotional outbursts than did other aphasics (Wernicke's did not weep at all), while the amnesic aphasics showed a different pattern of anxiety reaction that seemed to reflect greater awareness and control. Wernicke's aphasics were also quite different from nonaphasics and patients with right brain damage in the frequent use of emotional language (swearing, cursing, religious imprecations), though in this they were almost matched by Broca's aphasics. The latter group showed the highest incidence of aggressive behavior of all (25% as compared to about 10% for most of the other groups). Twenty-five percent of the fluent aphasics seemed unaware of their language problem, matching the proportion of right hemisphere patients who were anosognosic, but the fluent aphasics did not manifest other characteristics of "belle indifference" as did the right brain damaged patients. In fact, Wernicke's aphasics expressed discouragement in greater numbers than did all other groups and matched others in drawing attention to their failures, clear evidence of some degree of awareness of and concern about their deficits.

How can one interpret the affective differences among these groups? This continues to be a matter for discussion, for there is no basis at this time for an authoritative statement. Though a detailed analysis of the problem is not appropriate here, the following is suggested: The indifference of right hemisphere damaged patients probably represents an aberration in the basic emotional processing structure, of which the right hemisphere seems to be an integral part. In left hemisphere damaged individuals, emotionality is more or less intact, but control over its manifestations is impaired. Among aphasics, however, there are further differences that probably relate to both the extent and the locus of damage and that appear to be on a rough continuum. Amnesic aphasics are most aware of their deficits and retain the greatest degree of control over their emotional reactions. Broca's aphasics appear to be quite aware, but the quality of their anxiety and depression reflects less control than is available to the amnesics. Fluent aphasics are the most complicated; Gainotti's data suggest that they, too, are anxious and depressed but present a confusing pattern of awareness and control. The inappropriateness of the Wernicke's aphasic is well known to clinicians, and the intimations of psychosis is now a classical observation (Benson, 1980; Horenstein, 1970). We would suggest that the parapsychotic behavior of some fluent aphasics may be a function of both affective and cognitive incompetence resulting from the pathological lesion rather than a disorder that has its roots in aberrant emotionality alone. Smythies (1970) has suggested that psychoses are the result of QUALITATIVE changes in brain physiology (as opposed to quantitative ones in the neuroses) that in schizophrenia, for example, may be the result of a biochemical aberration. It is within the realm of possibility that the qualitative changes (cognitive and/or affective) are of significant magnitude in the Wernicke's aphasic to produce a picture that sometimes mimics that of a classical psychosis. Indeed, Wint in his personal account (1967) describes hallucinatory phenomena quite clearly, and his was not a very severe lesion nor was he a fluent aphasic. The frequent involvement of the temporal lobe in Wernicke's aphasics lends further credence to a special affective deficit because of the association of that area with emotional processes (Geschwind, 1977; Klüver & Bucy, 1939; Papez, 1937).

Further complicating the picture for the fluent aphasic are suggestions that deficits in auditory processing lead to paranoid ideas in the patient (Benson, 1980) and confusion in the mind of the examiner (Ziegler, 1952). Finally, the jargon of these patients has sometimes resulted in a diagnosis of schizophrenia, occasionally leading to psychiatric hospitalization.

If one follows the philosophic tendencies of Jackson, Goldstein, Luria, and more recently Brown (1977), the interaction and interdependence of all neural systems at multiple levels and loci may invalidate the concept of separate systems functioning independently. Whether one assigns it to the sphere of cognition or emotionality, the quality of the deficit in a fluent aphasic may be responsible for the distinctive picture one sees.

Closed Head Injury

Aside from stroke, one of the most frequent causes of brain damage, and often of aphasia, are those injuries resulting from high-velocity accidents that have become so common in modern society. The trauma to the brain takes multiple forms, including laceration of cerebral tissue, loss of substance, compression by bone, hemorrhage within and on the surface of the brain, and, perhaps the most subtle and pervasive of all, contusion of brain tissue. The last has been a rather inexact designation until recently. Ommaya and Gennarelli (1974) suggested that cortical–subcortical disconnection phenomena were the result of what they termed ACCELERATIVE TRAUMA TO THE HEAD and that the presence of coma, signaling damage to the least vulnerable areas of the brain (i.e., mesencephalic and caudal diencephalic structures) would invariably be associated with significant injury and dysfunction of the more peripheral parts of the brain.

In a report on the results of autopsy studies of 151 patients who sustained immediate impact damage to the brain, Adams, Mitchell, Graham, and Doyle (1977) stated that "diffuse damage to white matter" was the primary factor determining outcome in patients with nonmissile brain injury. They, too, indicated that damage to the rostral brain stem was invariably accompanied by diffuse hemispheric pathology.

These studies suggest that brain damage severe enough to produce coma will usually result in dysfunction in multiple brain systems because of the diffuse nature of the pathology.

Apropos of this, there is evidence that language dysfunction to some degree occurs in virtually every patient rendered comatose from closed head injury. In a population of these patients studied at a rehabilitation facility, Sarno (1980) has reported that 32% were frankly aphasic but that the rest of the group showed some evidence of a linguistic processing deficit when tested with a standard aphasia battery.

Lishman (1973) reviewed the psychiatric sequelae in the closed head injured and indicated that they were almost universal. While there was a correlation between the degree and type of damage to the brain and subsequent psychiatric phenomena, he found that this factor was statistically significant but contributed to a very small part (1/15) of the total causation of psychiatric disability. The left hemisphere was found to be more closely associated with psychiatric sequelae then the right, and temporal injuries were more important than those in frontal, parietal, or occipital areas. Other etiologic factors that were significant were the development of epilepsy, the patient's response to being intellectually impaired, environmental factors, compensation and litigation, emotional impact and repercussions of the injury, premorbid personality, and mental constitution.

In assessing the factor of intellectual impairment, Lishman (1973) indicates that permanent dementia is relatively rare and suggests that in the early stages of recovery coincident affective disorders and motivational defects may contribute to the appearance of a more severe dementia than in fact exists.

Of the psychiatric sequelae, which include changes in personality and temperament, psychoses, and neurotic disabilities, Lishman (1973) found the neurotic disabilities to be the most common. They included depressive reactions, anxiety states (some with phobias), neurasthenic reactions, conversion hysterias, obsessional neuroses, and a variety of somatic complaints.

In an attempt to identify the importance of physiogenic and psychogenic factors in the various psychiatric groups, Lishman concluded that there was almost always a mix but that psychogenic factors were most prominent in patients with neurotic symptoms and that stress in the predisposed individual appeared to be responsible for the functional psychoses, though he acknowledged the developing evidence of the importance of organic factors in schizophrenia.

For the purpose of this chapter, the foregoing section dealing with traumatic head injuries points up the importance of considering the type of pathology in studying the psychiatric sequelae of brain damage and establishes the concept, probably applicable to all categories of brain damage, that both physiological and psychological factors, often working synergistically, are to be considered in the assessment of the emotional concomitants of brain injury. More specific to the problem of aphasia is the observation that left brain damage appears to be more frequently associated with psychiatric phenomena and the fact that all individuals suffering catastrophic neurological sequelae, among which aphasia is prominent, can be expected to manifest serious emotional responses of a reactive nature.

The Ullman Monograph

Ullman (1962) published the results of the systematic observation of behavioral changes in 300 patients admitted to a stroke study over a period of 3 years. No attempt was made to categorize emotional responses on the basis of the site or extent of the lesion. Some of his conclusions are relevant to the purposes of this chapter. In analyzing reactive responses to the stroke, leaving aside the patient with diffuse impairment of brain function, he found that the severity and duration of "physical disability," in which category aphasia was included, was the most important determinant of the nature of the patient's response, where persistence of a deficit led to depression, hopelessness, and feelings of futility. Next in order of importance was the life situation to which the patient was returning. Premorbid personality was characterized as being "all important" but resisted classification that would predict whether a given patient would respond well or not.

Depression was described as reactive but differing from that seen in the usual psychiatric population. He found that the real problems confronting these patients often made it difficult to distinguish between appropriate feelings of despair, loneliness, etc. and depression attributable to the patient's premorbid personality. High on his list of reasons for psychiatric hospitalization of the stroke patient was depression secondary to aphasia. Other factors, not specifically related to aphasia, were antisocial behavior, inability to adapt to altered life circumstances, and latent psychosis precipitated by the stroke. Sexual sequelae, most particularly impotence, were found to be a reaction to psychological conflict, rather than the result of pathophysiological alterations.

Espmark's Study

Another formal study is that of Espmark (1973), published as a supplement in the *Scandinavian Journal of Rehabilitation Medicine*. Its limitations with regard to this chapter are that it pertains to a population of patients who sustained strokes before age 50, does not focus on aphasia specifically, and does not generally distinguish between those with left and right brain damage. The purpose of the project was to study the vocational and psychological adjustment of a group of 72 patients. It is worthy of study in that it systematically records psychological phenomena in both the early and long-term phases of rehabilitation (recording data collected as much as 8 years poststroke), engages the question of how to approach the study of the subject (i.e., "neurological–organic" versus "psychodynamic"), employs psychiatric interviews as a data collecting strategy, and studies coping processes. With respect to coping processes, the author concludes that the individual's manner of coping is determined by the integrated effect of premorbid personality, mental changes due to the lesion, and situational and social factors. The long-term emotional reactions were of great interest: 75% of a group of 52 patients were depressed, 63% had phobias or phobia-like reactions, 52% still expressed fears of a relapse, 13% experienced anxiety attacks, 12% reported jitteriness, 27% had feelings of inferiority, 12% manifested paranoid reactions, and 17% had sleep problems.

A Psychodynamically Oriented Report

In 1961 Friedman reported systematic observations of a group of aphasic patients in a group therapy setting over a period of 7½ months. He found that all of the patients expressed feelings of isolation, loneliness, sensitivity, and psychological impoverishment; almost all suffered feelings of lowered self-esteem that caused them to avoid and reject people, in fear of rejection. These feelings persisted even in the group therapeutic setting, from which they tended to withdraw. Behavior was generally regressive, as exemplified by the defensive use of dependency needs, projection, denial, and exaggeration of their deficits. The importance of language as a mechanism for exerting mastery over the environment was demonstrated in problems with reality testing experienced by these patients.

Horenstein's Review

Horenstein (1970) reviewed the effects of cerebrovascular disease on personality and emotionality, drawing attention to a number of important clinical phenomena that accompany or are the result of stroke. Of these, he singled out depression as representing a grief reaction—its existence and severity relating to the type and severity of the neural deficits, the patient's awareness of his illness, his premorbid capacity for adaptation, intellectual level, and feelings of self-worth. Horenstein notes, however, that the reaction is not specific to stroke but occurs with any catastrophic illness. Other determinants of severity and duration of depression are the personal and social situation of the patient—

for example, the loss of an accustomed role at home, in the community, or vocationally; the quality of family relationships; and the adequacy of plans for the posthospitalization period. Because of the importance of the severity and extent of neural deficits, Horenstein emphasized the therapeutic program as a practical means of combatting depression; to the same end, he stressed the need for careful and effective planning for the patient's future. The development of independence is paramount both for practical purposes and for its contribution to the patient's feelings of self-esteem. These observations are all particularly relevant to the patient with significant aphasia. In his review, Horenstein also considered denial of illness (or its manifestations) in a psychological context (distinct from the perceptual phenomenon). This reaction has been discussed by a number of authors (Baretz & Stephenson, 1976; Gainotti, 1972; Ullman, 1962; Weinstein & Kahn, 1955) and is often encountered in the patient with aphasia. Logically, it is related to the patient's prior personality; those who had difficulty facing reality in the past will surely react in the same way to problems posed by aphasia. Baretz and Stephenson (1976) see it as a necessary stage for many patients, serving the purpose of "buying time" as they struggle to adapt to their new reality but probably only temporarily staving off the depression that must inevitably come. Baretz and Stephenson and Horenstein call attention to the effect of denial in its various forms on the professionals who work with patients. We shall return to this in a later section.

Most of those who have written on the subject of denial explicitly or implicitly suggest the need for psychiatric help for such patients, particularly when the degree of denial interferes with rehabilitation progress or is clearly leading to a deep depression.

Horenstein (1970) includes in his review a discussion of the pseudobulbar state as possibly being confused with depression. In addition to inappropriate laughing and crying, there may be other symptoms, including a fixed facial expression, nonspastic articulatory and swallowing problems, partial mutism, and motor compulsions—all rather dramatic manifestations of anatomicophysiological aberrations and much more than one commonly sees with the aphasic, who cries easily when exposed to emotionally laden material, either happy or sad in content. The emotional lability of the aphasic patient does not have the distinctly "organic" flavor of the pseudobulbar state described by Horenstein. Indeed, he states that in almost all cases that have been documented there are bilateral corticobulbar lesions that are generally symmetrical and widespread. On the other hand, though the most frequent stroke lesion is unilateral, one does have the impression that there has been a loss of inhibition or control in the labile aphasic patient, suggesting a physiogenic process but reinforcing the concept that the left hemisphere plays a monitoring rather than a generative role in emotional expression (Lamendella, 1977).

Personal Reports

There is a fairly substantial literature consisting of the personal reports of people who have experienced aphasia that should be mentioned, not because these accounts contain the most pertinent information, but because it is appropriate to include material that may heighten one's awareness of the magnitude of the emotional devastation suffered by the person with aphasia.

Eric Hodgins (1964), a writer of great talent, is painfully successful in conveying his terror in the immediate poststroke period and the great frustration, panic, and despair that characterized his life in the months following his stroke. Guy Wint (1967), who was a journalist and historian and an excellent writer, succeeds in portraying a sense of utter desolation and isolation. One almost experiences his loss of the flavor of life, his fanatic need at first to find a cure for his illness somewhere in the world, and, failing this, his withdrawal into a gray, people-less existence.

Wint and other writers describing their aphasia (Dahlberg, 1977; Moss, 1976; Segre, 1976), mention memory problems. One has the sense that they are not talking about word-finding problems. Another recurrent report is the loss of the ability to dream (Moss, 1976; Wint, 1967), which has not been explained, to the best of my knowledge.

Wint's (1967) writing is so captivating that it can lead to unjustified generalizations. It is likely that his emotional reactions, though not rare by any means, particularly reflected his own personality. However, the loss of the ability to manipulate language in someone whose life was the written word, who was no doubt equally proud of his ability to discourse on subjects of great moment, must have been almost unbearable. This can lead to an appropriate generalization: that language is so much a part of the personality of each of us that its loss goes far beyond the practical inconveniences of impaired communication, whether mild or severe. We are verbal animals, and our capacity for communication is very likely inextricably entwined with both emotional and intellectual function. Lenneberg (1967) has made this point in part, suggesting that the biologic roots of language may reside in a person's emotional apparatus.

Wint appears to have possessed an unusual capacity for psychological insight and the ability to describe his feelings. His description of hallucinatory experiences (pp. 88, 89), including olfactory ones, gives one the impression that these are "organic" rather than psychodynamic in origin, that they are the result of sensory processes gone awry as a result of specific brain damage. This is in consonance with current thinking that attributes the psychoses to substantive changes in brain physiology (Smythies, 1970). The subject of hallucinosis and delusional phenomena has been well reviewed by Horenstein (1970); though, as with many other studies, the discussion does not pertain specifically to the aphasic patient. His review supports the impression gained from reading Wint (1967) that disordered sensory processes are probably responsible for hallucinations.

Returning to a review of personal accounts, there are two that refer specifically to aphasia (Moss, 1976; Segre, 1976) that should be noted. Moss was 43 years of age at onset and indicates that his aphasia was global in the early stages and secondary to a "permanent blockage of the left internal carotid artery." Both he and Segre placed a great deal of emphasis on the loss of intellectual ability (memory loss, concreteness, loss of the ability to abstract). Moss describes the inability to use words "internally" early in the course of his illness. Regarding emotional phenomena, he stresses the importance of premorbid personality; he apparently had struggled with feelings of inferiority prior to his stroke and found that he used the same compensatory behavior patterns after the stroke as he had before. He concludes that the basic personality does not change.

Segre (1976) does not give us a clear picture of the site of his lesion, although he mentions an embolus of cardiac origin, and indeed it is not certain that he was aphasic, though he probably was. Nevertheless, for our purposes there is an excellent review of his psychic and cognitive reactions early in the paper that includes many of the reactions that have been mentioned thus far. He draws attention to the importance of the attitude of the patient's family, that it be neither overprotective nor anxious, and states that when the aphasic is encouraged by family and others with an overly optimistic prognosis he may react with feelings of anxiety, depression, and the "complex of inferiority" when confronted with the reality of his situation.

One must be impressed with the aphasic's feelings of isolation and loneliness, of traversing a path unknown to the healthy, and of being unable to share the experience with anyone, primarily because of the impaired ability to communicate. Those of us who work with aphasic patients can probably serve them well by demonstrating our awareness of their emotional turmoil through verbalizing for them what they are experiencing. It is a clinical observation that patients prefer commiseration to expressions of optimism. If, in addition, as suggested by Baretz and Stephenson (1976), we employ strategies designed to help the patient live through his dark days, we will have discharged our clinical responsibilities consonant with the best principles of the healing arts.

Summary

Is it possible, then, to catalog the emotional concomitants of aphasia? To be sure, the material lacks the validity of carefully constructed prospective studies, but clinical imperatives suggest that some sort of summary is desirable.

In the immediate period postonset patients are often confused and apathetic, some expressing a kind of indifference ("I thought I might die, but it didn't seem to bother me"). There are some who are even euphoric during this stage. In many, this is rapidly followed by fear, to the point of terror, and anxiety. It is probably fair to say that, except in the demented, some degree of anxiety is universal. A variety of reactions may then ensue, depending upon previous personality characteristics to the largest extent but also upon the nature of the patient's close personal relationships, the personalities of his intimates, his financial and social status, and the availability of good treatment facilities and other support systems. These reactions will be modified by degrees of cognitive and perceptual loss as well as defects in the normal mechanisms of affective generation and control. They include:

1. Continuing anxiety manifested by one or more of the following: inattentiveness, insomnia, psychosomatic phenomena, phobias, obsessional states, or neurasthenia.
2. Depression, primarily as a grief reaction but reflecting premorbid inclinations in some.
3. Denial, which may be complete or manifest as overoptimism, withdrawal, or an inaccurate assessment of the dimensions of the illness.
4. Anger to the point of fury and assaultive behavior.
5. Loss of self-esteem, primarily based on premorbid tendencies.
6. Feelings of isolation and loneliness, often associated with listlessness and inertia; hopelessness; and futility.
7. Emotional regression manifesting as dependency, projection, exaggeration of deficits, reduced accuracy of reality testing, and withdrawal.

In a separate category, one must list the affective phenomena that are more or less physiogenic in origin; these may be modified by reactive factors, the reverse of the situation just described. They are emotional lability, paranoid and delusional states and hallucinosis, and frank psychoses including schizophrenia and manic–depression.

With the passage of time, there may or may not be a modification of these phenomena. As noted earlier, long-term data suggest that most of them can persist, outcome being dependent on a large number of variables.

About Treatment

Logically, treatment reflects what is known about the disorder to be treated. The material presented thus far suggests that the emotional concomitants of aphasia are more than likely primarily reactive in nature, either purely or in combination with physiological alteration of brain mechanisms subserving emotion, cognition, and perception.

Reactive responses to aphasia may be said to fall into roughly three categories: the normal reaction of an individual to an event that profoundly changes his or her life; a "neurotic" reaction to this event, reflecting a premorbid personality structure that is less capable of adaptation and/or prone to the expression of psychological distress through aberrant affective or psychophysiological manifestations; and a psychotic reaction, suggesting the presence of an underlying disorder that becomes overt as a result of the stress of the event (Lishman, 1973). These are ameliorated or worsened by the quality of the patient's interpersonal relationships as well as by other environmental factors (financial, community support, vocational and avocational opportunities if feasible, availability of adequate therapeutic facilities, etc.).

Whether or not the preceding is completely accurate, the patient's psychological reaction to the illness is one of the phenomena that may be capable of modification, and it follows that the participation of a psychiatrist, psychologist, or other competent psychotherapist would be highly desirable in every case. At the moment, this is probably somewhat utopian, but the spectrum of adverse emotional reactions is so broad and the incidence so high that it is difficult to escape the conclusion that psychotherapy is indicated. Were it not for the stigma that continues to be attached to psychotherapy, it is likely that either patient or family would demand it in every case as part of the therapeutic regimen, as they now demand speech therapy. That they do demand speech therapy is fortunate, since it is likely that one of the great virtues of speech therapy is its psychotherapeutic value.

Having made this suggestion, we must quickly refer to the injunctions of Eisenson (1973) regarding psychotherapy. Because the major vehicles of psychotherapy are language and intellect, if one or both are impaired, the patient may not only not profit from the process but find it a source of additional distress. Eisenson further suggests that people who would not have required psychotherapy premorbidly ought not to be so treated after having acquired aphasia. One can agree with this conclusion generally, but it is possible to adopt a broader view of psychotherapy to include supportive techniques, counseling for both patient and family, behavior modification techniques in selected situations, and group therapy—all of these beyond the usual analytically oriented techniques that are employed. In other words psychotherapy for the aphasic should be widely eclectic, reflecting the full range of psychological aberrations as well as the severity of aphasia in the individual patient.

If one uses the term PSYCHOTHERAPY broadly, it is fair to say that all health professionals who interact with the patient have an opportunity, and perhaps ought to assume the responsibility, to incorporate psychotherapeutic principles in these interactions. This is probably most true of the aphasia therapist and is undoubtedly widely practiced by experienced speech pathologists.

Continuing this same line of thought, the participation on the aphasia treatment team of someone trained in the psychological sciences is important for the guidance of the other members of the team. This is exemplified in the management suggestions of Baretz and Stephenson (1976) in their paper dealing with the subject of denial and depression in the disabled, which are clearly applicable to the patient with aphasia. They suggest that the psychiatrist (psychologist, psychotherapist) consultant can assist both staff and patient by helping to clarify the complex issue of what is realistic and what is unrealistic in expectations of recovery and benefits to be derived from treatment. The authors describe a number of practical management guidelines:

1. Provide information about the disorder to patient and family to allay fear, banish misconceptions, stress positive aspects, and provide the basis for a slowly developing recognition of the realities of the situation and a reasonable adjustment.
2. To staff, permit the patient to express unrealism during that period when denial is being used as a psychological strategy to avoid being overwhelmed by depression and frustration.
3. To staff, help the patient focus on function rather than recovery as a more realistic means of achieving independence, while at the same time allowing some expression of hope that there will be complete recovery.

4. To staff, try to build measures into the therapeutic regimen that will give the patient some sense of control and success.
5. To staff, beware of imposing personal biases on the patient.

Intrinsic to management suggestions is an accurate interpretation of the patient's reactions, something that often requires special knowledge and cannot always be appreciated by observing surface behaviors; this reinforces the need for a psychiatric consultant.

Another treatment philosophy, implied in the preceding, is the desirability of a "rehabilitation team," because the complexity of dealing with an aphasic patient requires people trained in different fields; professionals with training in medicine, speech pathology, psychology, and social work are basic for treating the patient with aphasia. Though this may pose problems in health care financing, it is clearly medically desirable.

It is one's hope that the participation of a multidiscipline team attending to all aspects of the problem will speed the development of independence, restore some of the lost feelings of self-esteem and dignity, and help the patient and family cope with the real decisions that must be made.

The use of drugs falls within the purview of the physician and need not be considered here. The dramatic case described by Robinson (1976), to which reference was made earlier, suggests an important role for drugs in some cases.

A Final Word

This chapter began with reference to the paucity of research in matters relating emotions and aphasia. This is understandable, for a "science of the emotions" is only now being born. In the meantime, clinical studies such as that of Gainotti (1972) are very helpful if certain ground rules are observed. One should strive for a pathologically and demographically homogeneous patient sample. The major groups that come to mind are patients with unilateral stroke (with the lesion in the distribution of one vessel only), space-occupying tumors, invasive tumors, missile wounds, head trauma with focal lesions (laceration, loss of substance, intracerebral hemorrhage, peridural hemorrhage), head trauma without focal lesions and with coma. The sample should, of course, exclude patients without aphasia.

There are limitations in studying groups because of the large number of variables even with a pathologically homogeneous sample. Personality patterns and genetic and socioeconomic factors, to name some of the most prominent sources of variation, make it difficult to generalize from statistically significant results, even when sophisticated statistical methods are employed. Though anecdotal evidence has always been suspect, careful in-depth study of individual cases can produce valuable information for clinical application. Lacking an animal model, research in human emotions has unique problems, and, until a great deal more is known about the physiology of emotional processes, as well as of communication processes, one must be content with approximations of the truth.

It will not be enough to identify the chemical and physical processes involved in this physiology; we have known a good bit about the chemistry and physics of the sensorimotor system for many years but still do not fully understand how that most basic of neural systems works. Emotion and communication are higher-order processes and therefore much more complex.

Another possible misconception concerning emotional processes is the idea that once their physiology is understood they can be easily modified. There must be a great deal of that kind of thinking in neuropharmacologic circles, but it may not follow that identifying the mechanism of an emotion will render it capable of such modification. The evidence is not conclusive that the psychological modification of behavior from without is permanently effective or that the end results are uniformly desirable.

These thoughts are presented as support for the idea that there may be merit in carefully conducted clinical studies that deal with observable emotional behaviors of aphasic patients, with the twin goals of learning more about their pathophysiology and developing more effective management methods. Among others, analytically oriented psychological techniques would appear to have a great deal to offer in the evaluation of the individual case and in selected cases requiring psychotherapy.

Although human emotions may be much more difficult to work with than measurable entities in the laboratory, the scientific method can be applied to them as to any other natural phenomenon.

To conclude on a clinical note, many workers with long experience in the management of patients with aphasia believe that eventual outcome in terms of meaningful rehabilitation is primarily determined by the patient's emotional state. The very best therapeutic efforts will be ultimately unsuccessful if the aphasic patient does not arrive at some point of reasonable adaptation to the disorder. If this be true, the emotional concomitants of aphasia deserve the most intense clinical and investigative attention.

References

Adams, J. H., Mitchell, D. E., Graham, D. I., & Doyle, D. 1977. Diffuse brain damage of immediate impact type. *Brain, 100,* 489–592.

Bard, P., & Montcastle, V. B. 1947. Some forebrain mechanisms involved in expression of rage with special reference to the suppression of angry behavior. *Research Publications, Association for Research in Nervous and Mental Disease, 27,* 362–404.

Baretz, R. M., & Stephenson, G. R. 1976. Unrealistic patient. *New York State Journal of Medicine, 76,* 54–57.

Bay, E. 1964. Principles of classification and their influence on our concepts of aphasia. In A. V. S. DeReuck & M. O'Connor (Eds.), *Disorders of language.* CIBA Symposium. London: Churchill.

Benson, D. F. 1979. *Aphasia, alexia and agraphia.* New York: Churchill Livingstone.

Benson, D. F. 1980. Psychiatric problems in aphasia. In M. T. Sarno & O. Hook (Eds.), *Aphasia: Assessment and treatment.* Stockholm: Almquist & Wiksell; and New York: Masson.

Brodal, A. 1947. The hippocampus and the sense of smell: A review. *Brain, 70,* 179–222.

Brown, J. 1977. *Mind, brain and consciousness: The neuropsychology of cognition.* New York: Academic Press.

Critchley, M. 1970. *Aphasiology and other aspects of language.* London: Arnold.

Dahlberg, C. C. 1977. Stroke. *Psychology Today, 2,* 121–128.

Eisenson, J. 1973. *Adult aphasia: Assessment and treatment.* Englewood Cliffs, N. J.: Prentice-Hall.

Espmark, S. 1973. Stroke before 50: A follow-up study of vocational and psychological adjustment. *Scandinavian Journal of Rehabilitation Medicine,* Suppl. no. 2.

Friedman, M. H. 1961. On the nature of regression in aphasia. *Archives of General Psychiatry, 5,* 60–64.

Gainotti, G. 1972. Emotional behavior and hemispheric side of the lesion. *Cortex, 8,* 41–55.

Geschwind, N. 1977. Behavioral changes in temporal lobe epilepsy. *Archives of Neurology, 34,* 453.

Goldstein, K. 1942. *After effects of brain injuries in war.* New York: Grune & Stratton.

Goldstein, K. 1952. The effect of brain damage on the personality. *Psychiatry, 15,* 245–260.

Goldstein, K. 1959. Functional disturbances in brain damage. In S. Arieti (Ed.), *American handbook of psychiatry.* New York: Basic Books.

Head, H. 1926. *Aphasia and kindred disorders of speech.* Cambridge: Cambridge Univ. Press.

Hodgins, E. 1964. *Episode.* New York: Atheneum.

Horenstein, S. 1970. Effects of cerebrovascular disease on personality and emotionality. In A. L. Benton (Ed.), *Behavioral change in cerebrovascular disease.* New York: Harper.

Jackson, J. H. 1932. On the nature of duality of the brain. In J. Taylor (Ed.), *Selected writings of John Hughlings Jackson.* London: Hodder & Stroughton.

Klüver, H., & Bucy, P. 1939. Preliminary analyses of functions of the temporal lobes in monkeys. *Archives of Neurology and Psychiatry, 42,* 979–1000.

Lamendella, J. T. 1977. The limbic system in human communication. In H. Whitaker & H. A. Whitaker (Eds.), *Studies in neurolinguistics* (Vol. 3). New York: Academic Press.

Lenneberg, E. H. 1967. *Biological foundations of language.* New York: Wiley.

Lishman, W. A. 1973. The psychiatric sequelae of head injury: A review. *Psychological Medicine, 3,* 304–318.

Luria, A. R. 1963. *Restoration of function after brain injury.* New York: Macmillan.

Luria, A. R. 1970. *Traumatic aphasia.* The Hague: Mouton.

MacLean, P. D. 1952. Some psychiatric implications of physiologic studies on frontotemporal portion of limbic system (Visceral brain). *Electroencephalography and Clinical Neurophysiology, 4,* 407–418.

Moss, S. 1976. Notes from an aphasic psychologist, or different strokes for different folks. In Y. Lebrun & R. Hoops (Eds.), *Recovery in aphasics.* Amsterdam: Swetz & Zeitlinger, B. V.

Ommaya, A. K., & Gennarelli, T. A. 1974. Cerebral concussion and traumatic unconsciousness. *Brain, 97,* 633–654.

Papez, J. W. 1937. A proposed mechanism of emotion. *Archives of Neurology and Psychiatry, 38,* 725–743.

Pribram, K. M. 1971. *Languages of the brain: Experimental paradoxes and principles of neuropsychology.* Englwood Cliffs, N.J.: Prentice-Hall.

Pribram, K. M., & Kruger, L. 1954. Functions of the "olfactory brain." *Annals of the New York Academy of Sciences, 58,* 109–138.

Robinson, B. W. 1976. Limbic influences on human speech. In Origins and evolution of language and speech. *Annals of the New York Academy of Sciences, 280,* 761–771.

Sarno, M. T. 1980. The nature of verbal impairment after closed head injury. *Journal of Nervous and Mental Disease, 168,* 685–692.

Schuell, H. M., Jenkins, J., & Jiménez-Pabón, E. 1964. *Aphasia in adults.* New York: Harper.

Segre, R. 1976. Autobiographical considerations on aphasic rehabilitation. *Folia Phoniatrica, 28,* 129–140.

Smythies, J. R. 1970. *Brain mechanisms and behavior.* New York: Academic Press.

Ullman, M. 1962. *Behavioral change in patients following strokes.* Springfield, Ill.: Thomas.

Weinstein, E., & Kahn, R. 1955. *Denial of illness.* Springfield, Ill.: Thomas.

Wepman, J. M. 1951. *Recovery from aphasia.* New York: Ronald Press.

Wint, G. 1967. *The third killer.* New York: Abelard-Schuman.

Ziegler, D. W. 1952. Word deafness and Wernicke's aphasia. *Archives of Neurology and Psychiatry, 67,* 323–331.

17

Recovery and Rehabilitation in Aphasia

MARTHA TAYLOR SARNO

At the first meeting of the Academy of Aphasia in Chicago in 1963, Arthur Benton aptly stated that the history of aphasia "begins at the beginning," for as long as humans have enjoyed the gift of language they have been subject to language disturbances through injury or disease. Informal attempts to "retrain" individual aphasic patients have probably occurred throughout history as a consequence of the seemingly natural inclination of humans to heal. Noting that language disturbances were of at least sufficient interest to physicians to be recorded as early as 3500 B.C. (Benton, 1964), Benton and Joynt (1960) cite some of the first recorded instances of both natural recovery and intervention. These include the patients of Nicolo Massa and Francisco Arceo in 1558 who recovered language completely after surgical intervention following head trauma as well as the work of Johann Schmidt (1624–1690), who reported on two apoplectic patients with language disturbances. In one case the patient recovered letter recognition, and in another case full recovery of reading skills was realized with training (Benton & Joynt, 1960). Professor Lordat reeducated himself in speech and writing until he resumed his chair of medicine at Montpellier, thereby providing support for his preconceived ideas about the dissociation of speech from thought. Later his auto-observations raised questions about whether he did, indeed, suffer from aphasia (Bay, 1969; Lordat, 1843).

In a paper published in 1904 (Mills, 1904), Charles K. Mills, founder of the neurology service at Philadelphia General Hospital, reported the training of a poststroke aphasic patient whom he and Donald Broadbent saw in a London Hospital and described in 1879 (Broadbent, 1879) and 1880 (Mills, 1904/1880). The training methods employed were largely

485

ACQUIRED APHASIA

determined by the patient, who began by systematically repeating letters, words, and phrases. Henry Head later commended Mills's work because it was not based on the more artificial methods of training then widely advocated and it acknowledged that the aphasic, because of prior experience and already organized brain function, presented a different teaching problem from the child (Weisenburg & McBride, 1935). Mills also described an experience retraining a 45-year-old physician whom he with T. Weisenberg and the patient's secretary systematically retrained at the patient's home over a period of 2 years. In this case the "physiological alphabet" designed by Wyllie (1894), essentially an articulatory–phonetic approach, was used as the basis for training.

Mills's paper is notable in that it discusses some of the methods used with aphasic patients at the turn of the century and shows concern with nonlinguistic aspects of the patient's rehabilitation management (i.e., emotional factors, premorbid intelligence, and education). He discusses the possible influence of semantic, lexical, and cognitive factors in recovery and suggests that different methods are appropriate for different patients and syndromes. He also noted that aphasia after trauma has a better outcome than after cerebrovascular accident (CVA) and that not all patients benefit from retraining to the same degree. He acknowledged that spontaneous recovery may influence the course and extent of recovery. Although Mills's work was done over a century ago, his observations and approach to aphasia rehabilitation are remarkably similar to much present-day practice and thought.

Although Bateman had suggested in 1890 that there was "sufficient evidence that re-education is a valuable means to re-establish man's noblest prerogative—the faculty of articulate language [p. 229]," Mills's paper was the first in English to address recovery and rehabilitation in aphasia. When the paper was published in 1904, there was a small German literature concerning the retraining of the aphasic patient.

During World War I several hospitals for the treatment of the brain-injured were established in various parts of the world, particularly in Germany. This occurred in spite of the fact that the treatment of aphasia was not popular among neurologists and securing their cooperation in establishing retraining programs was therefore difficult (Goldstein, 1942).

In Vienna Emil Froeschels treated approximately 2000 brain-injured patients between 1916 and 1925 (Schuell, Jenkins, & Jiménez-Pabón, 1964). Isserlin (1929) had a program in Munich, and Poppelreuter (1915) in Cologne. Henry Head's (1926) two-volume treatise on aphasia was based on his experiences in England with 26 posttraumatic patients, primarily the victims of gunshot wounds in World War I. Nielsen (1936) reported residual language impairments in 16 of 200 head-injured patients who were treated at Hospital #1 at Cape May from 1918 to 1919. Frazier and Ingham (1920), Gopfert (1922), and Franz (1924) also reported experiences retraining aphasic patients during this period.

Goldstein's extensive and intensive experiences in Frankfurt during both world wars, especially at the Institut Zur Erforschung der Folgeerscheinungen von Hirnverletzungen, provided one of the most comprehensive descriptions of the systematic treatment of approximately 2000 head-injured patients, of whom 90–100 were followed for a 10-year period (Goldstein, 1942). The Frankfurt facilities included a hospital, psychological laboratory, school, workshop, and research institute. Goldstein's work constitutes some of the most detailed early observations of attempts to retrain large numbers of aphasic patients (Goldstein, 1942, 1948).

Except for the Mills report (1904), knowledge of aphasia rehabilitation before World War II was based primarily on the literature that emerged from wartime experiences. There were only occasional reports of retraining poststroke aphasic civilians. Notable among these was the detailed description of Mills (1904), and in 1933, Singer and Low reported the case of a 39-year-old woman who suffered an apparent vascular infarct after a full-term delivery and showed continuous language improvement with consistent training over a 10-year period. Two years after onset, the patient's only verbal responses were the reiterative *o de—dar*, and she could neither read nor write. She reportedly used a vocabulary of 500 words freely and intelligibly with those who knew her well after 10 years. Autopsy findings 25 years later revealed complete absence of the hinder parts of the second and third frontal convolutions (Singer & Low, 1933).

During World War II several army hospitals established special programs for aphasic brain-injured soldiers, which provided a basis for the literature that began to emerge concerning recovery and rehabilitation. Programs were established at Percy Jones General Hospital in Battle Creek, Michigan (Sheehan, 1946), Halloran General Hospital in Staten Island (Huber, 1946), the Aphasia Clinic at the University of Michigan (Backus, 1945; Backus, Henry, Clancy, & Dunn, 1947), and McGuire General Hospital in Richmond, Virginia (Peacher, 1945). Eisenson (1949) reported on aphasic patients he studied at Halloran and Cushing General Hospital in 1947. At the Thomas M. England General Hospital in Atlantic City, Louis Granich, following the retraining model set forth by Kurt Goldstein, published a book-length report detailing the retraining of eight aphasic patients (Granich, 1947).

In England, Butfield and Zangwill (1946) followed the recovery course of 66 aphasic patients, the majority of whom were posttrauma. After reeducation, speech was judged to be significantly improved, both in patients who began therapy less than 6 months after onset (half of group) and in patients who began therapy more than 6 months after onset (third of group). The authors also reported that the best outcome was obtained in those with aphasia due to trauma rather than other causes.

Weisenburg and McBride's 5-year study concerned the general topic of aphasia without special reference to recovery, but the authors did comment on the effectiveness of reeducation in a study of 60 patients of less than 60 years of age, a majority of whom had suffered strokes. They concluded that reeducation increased the rate of recovery, assisted in facilitating the use of compensatory means of communication, and improved morale (Weisenburg & McBride, 1935).

One of the first comprehensive reports emerging from World War II was Joseph Wepman's book based on data obtained at the Aphasia Center of DeWitt General Hospital in Auburn, California. Wepman described the retraining of a population of 68 aphasic patients with a mean age of 25.8 years who began treatment 6 months posttrauma. He utilized training methods modeled after traditional language educational techniques. Aphasic patients made a gain of better than five school grades on language skills. It was Wepman's conviction that premorbid personality had a profound influence on outcome, and he concluded that aphasia after brain trauma is amenable to improvement with training. Specifically he found that expressive aphasics recovered the highest levels of language performance, followed by receptive and global aphasics (Wepman, 1951).

Luria (1948) reported the results of a large series of traumatic aphasic patients treated at the Institute of Neurology, Academy of Medical Sciences. He concluded that systematic retraining based on a careful analysis of the psycholinguistic breakdown and aimed at compensatory function provides the foundation for the successful restoration of verbal skills.

Until World War II aphasia and its concomitant neurological deficits in the stroke patient were viewed as a natural and necessary state in the aging process. The aphasic patient, generally elderly, could count on his extended family to meet his daily needs. In that era the civilian population did not consider treatment for aphasia as an option. Wepman (1951) drew attention to the large population of untreated civilians who, like the war veterans, could benefit from therapy.

Even in the period immediately following World War II, the word STROKE still carried the highly charged meaning "stricken by God," which surely delayed its adoption into everyday usage. In the preface to Wepman's *Recovery from Aphasia* (1951), Wendell Johnson used PARALYTIC STROKE to refer to those who suffered cerebrovascular impairment. Wepman also put quotation marks around STROKE.

Several historical factors stand out as having had an important influence in making the treatment of aphasia the common practice that it is today. These include the advent of speech pathology as a health profession, the emergence of rehabilitation medicine as a medical specialty, the mass media explosion, a larger and more affluent middle class, and a climate of increased expectations of medicine in an age of technology.

The latter has been particularly true in the industrialized areas of the world, where it is widely believed that there is a treatment for every human ill. Further, whereas talk of chronic disease was once considered taboo, it is now openly and widely discussed.

While social and attitudinal changes were taking place, the field of speech pathology grew rapidly. Membership in the American Speech and Hearing Association increased from 1623 to 35,000 in the period from 1950 to 1980. During that same period, the medical specialty of rehabilitation medicine burgeoned and is now an integral part of the health system.

Changing attitudes about chronic disease, the hope of modern medicine, and a more vocal lay press in the United States continued to sharpen interest in the subject of aphasia. Material appeared in the press about public figures who incurred strokes with aphasia, such as Sir Winston Churchill in 1953, President Dwight D. Eisenhower in 1957, and Ambassador Joseph Kennedy in 1962. In connection with President Eisenhower's stroke, Eugene J. Taylor, a medical writer long associated with Howard A. Rusk, wrote a series of articles that appeared on the front page of *The New York Times* describing stroke, particularly aphasia, to the lay public.

Several informational publications designed for use by the families and friends of aphasic patients also appeared in the post-World War II period (American Heart Association, 1969; Backus *et al.*, 1947; Boone, 1965; J. Sarno & M. T. Sarno, 1969b; Taylor, 1958; Simonson, 1971). One of these, *Understanding Aphasia* (Taylor, 1958), is still widely read in its original version and has been published in nine languages.

Workbooks, manuals, and other treatment guides for home use, as well as personal accounts by individuals who were aphasic after stroke, attested to strong public interest in the problem of aphasia. The treatment materials include Longerich and Bordeaux (1954), Taylor and Marks (1955, 1959), Keith (1972, 1977), Stryker (1975), and Brubaker (1978). Most notable of the personal accounts were those of Ritchie

(1961), Hodgins (1964), Wint (1967), Buck (1968), Moss (1972), Cameron (1973), Wulf (1973), and Dahlberg and Jaffee (1977).

After World War II the University of Michigan Aphasia Clinic (established during the war by Ollie Backus and Harlan Bloomer), the Speech Pathology Section of the Mayo Clinic under Josephine Simonson and Joe Brown, and the Speech Pathology Services of the Institute of Rehabilitation Medicine, New York University Medical Center, under Martha Taylor Sarno were among the few civilian programs where significant numbers of aphasic patients were treated.

Many programs at Veterans Adminstration hospitals, originally organized to treat traumatic aphasia, continued to provide service to stroke patients in peacetime. The Aphasia Section of the Neurology Service at the Minneapolis VA Hospital under Hildred Schuell is a notable example of a VA program that led to major contributions in the aphasia rehabilitation literature. Schuell and her colleagues studied an aphasic population of 155 patients, 75 of whom were available for follow-up testing; these patients provided a rich data base for Schuell's major publication (Schuell *et al.*, 1964).

Critical Factors in the Evaluation of Recovery and Treatment

Before reviewing the literature on contemporary methods and the value of treatment, it is essential to consider some inherent limitations in investigating treatment in aphasia. Chief among these is the question of what is meant by RECOVERY. No one disputes the idea that, at the least, RECOVERY refers to improvement in communication, but problems arise when one attempts to characterize RECOVERY in qualitative and quantitative terms. If complete recovery is to occur, it usually happens spontaneously, within a matter of hours or days following onset. Once aphasia has persisted for weeks and months, a complete return to a premorbid state is usually the exception.

There is often a discrepancy between a patient's perception of "recovery," performance on aphasia tests, and the clinical manifestations of aphasia. Patients show a wide range of interpretations of recovery. Most do not consider themselves "recovered" unless they have fully returned to previous levels of language competence (Yarnell, Monroe, & Sobel, 1976). When an unrecovered patient is content with his level of competence and considers himself "recovered," this is a psychological dimension and should not be confused with an objective evaluation of communication abilities.

Following this line of thought, it is reasonable and probably desirable to distinguish between two separate recovery dimensions: one that is totally objective and attempts to identify, as far as it is possible, whether the patient has regained his previous language abilities, and to what degree; and a second, which in humanistic terms may be more important, that measures the degree of functional recovery experienced by a patient. Few, if any, investigators have considered in their research this most relevant dimension of the patient's subjective perception of his "recovery." J. Sarno, M. T. Sarno, and Levita (1971) addressed themselves to a second recovery dichotomy and demonstrated that improvement in quantitative measures of language performance did not necessarily represent functional improvement.

If one wishes to do research on recovery and treatment, the problem becomes more complicated. Not only must one keep in mind the dichotomies noted, but difficult problems arise revolving around how one classifies patients, establishes levels of severity, and accounts for previous language competence, age, education, socioeconomic status, intellectual level, personality features, and, of critical importance, the therapist as a variable. The virtual impossibility of finding homogeneous groups of patients on whom to try a variety of treatment methods limits the validity of all studies. To further complicate the problem, it is now very difficult, if not impossible, to have a comparable control group of patients since it has become a cultural imperative in many settings that all patients have treatment.

These comments are not intended to discourage but rather to point up the factors that should be considered when designing research in this area. The student will do well to keep them in mind as he or she reads the aphasia literature.

It is clear that recovery and treatment are important topics. There are about 84,000 new aphasic patients in the United States each year, the majority of whom will demand treatment (Brust, Shafer, Richter, & Bruun, 1976). It is predicted that there will be 31 million people over the age of 65 by the year 2000 (U.S. Census Bureau, 1975, p. 25). Hence, it becomes increasingly important to establish scientifically valid treatment principles.

Studies on the Efficacy of Therapy in the Poststroke Aphasic Patient

In view of the limited literature on aphasia rehabilitation after stroke, those who pioneered attempts to rehabilitate civilian aphasic patients after World War II had to rely on knowledge obtained from experiences with earlier wartime casualties. Evidence emerged from the posttraumatic literature that suggested that (*a*) retraining was effective; (*b*) the posttraumatic aphasic enjoys a better outcome than the poststroke patient; (*c*) the early initiation of speech therapy enhances recovery; and (*d*) younger patients fare best (Butfield & Zangwill, 1946; Eisenson, 1949; Wepman, 1951). Eventually studies of the effectiveness of speech therapy with the post-CVA patient began to appear.

One of the first studies of reeducation in the poststroke population presented an analysis of 203 aphasic patients who received speech therapy and comprehensive rehabilitation services in a rehabilitation setting (Marks, Taylor, & Rusk, 1957). Aphasia was secondary to stroke in 93% of the group. Rehabilitation outcome was based primarily on clinical judgments of whether patients moved from lower to higher diagnostic or functional groups. Functional categories ranged from "institutional adequacy" to "vocational adequacy." The results supported the idea that there is significant functional benefit for aphasic patients who are exposed to language training in a rehabilitation setting, especially those with expressive aphasia.

In a retrospective study of 69 patients, Vignolo (1964) categorized patients into two groups: 42 patients received speech therapy and 27 were untreated. He concluded that there is a spontaneous evolution in the direction of recovery of function and that reeducation had a specific effect if it was adminstered for more than 6 months.

Sands, Sarno, and Shankweiler (1969) studied 30 treated poststroke aphasic patients in a rehabilitation medicine setting. Improvement in language function was measured by the Functional Communication Profile (FCP) (M. T. Sarno, 1969; Taylor, 1965), a functional rating scale. The median gain for all patients was 10 percentage points. Only three patients did not improve.

In another study (M. T. Sarno, Silverman, & Sands, 1970), 31 patients who were at least 3 months poststroke and classified as alert global aphasics were randomly assigned to three treatment conditions: programmed instruction, "traditional" speech therapy, and no treatment. Though the groups were equated for time since onset, there was a wide range of duration of symptoms in the sample from 3 months to 10 years poststroke. All patients showed small gains, but there were no significant differences in gains for any of the groups.

A. Smith (1971, 1972) studied 80 relatively young (mean age of 51.3 years) treated aphasic patients. Sixty-seven patients had a vascular etiology, and 13 patients were posttraumatic. Moderate or marked improvement in speech was noted in 55% of the group, in comprehension in 67%, in reading in 61%, and in writing in 54%.

Hagen (1973) studied the effects of treatment in 20 males with communication disorders after stroke, with a mean age of 52.6 years. Ten patients received therapy for 1 year, while the other group did not. Although both groups exhibited spontaneous improvement during the first 3 months, only those receiving treatment continued to improve beyond what is generally considered the spontaneous recovery period.

Basso, Faglioni, and Vignolo (1975) studied 185 subjects primarily poststroke; 91 received therapy (three sessions per week for 6 consecutive months) and 94 were untreated. The mean age of the group was 48.1 years. A positive effect of treatment on oral expression was reported even if undertaken 6 months after onset of aphasia.

Kertesz and McCabe (1977) reported findings on 93 post-CVA aphasics controlled for time since onset. The degree of improvement was greatest in the period between 1.5 and 3 months poststroke. Traumatic aphasics had a better overall prognosis than aphasics secondary to vascular disease. Where comparisons were possible, no significant differences were found between treated and untreated patient groups.

Levita (1978) compared Functional Communication Profile (M. T. Sarno, 1969; Taylor, 1965) results for 17 treated and 18 untreated aphasic patients. Treated patients received therapy during the period between 4 and 12 weeks postonset. No significant differences were found between the groups. The results suggested that patients who received traditional speech therapy could not be differentiated from untreated controls.

In a major treatment study of 162 treated patients and 119 untreated controls conducted in Milan (Basso, Capitani, & Vignolo, 1979), Basso and her co-workers addressed themselves to the relationship of time since onset, type of aphasia, overall initial severity, and presence or absence of treatment and improvement. A significant positive effect on improvement in all language skills was found for those patients who were treated. Some of the treated patients who began rehabilitation after the presumed spontaneous recovery period showed gains with therapy.

Specific Variables

Some investigators have focused on certain variables as particularly relevant to recovery from aphasia. This section identifies these and cites some of the studies that have drawn conclusions regarding their relative influence on recovery course and outcome.

SPONTANEOUS RECOVERY

There is general agreement that some natural recovery takes place in the majority of patients with or without intervention, and this is usually in the period immediately following onset. However, there is a lack of consensus about the duration of the spontaneous recovery period (Darley, 1970; Reinvang & Engvik, 1980; M. T. Sarno, 1980d).

Luria referred to a period of 6–7 months postonset as the time when spontaneous restitution takes place. Forty-three percent of his posttraumatic group showed residual signs requiring reeducation or psychotherapy after that period (Luria, 1963).

Culton (1969) found that rapid spontaneous recovery of language function as well as spontaneous recovery in intellectual function occurred in the first month following the onset of aphasia in a group of 21 untreated poststroke aphasic patients. These increases were not evident in the second month postonset.

Vignolo (1964), Basso *et al.* (1975), Kertesz and McCabe (1977), and Demeurisse, Demol, Derouck, deBeuckelaer, Coekaerts, and Capon (1980) concluded that the greatest improvement occurs in the first 2–3 months postonset. Butfield and Zangwill (1946), Sands *et al.* (1969), and Vignolo (1964) found that the recovery rate dropped significantly after 6 months. Some believe that spontaneous recovery does not occur after 1 year (Culton, 1969; Kertesz & McCabe, 1977).

Sarno and Levita (1971) studied 28 untreated poststroke patients with severe aphasia in the first 6 months poststroke and found that greater change took place within a 3-month than a 6-month post period.

Brust *et al.* (1976) surveyed 850 acute (first month post) stroke patients and found aphasia present in 177 patients (21% of the group) during the acute phase; 32% (N-57) were classified as fluent and 68% (N-120) as nonfluent. In the period 4–12 weeks poststroke, the aphasia improved in 74% of the patients and cleared in 44%. At 3 months poststroke, 12% in the fluent group and 34% in the nonfluent group were still considered impaired. In this study, the patient with fluent aphasia in the first month poststroke had the best chance of improving before the end of the spontaneous recovery period.

Lomas and Kertesz (1978) tested 31 aphasic stroke patients within 30 days (mean of 11.5 days) and at 3 months (mean of 97 days) poststroke. Eight language tests (i.e., yes–no responses, repetition and imitation, naming, Token Test, spontaneous speech in picture description and conversational questions, word fluency, sentence completion, responsive speech) were administered. Improvements on the eight comprehension, repetition, and expression tasks were documented for all aphasics, which supports the notion of spontaneous recovery in the first 3 months.

AGE AND RECOVERY

Generally speaking, reports of recovery outcome in groups of post-traumatic aphasics in wartime conclude that younger patients do better than older patients (Eisenson, 1949; Wepman, 1951). In peacetime, however, the largest number of patients with aphasia are those secondary to stroke, who usually fall into the older age group (M. T. Sarno, 1968, 1975; Schuell *et al.*, 1964). Yet some investigators have limited studies to younger aphasic patients. For example, in the now classic study of Weisenburg and McBride (1935), patients over the age of 60 were excluded "to prevent a picture complicated by senile changes [p. 119]."

Aphasiologists generally consider age an important variable in recovery outcome (Darley, 1972; Sands *et al.*, 1969; M. T. Sarno, 1976; Vignolo, 1964). However, the effects of age on recovery are not consistent (Basso *et al.*, 1979; M. T. Sarno, 1976; Yarnell, Monroe, & Sobel, 1976). Age is reported as both a decisive (Sands *et al.*, 1969; Vignolo, 1964) and weak factor (Basso *et al.*, 1979; Culton, 1969, 1971; Messerli, Tissot, & Rodriquez, 1976; Rose, Boby, & Capildeo, 1976; M. T. Sarno & Levita, 1971). Kertesz and McCabe (1977) found that younger patients had a higher initial recovery rate. The discrepancy in findings may be related to such methodological variables as sampling, the nature of the verbal measures used for assessment, and the procedures selected for data analyses.

In a study designed specifically to investigate the influence of chronological age on recovery in the adult poststroke aphasic patient, M. T. Sarno (1980b) concluded that chronological age had no effect on recovery on communication function. The results were based on data derived from 63 aphasic patients between the ages of 50 and 77 who were systematically followed for the first poststroke year.

TYPE AND SEVERITY OF APHASIA AND RECOVERY

Some investigations have concluded that patients with different types of aphasia syndromes recover differently. It has been observed that conduction and anomic aphasics have a good prognosis for recovery (Benson, 1970; Kertesz, 1979a, 1979b). In the Kertesz and McCabe study (1977), Broca's aphasics had the highest rate of recovery. The lowest rate of recovery occurred in the untreated global aphasic and anomic groups. There was a high correlation between initial severity and outcome. Lomas and Kertesz (1978) reported significant differences in recovery between different types of aphasia during the first 3 months poststroke.

Vignolo (1964) concluded that expressive disorders had a negative effect on recovery. In contrast, Marks *et al.* (1957) found that expressive type aphasics benefited most from speech therapy. Basso *et al.* (1975) found no significant differences in rate of recovery between Broca's and Wernicke's aphasics. Benson (1979b) and Kertesz and McCabe (1977) found that patients with mixed transcortical aphasia show little if any recovery.

There were no qualitative or quantitative differences between groups (fluent, mixed, nonfluent, severely nonfluent) in the study of Prins, Snow, and Wagenaar (1978), despite differences in severity. Using fluency alone as the basis for classification, there was a lack of differentiation among types of aphasia. Even though fluency had a high correlation with degree of severity, the pattern of change over the course of 1 year—that is, the relatively greater improvement in comprehension than in spontaneous speech—was the same for all types of aphasia.

Hildred Schuell (Schuell *et al.*, 1964) reported the best recovery in those patients whom she classified as Group 1 and the poorest outcome in the group designated as Group 5: irreversible syndrome.

In the M. T. Sarno and Levita study (1979), data were systematically obtained on 34 patients from 8 to 52 weeks poststroke. Fluent aphasics reached the highest level of functional communication and made the greatest gain (FCP overall percentage 36 points), whereas nonfluent and global aphasic patients made smaller gains (24 and 25 FCP overall percentage points, respectively). Prins (Prins *et al.*, 1978) found that some global aphasic patients recovered sufficiently to be reclassified as nonfluent.

To date, all investigators have reported that the more severe aphasias do not recover as well as milder forms (Kertesz & McCabe, 1977; Sands *et al.*, 1969; Schuell *et al.*, 1964). This finding has also been confirmed in studies where outcome in untreated global aphasics was compared to outcome in a treated group (M. T. Sarno & Levita, 1971; Sarno, Silverman, & Sands, 1970).

Sands, Freeman, and Harris (1978) studied recovery in a treated Broca's aphasic patient with speech dyspraxia by analyzing and comparing errors that prevailed in the first year poststroke with those manifest 10 years after onset. The features of place and manner improved, though voicing and addition errors persisted. (Errors of omission had virtually been eliminated.)

ETIOLOGY AND RECOVERY

It is generally agreed that posttraumatic aphasics recover more than patients with aphasia after vascular lesions. In fact, some cases of aphasia after closed head injury have been reported to recover completely (Kertesz 1979a; Kertesz & McCabe 1977). In the Kertesz series (1979a), some of the most severe instances of jargon and global aphasia occurred in patients with ruptured middle cerebral aneurysms. Kertesz (1979b) also noted that global aphasics after closed head injury may improve to a mild anomic state; a similar evolution is not observed in patients with vascular lesions with a similar degree of initial impairment.

In Schuell's series, the least recovery occurred in the most seriously impaired patient group (Group 5), which also had the highest incidence of complete thrombosis of the internal carotid and middle cerebral arteries and of the middle cerebral artery alone (Schuell *et al.*, 1964).

NEURORADIOLOGIC CORRELATES OF RECOVERY

Yarnell *et al.* (1976) systematically analyzed CAT scans in 14 aphasic patients up to 8 months poststroke and concluded that the size, location, and number of lesions documented by the scans showed a high degree of correlation with aphasia outcome. Those patients with large dominant hemisphere lesions, either one large or many small ones, fared poorly, whereas those with lesser lesions did better. Bilateral lesions, at times unrecognized clinically, helped to account for significant aphasia residuals. Bilateral, in part temporal, or large single-dominant hemisphere lesions correlated with acute severe global aphasic states. Fluent aphasics showed predominantly left posteroparietal lesions.

Kertesz (1979a) had similar CAT scan correlations for global aphasics in his study. He also reported that CT scans of patients reclassified as Broca's from global at 3–6 months had the greatest amount of temporoparietal damage (Kertesz, 1979a). Yarnell and his co-workers reported little prognostic value in angiographic and radioscintigram findings. CT scans did not help in predicting who might profit from language retraining in Reinvang's study (1980).

Pieniadz, Naeser, and Koff (1979) studied the relationship between CT scan hemispheric asymmetries and recovery from stroke in 14 right-handed global aphasic patients more than 7 months poststroke. Increased recovery in auditory comprehension was significantly correlated with atypical increased right occipital widths. The degree of right occipital width—more frequently observed in left handers in the LeMay (1977) control population—correlated $-.63$, $p < .02$, with Token Test scores (Spreen & Benton, 1969). The degree of atypical right occipital and atypical left frontal width asymmetries combined correlated $-.53$, $p < .05$, with naming ability on the Boston Diagnostic Aphasia Examination (Goodglass & Kaplan, 1972).

RECOVERY OF LINGUISTIC RULES

Ludlow (1977) used a taped sample of free speech and selected language tasks with 10 treated aphasics, 5 untreated aphasics, and 5 normal controls during the first 3 months post-CVA. The measures were administered nine times to each study subject. Analyses included a measurement of sentence length, an index of grammaticality, an index of sentence production, and a tabulation of transformations. In this study, the aphasic patients did not develop a new and simplified language system in connected speech but tended to recover the same structures used premorbidly. The relative frequency of the use of grammatical structures was similar to that of normal speakers. A common pattern of syntactic sequence was observed in the course of recovery for both treated and untreated patients. Ludlow noted no changes in language competence and concluded that recovery can be interpreted as an increase in the proficiency of language use (language performance). Further, there was no difference in the sequence of recovery with respect to type of aphasia (fluent and nonfluent).

Reinvang (1976) investigated sentence recovery in two aphasics: a 44-year-old man with Broca's aphasia secondary to stroke and a 73-year-old head-injured patient with Wernicke's aphasia. An analysis of spontaneous speech and tasks of sentence repetition and sentence judgment comprised the bases for his findings. Reinvang concluded that syntactically normal utterances were produced with regularity in the patients' speech samples and that an increase in utterance length was a dominant feature in recovery. The main form of deviant utterances were incomplete sentences.

RECOVERY PATTERNS

The idea that comprehension improves more than expression has been supported by a number of studies (Kenin & Swisher, 1972; Lebrun, 1976; Prins *et al.*, 1978; Vignolo, 1964). Recovery patterns of auditory comprehension are discussed in Chapter 8.

Vignolo (1964) noted that the receptive aspect tends to improve more than expression. In Vignolo's study, the initial level of auditory comprehension did not influence improvement in oral expression. Prins *et al.* (1978) analyzed, transcribed, and scored a taped speech corpus based on a linguistic paradigm, the Token Test, and a sentence comprehension test, on 54 aphasic patients (fluent, mixed, nonfluent, severely nonfluent) across the first year poststroke. The tests were administered at three specified time intervals (6-month intervals) in the course of 1 year. There was no overall clinical improvement in spontaneous speech in any group. On the sentence comprehension tests, all four groups did show considerable, significant improvement. There were no qualitative or quantitative differences among the groups in the course of recovery, despite the fact that the groups differed in severity of aphasia as well as on the fluency dimension.

Kenin and Swisher (1972) concluded that the greatest improvement occurs on imitative tasks and that auditory comprehension improves more than expressive language in nonfluent aphasics.

Lomas and Kertesz (1978) analyzed recovery patterns in 31 aphasic patients and found equal improvement on all language tasks for patients with good comprehension and more selective improvement largely in comprehension and imitative tasks for patients with severely impaired auditory comprehension.

Reinvang and Engvik (1980) concluded that the profile of linguistic impairment tended to be maintained during the 2–6-month period. Half of the patients showed a global impairment, and half showed a pattern of specific impairment. The most significant improvement was noted on oral language and a clinical rating of communication ability. Patients made only moderate improvement in writing. With regard to auditory comprehension, patients showed improvement in following commands, but there was not a significant agnosic or conceptual improvement.

In a small group of treated patients who were still classified as global aphasics at 3 months poststroke, the greatest improvement was noted in auditory comprehension and the least in propositional speech (M. T. Sarno & Levita, 1981).

TIME SINCE ONSET AND RECOVERY

In a retrospective study of the evolution of aphasia, Vignolo (1964) reported that as the time interval from onset increased, the number of patients improving decreased. Patients who received training for more than 6 months were compared with those who received training for less than 6 months, and the findings showed that the long-term group improved to a greater degree. Time since onset emerged as an important prognostic factor: 2 and 6 months from onset seemed to be important milestones. Sands *et al.* (1969) reported greater improvement in a group of patients who began treatment up to 2 months poststroke than in a group that started treatment after 4 months poststroke. The influence of early treatment on gains in language function were also demonstrated in A. Smith's (1972) study. Basso *et al.* (1975) found the least recovery in patients with the longest duration of symptoms.

Reinvang and Engvik (1980) reported a significant degree of improvement in the period 2–6 months postonset. Prins *et al.* (1978) noted

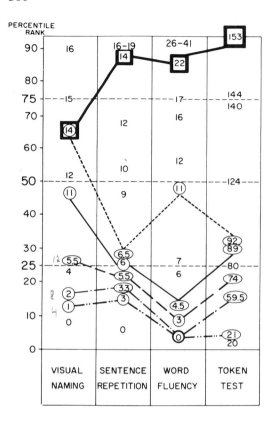

FIGURE 17.1. *Median raw scores for total group, Neurosensory Center Comprehensive Examination for Aphasia.* –··–·· = *4 weeks poststroke;* –·–·–· = *8 weeks poststroke;* – – – = *12 weeks poststroke;* ——— = *26 weeks poststroke;* ···· = *52 weeks poststroke;* ——— = *8th percentile rank normal.* [*From Sarno & Levita, 1979. Reproduced by permission of the American Heart Association, Inc.*]

significant time changes in spontaneous speech variables in the first year poststroke. Changes after the first year poststroke were noted by Marks *et al.* (1957) and Sands *et al.* (1969). On the other hand, Kertesz and McCabe (1977) reported little or no change after the first year.

In the M. T. Sarno and Levita study (1979), 34 treated aphasic patients were systematically examined during the first year poststroke. Patients were evenly distributed across fluent, nonfluent, and global diagnostic categories. Scores on the Neurosensory Center Comprehensive Examination for Aphasia (NCCEA) (Spreen and Benton, 1969) and clinical ratings on the Functional Communication Profile (FCP) (Taylor, 1965; Sarno, 1969) provided the data base. In the 4–8-week period, little change was observed on any of the measures administered. However, in the 12–26-week period, all diagnostic groups, particularly those designated as fluent, made gains on all measures.

As shown in Figure 17.2, fluent and nonfluent groups were similar in their performance and essentially equidistant from normal performance levels on the FCP at 12 weeks poststroke. Figure 17.1 shows changes over time for NCCEA subtests, where each graph shows the pattern of subtest performance at given time intervals. As was the case with the FCP it can be seen from Figure 17.2 that for the whole group performances generally improved during the 6–12-month period. The greatest changes on the NCCEA subtests from 6 to 12 months were made by the global group and the smallest gains by the fluent group, which was the reverse of the findings in the 3–6-month period. The most remarkable finding for this period was the magnitude of improvement on the Token Test achieved by the global group. In the all-inclusive period from 1 month to 1 year, the general trend indicated improvement in all areas.

The primary finding of the study was the persistence of improvement in all patients up to 1 year poststroke, which agrees with the long-term reports of other investigators and personal accounts of aphasic patients (Dahlberg & Jaffee, 1977; Moss, 1972; Sands *et al.*, 1969; Smith, 1971; Vignolo, 1964).

In spite of the fact that the global aphasic patients showed the greatest

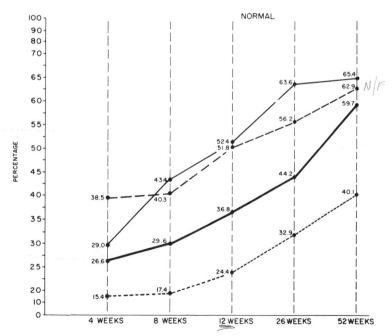

FIGURE 17.2. *Overall scores over time poststroke, based on median scores by group, Functional Communication Profile.* · · · · = *global;* —— = *fluent;* - - - = *nonfluent;* —— = *total group.* [*From Sarno & Levita, 1979. Reproduced by permission of the American Heart Association, Inc.*]

improvement in the latter part of the first poststroke year, these patients failed to evolve to another type of aphasia by the end of the year. No member of the global aphasic group exceeded a 40% overall FCP score. In contrast to the finding of Lomas and Kertesz (1978) and Kertesz and McCabe (1977), the group that showed the least change in the 3 months to 1 year poststroke was the nonfluent category. The discrepancy between changes observed on structured language tasks (NCCEA) and functional ratings was striking and is probably at least in part accounted for by extralinguistic compensatory mechanisms, not specific changes in linguistic processing. In this study, time since onset emerged as a potent variable in recovery.

PSYCHOSOCIAL AND OTHER FACTORS

A. Smith (1971) and M. T. Sarno *et al.* (1970) found no relationship between educational level, occupational status before illness, and recovery. In a retrospective study, Keenan and Brassell (1974) reported that health and employment had little if any prognostic value. Rose *et al.* (1976) found that sex, length of stay in a hospital, speech diagnosis, and presence of hemiplegia were not significant prognostic factors. In a study by M. T. Sarno and Levita (1971), individuals who were employed at the time of stroke recovered more than those who were unemployed. Subirana (1969) and Gloning, Gloning, Haub, and Quatember (1969) reported that left handers have a better prognosis for recovery than right handers.

Several aphasiologists have cited the presence of certain psychological symptoms, such as depression, anxiety, and paranoia, as factors that have a negative effect on outcome (Benson, 1979a, 1979b, 1980; Lebrun, 1980). Some have emphasized a patient's psychological state and premorbid personality as important prognostic factors (Eisenson 1973; Wepman 1951). The influence of fatigue (R. Marshall & King, 1973; R. Marshall & Watts, 1976), discouraging instructions, and nonverbal negative messages (Chester & Egolf, 1974) on task performance (Stoicheff, 1960) have also been studied.

Eisenson (1949, 1964, 1973) felt that patients with outgoing personalities are likely to recover more than those with introverted, dependent, rigid personalities.

SUMMARY

Until the early 1950s, the reeducation of aphasic patients was largely limited to wartime experiences. Since then, poststroke aphasic patients, who are genrally older than posttraumatics, have been seeking and receiving training. Reports of the efficacy of aphasia rehabilitation are generally positive. However, the limits of spontaneous recovery and the relative influence of many variables on outcome is still not definitive.

Approaches to the Treatment of Aphasia

The preceding section reviewed certain aspects of recovery and treatment in aphasia and the social and medical currents that led directly to the demand for aphasia remediation. This demand has grown steadily over the years, and with it there has been a proliferation of treatment methods. As noted earlier large numbers of aphasic patients have been treated, especially since World War II, in hospitals, rehabilitation medicine centers, and other facilities. The provision of speech therapy services is generally implemented by speech pathologists. As with aphasia classification and testing, therapeutic approaches have been based on theoretical concepts of the nature of language and pathology of aphasia. The following will outline some of the main currents in treatment.

Literally hundreds of specific techniques are cited in the literature. Aphasia therapy is rarely the same in any two treatment settings. This lack of therapeutic uniformity has undoubtedly impeded carefully controlled studies on the effects of language retraining (Taylor, 1964a). Most of these derive essentially from traditional pedagogic practices, relying heavily on repetition (Darley, 1975; M. T. Sarno, 1974, 1975, 1980a). For a detailed elaboration of therapeutic techniques, the reader will want to consult Chapey's volume (Chapey, 1981).

In general, treatment methods can be categorized as those that are largely stimulation–facilitation and those that are essentially direct–structured–pedagogic (Benson, 1979b; Darley, 1975; Kertesz, 1979a; M. T. Sarno, 1980a; Taylor, 1964a).

The two principles that underlie most treatment methods reflect contrasting views of aphasia as either impaired access to language or a "loss" of language. The stimulation methods generally follow an impaired access theory and pedagogic approaches are based on a theory of aphasia as a language loss.

Following a behavioral model, Luria (1963, 1966) put forth the view that aphasia treatment promotes the reorganization of the brain. He considered that both premorbid personality and differences in lesion might have an effect on this process and identified three types of restoration: (*a*) de-inhibition of temporarily depressed functions; (*b*) substitution of the opposite hemisphere; and (*c*) radical reorganization of functional systems.

Both Goldstein (1948) and Lenneberg (1967) felt that the aphasia therapist might help the patient compensate for impaired function. In fact, they suggested that compensatory adjustments were intrinsic to the hemeostatic tendencies of the organism.

In an experiment that focused on stimulating a patient's access to a lexicon rather than on the lexicon itself, Seron, Deloche, Bastard, Chassin, and Hermand (1979) found it more efficient to restore the access process rather than to restore specific lexical items, as in the traditional method. These findings were consonant with those of Holland (1970) and Weigel-Crump and Koenigsknecht (1973).

Stimulation–Facilitation Approaches

Wepman (1951, 1953) believed that the primary role of the aphasia therapist was to "stimulate" language in order to facilitate language performance. He suggested that the manner of stimuli presentation was of paramount importance and that it was not the role of the therapist to "teach" vocabulary or syntax. One technique he suggested was the presentation of filmstrips selected for individual patients according to their levels of interest and competence (Wepman & Morency, 1963).

Schuell and her associates (1964) also felt that the speech clinician's role was not as teacher, and they too developed stimulation techniques, especially in the auditory mode. They viewed the aphasia therapist as someone who tries to stimulate disrupted processes to function maximally and called language stimulation the "backbone of aphasia therapy." Basic to their approach was the notion that sensory stimulation is the only method available for making complex events happen in the brain.

Schuell's approach to aphasia rehabilitation was based on the premise that auditory processing impairments underlie aphasia. She stressed adequate stimulation, carefully controlled for length, rate, and loudness. She saw individual therapy as more effective than group therapy because of the individual differences among patients. Within this framework, one language modality is used to stimulate another in a program carefully graded for complexity. She stressed the importance of repetition and overt responses from patients, with a minimum of correcting or explaining on the part of the therapist. Schuell also considered the treatment atmosphere as important in its influence on a patient's self-esteem. She believed that establishing rapport with the aphasic patient is also an important treatment variable. The details of Schuell's rationale and approach to aphasia therapy are elaborated in her book (Schuell *et al.*, 1964).

Wepman held to the view that there was no specific formula to be followed in administering treatment for aphasia and that the efforts should be stimulating, indirect, and not focused on specific behaviors. He believed that therapeutic intervention should consider using topics known to be of interest to the patient in his premorbid life and should be elaborated largely through an increased focus on visualization. Wepman viewed stimulation as the core of therapy and objected to attempts to have the patient produce specific words or syntax. Whatever the patient produced should be accepted as "his best possible response at the moment" (Wepman, 1976).

More recently Wepman proposed the thesis that language is inextricably related to thought but not identical with it, that it is the product of thought and the servant of the highest human mental processing. He saw the process of stimulation in speech therapy as an "embellishment of thought," removing the implied criticism of corrective therapy and never asking for or trying in any way to elicit verbal expression (Wepman, 1976).

Wepman (1951) continued to reject the notion of aphasia as a specific speech or language disorder and interpreted the disturbance as a "disorder affecting the patient's total reaction pattern due to a disturbance of the integrating capacity of the cortex [p. 85]." His "indirect" stimulation approach was the natural result of his views on the nature of the disorder. He saw direct psycholinguistic attacks on the aphasic manifestation as most likely to become rigid language approaches and placed a premium on innovation, ingenuity, and individual creativity in therapy with aphasic patients.

In the case of patients with phonetic impairment, Wepman (1976) and many others (Millikan & Darley, 1967; J. Sarno & M. T. Sarno, 1969a, 1969b, 1979; Schuell *et al.*, 1964) have recommended direct methods of articulation therapy along traditional lines in which the basis is primarily imitation practice with visual and kinesthetic cues.

The possibility that linguistic principles might apply to reeducation in aphasia has been raised by a number of authors (Jakobson, 1955; Morley, 1960; Pincas, 1965; Scargill, 1964; Taylor, 1964b) who have presented a theoretical orientation toward language reacquisition in aphasia on the basis of what is known about neurological, linguistic, and psycholinguistic aspects of natural language. Ludlow (1977) reported a common order of recovery of syntactic structures in the aphasics she studied, which was unrelated to type of aphasia or whether or not patients were treated. She suggested that this sequence of syntactic recovery might provide a logical basis for a treatment regimen.

Using a programmed instruction approach, Naeser (1975) succeeded in showing an average 10% improvement in the production of three basic declarative sentence types in four male aphasic patients. Naeser also reported a carryover of 36% improvement in untrained sentences of the same type.

Wiegel-Crump (1976) studied two treatment methods (programmed and nonstructured) with the goal of increasing syntax retrieval. After 4 weeks of highly structured therapy, improvement in syntax generation did not generalize from specific items drilled on in therapy to additional nondrilled items. The level of improvement on nondrilled items did not significantly differ from the level of improvement on drilled items.

Weniger, Huber, Stachowiak, and Poeck (1980) also reported on a therapeutic regimen based on linguistic principles, which they concluded is superior to conventional methods.

Hatfield and Zangwill (1974) employed a picture story method in which the capacity of aphasic patients to communicate a sequence of events by drawing was explored. The underlying notion was that ideational processes in aphasia may be substantially intact in spite of severe defects in speaking and writing.

Luria (1966) used a "card index plan" to train a posttraumatic, mildly impaired aphasic who had difficulty in producing fluent narrative speech. The patient was trained to write down, on separate cards, fragments of the theme he was to relate and to speak from them. Luria's idea was that a defective internal system can be replaced by an external aid, and in this instance writing was used to facilitate speech.

Beyn and Shokhor-Trotskaya (1966) reported on the effect of a specific plan of therapy with 25 poststroke patients. They attempted to "prevent the appearance of some of the speech defects of aphasic patients which, up to now, seemed to be inevitable [p. 98], specifically "telegraphic style" of responses. They avoided teaching nominative words, teaching at first only simple words that could function as a whole sentence, such as *no, there, here, give, tomorrow,* and *thanks.* Only when words appeared spontaneously in a patient's speech were nouns introduced into therapy. These were never introduced in the nominative case but only in one of the other five Russian cases involving some inflection. "The results of the rehabilitation of active speech varied; but the most important fact is that telegraphic style, which is inevitable with other methods of rehabilitation, did not emerge in any of our patients [p. 104]."

Behavior Modification

The application of behavior modification principles to aphasia therapy is a good example of method following theoretical concept. It was perhaps inevitable than an attempt would be made to apply the work of B. F. Skinner to aphasia therapy. Let us first consider operant conditioning. The use of operant conditioning rests on the assumption that the desired behavior, or a behavior similar to it, exists in the patient's behavioral inventory and can be manipulated so that it will occur in a specifiable manner in response to a specific stimulus. The assumption is supported by several studies, although Lenneberg (1967) thought that aphasia was not a learning impairment and that conditioning procedures should not be effective in restoring language to a patient with a well-established aphasia.

Tikofsky and Reynolds (1963) found that conditioning occurred in aphasic subjects more slowly than in normal subjects. Goodkin (1968) reported that verbal perseveration and inappropriateness were altered in two aphasic subjects using a conditioning protocol. Lane and Moore (1962) successfully conditioned aphasics who could not discriminate between the phonemes /t/ and /d/.

M. Smith (1974) applied operant conditioning in a 32-year-old aphasic patient who was 6 months poststroke and a 65-year-old patient 11 months poststroke. Using an informal operant conditioning technique that did not require the patient to speak and a two-stage training procedure, the subjects were taught to use prepositions and word order to convey the nature and direction of a spatial relationship. The two patients learned to choose prepositions that correctly identified spatial relationships among objects. They learned a sequencing strategy that enabled them to arrange three word cards to describe an object display that they could not describe spontaneously. The experimental results suggested that conditioning techniques might enable nonlanguage mechanisms to solve, or help solve, language problems.

Holland (1969) discusses the nature of reinforcers and the need for careful attention to gradually changing either the topography of the behavior in question or to systematically altering the stimulus conditions in which the desired behavior is supposed to occur—the process of successive approximation in clinical application. A programmed instruction approach views language rehabilitation as an educative process and rigorously applies operant conditioning methods drawn from learning theory and principles drawn from psycholinguistic analysis to guide the content and order of presentation of the linguistic elements taught (Boone, 1967; Holland, 1969, 1970; Taylor, 1964b). It is based on the belief that there are several distinguishable stages of learning, including recognition, imitation, repetition of the model based on memory of the echoed performance, and finally spontaneous selection of a response from a repertoire of learned responses.

Several experiments requiring aphasics to perform a variety of tasks on automated devices have suggested that even severely impaired aphasics can learn to match visual configurations, to perform visual oddity tasks, and to write their names. Rosenberg (1965) used automated training procedures in an experiment designed to assess and train aphasics to make perceptual discriminations basic to reading. The programs were effective in teaching certain discriminations as well as in increasing the rate of response and retention of the material. Edwards (1965) investigated differential responses to tasks involving the matching of visual stimuli by more than 100 severely impaired aphasics and found that all but 4 of the patients successfully completed the program. In still another study, Filby and Edwards (1963) taught form discrimination to 12 severely impaired aphasics and 10 normal subjects. In the optimal learning conditions of the experiment, the aphasic group did not differ significantly from the controls and also did not exhibit catastrophic reactions or other forms of disruptive responses.

Holland and Levy (1971) have expressed the view that aphasics learn by having consequences applied to their behavior and that the clinician's primary concern should be to screen subject matter and control reinforcement. Making this possible is the outgrowth of operant conditioning called programmed instruction. Based on the premise that aphasic patients need smaller steps, more than an average number of repetitions, and a more systematically structured teaching procedure (Taylor, 1964a; Taylor & Marks, 1959; Taylor & Sands, 1966), the technology of programmed instruction lends itself to experimentation with these patients.

Holland and Sonderman (1974) attempted to teach 24 aphasic patients tasks from the Token Test in a programmed approach. Patients had a mean age of 54.45 years and a mean time since onset of 5.6 years. All exept two head trauma patients had aphasia secondary to CVA. Patients were rated on a severity scale as follows: 4 mild, 6 mild-moderate, 5 moderate, 3 moderate-severe, and 6 severe. They were divided into low and high groups according to Token Test scores. The mild and mild-moderate patients demonstrated significant improvement as a result of training, whereas the moderate and severe patients did not. In addition, the high group was more receptive than the low group to the program. Training was most effective for those who initially did well; however, no patient was error free. In general, the patients did not easily transfer language skills acquired in the program to similar untrained tasks.

In a kind of revamping of a traditional approach, Weigl (1961) developed an approach to therapy called DEBLOCKING, which is based on the factor of context. It is essentially a systematic use of a patient's intact modalities. For example, if a patient is having trouble with auditory recognition, he may be helped in his recognition of a given word by having prestimulation with the same stimulus through the visual channel. Deblocking seems to be naturally in tune with clinical approaches that build new responses upon a patient's most intact language skill. The clearest clinical description of deblocking therapy is the longitudinal single-case report of Ulatowska and Richardson (1974), which provides a detailed description of the use of a deblocking technique to reintegrate the mechanisms for correlating sound and meaning in an aphasic patient with a severe impairment of auditory comprehension. The visual mode of presentation of linguistic material was used both to provide a stable representation of speech units and to allow reinforcement of auditory representations. The patient was given tasks of repetition, reading aloud, and sequencing, using progressively more complex material.

Treatment of the Patient with Speech Dyspraxia

The disorder of articulation referred to as speech dyspraxia seldom, if ever, is manifest in the absence of a coexisting Broca's aphasia, however mild. The speech dyspraxic component of this multifaceted communication disorder appears to be especially amenable to direct therapeutic intervention using approaches adapted primarily from the traditional articulation therapy techniques, including stress and intonation drills. These approaches designed to improve phonemic accuracy typically depend on imitation, progressive approximation, phonetic placement, and stress, which are drilled using kinesthetic, visual, and auditory cues. Generally, the stimuli used as the bases of exercises are selected in a presumed order of difficulty, beginning with nonoral imitation, followed by sounds, words, and finally utterances.

The techniques have been specified by many clinicians (Deal & Florance, 1978; Halpern, 1981; Rosenbek, 1978; Rosenbek, Lemme, Ahern, Harris, & Wertz, 1973; Wiedel, 1976). Various rhythmic techniques in which the patient generates the rhythm have also been reported as facilitory methods to increase articulation accuracy (Rosenbek, Hansen, Baughman, & Lemme, 1974; Schuell *et al.*, 1964; Yoss & Darley, 1974). In contrast, Shane and Darley (1978) found that articulation precision tended to deteriorate under externally imposed rhythmic stimulation. Melodic intonation therapy and Amerind have also been employed as facilitory techniques in the treatment of the patient with speech dyspraxia (see following sections).

In the Sands *et al.* study (1978), the phonemic errors made by a Broca's aphasia patient with speech dyspraxia who received speech therapy for 10 years were analyzed and compared. They reported that speech therapy had been effective in improving place and manner production and had virtually eliminated omission errors.

Visual Communication Therapy (VIC)

Visual communication therapy (VIC) (Gardner, Zurif, Berry, & Baker, 1976) is an experimental technique designed for the global aphasic. It follows earlier work done by Premack (1971), who reported an experiment in which a chimpanzee was taught a simple communication system, and Velletri-Glass, Gazzaniga, and Premack (1973), who trained global aphasic patients to use an artificial language system using cut out paper symbols. VIC employs an index card system of arbitrary symbols representing syntactic and lexical components. Patients learn to recognize the symbols and manipulate them so as to (*a*) respond to a command; (*b*) answer a question relative to the circumstance; (*c*) describe actions; or (*d*) express needs, wishes, or other emotions. The system attempts to circumvent the use of natural oral language, which is so severely impaired in the global aphasic patient.

The program included two levels of communicative functions. At Level 1, patients carry out commands, answer questions, and describe actions; at Level 2, they employ the system spontaneously to express desires and feelings. Of eight patients given sufficient opportunity to master VIC, five completed Level 1, and two of these also satisfied the criteria for Level 2. Among these five patients, performance in VIC far surpassed performance on matching tasks in English, error rates were quite low, and the pattern of errors was remarkably similar. An inverse correlation was obtained between ability in English and in the use of VIC.

The authors concluded that the evidence supports the notion that some severely aphasic patients can master the basics of an artificial language. Moreover, several indexes suggested that the communication effectiveness of the system was appreciated and that some of the cognitive operations entailed in natural language are preserved despite severe aphasia.

In personal communication with these experimenters, they have expressed the idea that the method may have greater relevance as a means of exploring residual mental function in global aphasics than as a system of therapy.

Melodic Intonation Therapy (MIT)

Sparks, Helm, and Albert (1974) have elaborated a programmed therapeutic regimen called melodic intonation therapy (MIT) based on the observation that language that is unavailable in spontaneous speech can sometimes be produced in association with a sung melody. The system presumes an intact right hemisphere, thought to be the locus of melodic production. It proceeds on the assumption that functional language can be developed if it is "taught" in association with rhythm and melody. In a series of carefully graded steps, the therapist slowly introduces melody, rhythm, and verbal content, gradually including the patient in the process and eventually leaving the patient as the sole "performer."

The MIT program uses a number of probability phrases and sentences that are sung instead of spoken. The first level of the program includes the following five steps:

1. The clinician begins by singing (intoning) the target phrase to the patient. No response is required.
2. The clinician and the patient sing the phrase in unison.
3. The clinician and the patient sing the initial part of the phrase in unison, but about the halfway point, the clinician fades out and the patient completes the phrase alone.
4. The patient repeats the sung phrase after the clinician.
5. The patient sings the target phrase in response to a question that is sung by the clinician.

In this procedure the patient's hand is held by the clinician, who taps out each syllable in a rhythmic fashion.

In the experience of the authors, success is more likely in patients who have good auditory comprehension, facility for self-correction, markedly limited verbal output, reasonably good attention span, and good emotional stability (Helm, 1976; N. Marshall & Holtzapple, 1976).

Visual Action Therapy (VAT)

Visual action therapy (VAT) was designed and tested in a pilot study at the Boston Veterans Administration Medical Center (Helm & Benson, 1978). The goal of the technique is to train the global aphasic patient to associate ideographic forms with specific objects and actions. Using real objects (e.g., cup, razor) and following rigorously specified steps, the patient is taught to appreciate the symbolic representation of drawings and gestures and later to produce symbolic gestures.

Amerind

In an attempt to utilize systematized gestural language to facilitate oral production, Skelly, Schinsky, Smith, and Fust (1974) have modified

American Indian sign language in a method that combines gestural sign with oral speech production (Amerind). The technique was systematically studied in six patients with long-standing severe speech dyspraxia (cortical dysarthria). Three of the six patients progressed to two-word sentences and another to single-word usage. The sixth patient remained unable to speak intelligibly.

Summary

It will be appreciated that it is not possible to summarize or synthesize the foregoing review of therapeutic approaches. Clearly each is based upon theoretical concepts of the nature of aphasia and its remediation. Until the definitive physiology of communication has been described, there is no recourse but to continue the process of experimentation, and clinicians should adopt the system with which they are most comfortable.

It is probably appropriate that there have been few studies comparing treatment methods in view of the seemingly insurmountable methodological problems associated with such research and our present state of knowledge. Though we cannot be certain of the basis for therapy, there are large numbers of patients requiring management.

The following section represents an approach to that problem.

Toward a Comprehensive Approach to Aphasia Rehabilitation

A critical factor in aphasia rehabilitation is the fact that once the condition is stabilized very few patients recover normal communication function, with or without speech therapy. This unfortunate reality requires that aphasia rehabilitation be viewed as a process of patient management in the broadest sense of the word, for the task then becomes primarily one of helping the patient and his intimates adjust to the alterations and limitations imposed by the disability. Many experienced clinicians have addressed themselves to this probelm, citing a variety of contributory factors. These include the type and severity of the aphasic deficit, physical disability, premorbid personality patterns, cognitive status, time since onset, cultural and educational background, associated neuropsychological deficits, and general physical condition (Benson, 1979b; Darley, 1970, 1972, 1975; Eisenson, 1973; Reinvang, 1980; M. T. Sarno, 1980a; Schuell *et al.*, 1964; Wepman, 1951). This complexity suggests that effective rehabilitation requires the participation of a variety of disciplines, including medicine, psychology, physical and occupational therapy, social work, vocational counseling and, most critical, aphasia therapy. Any therapeutic setting providing all of the necessary services can implement an effective program. In this regard the advent of rehabilitation medicine as a speciality has been fortuitous, for it provides a well-organized setting in which all these services can be mobilized for the benefit of the aphasic patient. The greatest responsibility in this process falls to the aphasia therapist. We shall return later to a description of how the therapist works with an aphasic. Let us first look at the patient and catalog some of the important clinical–behavioral features of the disorder.

The Aphasia Patient

Ullman (1962) observed that the variability of psychological reactions is rarely determined by the type or location of the lesion but is an expression of the whole life experience of the person who has had a stroke. Regarding this Ullman wrote:

> ... the need to focus not on an abstract appraisal of psychopathological patterns but on understanding the current life situation and the consequent meaning of the stroke to the patient at this particular moment in his life. Repeatedly one gets the feeling in talking with these patients that had the stroke occurred a year or two earlier or a year or two later, their reactions would have been quite different. At times it climaxes a process of resignation and surrender set in motion years before; at other times it initiates such a process. In some patients it touches off a last-ditch stand dedicated to the pursuit of unattained life goals and ambitions. Occasionally it opens up new vistas for the elaboration of secondary gain from illness. Unrealistic strivings for independence and unrealistic dependency are perhaps the two main channels into which irrational modes of adaptation flow [From Ullman, M. 1962. *Behavioral Changes in Patients following Stroke.* Courtesy of Charles C Thomas, publisher, Springfield, Illinois.]

In a study of aphasic patients participating in a group psychotherapy program, Friedman (1961) investigated the nature of psychological regression in aphasia. Beyond the communication difficulties posed by aphasia, Friedman observed that each patient remained psychologically an individual island. Patients did not maintain a consistent level of group participation and expressed intense feelings that they were very different from other people. Both withdrawal and projection were apparent as each patient acted in isolation and yet complained of this characteristic in others. His study suggested that aphasia can result in regressive behavior with impaired reality testing. Patients made a defensive use of dependence, as manifested in a recurring demand that they be given more help by the therapist and preferably in smaller groups where individualized attention would be provided (Friedman, 1961).

The work of Ullman and Friedman provides some insight into the magnitude and complexity of the psychological and social consequences of aphasia. Responding to this, individual psychotherapy (Aronson, Shatin, & Cook, 1956; Blackman, 1950) and family counseling (Linell & Steg, 1980; Malone, 1969; J. Sarno & M. T. Sarno, 1979) have been suggested to alleviate these aspects of the problem.

An effective management tool is the selective and discriminating use of speech therapy to stimulate and support the patient through the various stages of recovery (Brumfitt & Clarke, 1980; M. T. Sarno, 1980a; Tanner, 1980). The experienced therapist recognizes that while working on a specific communication deficit he is simultaneously dealing psychotherapeutically with a readjusting personality (Wepman, 1951). Hence, speech therapy serves different purposes at different points along the way. Sometimes it allows the patient to "borrow time," as Baretz and Stephenson (1976) have aptly stated. Other times it helps him to a realistic assessment of language capacity, which he needs at that moment. Occasionally depression lifts after speech therapy has been initiated, reflecting the supportive and nurturing nature of the therapeutic relationship rather than an objective improvement in speech (Ullman, 1962).

Viewed in this way, aphasia rehabilitation can be understood as a dynamic process consisting of a series of stages through which the majority of patients evolve. Some of course, never emerge from the first stage and remain severely depressed (Espmark, 1973).

In her classic characterization of the stages of death and dying Elizabeth Kubler-Ross (1969) provides a model that can be applied to the reactions to loss manifested by the aphasic patient. She specified five stages: denial and isolation, anger, bargaining, depression, and acceptance. Both real and symbolic loss can be experienced by aphasic patients. Loss of the ability to communicate has real meaning because speech is such a vital human function. But aphasics may experience symbolic loss as well because of altered perceptions of their familial, social, and vocational roles.

The perception of loss leads to grief, which is not a single reaction but a complex progression involving many emotions and attempts to adjust to and cope with loss. A number of authors have suggested a sequence of phases in grieving. Engle (1964) listed shock and disbelief, awareness, and restitution–recovery. Schneider (1974) suggested that the stages proposed by Kubler-Ross and other authors could be categorized as attempts to overcome loss, which include denial, rage, and bargaining;

awareness of the loss; and acceptance of the loss. The stages of grief are universal but many vary with respect to their order and progress. Those who make an adequate adjustment have passed through all stages.

Based on all the above, one may postulate three stages through which the aphasic patient passes: depression–denial, anger, and adaptation. In the first stage patients usually withdraw from friends and social situations. Some patients experience a vague, dreamlike state, with a lack of interest in surroundings and no apparent concern over what has happened. They may be lethargic, often complaining of chronic fatigue and manifesting the universal signs of helplessness. They often make unrealistic plans based on complete recovery, set deadline dates for recovery, or otherwise stall for time while the depression resolves. Health professionals are generally unaccepting of these behaviors and tend to express anger at the patient's "unrealistic attitude," reflecting their own biases and needs for success. As a consequence of these dynamics, therapists are not generally kindly disposed to patients who are preoccupied, self-involved, or seclusive, or who express hopeless attitudes.

Speech therapy can serve an important purpose during this stage. By directly addressing the patient's linguistic deficits and channeling attention and energies toward constructive ends, speech therapy may produce a noticeable reduction in depression. Speech therapy, in this instance, acts as an equivalent for work, which has long been recognized as an antidote for depression. The title of a chapter written in a personal account of a stroke patient (Wulf, 1973), "My Lifeline to Sanity, The Marvels of Speech Therapy," is a testament to the positive psychological impact of speech therapy.

In his *Autobiographical Considerations on Aphasia Rehabilitation,* Renato Segre suggests that there is value in allowing the aphasic patient to delay speaking and to economize on the length and complexity of utterances. He says, "It is important not to interrupt these resting periods because they represent a defense and compensation measure... some aphasics enjoy their verbal silence. It is a kind of spiritual rest, of quiet criticism of other people's opinions; a kind of personal formula to reach a better optimism [Segre, 1976, p. 136]."

In the second stage, the expression of anger that the severely impaired patient originally internalized—in particular, the expression of anger by nonverbal means—may be difficult to interpret. Some patients act out physically or precipitate confrontations with family or staff members. During this stage the patient is particularly difficult to manage. By understanding this phase as a natural and necessary part of the recovery course, those around the patient can continue to provide a supportive environment.

The third and last stage is a period of adaptation that continues for the remainder of the patient's life. It is in this period that the patient mobilizes and brings to bear all his strengths and begins to compensate for deficits. In the poststroke patient, the pattern of linguistic impairment is generally stabilized by 1 year, and, although some improvement may continue indefinitely beyond this period, full recovery is rare if not achieved by this time.

There is a great tendency to overestimate the capacity of an aphasic to return to work, particularly if the verbal deficits are mild. If the patient's work depends upon cognitive and verbal skills, even at fairly low levels, great caution should be exercised since it is impossible to correctly evaluate a patient's performance except on the job and premature attempts to return to work may be psychologically devastating. Generally, it is advisable to postpone such plans for as long as possible.

The process of finding acceptable vocational alternatives is very difficult and time consuming and often unsuccessful. Vocational counseling is frequently best employed to help the patient adjust to the reality of his problem. A professional rehabilitation counselor is best equipped to do this and to carry out the long and arduous process of evaluating work performance and job requirements for those patients for whom an alternative vocation is feasible.

Many experienced aphasia clinicians have stressed the importance of the patient's family in the rehabilitation process (Boone, 1967; Godfrey & Douglass, 1959; Malone, 1969; J. Sarno & M. T. Sarno, 1979; Schuell *et al.*, 1964; Wepman, 1951). Some of the potentially negative reactions of the family include overprotectiveness, hostility, anger, unrealistic expectations, overzealousness, lack of knowledge of the dimensions of the disorder, and inability to cope with practical difficulties. Also, the apparently natural tendency of family members to minimize the patient's communication impairment, particularly in the early stages of recovery (Buxbaum, 1967; Helmick, Watamori, & Palmer, 1976; M. T. Sarno, 1971), requires understanding and management.

In general, the quality of premorbid relationships tends to be intensified in the aftermath of a catastrophic event; those that were problematic may deteriorate further, whereas the bond between a loving couple, for example, often becomes stronger. The reversal of roles, changes in levels of dependency, and a changed economic situation, which is so often a consequence of chronic disability, can have a critical negative impact on the patient and his family. One must utilize all available resources in negative situations to minimize deleterious effects on the patient. Formal programs designed to educate and counsel have been reported and strongly support the need for similar programs as an integral part of the service provided by agencies that treat aphasic patients (Boone, 1967; Crewe, 1969; Derman & Manaster, 1967; Newhoff & Davis, 1978; Rolnick, 1969; Strauss, Burrucker, Cicero, & Edwards, 1967; Turnblom & Meyers, 1952; Watzlawick & Coyne, 1980).

In a positive family milieu, the patient is encouraged to develop a regular daily routine as close to his premorbid pattern as possible and is treated as a contributing member of the family. He is allowed to progress at his own speed, and the family facilitates participation in avocational activities that suit the patient's interests and abilities. A great deal of patience, understanding, and information are essential to achieve these difficult goals.

Experience suggests additional guidelines. Patients need to be allowed some sense of control. Allowing them to participate in some of their own rehabilitation planning helps to restore feelings of self-worth. In this regard, the emphasis on function rather than complete recovery, pointing up success rather than performance failure, adds to the patient's sense of himself as a person (Baretz & Stephenson, 1976; Tanner 1980).

It is essential to listen to the patient, particularly to his expressions of loss. Commiseration is often more comforting than optimistic prognostic statements.

In an analysis of the frequency of individual speech therapy sessions in a rehabilitation medicine setting, the amount of treatment ranged from three to five sessions per week in the first 3 months poststroke, with over half of the patients receiving inpatient services. Except for the very severe, who were also physically disabled, patients tended to become outpatients after 3 months, and by the end of 6 months all patients were outpatients. The frequency of fluent and nonfluent patients receiving daily speech therapy decreased significantly, while the majority of the global patients continued to receive daily speech therapy. By the end of the first year poststroke, all patients were receiving from two to three individual sessions weekly (M. T. Sarno & Levita, 1979).

Group speech therapy, stroke clubs, and other social groups are techniques frequently employed to good effect in the management of some patients with chronic aphasia. They generally serve their best function after the acute and spontaneous recovery periods, when the patient is more aware of his deficits and less preoccupied with symptoms. By this time the patient may be more interested in and capable of interacting with others and can gain support by sharing feelings with those who have gone through the same experience. Knowledge that one is not alone often helps to reduce depression and loneliness (Benson, 1979a; M. T. Sarno, 1980a). Group therapy also provides a permissive

atmosphere with peers where patients can meet new friends and venti-
late feelings. Not all aphasic patients can benefit from group therapy. A
positive effect seems related to level of comprehension, time since onset,
and personality factors. While group therapy plays an important role in
aphasia rehabilitation, it should be noted that its effectiveness is dependent on the skill of the group leader. Since group dynamics can be
volatile and emotionally loaded, the inexperienced, untutored aphasia
therapist would do best to avoid this therapy format.

The foregoing briefly describes a philosophy of rehabilitation that
takes into account the broad spectrum of problems and residuals presented by aphasic patients. It is based primarily on experiences with the
poststroke patient. However, the principles apply as well to the closed
head injured aphasic patient, with some exceptions regarding the recovery timetable. The picture is somewhat more complicated in that the
closed head injured patient often presents a greater number of behavioral, cognitive, and perceptual deficits, and he is generally younger,
posing a great many problems that do not exist in the elderly aphasic (M.
T. Sarno, 1980c).

The late Hildred Schuell (Schuell *et al.*, 1964) had great concern for
the humanitarian aspects of aphasia rehabilitation. Some of her
thoughts are an apt conclusion for this section.

> There has always been a good deal of discussion about the art and the
> science of professions that include clinical practice as well as laboratory
> research. If by art one means appreciation of the fact that one is dealing
> with human life, and by science one means precise information, both are
> necessary and must go hand in hand. In a sense they have always done so.
> This is to say that asking questions and making observations is not the
> exclusive domain of either art or science, or the clinic or the laboratory.
> The dichotomy seems to reflect the either-orishness that Aristotelian lan-
> guage habits have tended to impose on our thinking.
>
> What the clinician cannot get along without, and what great artists and
> scientists alike have always had, is a kind of reverence for human
> life . . . . The great literature of all times and places has had something to say
> about the human condition as searching and as probing as the questions
> scientists have asked about the nature of the universe and the nature of
> man. Scientists have learned that one cannot leave the observer out of the
> equation, and clinicians know one cannot leave the laboratory out of the
> clinic [p. 347].

The Aphasia Therapist

The aphasia therapist may be the most critical variable in the patient's
rehabilitation. No approach or treatment technique can be effective unless it is implemented by an experienced, sophisticated, mature
therapist.

To the experienced clinician, it is clear that no single technique is adequate to produce normal communication function in the aphasic and the ideal approach, given our present state of knowledge, remains eclectic and specific to the individual patient's needs. Fundamental to this therapeutic philosophy is the acknowledgment and appreciation of the uniqueness of the individual. This is not simply to pay lip service to the humanistic idea that we are all created differently but to recognize in the most practical sense that no two aphasic persons are exactly alike in pathology, personality, linguistic deficits, reactions to catastrophic illness, life experience, spiritual values, etc.; that the influence of these factors assumes different characteristics and strengths at different stages of recovery; and that they are all inextricably related to recovery outcome.

There are a number of principles that underlie daily practice. The first of these was stated by Brumfitt and Clarke (1980), that speech therapy is a "special case of the general art of psychotherapy [p. 2]." Basic to each therapeutic technique is the concept that it must contribute to the patient's phychological comfort and, conversely, should never feed into depression, frustration, anger, feelings of low self-esteem, etc. This is uppermost in the mind of the experienced, enlightened therapist and dictates the selection of therapeutic activity. At the outset the therapist chooses those techniques or exercises that allow the patient to use preserved skills, thereby increasing the chances for a successful performance. As the therapist comes to know the patient better, he or she learns which activities facilitate the most successful performance and employs these as much as possible. These early therapeutic sessions should foster the growth of a trusting relationship between patient and therapist and lead to the therapist's image as a forgiving, accepting, approving ally. A strictly pedagogic approach based upon preconceived notions of what is to be taught, except in the patient with mild aphasia or speech dyspraxia, must lead to failure. For what the therapist is attempting to do is help the patient toward an acceptance of himself as he is. This is difficult and requires much time and patience, for the aphasic sees himself as inferior and altered in the profoundest sense. A strong ego is required if the aphasic can continue to feel important, worthy of respect, etc. Unfortunately, few people possess such psychological equipment. The therapist, then, becomes the patient's advocate while at the same time learning in greater detail what he can and cannot do.

Experience has revealed that the choice of teaching technique is far less important than how it is applied. Any language-teaching method may be used in aphasia therapy providing, of course, that it is adapted to the individual patient. One must be careful to keep the material at a level commensurate with the patient's ability to perform successfully. The choice of vocabulary, length of phrase or sentence, and grammatical or semantic complexity must often be restricted, though material should never be presented in anything other than an adult context. The effective therapist never pursues treatment activities that the patient perceives as meaningless. As in all teaching settings, repetition and reinforcement are important. It is essential as well that the therapist construct a program that makes use of cues that appear to enhance the possibility of evoking correct responses. For example, if a patient seems to be capable of completing words if the first letter is provided, this might be the basis for a sequence of drills; or if a patient is able to produce a word verbally if he writes it first, then this is a perfectly legitimate therapeutic strategy.

Kindness and good intentions are insufficient for effective aphasia therapy. The competent therapist must have a thorough knowledge of aphasia so as to be able to explain to the patient (and often his family as well) the meaning of symptoms, reactions, etc. Sometimes these explanations require endless repetition before they can be incorporated by the patient.

The subject of motivation always arises in the treatment of disabling neurological disorders. Experience suggests that, except for severely depressed individuals, who are unable to put forth much effort, patients generally produce everything they are capable of producing. The therapist must not allow his or her expectations to predominate in the therapeutic interaction; this is not uncommon and is usually motivated by laudatory aspirations, for one wants to see one's patient improve. Patients with involvement of subcortical areas may have low levels of activation, a purely physiological process having nothing to do with psychological motivation.

A clinical observation with particular relevance to aphasia therapy is the fact that anxiety invariably deteriorates performance. This is true whether or not an individual is suffering from a neurological disorder and has special significance in the brain-damaged. The therapeutic setting and the quality of interaction between patient and therapist should be relaxed, quiet, and comfortable in order to elicit the best performance the patient is capable of producing. This may be the basis for the common report that patients often do better at home than in therapeutic sessions. The report should always be given credence.

One of the tasks requiring very great skill is the management of the patient during the process of treatment termination. The criteria for this cannot be reduced to a simple formula, for it depends upon multiple factors, some of the most important of which are the patient's level of linguistic ability, psychological state (including adjustment to disability, levels of anxiety or depression, dependency needs, ego strength, feelings of self-esteem), family situation, opportunity for social contact, and vocational status. For some patients speech rehabilitation need not go beyond a 2- or 3-week period during which they participate in selected language exercises and receive information about their condition. Others may require some form of speech rehabilitation (group and/or individual) indefinitely. Most fall somewhere between these two extremes, and the skill of the therapist is in evaluating and balancing linguistic skill, patient expectations, adequacy of support systems, etc. Successful interaction with the patient once decisions have been made also requires tact and experience.

Experienced aphasia therapists evoke much respect and admiration, for they engage in work that is always difficult and frequently unrecognized for the skill, wisdom, patience, and understanding that are required. Through knowledge of aphasic deficits, specific treatment techniques, and the needs of the patient, they make ever changing judgments and decisions about the requirements of the moment, often balancing a patient's need for nurturance with the reality of his limitations.

A Concluding Comment

Historical realities suggest that the realm of recovery and rehabilitation in aphasia does not yet enjoy a firm basis in objective data. A great deal of what is known and practiced depends upon clinical experience and the slow accumulation of maturity and skill in those who undertake this difficult work. Systematic investigation to date has not clarified the physiology and pathophysiology of communication or provided a therapeutic blueprint for persistent disorders such as aphasia. To a large extent, successful treatment is compensatory in nature and the effective therapist is one who has learned from experience how to maximize this process.

Given the reality of anatomical and physiological pathology, we may never progress beyond this point. This is a possibility familiar to all who have studied the problem of aphasia, and it is not likely to deter those who engage in this work in the future. The study of human brain mechanisms is one of the last frontiers of biology and as such will continue to be an irresistible challenge.

References

American Heart Association. 1969. *Aphasia and the family.* American Heart Association, Publication EM 359.

Aronson, M., Shatin, L., & Cook, J. 1956. Socio-psychotherapeutic approach to the treatment of aphasic patients. *Journal of Speech and Hearing Disorders, 21,* 352–364.

Backus, O. 1945. Rehabilitation of aphasic veterans. *Journal of Speech Disorders, 10,* 149–153.

Backus, O., Henry, L. Clancy, J., & Dunn, H. 1947. *Aphasia in adults.* Ann Arbor: Univ. of Michigan Press.

Baretz, R., & Stephenson, G. 1976. Unrealistic patient. *New York State Journal of Medicine, 76* (Pt. 1), 54–57.

Basso, A., Capitani, E., & Vignolo, L. 1979. Influence of rehabilitation on language skills in aphasic patients: A controlled study. *Archives of Neurology, 36,* 190–196.

Basso, A., Faglioni, P., & Vignolo, L. 1975. Étude controlée de la rééducation du language dans l'aphasie: Comparaison entre aphasiques traités et non-traités. *Revue Neurologique* (Paris), *131,* 607–614.

Bateman, F. 1890. *On aphasia and the localization of the faculty of speech.* (2nd edition) London: Churchill.

Bay, E. 1969. The Lordat case and its import on the theory of aphasia. *Cortex, 5,* 302–308.

Benson, D. F. 1970. Language rehabilitation: Presentation 10. In A. Benton (Ed.), *Behavioral change in cerebrovascular disease.* New York: Harper.

Benson, D. F. 1979. Aphasia. In K. M. Heilman & E. Valenstein (Eds.), *Clinical neuropsychology.* New York: Oxford Univ. Press. (a)

Benson, D. F. 1979. *Aphasia, alexia, and agraphia.* New York: Churchill Livingstone. (b)

Benson, D. F. 1980. Psychiatric problems in aphasia. In M. T. Sarno & O. Hook (Eds.), *Aphasia: Assessment and treatment.* Stockholm: Almquist & Wiksell; and New York: Masson.

Benton, A. L. 1964. Contributions to aphasia before Broca. *Cortex, 1,* 314–327.

Benton, A. L., & Joynt, R. J. 1960. Early descriptions of aphasia. *Archives of Neurology, 3,* 109–126.

Beyn, E., & Shokhor-Trotskaya, M. 1966. The preventive method of speech rehabilitation in aphasia. *Cortex 2,* 96–108.

Blackman, N. 1950. Group psychotherapy with aphasics. *Journal of Nervous and Mental Disease, 111,* 154–163.

Boone, D. 1965. *An adult has aphasia.* Danville, Ill.: Interstate.

Boone, D. 1967. A plan for rehabilitation of aphasic patients. *Archives of Physical Medicine and Rehabilitation, 48,* 410–414.

Broadbent, D. 1879. A case of peculiar affection of speech, with commentary. *Brain, 1,* 484–503.

Brubaker, S. 1978. *Workbook for aphasia: Exercises for the re-development of higher level language.* Detroit: Wayne State Univ. Press.

Brumfitt, S., & Clarke, P. 1980. An application of psychotherapeutic techniques to the management of aphasia. Paper presented at Summer Conference: Aphasia Therapy, Cardiff, England, July 19.

Brust, J., Shafer, S., Richter, R., & Bruun, B. 1976. Aphasia in acute stroke. *Stroke, 7,* 167–174.

Buck, M. 1968. *Dysphasia: Professional guidance for family and patient.* Englewood Cliffs, N. J.: Prentice-Hall.

Butfield, E., & Zangwill, O. 1946. Re-education in aphasia: A review of 70 cases. *Journal of Neurology, Neurosurgery and Psychiatry, 9,* 75–79.

Buxbaum, J. 1967. Effect of nurturance on wives' appraisals of their marital satisfaction and the degree of their husband's aphasia. *Journal of Counseling Psychology, 31,* 240–243.
Cameron, C. 1973. *A different drum.* Englewood Cliffs, N. J.: Prentice-Hall.
Chapey, R. 1981. *Language intervention strategies in adult aphasia.* Baltimore: Williams & Wilkins.
Chester, S., & Egolf, D. 1974. Nonverbal communication and aphasia therapy. *Rehabilitation Literature, 35,* 231–233.
Crewe, M. 1969. Training course: Stroke in your family. *Rehabilitation Record,* Jan.–Feb., 32–34.
Culton, G. 1969. Spontaneous recovery from aphasia. *Journal of Speech and Hearing Research, 12,* 825–832.
Culton, G. 1971. Reaction to age as a factor in chronic aphasia in stroke patients. *Journal of Speech and Hearing Disorders, 36,* 563–564.
Dahlberg, C., & Jaffee, J. 1977. *Stroke: A physician's personal account.* New York: W. W. Norton.
Darley, F. 1970. Language rehabilitation: Presentation 8. In A. Benton (Ed.), *Behavioral change in cerebrovascular disease.* New York: Harper.
Darley, F. 1972. The efficacy of language rehabilitation in aphasia. *Journal of Speech and Hearing Disorders, 37,* 3–21.
Darley, F. 1975. Treatment of acquired aphasia. In W. J. Friedlander (Ed.), *Advances in neurology* (Vol. 7). New York: Raven.
Deal, J., & Florance, C. 1978. Modification of the eight-step continuum for treatment of apraxia of speech in adults. *Journal of Speech and Hearing Disorders, 43,* 89–95.
Demeurisse, G., Demol, O., Derouck, M., deBeuckelaer, R., Coekaerts, M.-J., & Capon, A. 1980. Quantitative study of the rate of recovery from aphasia due to ischemic stroke. *Stroke, 11,* 455–458.
Derman, S., & Manaster, A. 1967. Family counseling with relatives of aphasic patients at Schwab Rehabilitation Hospital. *Journal of the American Speech and Hearing Association, 9,* 175–177.
Edwards, A. 1965. Automated training for a "matching-to-sample" task in aphasia. *Journal of Speech and Hearing Research, 8,* 39–42.
Eisenson, J. 1949. Prognostic factors related to language rehabilitation in aphasic patients. *Journal of Speech and Hearing Disorders, 14,* 262–264.
Eisenson, J. 1964. Aphasia: A point of view as to the nature of the disorder and factors that determine prognosis for recovery. *International Journal of Neurology, 4,* 287–295.
Eisenson, J. 1973. *Adult aphasia: Assessment and treatment.* Englewood Cliffs, N. J.: Prentice-Hall.
Engle, G. 1964. Grief and grieving. *American Journal of Nursing, 64,* 93.
Espmark, S. 1973. Stroke before 50: A follow-up study of vocational and psychological adjustment. *Scandinavian Journal of Rehabilitation,* Suppl. No. 2.
Filby Y., & Edwards, A. 1963. An application of automated-teaching methods to test and teach form discrimination to aphasics. *Journal of Programmed Instruction, 2,* 25–33.
Franz, S. 1924. Studies in re-education: The aphasics. *Journal of Comparative Psychology, 4,* 349–429.
Frazier, C., & Ingham, S. 1920. A review of the effects of gunshot wounds of the head. *Archives of Neurology and Psychiatry, 3,* 17–40.
Friedman, M. 1961. On the nature of regression. *Archives of General Psychiatry, 5,* 60–64.
Gardner, H., Zurif, E., Berry, T., & Baker E. 1976. Visual communication in aphasia. *Neuropsychologia, 14,* 275–292.

Gloning, I., Gloning, K., Haub, G., & Quatember, R. 1969. Comparison of verbal behavior in right-handed and non-right-handed patients with anatomically verified lesions of one hemisphere. *Cortex, 5,* 43–52.

Godfrey, C., & Douglass, E. 1959. Recovery in aphasia. *Canadian Medical Association Journal, 80,* 618–624.

Goldstein, K. 1942. *After-effects of brain injuries in war: Their evaluation and treatment.* New York: Grune & Stratton.

Goldstein, K. 1948. *Language and language disturbances.* New York: Grune & Stratton.

Goodglass, H., & Kaplan, E. 1972. *The assessment of aphasia and related disorders.* Philadelphia: Lea & Febiger.

Goodkin, R. 1968. Use of concurrent response categories in evaluating talking behavior in aphasic patients. *Perceptual Motor Skills, 26,* 1035–1040.

Gopfert, H. 1922. Beitrage zur Frage der Restitution nach Hirnverletzung. *Zeitschrift fur die Gesamte Neurologie und Psychiatrie, 75,* 411–459.

Granich, L. 1947. *Aphasia: A guide to retraining.* New York: Grune & Stratton.

Hagen, C. 1973. Communication abilities in hemiplegia: Effect of speech therapy. *Archives of Physical Medicine and Rehabilitation, 54,* 454–463.

Halpern, H. 1981. Therapy for agnosia, apraxia, and dysarthria. In R. Chapey (Ed.), *Language intervention strategies in adult aphasia.* Baltimore: Williams & Wilkins.

Hatfield, F., & Zangwill, O. 1974. Ideation in aphasia: The picture story method. *Neuropsychologia, 12,* 389–393.

Head, H. 1926. *Aphasia and kindred disorders of speech* (Vols. 1 & 2). London: Cambridge Univ. Press. (2nd ed.—New York: Hafner, 1963).

Helm, N. 1976. Assessing candidacy for melodic intonation therapy. Paper presented at American Speech and Hearing Association Convention, Texas.

Helm, N., & Benson, D. F. 1978. Visual action therapy for global aphasia. Presentation at the 16th Annual Meeting of the Academy of Aphasia, Chicago, Illinois.

Helmick, J., Watamori, T., & Palmer, J. 1976. Spouses understanding of the communication disabilities of aphasic patients. *Journal of Speech and Hearing Disorders, 41,* 238–243.

Holland, A. 1969. Some current trends in aphasia rehabilitation. *Journal of the American Speech and Hearing Association, 11,* 3–7.

Holland, A. 1970. Case studies in aphasia rehabilitation using programmed instruction. *Journal of Speech and Hearing Research, 35,* 377–390.

Holland, A., & Levy, C. 1971. Syntactic generalization in aphasics as a function of relearning an active sentence. *Acta Symbolica, 2,* 34–41.

Holland, A., & Sonderman, J. 1974. Effects of a program based on the Token Test for teaching comprehension skills to aphasics. *Journal of Speech and Hearing Research, 17,* 589–598.

Hodgins, E. 1964. *Episode.* New York: Atheneum.

Huber, M. 1946. Linguistic problems of brain-injured servicemen. *Journal of Speech and Hearing Disorders, 11,* 143–147.

Isserlin, M. 1929. Die pathologische Physiologie der Sprache. *Ergebnisse der Psysiologie, Biologischene Chemie und Experimentellen Pharmakologie, 29,* 129.

Jakobson, R. 1955. Aphasia as a linguistic problem. In H. Werner (Ed.), *On expressive language.* Worcester, Mass., Clark Univ. Press.

Keenan, J., & Brassell, E. 1974. A study of factors related to prognosis for individual aphasic patients. *Journal of Speech and Hearing Disorders, 39,* 257–269.

Keith, R. 1972. *Speech and language rehabilitation: A workbook for the neurologically impaired* (Vol. 1). Danville, Ill.: Interstate.

Keith, R. 1977. *Speech and language rehabilitation: A workbook for the neurologically impaired* (Vol. 2). Danville, Ill.: Interstate.

Kenin, M., & Swisher, L. 1972. A study of pattern of recovery in aphasia. *Cortex, 8,* 56–68.

Kertesz, A. 1979. *Aphasia and associated disorders: Taxonomy, localization and recovery.* New York: Grune & Stratton. (a)

Kertesz, A. 1979. Recovery and treatment. In K. M. Heilman & E. Valenstein (Eds.), *Clinical neuropsychology.* New York: Oxford Univ. Press. (b)

Kertesz, A., & McCabe, P. 1977. Recovery patterns and prognosis in aphasia. *Brain, 100,* 1–18.

Kubler-Ross, E. 1969. *On death and dying.* New York: Macmillan.

Lane, H., & Moore, D. 1962. Reconditioning a consonant discrimination in an aphasic: An experimental case history. *Journal of Speech and Hearing Disorders, 27,* 232–241.

Lebrun, Y. 1976. Recovery in polygot aphasics. In Y. Lebrun & R. Hoops (Eds.), *Recovery in aphasics.* Amsterdam: Swets & Zeitlinger, B. V.

Lebrun, Y. 1980. The aphasic condition. In M. T. Sarno & O. Hook (Eds.), *Aphasia: Assessment and treatment.* Stockholm: Almquist & Wiksell; and New York: Masson.

LeMay, M. 1977. Asymmetries of the skull and handedness. *Journal of Neurological Sciences, 32,* 243–253.

Lenneberg, E. 1967. *Biological foundations of language.* New York: Wiley.

Levita, E. 1978. Effects of speech therapy on aphasics' responses to the Functional Communication Profile. *Perceptual and Motor Skills, 47,* 151–154.

Linell, S., & Steg, G. 1980. Family treatment in aphasia- experience from a patient association. In M. T. Sarno & O. Hook (Eds.), *Aphasia: Assessment and treatment.* Stockholm: Almquist & Wiksell; and New York: Masson.

Lomas, A., & Kertesz, A. 1978. Patterns of spontaneous recovery in aphasic groups: A study of adult stroke patients. *Brain and Language, 5,* 388–401.

Longerich, M., & Bordeaux, J. 1954. *Aphasia therapeutics.* New York: Macmillan.

Lordat, J. 1843. Analyse de la parole pour servir a la théorie de divers cas d'alalie et de puralie (de mutisme et d'imperfection du parler) que les nosologistes ont mal connus. (Lecons tirées du cours de physiologie de l'anée scolaire, 1842–1843). *Journal de la Société de Médecine Pratique de Montpellier, 7,* 333 & 417; *8,* 1.

Ludlow, C. 1977. Recovery from aphasia: A foundation for treatment. In M. Sullivan & M. Krommers (Eds.), *Rationale for adult aphasia therapy.* Omaha: University of Nebraska Medical Center.

Luria, A. R. 1948. *Rehabilitation of brain functioning after war traumas.* Moscow: Academy of Sciences Press.

Luria, A. R. 1963. *Restoration of function after brain injury.* New York: Macmillan.

Luria, A. R. 1966. Human brain and psychological processes. New York: Harper.

Malone, R. 1969. Expressed attitudes of families of aphasics. *Journal of Speech and Hearing Disorders, 34,* 146–151.

Marks, M., Taylor, M. L., & Rusk, H. 1957. Rehabilitation of the aphasic patient: A survey of three years experience in a rehabilitation setting. *Neurology, 7,* 837–843.

Marshall, N. & Holtzapple, P. 1976. Melodic intonation therapy: Variations on a theme. In R. Brookshire (Ed.), *Clinical aphasiology—Conference Proceedings.* Minneapolis: BRK Publications.

Marshall, R., & King, P. 1973. Effects of fatigue produced by isokinetic exercise on the communication ability of aphasic adults. *Journal of Speech and Hearing Research, 16,* 222–230.

Marshall, R., & Watts, M. 1976. Relaxation training: Effects on the communicative ability of aphasic adults. *Archives of Physical Medicine and Rehabilitation, 57,* 464–467.

Messerli, P., Tissot, A., & Rodriguez, J. 1976. Recovery from aphasia: Some factors of prognosis. In Y. Lebrun & R. Hoops (Eds.), *Recovery in aphasics.* Amsterdam: Swets & Zeitlinger, B. V.

Millikan, C., & Darley, F. L. 1967. *Brain mechanisms underlying speech and language.* New York: Grune & Stratton.

Mills, C. K. 1880. *Medical Bulletin,* May. [Cited in Mills, 1904]

Mills, C. 1904. Treatment of aphasia by training. *Journal of the American Medical Association,* 43, 1940–1949.

Morley, H. 1960. Applying linguistics to speech and language therapy for aphasics. *Language and Learning,* 10, 135–149.

Moss, C. 1972. *Recovery with aphasia: The aftermath of my stroke.* Urbana: Univ. of Illinois Press.

Naeser, M. 1975. A structured approach teaching aphasics basic sentence types. *British Journal of Disorders of Communication,* 10, 70–76.

Newhoff, M., & Davis, G. 1978. A spouse intervention program: Planning, implementation, and problems of evaluation. In R. H. Brookshire (Ed.), *Clinical aphasiology: Conference proceedings.* Minneapolis; BRK Publishers.

Nielsen, J. 1936. *Agnosia, apraxia, aphasia: Their value in cerebral localization.* (Copyright 1936 by J. M. Nielsen, Los Angeles, California and 1946 by Hoeber, New York).

Peacher, W. G. 1945. Speech disorders in World War II. *Journal of Speech Disorders,* 10, 155–161, 287–291.

Pieniadz, J., Naeser, M., & Koff, E. 1979. CT scan reversed cerebral hemispheric asymmetries and improved recovery in aphasia. Paper presented at the Academy of Aphasia, San Diego, California, October. Manuscript submitted for publication.

Pincas, A. 1965. Linguistics and aphasia. *Australian Journal of the College of Speech Therapists,* 15, 20–28.

Poppelreuter, W. 1915. Ueber psychische ausfall serscheinungen nach hirnverletzungen. *Munchener Medizinische Wochenschrift,* 62, 489–491.

Premack, D. 1971. Language in chimpanzee? *Science,* 172, 808–822.

Prins, R., Snow, C., & Wagenaar, E. 1978. Recovery from aphasia: Spontaneous speech versus language comprehension. *Brain and Language,* 6, 192–211.

Reinvang, I. 1976. Sentence production in recovery from aphasia. In Y. Lebrun & R. Hoops (Eds.), *Recovery in aphasics.* Amsterdam: Swets & Zeitlinger, B. V.

Reinvang, I. 1980. A plan for rehabilitation of aphasics. *Scandinavian Journal of Rehabilitation Medicine,* Suppl. No. 7, 120–129. In A. R. Fugl-Meyer (Ed.), *Stroke with hemiplegia.* Proceedings of a Symposium in Umea, Sweden, May 5–7, 1978.

Reinvang, I., & Engvik, E. 1980. Language recovery in aphasia from 3–6 months after stroke. In M. T. Sarno & O. Hook (Eds.), *Aphasia: Assessment and treatment.* Stockholm; Almquist & Wiksell; and New York: Masson.

Ritchie, D. 1961. *Stroke: A study of recovery.* New York: Doubleday.

Rolnick, I. 1969. Speech pathology services in a home health agency: The visiting nurse association of Detroit. *Journal of the American Speech and Hearing Association,* 11, 462–463.

Rose, C., Boby, V., & Capildeo, R. 1976. A retrospective survey of speech disorders following stroke, with particular reference to the value of speech therapy. In Y. Lebrun & R. Hoops (Eds.), *Recovery in aphasics.* Amsterdam: Swets & Zeitlinger, B. V.

Rosenbek, J. 1978. Treating apraxia of speech. In D. F. Johns (Ed.), *Clinical management of neurogenic communication disorders.* Boston: Little, Brown.

Rosenbek, J. Hansen, R., Baughman, C., & Lemme, M. 1974. Treatment of developmental apraxia of speech: A case study. *Language, Speech and Hearing Services in the Schools,* 5, 13–22.

Rosenbek, J., Lemme, M., Ahern, M., Harris, E., & Wertz, R. 1973. A treatment for apraxia of speech in adults. *Journal of Speech and Hearing Disorders,* 38, 462–472.

Rosenberg, B. 1965. The performance of aphasics on automated visuo-perceptual discrimination, training and transfer tasks. *Journal of Speech and Hearing Research, 8,* 165–181.

Sands, E., Freeman, F., & Harris, K. 1978. Progressive changes in articulatory patterns in verbal apraxia: A longitudinal case study. *Brain and Language, 6,* 97–105.

Sands, E., Sarno, M. T., & Shankweiler, D. 1969. Long-term assessment of language function in aphasia due to stroke. *Archives of Physical Medicine and Rehabilitation, 50,* 203–207.

Sarno, J. E., & Sarno, M. T. 1969. The diagnosis of speech disorders in brain damaged adults. *Medical Clinics of North America, 53,* 561–573. (a)

Sarno, J., & Sarno, M. T. 1969. *Stroke: The condition and the patient.* New York: McGraw-Hill. (b)

Sarno, J., & Sarno, M. T. 1979. *Stroke: A guide for patients and their families* (Rev. ed.). New York: McGraw-Hill.

Sarno, J., Sarno, M. T., & Levita, E. 1971. Evaluating language improvement after completed stroke. *Archives of Physical Medicine and Rehabilitation, 52,* 73–78.

Sarno, M. T. 1968. Method for multivariant analysis of aphasia based on studies of 235 patients in a rehabilitation setting. *Archives of Physical Medicine and Rehabilitation, 49,* 210–216.

Sarno, M. T. 1969. *The Functional Communication Profile: Manual of directions.* New York: Institute of Rehabilitation Medicine, New York University Medical Center.

Sarno, M. T. 1971. The role of the family in aphasia. In T. D. Hanley (Ed.), *The family as supportive personnel in speech and hearing remediation. Proceedings of a Post-Graduate Course.* Santa Barbara: University of California.

Sarno, M. T. 1974. Aphasia rehabilitation. In S. Dickson (Ed.), *Communication disorders: Remedial principles and practices.* Glenview, Ill.: Scott, Foresman.

Sarno, M. T. 1975. Disorders of communication in stroke. In S. Licht (Ed.), *Stroke and its rehabilitation.* Baltimore: Williams & Wilkins.

Sarno, M. T. 1976. The status of research in recovery from aphasia. In Y. Lebrun & R. Hoops (Eds.), *Recovery in aphasics.* Amsterdam: Swets & Zeitlinger, B. V.

Sarno, M. T. 1980. Aphasia rehabilitation. In M. T. Sarno & O. Hook (Eds.), *Aphasia: Assessment and treatment.* Stockholm: Almquist & Wiksell; and New York: Masson. (a)

Sarno, M. T. 1980. Language rehabilitation outcome in the elderly aphasic patient. In L. K. Obler & M. L. Albert (Eds.), *Language and communication in the elderly: Clinical, therapeutic, and experimental issues.* Lexington, Mass.: D. C. Heath. (b)

Sarno, M. T. 1980. The nature of verbal impairment after closed head injury. *Journal of Nervous and Mental Disease, 168,* 685–692. (c)

Sarno, M. T. 1980. Review of research in aphasia: Recovery and rehabilitation. In M. T. Sarno & O. Hook (Eds.), *Aphasia: Assessment and treatment.* Stockholm: Almquist & Wiksell; and New York: Masson. (d)

Sarno, M. T., & Levita, E. 1971. Natural course of recovery in severe aphasia. *Archives of Physical Medicine and Rehabilitation, 52,* 175–179.

Sarno, M. T., & Levita, E. 1979. Recovery in treated aphasia during the first year poststroke. *Stroke, 10,* 663–670.

Sarno, M. T., & Levita, E. 1981. Some observations on the nature of recovery in global aphasia. *Brain and Language, 13,* 1–12.

Sarno, M. T., Silverman, M., & Sands, E. 1970. Speech therapy and language recovery in severe aphasia. *Journal of Speech and Hearing Research, 13,* 607–623.

Scargill, M. 1964. Modern linguistics and recovery from aphasia. *Journal of Speech and Hearing Disorders, 19,* 507–513.

Schneider, J. 1974. The stresses of living: Loss. Paper presented at Michigan State University. (Cited in Tanner, D. 1980. Loss and grief: Implications for the speech-language pathologist and audiologist. *Journal of the American Speech and Hearing Association, 22,* 916–928.)

Schuell, H., Jenkins, J., & Jiménez-Pabón, E. 1964. *Aphasia in adults.* New York: Harper.

Segre, R. 1976. Autobiographical considerations on aphasic rehabilitation. *Folia Phoniatrica, 28,* 129–140.

Seron, X., Deloche, G., Bastard, V., Chassin, G., & Hermand, N. 1979. Word-finding difficulties and learning transfer in aphasic patients. *Cortex, 15,* 149–155.

Shane, H., & Darley, F. L. 1978. The effect of auditory rhythmic stimulation on articulatory accuracy in apraxia of speech. *Cortex, 14,* 444–450.

Sheehan, V. 1946. Rehabilitation of aphasics in an army hospital. *Journal of Speech and Hearing Disorders, 11,* 149–157.

Simonson, J. 1971. *According to the aphasic adult.* Texas: University of Texas Southwestern Medical School.

Singer, H., & Low, A. 1933. The brain in a case of motor aphasia in which improvement occurred with training. *Archives of Neurology and Psychiatry, 29,* 162–165.

Skelly, M., Schinsky, L., Smith, R., & Fust, R. 1974. American Indian sign (AMERIND) as a facilitator of verbalization for the oral verbal apraxic. *Journal of Speech and Hearing Disorders, 39,* 445–456.

Smith, A. 1971. Objective indices of severity of chronic aphasia in stroke patients. *Journal of Speech and Hearing Disorders, 26,* 167–207.

Smith, A. 1972. *Diagnosis, intelligence and rehabilitation of chronic aphasics.* Ann Arbor: University of Michigan, Department of Physical Medicine and Rehabilitation.

Smith, M. 1974. Operant conditioning of syntax in aphasia. *Neuropsychologia, 12,* 403–405.

Sparks, R., Helm, N., & Albert, M. 1974. Aphasia rehabilitation resulting from melodic intonation therapy. *Cortex, 10,* 303–316.

Spreen, O., & Benton, A. 1969. *Neurosensory Center Comprehensive Examination for Aphasia.* Victoria, B. C.: Department of Psychology, University of Victoria.

Stoicheff, M. 1960. Motivating instructions and language performance of dysphasic subjects. *Journal of Speech and Hearing Research, 3,* 75–85.

Strauss, A., Burrucker, J., Cicero, J., & Edwards, R. 1967. Groupwork with stroke patients. *Rehabilitation Record,* Nov–Dec., 30–32.

Stryker, S. 1975. *Speech after stroke: A manual for the speech pathologist and the family member.* Springfield, Ill.: Thomas.

Subirana, A. 1969. Handedness and cerebral dominance. In P. Vinken & G. Bruyn (Eds.), *Handbook of clinical neurology* (Vol. 4). New York: Am. Elsevier.

Tanner, D. 1980. Loss and grief: Implications for the speech-language pathologist and audiologist. *Journal of the American Speech and Hearing Association, 22,* 916–928.

Taylor, M. L. 1958. *Understanding aphasia: A guide for family and friends.* New York: Institute of Rehabilitation Medicine, New York University Medical Center.

Taylor, M. L. 1964. Language therapy. In H. Burr (Ed.), *The aphasic adult: Evaluation and rehabilitation.* Charlottesville, Va.: Wayside Press. (a)

Taylor, M. L. 1964. Linguistic considerations of the verbal behavior of brain damaged adults. *Linguistic Reporter, 6,* 1–2. (b)

Taylor, M. L. 1965. A measurement of functional communication in aphasia. *Archives of Physical Medicine and Rehabilitation, 46,* 101–107.

Taylor, M. L., & Marks, M. 1955. *The basic 100 words: Aphasia rehabilitation manual and workbook.* New York: Institute of Rehabilitation Medicine, New York University Medical Center.

Taylor, M. L., & Marks, M. 1959. *Aphasia rehabilitation manual and therapy kit.* New York: Institute of Rehabilitation Medicine, New York University Medical Center.

Taylor, M. L., & Sands, E. 1966. Application of programmed instruction techniques to the language rehabilitation of severely impaired aphasic patients. *Journal of the National Society of Programmed Instruction, 5,* 10–11.

Tikofsky, R., & Reynolds, G. 1963. Further studies of non-verbal learning and aphasia. *Journal of Speech and Hearing Research, 6,* 133–143.

Turnblom, M., & Meyers, J. 1952. A group discussion program with the families of aphasic patients. *Journal of Speech and Hearing Disorders, 17,* 393–396.

Ulatowska, H., & Richardson, S. 1974. A longitudinal study of an adult with aphasia: Considerations for research and therapy. *Brain and Language, 1,* 151–166.

Ullman, M. 1962. *Behavioral changes in patients following strokes.* Springfield, Ill.: Thomas.

U.S. Census Bureau. 1975. *Current Population Report,* (Publication No. 541). Washington, D.C.: Government Printing Office, February.

Velletri-Glass, A., Gazzaniga, M., & Premack, D. 1973. Artificial language training in global aphasics. *Neuropsychologia, 11,* 95–103.

Vignolo, L. 1964. Evolution of aphasia and language rehabilitation: A retrospective exploratory study. *Cortex, 1,* 344–367.

Watzlawick, P., & Coyne, J. 1980. Depression following stroke: Brief, problem-focused family treatment. *Family Process, 19,* 13–18.

Weigl, E. 1961. [The phenomenon of temporary deblocking in aphasia.] *Zeitschrift Fuer Phonetik, Sprachwissenschaft Und Kommunikationsforschung, 14* (Ht 4), 337–364.

Weisenburg, T., & McBride, K. 1935. *Aphasia: A clinical and psychological study.* New York: Commonwealth Fund. (2nd ed.—New York: Hafner, 1964.)

Weniger, D., Huber, W., Stachowiak, F. -J., & Poeck, K. 1980. Treatment of aphasia on a linguistic basis. In M. T. Sarno & O. Hook (Eds.), *Aphasia: Assessment and treatment.* Stockholm: Almquist & Wiksell; and New York: Masson.

Wepman, J. 1951. *Recovery from aphasia.* New York: Ronald Press.

Wepman, J. 1953. A comceptual model for the processes involved in recovery from aphasia. *Journal of Speech and Hearing Disorders, 18,* 4–13.

Wepman, J. 1972. Aphasia therapy: A new look. *Journal of Speech and Hearing Disorders, 37,* 201–214.

Wepman, J. 1976. Aphasia: Language without thought or thought without language? *Journal of the American Speech and Hearing Association, 18,* 131–136.

Wepman, J., & Morency, A. 1963. Filmstrips as an adjunct to language therapy for aphasia. *Journal of Speech and Hearing Disorders, 28,* 191–194.

Wiedel, I. M. H. 1976. The basic foundation approach for decreasing aphasia and verbal apraxia in adults (BFA). In R. H. Brookshire (Ed.), *Clinical aphasiology: Proceedings of the conference.* Minneapolis: BRK Publishers.

Wiegel-Crump, C. 1976. Agrammatism and aphasia. In Y. Lebrun & R. Hoops (Eds.), *Recovery in aphasics.* Amsterdam: Swets & Zeitlinger, B. V.

Wiegel-Crump, C., & Koenigsknecht, R. 1973. Tapping the lexical store of the adult aphasic: Analysis of the improvement made in word retrieval skills. *Cortex, 9,* 410–417.

Wint, G. 1967. *The third killer: Meditations on a stroke.* New York: Abelard.

Wulf, H. 1973. *Aphasia: My world alone.* Detroit: Wayne State Univ. Press.

Wyllie, J. 1894. *The disorders of speech.* Edinburgh: Oliver and Boyd.

Yarnell, P., Monroe, P., & Sobel, L. 1976. Aphasia outcome in stroke: A clinical neuroradiological correlation. *Stroke, 7,* 514–522.

Yoss, K., & Darley, F. L. 1974. Therapy in developmental apraxia of speech. *Language, Speech and Hearing Services in the Schools, 5,* 23–31.

Subject Index

A

Abstract attitudes, 466
Abstract reasoning deficits, 15, 17
Acalculia, 303, 308, 310, 311–312, 314, 453, 458, 460
Acquired aphasia in children, *see* Childhood aphasia
Affective phenomena, 470, 472, 478
Aging
    and aphasia, 386–389
    and type of aphasia, 387–389
Agnosia
    auditory, 243, 367
    finger, 303, 308, 312–313, 314, 458
    visual, 304
Agraphia, 6, 303, 304, 308, 309–310, 314, 458
Agrammatism, 18, 134, 236, 239–240, 309
Alexia, 2, 3, 52, 303, 304, 307, 435, 457, 458
    with agraphia, 62, 308–309
    without agraphia, 43–44, 63, 307, 457
    literal, 307
Alzheimer's disease, 335, 389–393
    language disturbance in, 389
    symptoms, 389–391
    and Wernicke's aphasia, 392
Amusia, 369
Anomia, 431, 435, 441–445, 457, 458
Anosognosia, 469, 475
Anterograde amnesia, 429
Aphasia, acquired in children, *see* Childhood aphasia

Aphasia, definition, 51–54
Aphemia, 8, 9, 303
Aphonia, 53
Apraxia, 303, 317–320
    afferent, 288
    constructional, 18, 344, 345–346
    ideational, 275, 279, 282, 286, 288
    ideokinetic, 277, 282
    ideomotor, 276, 281, 286, 457
    kinesthetic, 279
    kinetic, 278, 286
    limb, 280
    limb-kinetic, 275, 276, 277, 278, 287, 288–291, 292, 294, 297
    motor, 282
    oral, 280
    oral facial, 274, 278, 287, 288
    sympathetic, 285
Apraxia of speech, 271–298
    as comprehension deficit, 275
    and dysarthria, 298
    experimental studies, 291–297
    and hemiplegia, 285
    historical background, 271, 272–277, 286
    initiation of speech, 298
    and memory of movement, 282
    and repetition disturbance, 276, 282, 297
    in spontaneous speech, 281
    treatment, 320
    and vocal tract musculature, 272
Articulatory timing, 139, 140